CLINICAL COMPANION TO

MEDICAL-SURGICAL NURSING

Assessment and Management of Clinical Problems

D0111555

CLINICAL COMPANION TO
MEDICAL-SURGICAL NURSING

Assessment and Management of Clinical Problems

10th Edition

Prepared by
Debra Hagler, RN, PhD, ACNS-BC, CNE, CHSE, ANEF, FAAN
Clinical Professor
College of Nursing and Health Innovation
Arizona State University
Phoenix, Arizona

Acknowledgment: We acknowledge the contributions of
Shannon Ruff Dirksen, RN, PhD, FAAN, Associate Professor,
College of Nursing and Health Innovation, Arizona State
University, Phoenix, Arizona, for her work on past editions
of this book.

Sharon L. Lewis, RN, PhD, FAAN
Linda Bucher, RN, PhD, CEN, CNE
Margaret McLean Heitkemper, RN, PhD, FAAN
Mariann M. Harding, RN, PhD, CNE
Jeffrey Kwong, DNP, MPH, ANP-BC, FAANP
Dottie Roberts, RN, EdD, MACI, CMSRN, OCNS-C, CNE

ELSEVIER

ELSEVIER

3251 Riverport Lane
St. Louis, Missouri 63043

Notices

Knowledge and best practice in this field are constantly changing. As new research and experience broaden our understanding, changes in research methods, professional practices, or medical treatment may become necessary.

Practitioners and researchers must always rely on their own experience and knowledge in evaluating and using any information, methods, compounds, or experiments described herein. In using such information or methods they should be mindful of their own safety and the safety of others, including parties for whom they have a professional responsibility.

With respect to any drug or pharmaceutical products identified, readers are advised to check the most current information provided (i) on procedures featured or (ii) by the manufacturer of each product to be administered, to verify the recommended dose or formula, the method and duration of administration, and contraindications. It is the responsibility of practitioners, relying on their own experience and knowledge of their patients, to make diagnoses, to determine dosages and the best treatment for each individual patient, and to take all appropriate safety precautions.

To the fullest extent of the law, neither the Publisher nor the authors, contributors, or editors, assume any liability for any injury and/or damage to persons or property as a matter of products liability, negligence or otherwise, or from any use or operation of any methods, products, instructions, or ideas contained in the material herein.

Previous editions copyrighted 2014, 2011, 2007, 2004, 2000, 1996 by Mosby, Inc., an affiliate of Elsevier Inc.

Herdman, T.H. & Kamitsuru, S. (Eds.). (2014). *NANDA International Nursing Diagnoses: Definitions & Classification, 2015-2017.* Oxford: Wiley Blackwell.

Library of Congress Cataloging-in-Publication Data
Names: Hagler, Debra, author. | Complemented by (expression): Lewis, Sharon Mantik. Medical-surgical nursing. Tenth edition. | Preceded by (work): Dirksen, Shannon Ruff. Clinical companion to Medical-surgical nursing.
Title: Clinical companion to Medical-surgical nursing : assessment and management of clinical problems / prepared by Debra Hagler, Sharon L. Lewis, Linda Bucher, Margaret McLean Heitkemper, Mariann M. Harding, Jeffrey Kwong, Dottie Roberts.
Description: Tenth edition. | St. Louis, Missouri : Elsevier, [2017] | Complemented by Medical-surgical nursing / Sharon L. Lewis [and five others]. Tenth edition. [2017]. | Preceded by Clinical companion to Medical-surgical nursing / prepared by Shannon Ruff Dirksen, Sharon L. Lewis, Margaret McLean Heitkemper, Linda Bucher. Ninth edition. [2014]. | Includes bibliographical references and index.
Identifiers: LCCN 2016030243 | ISBN 9780323371179 (pbk.)
Subjects: | MESH: Perioperative Nursing | Nursing Process | Handbooks
Classification: LCC RT41 | NLM WY 49 | DDC 610.73–dc23 LC record available at https://lccn.loc.gov/2016030243

Senior Content Strategist: Jamie Blum
Content Development Manager: Jean Sims Fornango
Content Development Specialist: Jennifer Hermes, Melissa Rawe
Publishing Services Manager: Julie Eddy
Senior Project Manager: Mary G. Stueck
Design Direction: Ashley Miner

Printed in Canada

Working together
to grow libraries in
developing countries

www.elsevier.com • www.bookaid.org

Last digit is the print number: 9 8 7 6 5 4 3 2

PREFACE

The *Clinical Companion* to Lewis, Bucher, Heitkemper, Harding, Kwong, and Robert's *Medical-Surgical Nursing: Assessment and Management of Clinical Problems*, tenth edition, has been revised and updated as a condensed reference of essential information on almost 200 medical-surgical patient problems and clinically related topics. The tenth edition of this pocket-sized book provides nurses and nursing students with quick access to current, concise, and important information when caring for patients.

The *Clinical Companion* can be used separately as a reference or in conjunction with *Medical-Surgical Nursing: Assessment and Management of Clinical Problems*, tenth edition.

The book is divided into three sections. Part One contains commonly encountered medical-surgical patient problems that are arranged alphabetically and organized in an easy-to-use format. The disorders are extensively cross-referenced to *Medical-Surgical Nursing*, tenth edition, for the reader who desires additional information. Part Two contains brief explanations of common medical-surgical treatments and procedures (e.g., pacemakers, oxygen therapy) in which the role of the nurse is emphasized. Part Three contains reference material that is frequently used in clinical nursing practice (e.g., heart and breath sounds, medication administration, blood and urine laboratory values). An extensive index is provided for easy location of information. Content updates may be found at http://evolve.elsevier.com/Lewis/medsurg.

We strongly believe the *Clinical Companion* is an invaluable source of information that will serve as an important resource in helping nurses meet the challenges and opportunities in caring for patients and their caregivers during states of altered health and well-being.

Debra Hagler
Sharon L. Lewis

Our greatest weakness lies in giving up. The most certain way to succeed is to try just one more time.
Thomas Edison

CONTENTS

Part One: Disorders

Part Two: Treatments and Procedures

Part Three: Reference Appendix

Disorders

Disorders

ABDOMINAL PAIN, ACUTE

Description

Acute abdominal pain is pain of recent onset. It may signal a life-threatening problem and therefore requires immediate attention. Causes include damage to organs in the abdomen and pelvis, which may lead to inflammation, infection, obstruction, bleeding, or perforation. Common causes of acute abdominal pain are listed in Table 1.

Clinical Manifestations

Pain is the most common symptom of an acute abdominal problem. Patients may have nausea, vomiting, diarrhea, constipation, flatulence, fatigue, fever, rebound tenderness, and bloating.

Diagnostic Studies

Diagnosis begins with a complete history and physical examination. Description of the pain (frequency, timing, duration, location), accompanying symptoms, and sequence of symptoms (e.g., pain before or after vomiting) provide vital clues about the problem. Physical examination should include both rectal and pelvic examinations in addition to an abdominal examination.

- Complete blood count (CBC), urinalysis, abdominal x-ray, and an electrocardiogram (ECG) are done initially, along with an ultrasound or CT scan.
- A pregnancy test is performed in women of childbearing age to rule out ectopic pregnancy.

Interprofessional Care

The goal of management is to identify and treat the cause and monitor and treat complications, especially shock. Table 42-10 in

TABLE 1	Causes of Acute Abdominal Pain
• Abdominal compartment syndrome	• Pelvic inflammatory disease
• Acute pancreatitis	• Perforated gastric or duodenal ulcer
• Appendicitis	• Peritonitis
• Bowel obstruction	• Ruptured abdominal aneurysm
• Cholecystitis	• Ruptured ectopic pregnancy
• Diverticulitis	
• Gastroenteritis	

Lewis et al, *Medical-Surgical Nursing,* ed 10, p. 939, outlines emergency management of the patient with acute abdominal pain.

- A diagnostic laparoscopy may be performed to inspect the surface of abdominal organs, obtain biopsy specimens, perform laparoscopic ultrasounds, and remove organs.
- A laparotomy is used when laparoscopic techniques are inadequate. If the cause of the acute abdomen can be surgically removed (e.g., inflamed appendix) or surgically repaired (e.g., ruptured abdominal aneurysm), surgery is considered definitive therapy.

Nursing Management

Goals

The patient will have resolution of inflammation, relief of abdominal pain, freedom from complications (especially hypovolemic shock), and normal nutritional status.

Nursing Interventions

General care involves management of fluid and electrolyte imbalances, pain, and anxiety. Assess the quality and intensity of pain at regular intervals, and provide medication and other comfort measures. Maintain a calm environment and provide information to help allay anxiety. Conduct ongoing assessments of vital signs, intake and output, and level of consciousness, which are key indicators of hypovolemic shock.

Preoperative care includes the emergency care of the patient and general care of the preoperative patient (Chapter 17 and Table 42-10 in Lewis et al, *Medical-Surgical Nursing,* ed 10, p. 939).

Postoperative care depends on the type of surgical procedure performed. Laparoscopic procedures result in lower rates of postoperative complications (e.g., poor wound healing, paralytic ileus), earlier diet advancement, and shorter hospital stays compared with open surgical procedures. A general nursing care plan (eNursing Care Plan 19-1) for the postoperative patient is available on the website for Chapter 19.

A nasogastric (NG) tube with low suction may be used to empty the stomach and prevent gastric dilation. If the upper gastrointestinal (GI) tract was entered, drainage from the NG tube may be dark brown to dark red for the first 12 hours. Later it should be light yellowish brown or greenish. If a dark red color continues or if bright red blood is observed, notify the surgeon of the possibility of hemorrhage. "Coffee ground" granules in the drainage indicate blood that has been changed by acidic gastric secretions.

- Nausea and vomiting are common after a laparotomy and may result from the surgery, decreased peristalsis, or pain medication. Antiemetics such as ondansetron (Zofran), promethazine, and prochlorperazine may be ordered (see Nausea and Vomiting, p. 429).

- Monitor fluid and electrolyte status along with BP, heart rate, and respirations.
- Swallowed air and decreased peristalsis from decreased mobility, manipulation of abdominal organs during surgery, and anesthesia can lead to abdominal distention and gas pains. Early ambulation helps to restore peristalsis, expel flatus, and reduce gas pain.

▼ **Patient and Caregiver Teaching**

Preparation for discharge begins soon after surgery. Teach the patient and caregiver about any modifications in activity, care of the incision, diet, and drug therapy.

- Clear liquids are given initially after surgery, and if tolerated, the patient progresses to a regular diet.
- Normal activities should be resumed gradually, with planned rest periods.
- Both patient and caregiver should be aware of possible complications after surgery. Teach them to notify the surgeon immediately if fever is higher than 101° F (38.3° C) or if pain, weight loss, incisional drainage, or changes in bowel function occur.

ACUTE CORONARY SYNDROME

Description

Acute coronary syndrome (ACS) develops when myocardial ischemia is prolonged and not immediately reversible. ACS encompasses the spectrum of unstable angina (UA), non–ST-segment-elevation myocardial infarction (NSTEMI), and ST-segment-elevation myocardial infarction (STEMI) (Fig. 1).

Pathophysiology

ACS is associated with deterioration of an atherosclerotic plaque in a coronary artery. The previously stable plaque ruptures, releasing substances into the vessel. This stimulates platelet aggregation and thrombus formation. The unstable lesion may be partially occluded by a thrombus (manifesting as UA or NSTEMI) or totally occluded by a thrombus (manifesting as STEMI).

Unstable Angina

The patient with chronic stable angina may develop UA, or UA may be the first clinical manifestation of coronary artery disease (CAD). Unlike chronic stable angina, UA is unpredictable and must be treated immediately.

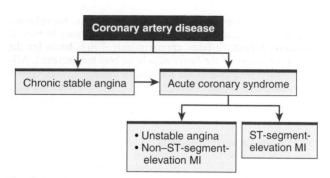

Fig. 1 Relationships among coronary artery disease, chronic stable angina, and acute coronary syndrome.

- The patient with previously diagnosed chronic stable angina describes a significant change in the pattern of angina. It occurs with increasing frequency and is easily provoked by minimal or no exertion, during sleep, or even at rest.
- The patient without previously diagnosed angina describes anginal pain that has progressed rapidly in the past few hours, days, or weeks, often culminating in pain at rest.

Myocardial Infarction: ST-Elevation (STEMI) and Non–ST-Elevation (NSTEMI)

- A *myocardial infarction* (MI) occurs because of abrupt stoppage of blood flow through a coronary artery from a thrombus caused by platelet aggregation. This causes irreversible myocardial cell death (necrosis). Most MIs occur in the setting of preexisting CAD. When a thrombus develops, blood flow to the heart muscle beyond the blockage stops, resulting in necrosis.
- A STEMI caused by an occlusive thrombus creates ST elevation in the electrocardiogram (ECG) leads facing the area of infarction. A STEMI is an emergency situation. To limit infarct size, the artery must be opened within 90 minutes of presentation. This can be done either by percutaneous coronary intervention (PCI) or with thrombolytic (fibrinolytic) therapy. PCI is the preferred treatment if a hospital is capable of performing PCI.
- NSTEMI, caused by a non-occlusive thrombus, does not cause ST elevation on the 12-lead ECG. Patients may or may not develop ST-T wave changes in the leads affected by the infarction. NSTEMI patients do not go to the catheterization laboratory emergently, but usually undergo the procedure within 12 to 72 hours if there are no contraindications. Thrombolytic therapy is not indicated for NSTEMI patients.

- Cardiac cells can withstand ischemic conditions for approximately 20 minutes before cellular death (necrosis) begins. If ischemia persists, it takes approximately 4 to 6 hours for the entire thickness of the heart muscle to become necrosed. MIs are usually described by the location of damage (anterior, inferior, lateral, or posterior wall). The location correlates with the involved coronary circulation. For example, inferior wall infarctions result from occlusions in the right coronary artery. The majority of MIs affect the left ventricle. Damage can occur in more than one location (e.g., anterolateral MI, anteroseptal MI).
- The degree of preestablished collateral circulation also influences the severity of the infarction. An individual with a long history of CAD may have developed good collateral circulation to provide the area surrounding the infarction site with a blood supply.

The body's response to cell death is the inflammatory process. Within 24 hours, leukocytes infiltrate the area. Enzymes are released from the dead cardiac cells and are important diagnostic indicators (markers) of MI. Proteolytic enzymes from neutrophils and macrophages remove necrotic tissue by the fourth day.

- The necrotic zone is identifiable by ECG changes (e.g., ST-segment elevation, pathologic Q wave) and by nuclear scanning after the onset of symptoms.

At 10 to 14 days after an MI, the new scar tissue is still weak. The myocardium is vulnerable to increased stress because of the unstable state of the healing heart wall. Changes in the infarcted heart muscle also cause changes in the unaffected areas. In an attempt to compensate for the damaged muscle, the normal myocardium hypertrophies and the ventricle dilates. This process of ventricular remodeling can lead to the development of late heart failure (HF), especially in a person with atherosclerosis of other coronary arteries and/or an anterior MI.

Clinical Manifestations

Unstable Angina

The chest pain associated with UA is new in onset, occurs at rest, or has a worsening pattern. Women seek medical attention for symptoms of UA more often than men. Despite national efforts to increase awareness, women's symptoms (fatigue, shortness of breath, indigestion, anxiety) often go unrecognized as related to heart problems.

Myocardial Infarction

Severe and persistent chest pain not relieved by rest or nitrate administration is the hallmark of an MI.

- Pain is usually described as a heaviness, pressure, burning, crushing, tightness, or constriction. The persistent pain is unlike any other pain.
- Common locations are epigastric, substernal, or retrosternal. The pain may radiate to the neck, jaw, and arms or to the back. It may occur while the patient is active or at rest, asleep or awake, and commonly occurs in the early morning hours.
- The pain usually lasts for 20 minutes or more and is more severe than usual anginal pain. When epigastric pain is present, the patient may take antacids without relief.
- Some patients may not have pain but may report having "discomfort," weakness, fatigue, nausea, indigestion, or shortness of breath. Women may experience atypical discomfort, shortness of breath, or fatigue.
- An older patient may experience a change in mental status (e.g., confusion), shortness of breath, pulmonary edema, dizziness, or a dysrhythmia.

Additional manifestations may include vomiting, and the patient's skin may be ashen, clammy, and cool (cold sweat). Fever occurs within the first 24 hours (up to 100.4° F [38° C]) and may continue for 1 week. BP and pulse rate are elevated initially. The BP may then drop, with decreased urine output, lung crackles, hepatic engorgement, and peripheral edema. Jugular veins may be distended, with obvious pulsations.

Complications

- *Dysrhythmias* are the most common complication after an MI and are the most common cause of death in patients in the prehospital period. Dysrhythmias are caused by any condition that affects the myocardial cell's sensitivity to nerve impulses, such as ischemia, electrolyte imbalances, and sympathetic nervous system stimulation. The intrinsic rhythm of the heart is disrupted, causing either a very fast heart rate (HR) (tachycardia), a very slow HR (bradycardia), or irregular HR. Life-threatening dysrhythmias occur most often with anterior wall infarction, heart failure, and shock. Complete heart block is seen in a massive infarction (see Dysrhythmias, p. 198).
- *Ventricular tachycardia and ventricular fibrillation* are lethal dysrhythmias that most often occur within the first 4 hours after the onset of pain. Premature ventricular contractions may precede ventricular tachycardia and fibrillation. Life-threatening ventricular dysrhythmias must be treated immediately.
- *Heart failure* (HF) occurs when the heart's pumping action is reduced. Left-sided HF occurs initially with subtle signs such as mild dyspnea, restlessness, agitation, or slight tachycardia.

Other signs indicating the onset of left-sided HF include pulmonary congestion on chest x-ray, S3 or S4 heart sounds on auscultation of the heart, crackles on auscultation of the lungs, paroxysmal nocturnal dyspnea (PND), and orthopnea. Signs of right-sided HF include jugular venous distention, hepatic congestion, and lower extremity edema. (See Heart Failure, p. 274.)

- *Cardiogenic shock* occurs when inadequate oxygen and nutrients are supplied to the tissues because of severe left ventricular (LV) failure, papillary muscle rupture, ventricular septal rupture, LV free wall rupture, or right ventricular infarction. Cardiogenic shock requires aggressive management, including control of dysrhythmias, intraaortic balloon pump therapy, and support of contractility with vasoactive drugs.

Diagnostic Studies

In addition to the patient's history of pain, risk factors, and health history, the primary diagnostic studies used to determine whether a person has UA or an MI include an ECG and serum cardiac markers. Other diagnostic measures can include coronary angiography, exercise stress testing, and echocardiogram.

ECG

- When a patient first presents with chest pain, ST elevations on the 12-lead ECG are most likely indicative of a STEMI. The ECG should be compared with a previous ECG whenever possible. For a patient with chest pain whose ECG does not show ST elevation or ST-T wave changes, it is difficult to distinguish between UA and NSTEMI until serum cardiac biomarkers are measured.
- A patient with STEMI tends to have a more extensive MI that is associated with prolonged and complete coronary occlusion. A pathologic Q wave develops on the ECG.
- A patient with UA or NSTEMI usually has transient thrombosis or incomplete coronary occlusion, and the ECG typically does not develop pathologic Q waves.
- Serial ECGs often reveal the evolution and time sequence of ischemia, injury, infarction, and resolution of the infarction.
- Even if the initial ECG is normal or nondiagnostic when the patient presents with chest pain, the ECG pattern may change within a few hours to reflect the infarction process.

Cardiac Biomarkers

Certain proteins, called *serum cardiac biomarkers,* are released into the blood from necrotic heart muscle after an MI.

- Cardiac-specific troponin has two subtypes: cardiac-specific troponin T (cTnT) and cardiac-specific troponin I (cTnI). These markers are highly specific indicators of MI and have greater sensitivity and specificity for myocardial injury than creatine kinase (CK)-MB.

- Myoglobin is released into the circulation within 2 hours after an MI and peaks in 3 to 15 hours. Although it is one of the first serum cardiac markers to appear after an MI, it lacks cardiac specificity.

Interprofessional Care

It is extremely important that a patient with ACS is rapidly diagnosed and treated to preserve cardiac muscle. Initial management of the patient with chest pain most often occurs in the emergency department (ED). Emergency care of the patient with chest pain is presented in Table 33-12, Lewis et al, *Medical-Surgical Nursing,* ed 10, p. 723.

- Establish an IV line and give sublingual nitroglycerin and chewable aspirin if not already given. IV morphine sulfate is given for pain unrelieved by nitroglycerin.
- Obtain a 12-lead ECG and start continuous ECG monitoring. Position patient in an upright position unless contraindicated, and initiate O_2 by nasal cannula to keep O_2 saturation above 93%.
- The patient usually receives ongoing care in a critical care or telemetry unit where continuous ECG monitoring is available and dysrhythmias can be treated.
- Monitor vital signs, including pulse oximetry, frequently during the first few hours after admission and closely thereafter. Maintain bed rest and limit activity for 12 to 24 hours, with a gradual increase in activity unless contraindicated.
- For a patient with UA or NSTEMI, aspirin and heparin (unfractionated heparin [UH] or low-molecular-weight heparin [LMWH]) are recommended. Dual antiplatelet therapy (e.g., with aspirin and clopidogrel) and heparin are recommended for NSTEMI. Cardiac catheterization with possible PCI is considered as treatment for both UA and NSTEMI once the patient is stabilized and angina is controlled, or if angina returns or increases in severity.
- For a patient with STEMI, reperfusion therapy is initiated. Reperfusion therapy can include emergent PCI (preferred) or thrombolytic therapy for STEMI. Thrombolytic therapy (e.g., reteplase [Retavase]) is given as soon as possible, ideally within the first hour after the onset of symptoms. The goal is to save as much heart muscle as possible. Contraindications and complications with thrombolytic therapy are described in Lewis et al, *Medical-Surgical Nursing,* ed 10, pp. 723 to 724. Dual antiplatelet therapy and heparin are also used.

Coronary artery bypass graft (CABG) surgery consists of the placement of conduits to transport blood between the aorta, or other major arteries, and the myocardium distal to the obstructed coronary artery (or arteries). It requires a sternotomy (opening of the chest cavity) and the use of cardiopulmonary bypass (CPB). It is a palliative treatment for CAD and not a cure. Newer techniques include minimally invasive direct coronary artery bypass, off-pump coronary artery bypass, totally endoscopic coronary artery bypass (TECAB), and transmyocardial laser revascularization. These surgical procedures and related nursing care are further discussed in Lewis et al, *Medical-Surgical Nursing*, ed 10, pp. 726 to 733.

Drug therapy includes IV nitroglycerin, aspirin, β-adrenergic blockers, and anticoagulation. Systemic anticoagulation may be achieved with LMWH given subcutaneously or IV UH. If PCI is anticipated, glycoprotein IIb/IIIa inhibitors may be used. Angiotensin-converting enzyme (ACE) inhibitors are added for some patients after an MI. Calcium channel blockers may be used if the patient is already taking adequate doses of β-blockers or does not tolerate these blockers.

Nursing Management
Goals
The patient with an MI will experience relief of pain, preservation of myocardium, immediate and appropriate treatment, effective coping with illness-associated anxiety, participation in a rehabilitation plan, and reduction of risk factors. See eNursing Care Plan 33-1 for the patient with ACS on the website.

Nursing Diagnoses
- Acute pain
- Decreased cardiac output
- Anxiety
- Activity intolerance
- Ineffective health management

Nursing Interventions
Priorities for nursing interventions in the initial phase include pain assessment and relief, physiologic monitoring, promotion of rest and comfort, alleviation of stress and anxiety, and understanding of the patient's emotional and behavioral reactions. Proper management of these priorities decreases the O_2 needs of a compromised myocardium. In addition, you should institute measures to avoid the hazards of immobility while encouraging rest.
- Provide nitroglycerin, morphine, and supplemental O_2 as needed to eliminate or reduce chest pain.

- Maintain continuous ECG monitoring while the patient is in the ED and intensive care unit (ICU) and after transfer to a step-down or general care unit. Dysrhythmias need to be identified quickly and treated.
- In addition to taking frequent vital signs, evaluate intake and output and perform physical assessment to detect deviations from the patient's baseline parameters. Assess lung and heart sounds and inspect for evidence of early heart failure (e.g., dyspnea, tachycardia, pulmonary congestion, distended neck veins).
- Assess oxygenation status frequently, especially if the patient is receiving O_2. In addition, check the nares for irritation or dryness (see Oxygen Therapy, p. 718).
- Plan nursing and therapeutic actions to ensure adequate rest periods free from interruption.
- Promote rest and comfort. Bed rest may be ordered for the first few days after an MI involving a large portion of the ventricle.
- Anxiety is present in various degrees in patients with ACS. Your role is to identify the source of anxiety and assist the patient in reducing it. If the patient is afraid of being alone, allow a care-giver to sit quietly by the bedside or check in frequently with the patient. If a source of anxiety is fear of the unknown, you should explore these concerns with the patient.

▼ **Patient and Caregiver Teaching**

Patient teaching needs to occur at every stage of the patient's hospitalization and recovery (e.g., ED, telemetry unit, home care). The purpose of teaching is to give the patient and caregiver the tools to make informed health decisions (Table 2).

- Anticipatory guidance involves preparing both patient and care-giver for the usual course of recovery and rehabilitation. By learning what to expect, the patient gains a sense of control over his or her life.
- Teach the patient the parameters within which to exercise and how to check pulse rate. Tell the patient the maximum HR that should be present at any point. If the HR exceeds this level or does not return to the rate of the resting pulse within a few minutes, instruct the patient to stop. Also instruct the patient to stop exercising if pain or shortness of breath occurs. Basic physical activity guidelines for after ACS are presented in Table 33-19, Lewis et al, *Medical-Surgical Nursing*, ed 10, p. 732.
- Discuss participation in an outpatient or home-based cardiac rehabilitation program.
- It is important to include sexual counseling for cardiac patients and their partners. Tell the patient that resumption of sex

TABLE 2 **Patient & Caregiver Teaching**	**A**

Acute Coronary Syndrome

Include the following information in the teaching plan for the patient with acute coronary syndrome and the caregiver.

- Signs and symptoms of angina and MI and what to do should they occur (e.g., take nitroglycerin)*
- When and how to seek help (e.g., contact ERS)
- Anatomy and physiology of the heart and coronary arteries
- Cause and effect of CAD
- Definition of terms (e.g., CAD, angina, MI, sudden cardiac death, heart failure)
- Identification of and plan to decrease risk factors* (see Tables 33-2, 33-3, and 33-4, Lewis et al, *Medical-Surgical Nursing*, ed 10, pp. 708 and 709)
- Reasons for tests and treatments (e.g., ECG monitoring, blood tests, angiography), activity limitations and rest, diet, and drugs*
- Appropriate expectations about recovery (anticipatory guidance)
- Resumption of work, physical activity, sexual activity
- Measures to promote recovery and health (e.g., cardiac rehabilitation)
- Importance of the gradual, progressive resumption of activity*

*Identified by patients as most important to learn before discharge.

depends on the emotional readiness of both the patient and partner and on the HCP's assessment of recovery. It is generally safe to resume sexual activity 7 to 10 days after an uncomplicated MI.

ACUTE RESPIRATORY DISTRESS SYNDROME

Description

Acute respiratory distress syndrome (ARDS) is a sudden and progressive form of respiratory failure in which the alveolar-capillary membrane becomes damaged and more permeable to intravascular fluid. The alveoli fill with fluid, resulting in severe dyspnea, hypoxemia refractory to supplemental O_2, reduced lung compliance, and diffuse pulmonary infiltrates.

Incidence of ARDS in the United States is estimated at more than 150,000 cases annually. Despite supportive therapy, mortality from ARDS is approximately 50%. Patients who have both

TABLE 3 Conditions Predisposing Patients to Acute Respiratory Distress Syndrome	
Direct Lung Injury	**Indirect Lung Injury**
Common Causes	
• Aspiration of gastric contents or other substances • Viral or bacterial pneumonia • Sepsis	• Sepsis (especially gram-negative infection) • Severe massive trauma
Less Common Causes	
• Chest trauma • Embolism: fat, air, amniotic fluid, thrombus • Inhalation of toxic substances • Drowning • O_2 toxicity • Radiation pneumonitis	• Acute pancreatitis • Cardiopulmonary bypass • Disseminated intravascular coagulation • Opioid drug overdose (e.g., heroin) • Severe head injury • Shock states • Transfusion-related acute lung injury (e.g., multiple blood transfusions)

gram-negative septic shock and ARDS have a mortality rate of 70% to 90%.

■ Table 3 lists conditions that predispose patients to the development of ARDS. The most common cause is sepsis. Patients with multiple risk factors are three or four times more likely to develop ARDS.

■ Direct lung injury may cause ARDS, or ARDS may develop as a consequence of systemic inflammatory response syndrome (SIRS). ARDS may also develop as a result of multiple organ dysfunction syndrome (MODS) (see Systemic Inflammatory Response Syndrome and Multiple Organ Dysfunction Syndrome, p. 617).

Pathophysiology

An exact cause for damage to the alveolar-capillary membrane is not known. However, many changes are thought to be caused by stimulation of the inflammatory and immune systems, which causes an attraction of neutrophils to the pulmonary interstitium. The neutrophils cause a release of biochemical, humoral, and

A

cellular mediators that produce changes in the lung, including increased pulmonary capillary membrane permeability, destruction of elastin and collagen, formation of pulmonary microemboli, and pulmonary artery vasoconstriction. Pathophysiologic changes in ARDS are divided into three phases: injury or exudative, reparative or proliferative, and fibrotic.

The *injury* or *exudative phase* occurs approximately 1 to 7 days (usually 24 to 48 hours) after the initial direct lung injury or host insult. The primary changes of this phase are interstitial and alveolar edema (noncardiogenic pulmonary edema) and atelectasis.

- Initially, the peribronchial and perivascular interstitial spaces become engorged, producing interstitial edema. An intrapulmonary shunt develops because the alveoli fill with fluid and blood passing through them cannot be oxygenated.
- Alveolar cells that produce surfactant are damaged by the changes caused by ARDS. This damage, in addition to further fluid and protein accumulation, results in surfactant dysfunction. Widespread atelectasis further decreases lung compliance, compromises gas exchange, and contributes to hypoxemia.
- Hyaline begins to line the alveolar membrane. Hyaline membranes contribute to fibrosis and atelectasis, leading to a decrease in gas exchange capability and lung compliance.
- Severe ventilation-perfusion (V/Q) mismatch and shunting of pulmonary capillary blood result in hypoxemia unresponsive to increasing concentrations of O_2 *(refractory hypoxemia).*

The *reparative* or *proliferative phase* begins 1 to 2 weeks after the initial lung injury. During this phase, there is an influx of granulocytes, monocytes, and lymphocytes and fibroblast proliferation.

- Increased pulmonary vascular resistance and pulmonary hypertension may occur in this stage because fibroblasts and inflammatory cells destroy the pulmonary vasculature.
- Lung compliance continues to decrease and hypoxemia worsens because of the thickened alveolar membrane.
- If this phase persists, widespread fibrosis results. If this phase is stopped, the lesions resolve.

The *fibrotic phase* occurs approximately 2 to 3 weeks after the initial lung injury. This phase is also called the chronic or late phase of ARDS. By this time, the lung is completely remodeled by collagenous and fibrous tissues. Diffuse scarring and fibrosis result in decreased lung compliance and decreased surface area for gas exchange. Pulmonary hypertension results from fibrosis.

The progression of ARDS varies. Some patients survive the acute phase of lung injury and complete recovery occurs in a few days. Others progress to the fibrotic phase, requiring long-term mechanical ventilation, with a poor chance of survival.

Clinical Manifestations

From the time of initial injury to 1 to 2 days later, the patient may
not exhibit respiratory symptoms.

- Later, the patient may exhibit tachypnea, dyspnea, cough, and
  restlessness. Chest auscultation may be normal or reveal fine,
  scattered crackles. Arterial blood gases (ABGs) usually indicate
  mild hypoxemia and respiratory alkalosis. Chest x-ray may be
  normal or exhibit evidence of minimal scattered interstitial infiltrates. Edema may not be apparent until there is a 30% increase
  in lung fluid content.

As ARDS progresses, symptoms worsen because of increased
fluid accumulation in the lungs and decreased lung compliance.
Tachycardia, diaphoresis, changes in sensorium with decreased
mentation, cyanosis, and pallor may be present. Chest auscultation
usually reveals scattered to diffuse crackles and wheezing.

- Hypoxemia, despite increased fraction of inspired O_2 concentration (FIO_2) delivered by mask, cannula, or endotracheal tube,
  is a hallmark of ARDS. Hypercapnia signifies respiratory
  muscle fatigue and hypoventilation.
- As ARDS progresses, profound respiratory distress requires
  endotracheal intubation and positive pressure ventilation (PPV).
  The chest x-ray reveals *whiteout* or *white lung* as consolidation
  and coalescing infiltrates pervade the lungs, leaving few recognizable air spaces.
- Pleural effusions may be present. Severe hypoxemia, hypercapnia, and metabolic acidosis, with symptoms of target organ or
  tissue hypoxemia, may develop if therapy is not promptly started.

Complications may develop as a result of ARDS itself or its
treatment. The primary cause of death in ARDS is MODS, often
accompanied by sepsis. The vital organs most commonly involved
are the kidneys, liver, and heart. The organ systems most often
involved are the central nervous system (CNS) and the hematologic
and gastrointestinal systems.

Diagnostic Studies

Findings that support a diagnosis of ARDS are refractory hypoxemia, new bilateral interstitial or alveolar infiltrates on chest x-ray,
and pulmonary artery wedge pressure of 18 mm Hg or less with
no evidence of heart failure.

Nursing and Interprofessional Management
Goals

The overall goals for the patient with ARDS include maintaining
a partial pressure of O_2 in arterial blood (PaO_2) of at least 60 mm Hg

and adequate lung volume to maintain normal pH. A patient recovering from ARDS will exhibit a PaO_2 within limits of normal for age or baseline values on room air, O_2 saturation in arterial blood (SaO_2) greater than 90%, a patent airway, and clear lungs on auscultation.

Nursing Diagnoses
Nursing diagnoses for the patient with ARDS may include, but are not limited to, those described under Respiratory Failure, Acute (p. 533).

Interprofessional Care
The interprofessional care for acute respiratory failure is applicable to ARDS (see Respiratory Failure, Acute, p. 533). Patients with ARDS are commonly cared for in critical care units.

O_2 Administration. The goal of O_2 therapy is to correct hypoxemia (see Oxygen Therapy, p. 718). Initially use a nasal cannula or face mask with high-flow systems that deliver higher O_2 concentrations. The general standard for O_2 administration is to give the lowest concentration that results in a PaO_2 of 60 mm Hg or greater. When FIO_2 exceeds 60% for more than 48 hours, the risk for O_2 toxicity is increased. Patients with severe ARDS and refractory hypoxemia need intubation with mechanical ventilation (see Artificial Airways: Endotracheal Tubes, p. 683) to maintain the PaO_2 at an acceptable level.

Mechanical Ventilation. Endotracheal intubation and positive pressure ventilation provide additional respiratory support. In patients with ARDS, positive expiratory-end pressure (PEEP) is often used. When PEEP is applied, the lung is kept partially expanded, which prevents the alveoli from totally collapsing. If hypoxemic failure persists despite high levels of PEEP, alternative modes and therapies may be used. These include airway pressure release ventilation, pressure-control inverse-ratio ventilation, high-frequency ventilation, and permissive hypercapnia (low tidal volumes that allow the positive pressure of CO_2 in arterial blood [$PaCO_2$] to increase slowly).

Extracorporeal membrane oxygenation (ECMO) and extracorporeal CO_2 removal pass blood across a gas-exchanging membrane outside the body and return oxygenated blood back to the body.

Positioning. Some patients with ARDS have a marked improvement in PaO_2 when turned from the supine to the prone position (e.g., PaO_2 70 mm Hg supine, PaO_2 90 mm Hg prone). The response may be sufficient to allow a reduction in inspired O_2 concentration or PEEP.

Another positioning strategy to consider for management of ARDS is continuous lateral rotation therapy, which provides continuous, slow, side-to-side turning of the patient by rotating the actual bed frame. Maintain the lateral movement of the bed for 18 of every 24 hours to stimulate postural drainage and help to mobilize pulmonary secretions. The bed may contain a vibrator pack that can provide chest physiotherapy to assist with secretion mobilization and removal.

Interprofessional Supportive Therapy

Patients on PPV and PEEP frequently experience decreased cardiac output. Hemodynamic monitoring is essential to see trends, detect changes, and adjust therapy as needed. An arterial catheter is inserted for continuous monitoring of BP and sampling of blood for ABGs. Use of inotropic drugs, such as dobutamine or dopamine, may also be necessary. Packed red blood cells are used to increase hemoglobin and O_2-carrying capacity, but the optimal hemoglobin level remains controversial.

Maintenance of nutrition and fluid balance is challenging in the patient with ARDS. Parenteral or enteral feedings are started to meet the high energy requirements of these patients. Increasing pulmonary capillary permeability results in fluid in the lungs and causes pulmonary edema. The patient is usually placed on fluid restriction, and diuretics are used as necessary. At the same time, the patient may be volume-depleted and therefore prone to hypotension and decreased cardiac output from mechanical ventilation and PEEP. Monitor fluid status carefully.

▼ Patient and Caregiver Teaching

The patient with ARDS may fear suffocation or death. Providing reassurance, spending time at the bedside, and ensuring that the patient can obtain assistance immediately (e.g., call light and tools for alternate communication strategy while intubated) may help to decrease the anxiety level. Anxiety also may be reduced through instruction in and use of progressive relaxation, guided imagery, and music therapy.

- Explain to the patient any expected sensations that may be encountered with each new experience (e.g., suctioning, drawing ABGs) so that coping strategies can be purposefully selected.

ADDISON'S DISEASE

Description

Addison's disease is a primary adrenocortical insufficiency in which all three classes of adrenal steroids—glucocorticoids, mineralocorticoids, and androgens—are reduced because of adrenal cortex hypofunction.

In secondary adrenocortical insufficiency, which is caused by a lack of pituitary adrenocorticotropic hormone (ACTH) secretion, corticosteroids and androgens are deficient, but mineralocorticoids rarely are.

Up to 80% of Addison's disease cases in the United States are caused by an autoimmune response. Autoimmune adrenalitis causes the adrenal cortex to be destroyed by antibodies. This results in loss of glucocorticoid, mineralocorticoid, and adrenal androgen hormones. Addison's disease can be present along with other endocrine disorders. This condition is known as autoimmune polyglandular syndrome.

Other causes of Addison's disease include amyloidosis, fungal infections (e.g., histoplasmosis), acquired immunodeficiency syndrome (AIDS), and metastatic cancer. Iatrogenic Addison's disease may be due to adrenal hemorrhage, often related to anticoagulant therapy, chemotherapy, ketoconazole therapy for AIDS, or bilateral adrenalectomy.

Clinical Manifestations

Manifestations have a slow (insidious) onset and include anorexia, nausea, progressive weakness, fatigue, and weight loss. Skin hyperpigmentation is seen primarily in sun-exposed areas of the body; at pressure points; over joints; and in the creases, especially palmar creases. Other manifestations include abdominal pain, diarrhea, headache, orthostatic hypotension, salt craving, and joint pain.

Patients with adrenocortical insufficiency are at risk for *addisonian crisis* (acute adrenal insufficiency), a life-threatening emergency caused by critically low levels of adrenocortical hormones.

- The most dangerous manifestation is hypotension, which may cause shock, especially during stress. Circulatory collapse is often unresponsive to the usual treatment (vasopressors and fluid replacement).
- Addisonian crisis may be triggered by stress (e.g., from infection, surgery, trauma, or psychologic distress), sudden withdrawal of corticosteroid hormone therapy (often by the patient lacking knowledge regarding replacement therapy), adrenal surgery, or sudden pituitary gland destruction.

Diagnostic Studies

- Plasma cortisol levels are subnormal or fail to rise over basal levels with an ACTH stimulation test. A positive response to ACTH stimulation indicates a functioning adrenal gland and points to pituitary disease rather than adrenal disease.

- Urine levels of free cortisol and aldosterone are low.
- Serum electrolytes show hyperkalemia, hypochloremia, and hyponatremia.
- CT and MRI are used to localize other causes including tumors, fungal infections, and tuberculosis.

Interprofessional Care

Treatment is focused on managing the underlying cause. The mainstay of treatment is lifelong hormone therapy with glucocorticoids and mineralocorticoids. Overall, patients who take their medications consistently can anticipate a normal life expectancy.

- Hydrocortisone, the most commonly used form of hormone therapy, has both glucocorticoid and mineralocorticoid properties. The dosage is increased in stressful situations to prevent addisonian crisis.
  - Mineralocorticoids are replaced with fludrocortisone and increased dietary salt intake.
- Women need androgen replacement with dehydroepiandrosterone (DHEA), because their only source of androgen production is the adrenal glands.

The patient in addisonian crisis requires immediate aggressive shock management and high-dose hydrocortisone replacement. Large volumes of 0.9% saline solution and 5% dextrose are administered to reverse hypotension and electrolyte imbalances until BP returns to normal.

Nursing Management

When the patient with Addison's disease is hospitalized, nursing management focuses on monitoring the patient while correcting fluid and electrolyte balance.

- Assess vital signs and signs of fluid volume deficit and electrolyte imbalance. Monitor trends in serum glucose, sodium, and potassium.
- Nursing interventions include daily weights, protection against exposure to infection, and assistance with daily hygiene.
- Protect the patient from noise, bright light, and environmental temperature extremes. The patient cannot cope with stress because corticosteroids cannot be produced.
- If hospitalization was due to an adrenal crisis, patients usually respond by the second day and can start oral corticosteroid replacement.
- Because discharge frequently occurs before the usual maintenance dose of corticosteroids is reached, the patient should be instructed on the importance of keeping scheduled follow-up appointments.

▼ **Patient and Caregiver Teaching**

The serious nature of Addison's disease and the need for lifelong hormone therapy necessitate a comprehensive teaching plan.

- Teach patients the signs and symptoms of corticosteroid deficiency and excess and to report these to their HCP so that the dosage can be adjusted.
- It is critical that the patient wear a medical identification (Medic Alert) bracelet and carry a wallet card stating the patient has Addison's disease, so that appropriate therapy can be initiated in case of an emergency.
- Patients should carry an emergency kit with 100 mg of IM methylprednisolone (Solu-Medrol), syringes, and instructions for use when hormone therapy cannot be taken orally. Have the patient verbalize instructions, practice IM injections with normal saline, and carry written instructions on when the dosage should be changed.
- Teach about conditions requiring increased medication (e.g., trauma, infection, surgery, emotional crisis).
- Teach prevention of infection and need for prompt and vigorous treatment of existing infections.
- Provide management instructions for patients who have diabetes and those who have elevated blood glucose levels when taking corticosteroids.

ALZHEIMER'S DISEASE

Description

Alzheimer's disease (AD) is a chronic, progressive, neurodegenerative disease of the brain. It is the most common form of dementia, accounting for about 60% to 80% of all cases of dementia (see Dementia, p. 165). Approximately 5.4 million people in the United States have AD. Ultimately the disease is fatal, with death typically occurring 4 to 8 years after diagnosis, although some patients live for 20 years. AD is the sixth leading cause of death in the United States.

Pathophysiology

The exact etiology of AD is unknown. Although age is the greatest risk factor, AD is not a normal part of aging, and age alone is not sufficient to cause the disease. When AD develops in someone younger than 60 years, it is referred to as *early-onset AD*. AD that becomes evident after the age of 60 years is called *late-onset AD*.

Characteristic findings in AD relate to changes in the brain's structure and function, including amyloid plaques, neurofibrillary tangles, loss of connections between neurons, and neuron death.

- *Amyloid plaques* consist of insoluble deposits of a protein called β-amyloid, other proteins, remnants of neurons, non-nerve cells such as microglia, and other cells. In AD, the plaques develop first in brain areas used for memory and cognitive function. Eventually the cerebral cortex, especially the areas responsible for language and reasoning, is affected.

- *Neurofibrillary tangles* are abnormal collections of twisted protein threads inside nerve cells. The main component of these structures is a protein called *tau*. Normally, tau proteins maintain cellular structure by holding intracellular microtubules together. In AD, the tau protein is altered, and as a result, the microtubules twist together in a helical fashion, ultimately forming neurofibrillary tangles.

Plaques and neurofibrillary tangles are not unique to patients with AD or dementia. They are also found in the brains of individuals without evidence of cognitive impairment. However, they are more abundant in the brains of individuals with AD.

The other features of AD are the loss of connections between neurons and neuron death. These processes result in structural damage. Affected parts of the brain begin to shrink in a process called *brain atrophy*. By the final stage of AD, brain tissue has shrunk significantly.

Genetic factors may play a critical role in the way that the brain processes the β-amyloid protein. Overproduction of β-amyloid appears to be an important risk factor for AD. Abnormally high levels of β-amyloid cause cell damage either directly or through eliciting an inflammatory response and ultimately neuron death.

Diabetes mellitus, hypertension, current smoking, hypercholesterolemia, obesity, and trauma are associated with an increased risk for dementia including AD.

Clinical Manifestations

Pathologic changes often precede clinical manifestations of dementia by 5 to 20 years. Early warning signs of AD are listed in Table 4. The rate of progression from mild to severe is highly variable, ranging from 3 to 20 years.

Initial manifestations are usually related to changes in cognitive functioning. Patients may have complaints of memory loss, mild disorientation, and/or trouble with words and numbers. Often it is a family member, in particular the spouse, who reports the patient's declining memory to the HCP.

TABLE 4 Patient & Caregiver Teaching

Early Warning Signs of Alzheimer's Disease (AD)

Include the following information in the teaching plan for the patient with AD and the caregiver.

1. Memory loss that affects job skills
   - Frequent forgetfulness or unexplainable confusion at home or in the workplace may signal that something is wrong.
   - This type of memory loss goes beyond forgetting an assignment, colleague's name, deadline, or phone number.
2. Difficulty performing familiar tasks
   - It is normal for most people to become distracted and to forget something (e.g., leave something on the stove too long).
   - People with AD may cook a meal but then forget not only to serve it but also that they made it.
3. Problems with language
   - Most people have trouble finding the "right" word from time to time.
   - People with AD may forget simple words or substitute inappropriate words, making their speech difficult to understand.
4. Disorientation to time and place
   - Most individuals occasionally forget the day of the week or what they need from the store.
   - People with AD can become lost on their own street, not knowing where they are, how they got there, or how to get back home.
5. Poor or decreased judgment
   - Many individuals from time to time may choose not to dress appropriately for the weather (e.g., not bringing a coat or sweater on a cold evening).
   - The person with AD may dress inappropriately in more noticeable ways, such as wearing a bathrobe to the store or a sweater on a hot day.
6. Problems with abstract thinking
   - For the person with AD, this goes beyond challenges such as balancing a checkbook.
   - The person with AD may have difficulty recognizing numbers or doing even basic calculations.

Continued

TABLE 4   Patient & Caregiver Teaching
Early Warning Signs of Alzheimer's Disease (AD)—cont'd
7. Misplacing things   • For many individuals, temporarily misplacing keys, purses, or wallets is a normal albeit frustrating event.   • The person with AD may put items in inappropriate places (e.g., eating utensils in clothing drawers) but have no memory of how they got there.   8. Changes in mood or behavior   • Most individuals experience mood changes.   • The person with AD tends to exhibit more rapid mood swings for no apparent reason.   9. Changes in personality   • As most individuals age, they may demonstrate some change in personality (e.g., become less tolerant).   • The person with AD can change dramatically, either suddenly or over time. For example, someone who is generally easygoing may become angry, suspicious, or fearful.   10. Loss of initiative   • The person with AD may become and remain uninterested and uninvolved in many or all of his or her usual pursuits.

Adapted from Alzheimer's Association: *Early warning signs,* Chicago, The Association. *www.alz.org/alzheimers_disease_know_the_10_signs.asp.*

- Memory loss initially relates to recent events, with remote memories still intact. With time and progression of AD, memory loss includes both recent and remote memory and ultimately affects the ability to perform self-care.
- Behavioral manifestations (e.g., agitation, aggression) result from changes that take place within the brain. The person's behaviors are neither intentional nor controllable by the individual with the disease. Some patients develop delusions and hallucinations.

As AD progresses, the individual may develop additional cognitive impairments such as *dysphasia* (difficulty comprehending language and oral communication), *apraxia* (inability to manipulate objects or perform purposeful acts), *visual agnosia* (inability to recognize objects by sight), and *dysgraphia* (difficulty communicating via writing).

- Later in the disease, long-term memories cannot be recalled, the person loses the ability to recognize family members, and eventually the ability to communicate and perform activities of daily living (ADLs) is lost.

- In the late or final stages, the patient is unresponsive and incontinent and requires total care.

Diagnostic Studies

The diagnosis of AD is primarily a diagnosis of exclusion. When all other possible conditions that can cause mental impairment have been ruled out and manifestations of dementia persist, the diagnosis of AD can be made.

- Comprehensive health history, physical examination, neurologic and mental status assessments, and laboratory tests are done.
- Brain imaging tests include CT or MRI scan, which may show brain atrophy in the later stages. However, this finding occurs in other diseases and in people without cognitive impairment.
- Positron emission tomography (PET) scanning can be used to differentiate AD from other forms of dementia.
- Definitive diagnosis of AD usually requires the presence of neurofibrillary tangles and neuritic plaques at autopsy.

Interprofessional Care

At this time there is no cure for AD. No treatment is available to stop the deterioration of brain cells in AD. Management of AD is aimed at controlling the undesirable behaviors that the patient may exhibit and providing support for the family caregiver. Table 59-11, Lewis et al, *Medical-Surgical Nursing,* ed 10, p. 1408, details drug therapy for AD. These drugs have no effect on overall disease progression.

- Cholinesterase inhibitors block cholinesterase, the enzyme responsible for the breakdown of acetylcholine in the synaptic cleft. Cholinesterase inhibitors include donepezil (Aricept), rivastigmine (Exelon), and galantamine (Razadyne). Rivastigmine is available as a patch.
- Memantine (Namenda) protects brain nerve cells by blocking the damaging effects of glutamate, which is released in large amounts by cells damaged by AD.
- Although antipsychotic drugs are approved for treating psychotic conditions (e.g., schizophrenia), they also have been used for the management of behavioral problems (e.g., agitation, aggressive behavior) that occur in patients with AD. However, these drugs have been shown to increase the risk of death in older patients with dementia.
- Treating the depression associated with AD may improve the patient's cognitive ability. These medications include selective

serotonin reuptake inhibitors (SSRIs) such as fluoxetine (Prozac), sertraline (Zoloft), fluvoxamine (Luvox CR), and citalopram (Celexa).

Nursing Management

Goals
The patient with AD will maintain functional ability for as long as possible, be maintained in a safe environment with a minimum of injuries, have personal care needs met, and have dignity maintained. Additional information on nursing diagnoses for the patient with AD is presented in eNursing Care Plan 59-1 (available on the website).

Nursing Diagnoses
- Impaired memory
- Self-neglect
- Risk for injury
- Wandering

Nursing Interventions
The diagnosis of AD is traumatic for both the patient and family.
- Assess family caregivers and their ability to accept and cope with the diagnosis. You are in an important position to assess for depression.
- Work collaboratively with the patient's HCP to manage symptoms effectively as they change over time. You are often responsible for teaching the caregiver to perform the many tasks required to manage the patient's care.
- Adult day care is one of the options available to provide respite for the family and a protective environment for the patient.
- As the disease progresses, the demands on the caregivers eventually exceed their resources. The person with AD may need to be placed in a special dementia unit of a long-term care facility.
- Support groups for caregivers and family members can provide an atmosphere of understanding and give current information about the disease itself and related topics such as safety, legal, ethical, and financial issues. The Alzheimer's Association has educational and support systems available to help family caregivers, including the booklet *Caring for a Person with Alzheimer's Disease* (*www.nia.nih.gov/Alzheimers/Publications/CaringAD*).

Hospitalization of the patient with AD can be a traumatic event and can precipitate a worsening of the disease. Patients with AD who are hospitalized in the acute care setting will need to be observed more closely because of concerns for safety, frequently oriented to place and time, and given reassurance. Anxiety or disruptive behavior may be reduced through the use of consistent nursing staff.

A family and caregiver teaching guide based on the disease stages is provided in Table 5.

AMYOTROPHIC LATERAL SCLEROSIS

Amyotrophic lateral sclerosis (ALS) is a rare, progressive neuro-muscular disease characterized by loss of motor neurons. This disease became known as Lou Gehrig's disease when the famous baseball player was stricken with it in 1939. The onset is between the ages of 45 and 75 years, and twice as many men as women are affected. This illness is devastating because the patient remains cognitively intact while wasting away. ALS usually leads to death within 2 to 5 years of diagnosis.

- For unknown reasons, motor neurons in the brainstem and spinal cord gradually degenerate in ALS. Consequently, chemical and electrical messages originating in the brain never activate the muscles.
- Early signs and symptoms of weakness vary but often include tripping, dropping things, abnormal fatigue of the extremities, slurred speech, and muscle cramps and twitches.
- Muscle wasting and fasciculations result from denervation of the muscles and lack of stimulation and use.
- Other manifestations include pain, sleep disorders, spasticity and hyperreflexia, drooling, emotional lability, depression, constipation, and esophageal reflux.
- There is no cure for ALS. Death usually results from respiratory infection secondary to compromised respiratory function.
- Riluzole (Rilutek) slows the progression of ALS by decreasing the amount of glutamate (an excitatory neurotransmitter) in the brain.

Nursing interventions include (1) facilitating communication, (2) reducing risk of aspiration, (3) facilitating early identification of respiratory insufficiency, (4) decreasing pain secondary to muscle weakness, (5) decreasing risk of injury related to falls, and (6) providing diversional activities such as reading and human companionship.

- Guide the patient in the use of moderate-intensity, endurance-type exercises for the trunk and limbs as this may help to reduce ALS spasticity.
- Help the patient and family manage the disease process, including grieving related to the loss of motor function and, ultimately, death. Discuss advance directives with the patient and caregivers.

TABLE 5   Family & Caregiver Teaching
Alzheimer's Disease

Include the following instructions when teaching families and caregivers the management of the patient with Alzheimer's disease.

Mild Stage
- Many treatable (and potentially reversible) conditions can mimic dementia (see Table 59-2, Lewis et al, *Medical-Surgical Nursing*, ed 10, p. 1400). Try to get a definitive diagnosis.
- Get the person to stop driving. Confusion and poor judgment can impair driving skills and potentially put others at risk.
- Encourage activities such as visiting with friends and family, listening to music, participating in hobbies, and exercising.
- Provide cues in the home, establish a routine, and determine a specific location where essential items (e.g., eyeglasses) need to be kept.
- Do not correct misstatements or faulty memory.
- Register with MedicAlert + Alzheimer's Association Safe Return, a program established by the MedicAlert Foundation and the Alzheimer's Association to locate individuals who wander from their homes.
- Make plans for the future in terms of advance directives, care options, financial concerns, and personal preference for care.

Moderate Stage
- Install door locks for patient safety.
- Provide protective wear for urinary and fecal incontinence.
- Ensure that the home has good lighting, install handrails in stairways and bathroom, and remove area rugs.
- Label drawers and faucets (hot and cold) to ensure safety.
- Develop strategies such as distraction and diversion to cope with behavioral problems. Identify and reduce potential triggers (e.g., reduce stress, extremes in temperature) for disruptive behavior.
- Provide memory triggers, such as pictures of family and friends.

Severe Stage
- Provide a regular schedule for toileting to reduce incontinence.
- Provide care to meet needs, including oral care and skin care.
- Monitor diet and fluid intake to ensure their adequacy.
- Continue communication through talking and touching.
- Consider placement in a long-term care facility when providing total care becomes too difficult.

ANAL CANCER

Anal cancer is uncommon in the general population, but the incidence is increasing. It mainly occurs in older adults. Human papillomavirus (HPV) is associated with about 80% of the cases of anal cancer. Those at high risk for anal cancer include smokers, men who have sex with men, women with cervical or vulvar cancer or precancerous lesions, and people who are immunocompromised (e.g., from posttransplantation immunosuppression) or human immunodeficiency virus (HIV)-positive.

- Frequently the initial manifestation is rectal bleeding. Other symptoms include rectal pain and sensation of a rectal mass. Some patients have no symptoms, which leads to delayed diagnosis and treatment.

It is especially important to screen high-risk individuals. A swab of the anal mucosa can be obtained during a digital rectal examination for identification of cell changes (e.g., dysplasia, neoplasia). High-resolution anoscopy allows visualization of the mucosa and obtaining a biopsy. An endoanal (endorectal) ultrasound also may be done.

Review with the patient the behavior practices used to reduce the risk of sexually transmitted infections. Encourage the use of condoms, avoiding unprotected anal sex, and limiting sexual partners. Two HPV vaccines—Gardasil and Gardasil 9—are available to help prevent cervical, vulvar, vaginal, and anal cancers and associated precancerous lesions. Both vaccines protect against HPV types 6, 11, 16, and 18. Gardasil 9 protects against five additional HPV types.

Treatment of anal cancer depends on the size and depth of the lesions. Topical therapy with bichloroacetic or trichloroacetic acid may be used to kill the HPV. Precancerous lesions may be surgically removed or treated with topical imiquimod (Aldara) and 5-fluorouracil (5-FU). Cancer therapy includes surgery, radiation, and chemotherapy. Chemotherapy may include combinations of mitomycin, cisplatin, and 5-FU.

ANEMIA

Description

Anemia is a deficiency in the number of red blood cells (RBCs), or erythrocytes, quantity of hemoglobin (Hgb), and/or volume of packed RBCs (hematocrit). It is a prevalent condition with many diverse causes such as blood loss, impaired production of erythrocytes, or increased destruction of erythrocytes.

- Because RBCs transport O_2, erythrocyte disorders can lead to tissue hypoxia. Hypoxia accounts for many of the signs and symptoms of anemia.
- Anemia is not a specific disease; it is a manifestation of a pathologic process.
- Anemia can result from primary hematologic problems or can develop secondary to disorders in other body systems.

The various types of anemias can be classified according to morphology (cell characteristics) or etiology. Although the morphologic system is the most accurate means of classifying anemia, it is easier to discuss patient care by focusing on the etiology of the anemia.

- *Morphologic classification* is based on erythrocyte size and color (Table 6).
- *Etiologic classification* is related to clinical conditions causing the anemia (Table 7).

Diagnostic Studies

- Anemia is diagnosed using a complete blood count (CBC), reticulocyte count, and peripheral blood smear. Once anemia is identified, further investigation may determine its specific cause.

TABLE 6 Morphologic Classification and Etiology of Anemia	
RBC Morphology	**Etiology**
Normocytic, normochromic (normal size and color) MCV 80-100 fL, MCH 27-34 pg	Acute blood loss, hemolysis, chronic kidney disease, chronic disease, cancers, sideroblastic anemia, endocrine disorders, starvation, aplastic anemia, sickle cell anemia, pregnancy
Microcytic, hypochromic (small size, pale color) MCV <80 fL, MCH <27 pg	Iron-deficiency anemia, vitamin B_6 deficiency, copper deficiency, thalassemia, lead poisoning
Macrocytic (megaloblastic), normochromic (large size, normal color) MCV >100 fL, MCH >34 pg	Cobalamin (vitamin B_{12}) deficiency, folic acid deficiency, liver disease (including effects of alcohol abuse)

MCH, Mean corpuscular hemoglobin; *MCV,* mean corpuscular volume.

TABLE 7   Etiologic Classification of Anemia

Decreased RBC Production

Decreased Hemoglobin Synthesis

- Iron deficiency
- Thalassemias (decreased globin synthesis)
- Sideroblastic anemia (decreased porphyrin)

Defective DNA Synthesis

- Cobalamin (vitamin B_{12}) deficiency
- Folic acid deficiency

Decreased Number of RBC Precursors

- Aplastic anemia and inherited disorders (e.g., Fanconi syndrome)
- Anemia of myeloproliferative diseases (e.g., leukemia) and myelodysplasia
- Chronic diseases or disorders
- Medications and chemicals (e.g., chemotherapy, lead)
- Radiation

Blood Loss

Acute

- Trauma
- Blood vessel rupture
- Splenic sequestration crisis

Chronic

- Gastritis
- Menstrual flow
- Hemorrhoids

Increased RBC Destruction (Hemolytic Anemias)

Hereditary (Intrinsic)

- Abnormal hemoglobin (sickle cell disease)
- Enzyme deficiency (G6PD)
- Membrane abnormalities (paroxysmal nocturnal hemoglobinuria, hereditary spherocytosis)

Continued

TABLE 7   Etiologic Classification of Anemia—cont'd
Acquired (Extrinsic)
• Physical destruction
• Prosthetic heart valves
• Extracorporeal circulation
• Disseminated intravascular coagulopathy (DIC)
• Thrombotic thrombocytopenic purpura (TTP)
• Antibodies against RBCs
• Infectious agents (e.g., malaria) and toxins

G6PD, Glucose-6-phosphate dehydrogenase.

- Although the Hgb level is decreased in all types of anemias, other laboratory results are characteristic of specific types of anemias (Table 8).

Clinical Manifestations

Manifestations of anemia are caused by the body's response to tissue hypoxia (Table 9). Specific manifestations vary depending on the rate at which the anemia has evolved, its severity, and any coexisting disease. Hgb levels may determine the severity of anemia.

- *Mild anemia* (Hgb 10 to 14 g/dL [100 to 140 g/L]) may not cause symptoms. If signs and symptoms develop, they are usually caused by an underlying disease or represent a compensatory response to heavy exercise. Manifestations may include palpitations, dyspnea, and mild fatigue.
- In *moderate anemia* (Hgb 6 to 10 g/dL [60 to 100 g/L]), cardiopulmonary signs and symptoms (e.g., increased heart rate) may be present with rest as well as activity.
- In *severe anemia* (Hgb <6 g/dL [60 g/L]), patients display many clinical manifestations involving multiple body systems.

Nursing Management

Goals

The patient with anemia will assume normal activities of daily living (ADLs), maintain adequate nutrition, and develop no complications related to anemia. See eNursing Care Plan 30-1 for the patient with anemia (available on the website).

Nursing Diagnoses

- Fatigue
- Imbalanced nutrition: less than body requirements
- Ineffective health management

TABLE 8 Laboratory Results in Anemias

Etiology of Anemia	Hgb/Hct	MCV	Reticulocytes	Serum Iron	TIBC	Transferrin	Ferritin	Bilirubin	Serum B₁₂	Folate
Iron deficiency	↓	↓	N or slight ↓ or ↑	↓	↑	N or ↓	↓	N or ↓	N	N
Thalassemia major	↓↓	N or ↓	↑	↑	↓ N	↓	N or ↑	↑	N	↓
Cobalamin deficiency	↓	↑	N or ↓	N or ↑	N	Slight ↑	↑	N or slight ↑	↓	N
Folic acid deficiency	↓	↑	N or ↓	N or ↑	N	Slight ↑	↑	N or slight ↑	N	↓
Aplastic anemia	↓	N or slight ↑	↓	N or ↑	N or ↑	N	N	N	N	N
Chronic disease	↓	N or ↓	N or ↓	N or ↓	↓ N	N or ↓	N or ↑	N	N	N
Acute blood loss	↓	N or ↓	N or ↑	N	N	N	N	N	N	N
Chronic blood loss	↓	↓ or N	N or ↑	↓	↓	N	N	N or ↓	N	N
Sickle cell anemia	↓	N	↓ or ↑	N or ↑	N or ↓	N	N or ↑	↑	N	↓
Hemolytic anemia	↓	N or ↑	↑	N or ↑	N or ↓	N	N or ↑	↑	N	N

Hgb/Hct, Hemoglobin/hematocrit; *MCV,* mean corpuscular volume; *N,* normal; *TIBC,* total iron-binding capacity.

A

TABLE 9 Manifestations of Anemia

BODY SYSTEM	SEVERITY OF ANEMIA		
	Mild (Hgb 10-12 g/dL [100-120 g/L])	Moderate (Hgb 6-10 g/dL [60-100 g/L])	Severe (Hgb <6 g/dL [<60 g/L])
Integument	None	None	Pallor, jaundice,* pruritus*
Eyes	None	None	Icteric conjunctiva and sclera,* retinal hemorrhage, blurred vision
Mouth	None	None	Glossitis, smooth tongue
Cardiovascular	Palpitations	Increased palpitations, "bounding pulse"	Tachycardia, increased pulse pressure, systolic murmurs, intermittent claudication, angina, heart failure, MI
Pulmonary	Exertional dyspnea	Dyspnea	Tachypnea, orthopnea, dyspnea at rest
Neurologic	None	"Roaring in the ears"	Headache, vertigo, irritability, depression, impaired thought processes
Gastrointestinal	None	None	Anorexia, hepatomegaly, splenomegaly, difficulty swallowing, sore mouth
Musculoskeletal	None	None	Bone pain
General	None or mild fatigue	Fatigue	Sensitivity to cold, weight loss, lethargy

*Caused by hemolysis.

Nursing and Interprofessional Management

The numerous causes of anemia require nursing interventions specific to the type of anemia and the patient's needs. General components of care for all patients with anemia may include:

- Dietary and lifestyle changes that may reverse some causes of anemia
- Acute interventions such as blood or blood product transfusions, drug therapy (e.g., erythropoietin, vitamin supplements), volume replacement, and O_2 therapy
- Assisting the patient in prioritizing activities and planning rest to accommodate energy levels and manage fatigue
- Assessing the patient's knowledge regarding adequate nutritional intake and adherence to safety precautions to prevent falls and injury

Specific types of anemias are listed under separate headings.

ANEMIA, APLASTIC

Description

Aplastic anemia is a disease in which the patient has peripheral blood *pancytopenia* (decrease in number of all blood cell types—red blood cells [RBCs], white blood cells [WBCs], and platelets) and hypocellular bone marrow. The spectrum of the anemia can range from a chronic condition managed with erythropoietin or blood transfusions to a critical condition with hemorrhage and sepsis.

Pathophysiology

Aplastic anemias, which are most often acquired and idiopathic, are thought to have an autoimmune basis. Causes include chemical agents and toxins (e.g., benzene, insecticides, arsenic, alcohol); drugs (e.g., alkylating agents, antiseizure drugs, antimetabolites, antimicrobials, gold, nonsteroidal antiinflammatory drugs, thyroid medications, allopurinol); radiation; and viral or bacterial infections.

Clinical Manifestations

Aplastic anemia can manifest abruptly over days or develop insidiously over weeks and months. It can range from mild to severe. Clinically the patient may have symptoms caused by suppression of any or all bone marrow elements.

- General manifestations of anemia such as fatigue and dyspnea, as well as cardiovascular and cerebral signs, may be seen (see Table 9).

- The patient with neutropenia (low neutrophil count) is susceptible to infection and at risk for development of septic shock and death. Even a low-grade temperature (>100.4°F [38°C]) should be considered a medical emergency.
- Thrombocytopenia may be manifested by a predisposition to bleeding (e.g., petechiae, ecchymoses, epistaxis).

Diagnostic Studies

Diagnosis is confirmed by laboratory studies.

- All marrow elements are affected (RBC, WBC, and platelet), with values often decreased (see Table 8). Reticulocyte count is low.
- Serum iron and total iron-binding capacity (TIBC) may be elevated as initial signs of erythroid suppression.
- Bone marrow examination is especially important in aplastic anemia. Findings include a hypocellular marrow with increased yellow marrow (fat content).

Nursing and Interprofessional Management

Management of aplastic anemia is based on identifying and removing the causative agent (when possible) and providing supportive care until pancytopenia reverses.

Nursing interventions appropriate for the patient with pancytopenia from aplastic anemia are presented in the nursing care plans (on the website) for patients with anemia (see eNursing Care Plan 30-1), thrombocytopenia (eNursing Care Plan 30-2), and neutropenia (eNursing Care Plan 30-3). Nursing actions are directed at preventing complications from infection and hemorrhage.

- The prognosis for severe untreated aplastic anemia is poor. However, advances in medical management, including hematopoietic stem cell transplantation (HSCT) and immunosuppressive therapy with antithymocyte globulin (ATG) and cyclosporine or high-dose cyclophosphamide, have significantly improved outcomes. Alemtuzumab (Campath) (a monoclonal antibody) and eltrombopag (Promacta) (an oral thrombopoietin receptor agonist) are options for select patients who do not respond other therapies.
- Treatment of choice for adults younger than 55 years of age who do not respond to immunosuppressive therapy and who have a human leukocyte antigen (HLA)–matched donor is HSCT. Best results are seen in younger patients who have not had previous blood transfusions. Prior transfusions increase the risk of graft rejection. For older adults without an HLA-matched donor, the treatment of choice is immunosuppression with ATG

or cyclosporine or high-dose cyclophosphamide. This therapy may be only partially beneficial.

ANEMIA, COBALAMIN (VITAMIN B_{12}) DEFICIENCY

Description

Anemia resulting from a cobalamin (vitamin B_{12}) deficiency is a type of megaloblastic anemia caused by impaired DNA synthesis. When DNA synthesis is impaired, defective red blood cell (RBC) maturation results in large, abnormal RBCs. Normally a protein known as *intrinsic factor* (IF) is secreted by parietal cells of the gastric mucosa. IF is required for cobalamin (extrinsic factor) absorption in the distal ileum. Therefore when IF is not secreted, cobalamin will not be absorbed.

- In *pernicious anemia,* the most common cause of cobalamin deficiency, the gastric mucosa does not secrete IF.

Pathophysiology

Cobalamin deficiency can occur in patients who have had GI surgery such as gastrectomy, gastric bypass, or small bowel resection involving the ileum, and in patients with Crohn's disease, ileitis, diverticula of the small intestine, and/or chronic atrophic gastritis. In these cases, cobalamin deficiency results from the loss of IF-secreting gastric mucosal surface or impaired absorption of cobalamin in the distal ileum. Cobalamin deficiency also is found in people who ingest excessive alcohol or hot tea, smokers, long-term users of histamine (H_2)-receptor blockers and proton pump inhibitors, and those who are strict vegetarians.

Pernicious anemia is caused by an absence of IF from either gastric mucosal atrophy or autoimmune destruction of parietal cells. Such changes decrease HCl acid secretion by the stomach.

Clinical Manifestations

Manifestations of anemia related to cobalamin deficiency develop as a result of tissue hypoxia (Table 9).

- GI manifestations include a sore red tongue, anorexia, nausea, vomiting, and abdominal pain.
- Neuromuscular manifestations include weakness, paresthesias of feet and hands, reduced vibratory and position senses, ataxia, muscle weakness, and impaired thought processes ranging from confusion to dementia.

Diagnostic Studies

Laboratory data reflective of cobalamin deficiency anemia are presented in Table 8.

- Erythrocytes appear large (macrocytic) with abnormal shapes. This structure contributes to erythrocyte destruction because the cell membrane is fragile.
- Serum cobalamin levels are reduced.
- Normal serum folate levels with low cobalamin levels suggest that megaloblastic anemia is due to a cobalamin deficiency.
- A serum test for anti-IF antibodies may be done that is specific for pernicious anemia.
- An upper GI endoscopy and biopsy of the gastric mucosa may also be done.

Interprofessional Care

Dietary management is not used for cobalamin replacement. Regardless of how much cobalamin is ingested, the patient is not able to absorb it when IF is lacking or if absorption in the ileum is impaired

- Lifelong administration of cobalamin is needed. It can be given parenterally (cyanocobalamin or hydroxocobalamin) or intranasally (Nascobal). A typical treatment schedule consists of 1000 mg cobalamin IM daily for 2 weeks, then weekly until hematocrit is normal, and then monthly for life.
- High-dose oral cobalamin and sublingual cobalamin also are available for patients in whom GI absorption is intact.
- Long-standing neuromuscular complications may not be reversible, but physical therapy may be warranted.

Nursing Management

- Nursing interventions for the patient with anemia also are appropriate for the patient with cobalamin deficiency (see Anemia, p. 29).
- Ensure that the patient is protected from burns and trauma, because of a diminished sensation to heat and pain as a result of neurologic impairment.
- Ongoing care is primarily related to ensuring patient compliance with treatment. Careful follow-up evaluation is essential to assess for neurologic difficulties that were not fully corrected by cobalamin replacement therapy. Because the potential for gastric cancer is increased in patients with atrophic gastritis–related pernicious anemia, the patient should have frequent and appropriate screening for gastric cancer.

ANEMIA, FOLIC ACID DEFICIENCY

A

Folic acid (folate) deficiency can cause megaloblastic anemia. Folic acid is required for deoxyribonucleic acid (DNA) synthesis leading to the formation and maturation of red blood cells (RBCs). Common causes of folic acid deficiency are (1) dietary deficiency, especially a lack of leafy green vegetables and citrus fruits; (2) malabsorption syndromes; (3) drugs that interfere with absorption/or use of folic acid (e.g., methotrexate); antiseizure medications (e.g., phenobarbital, phenytoin [Dilantin]); (4) chronic alcohol use and anorexia; and (5) chronic hemodialysis.

Clinical Manifestations

Clinical manifestations of folic acid deficiency are similar to those of cobalamin deficiency. The disease develops insidiously, and the patient's symptoms may be attributed to other coexisting problems, such as cirrhosis or esophageal varices.

- GI disturbances include dyspepsia and a smooth, beefy-red tongue.
- Absence of neurologic problems is an important diagnostic finding and differentiates folic acid deficiency from cobalamin deficiency.
- Laboratory findings in folic acid deficiency are presented in Table 8. The serum folate level is low (normal is 3 to 16 ng/mL [7 to 36 nmol/L]), and the serum cobalamin level is normal.

Nursing and Interprofessional Management

Folic acid deficiency is treated by replacement therapy, with a usual dosage of 1 mg/day by mouth. In malabsorption states, up to 5 mg/day may be required. The duration of treatment depends on the reason for the deficiency. Encourage the patient to eat foods containing large amounts of folic acid (e.g., leafy green vegetables, breakfast cereals, breads, pasta).

Nursing interventions for the patient with anemia are also appropriate for the patient with folic acid deficiency (see Anemia, p. 29).

ANEMIA, IRON-DEFICIENCY

Description

Iron-deficiency anemia is the most common nutritional disorder in the world. Those most susceptible to iron-deficiency anemia are the very young, those on poor diets, and women in their reproductive years.

Pathophysiology

Iron deficiency may develop from inadequate dietary intake, malabsorption, blood loss, or hemolysis. Dietary iron is adequate to meet the needs of men and older women, but it may be inadequate for those individuals who have higher iron needs (e.g., menstruating or pregnant women).

Iron absorption occurs in the duodenum, and absorption can be altered after surgical procedures that involve removal of or bypass of the duodenum. Malabsorption syndromes also may involve disease of the duodenum, affecting iron absorption.

Blood loss is a major cause of iron deficiency in adults. Major sources of chronic blood loss are from the GI and genitourinary (GU) systems.

- GI bleeding is often not apparent and may occur over a prolonged period before the problem is identified. A loss of 50 to 75 mL of blood from the upper GI tract is required to cause stools to appear black *(melena)*. This color results from iron in the red blood cells (RBCs).
- Common causes of GI blood loss are peptic ulcer, esophagitis, diverticula, hemorrhoids, and neoplasia. GU blood loss occurs primarily from menstrual bleeding. The average monthly menstrual blood loss is about 45 mL, which causes a loss of about 22 mg of iron.
- In addition to anemia of chronic kidney disease, dialysis treatment may induce iron-deficiency anemia because of the blood lost in the dialysis equipment and frequent blood sampling.

Clinical Manifestations

In the early course of iron-deficiency anemia, the patient may be free of symptoms. As the disease becomes chronic, general manifestations of anemia may develop (Table 9). In addition, specific clinical signs and symptoms related to iron-deficiency anemia may occur.

- Pallor is the most common finding, and glossitis (inflammation of the tongue) is the second most common; another finding is cheilitis (inflammation of the lips).
- In addition, the patient may report headache, paresthesia, and a burning sensation of the tongue, all of which are caused by lack of iron in the tissues.

Diagnostic Studies

Laboratory abnormalities characteristic of iron-deficiency anemia are presented in Table 8. Other diagnostic studies are done to determine the cause of iron deficiency. Endoscopy and colonoscopy may be used to detect GI bleeding.

Interprofessional Care

The main goal is to treat the underlying cause of reduced intake (e.g., malnutrition, alcoholism) or absorption of iron. Efforts are directed toward replacing iron.

- Teach the patient which foods are good sources of iron. If nutrition is adequate, increasing iron intake by dietary means may not be practical. Consequently, oral or occasionally parenteral iron supplements are used.
- Drug therapy with iron supplements requires special considerations related to administration and side effects (see Drug Therapy, Iron-Deficiency Anemia in Chapter 30, Lewis et al, *Medical-Surgical Nursing*, ed 10, p. 610).
- If iron deficiency is from acute blood loss, transfusion of packed RBCs may be required.

Nursing Management

Consider groups who are at increased risk for development of iron-deficiency anemia, including premenopausal and pregnant women, people from lower socioeconomic backgrounds, older adults, and individuals experiencing blood loss. Diet teaching, with an emphasis on foods high in iron and ways to maximize absorption, is important for these groups.

Appropriate nursing measures are presented in eNursing Care Plan 30-1, on the website.

▼ **Patient and Caregiver Teaching**

- Discuss the need for diagnostic studies to identify the cause of anemia. Reassess the hemoglobin (Hgb) level and RBC counts to evaluate response to therapy.
- Emphasize adherence with dietary and drug therapy. To replenish the body's iron stores, the patient needs to take iron therapy for 2 to 3 months after the Hgb level returns to normal.
- Monitor patients who require lifelong iron supplementation for potential liver problems related to the iron storage.

ANEURYSM, AORTIC

Description

An *aneurysm* is a localized outpouching or dilation of the blood vessel wall. About 1.1 million adults between 55 and 84 years of age have an *abdominal aortic aneurysm* (AAA). Aneurysms occur in men more often than in women.

Aneurysms may occur in more than one location. Aortic aneurysms may involve the aortic arch, thoracic aorta, and/or abdominal aorta. Most aneurysms are found in the abdominal aorta below the level of the renal arteries. Over time, the dilated aortic wall becomes lined with thrombi that can embolize, leading to acute ischemia in distal arteries.

Pathophysiology

A variety of disorders are associated with aortic aneurysms. The primary causes are classified as degenerative, congenital, mechanical (e.g., penetrating or blunt trauma), inflammatory (e.g., aortitis [Takayasu's arteritis]), or infectious (e.g., aortitis [*Chlamydia pneumoniae,* human immunodeficiency virus]). The larger the aneurysm, the greater the risk of rupture.

- Risk factors for aortic aneurysms include age, male gender, hypertension, coronary artery disease, family history, tobacco use, high cholesterol, lower extremity peripheral artery disease (PAD), carotid artery disease, previous stroke, and excess weight or obesity. Tobacco use is the most important modifiable risk factor.
- The development of aortic aneurysm and dissection has a strong genetic component. (Aortic dissection is discussed as a separate topic.) The familial tendency is related to congenital anomalies such as bicuspid aortic valve, coarctation of the aorta, Turner syndrome, and autosomal dominant polycystic kidney disease. Aneurysms are classified as true and false aneurysms.
- A *true aneurysm* is one in which the wall of the artery forms the aneurysm, with at least one vessel layer still intact. True aneurysms are further subdivided into fusiform and saccular dilations. A *fusiform aneurysm* is circumferential and relatively uniform in shape. A *saccular aneurysm* is pouchlike, with a narrow neck connecting the bulge to one side of the arterial wall.
- A *false aneurysm,* or *pseudoaneurysm,* is not an aneurysm but a disruption of all layers of all wall layers with bleeding that is contained by surrounding anatomic structures. False aneurysms may result from trauma, infection, after peripheral artery bypass graft surgery at the site of the graft-to-artery anastomosis, or arterial leakage after removal of cannulae (e.g., femoral artery catheters, intraaortic balloon pump devices).

Clinical Manifestations

Thoracic aortic aneurysms are usually asymptomatic. When symptoms present, the most common is deep, diffuse chest pain that may extend to the interscapular area.

Aneurysms in the ascending aorta and aortic arch can cause (1) angina from decreased blood flow to the coronary arteries; (2) transient ischemic attacks from decreased blood flow to the carotid arteries; and (3) coughing, shortness of breath, hoarseness, and/or dysphagia (difficulty swallowing) from pressure on the laryngeal nerve. Compression of the superior vena cava by the aneurysm can cause distended neck veins and face and arm edema.

AAAs are often asymptomatic and found during routine physical examination or on evaluation for an unrelated problem (e.g., abdominal x-ray). A pulsatile mass in the periumbilical area slightly to the left of midline may be present. Bruits may be auscultated over the aneurysm. Physical findings may be more difficult to detect in obese individuals.

- AAA symptoms may mimic pain associated with abdominal or back disorders. Compression of nearby anatomic structures and nerves may cause symptoms such as back pain, epigastric discomfort, altered bowel elimination, and intermittent claudication.
- Occasionally aneurysms spontaneously embolize plaque, causing "blue toe syndrome," in which patchy mottling of the feet and toes occurs despite the presence of peripheral pulses.

Complications

Smokers with an aortic aneurysm are most likely to experience the serious complication of aortic rupture.

- If rupture occurs into the retroperitoneal space, bleeding may be controlled by surrounding structures, preventing exsanguination and death. In this case, the patient has severe back pain and may have back and/or flank ecchymosis *(Grey Turner's sign)*.
- If rupture occurs into the thoracic or abdominal cavity, the patient can die from massive hemorrhage. For patients admitted with a ruptured AAA, in-hospital mortality is high at 53%.
- The patient who reaches the hospital will be in hypovolemic shock with tachycardia; hypotension; pale, clammy skin; decreased urine output; altered sensorium; and abdominal tenderness. Simultaneous resuscitation and immediate surgical repair are necessary.

Diagnostic Studies

- Chest x-rays reveal abnormal widening of the thoracic aorta. Abdominal x-rays may show calcification within the aortic wall.
- Echocardiography assesses the function of the aortic valve.
- Ultrasound is useful for aneurysm screening and to monitor aneurysm size.

- CT is the most accurate test to determine the length and cross-sectional diameter and the presence of thrombus in the aneurysm.
- MRI may be useful to diagnose and assess the location and severity of aneurysms.

Interprofessional Care

The goal of management is to prevent aneurysm rupture. Early detection and prompt treatment are essential. Conservative therapy of small, asymptomatic AAAs (4.0 to 5.5 cm) is the best practice.

- Risk factor modification is recommended (ceasing tobacco use, decreasing BP, improving lipid blood values, gradually increasing physical activity).
- Aneurysm size is monitored using ultrasound or CT every 6 to 12 months. Monitoring by ultrasound every 2 to 3 years is recommended for patients with AAAs smaller than 4.0 cm in diameter.
- Aneurysm growth may be slowed with β-blockers (e.g., propranolol [Inderal]), angiotensin-converting enzyme (ACE) inhibitors (e.g., captopril), angiotensin II receptor blockers (e.g., losartan [Cozaar]), statins (e.g., simvastatin [Zocor]), and antibiotics (e.g., doxycycline [Acticlate]).

Aneurysms 5.5 cm in diameter or larger are surgically repaired. Surgical intervention may occur sooner if the patient has a genetic disorder (e.g., Marfan's), if the aneurysm expands rapidly or becomes symptomatic, or if the risk of rupture is high.

- The open aneurysm repair (OAR) involves a large abdominal incision through which the surgeon (1) cuts into the diseased aortic segment, (2) removes any thrombus or plaque, (3) sutures a synthetic graft to the aorta proximal and distal to the aneurysm, and (4) sutures the native aortic wall around the graft to act as a protective cover.

Surgical repair of an AAA is presented in Fig. 37-6 in Lewis et al, *Medical-Surgical Nursing,* ed 10, p. 812.

- An alternative to OAR is the minimally invasive endovascular grafting technique. This procedure involves placement of a sutureless aortic graft into the abdominal aorta inside the aneurysm via a femoral artery cutdown.
- Endovascular aneurysm repair (EVAR) is less invasive than OAR.

The most common complication of aneurysm repair is *endoleak,* the seepage of blood back into the old aneurysm. This defect may be due to an inadequate seal at either graft end, a tear through the graft fabric, or leakage between overlapping graft segments.

Repair may require coil embolization (insertion of beads) for hemostasis.

Nursing Management

Goals
The patient undergoing aortic surgery will have normal tissue perfusion, intact motor and sensory function, and no complications related to surgical repair, such as infection, rupture, or thrombosis.

Nursing Diagnoses
- Ineffective peripheral tissue perfusion
- Risk for infection

Nursing Interventions
Encourage the patient to reduce cardiovascular risk factors, including controlling BP, smoking cessation, increasing physical activity, and maintaining normal body weight and serum lipid levels.

- During the preoperative period, provide emotional support and teaching to the patient and caregivers. Preoperative teaching includes a brief explanation of the disease process, the planned surgical procedure(s), preoperative routines, what to expect immediately after surgery (e.g., recovery room, tubes/drains), and usual postoperative timelines.
- In the postoperative period, in addition to the usual goals of care for a postoperative patient (e.g., maintaining adequate respiratory function, fluid and electrolyte balance, pain control), check for graft patency and renal perfusion. Also watch for and intervene to limit or treat dysrhythmias, ischemia, venous thromboembolism, infections, and neurologic complications.
- A potentially lethal complication in an emergency repair of a ruptured AAA is the development of intraabdominal hypertension (IAH) with associated abdominal compartment syndrome (ACS). Persistent IAH reduces blood flow to the viscera. ACS refers to the impaired organ perfusion caused by IAH with resulting multisystem organ failure. IAH is confirmed by measuring the patient's intraabdominal pressure indirectly through a catheter and transducer system.

▼ Patient and Caregiver Teaching
Instruct the patient and caregiver to gradually increase activities at home. Fatigue, poor appetite, and irregular bowel habits are common.

- Teach the patient to avoid heavy lifting for 6 weeks after surgery. Any redness, swelling, increased pain, drainage from incisions, or fever greater than 100°F (37.8°C) should be reported to an HCP.

- Teach patient and caregiver to observe for changes in color or warmth of the extremities and changes in peripheral pulses.
- Sexual dysfunction in male patients is common after aortic surgery. Referral to a urologist may be useful if erectile dysfunction occurs.

ANGINA, CHRONIC STABLE

Description

Chronic stable angina refers to chest pain that occurs intermittently over a long period with a similar pattern of onset, duration, and intensity of symptoms. Chronic stable angina is a clinical manifestation of coronary artery disease (CAD).

Angina, or chest pain, is a result of reversible myocardial ischemia that occurs when the demand for myocardial oxygen exceeds the ability of the coronary arteries to supply the heart muscle with oxygen. The primary cause of myocardial ischemia is insufficient blood flow to the myocardium through coronary arteries narrowed by atherosclerosis (see Coronary Artery Disease, p. 153).

Variants of chronic stable angina include:

- *Silent ischemia,* in which ischemia occurs in the absence of any subjective symptoms.
- *Prinzmetal's angina* (variant angina), which often occurs at rest, usually in response to spasm of a major coronary artery. This rare form of angina is seen in patients with a history of migraine headaches, Raynaud's phenomenon, or heavy smoking. It is usually due to spasm of a major coronary artery, with or without CAD.

Microvascular angina occurs in the absence of significant coronary atherosclerosis or coronary spasm, especially in postmenopausal women. In these patients, chest pain is related to myocardial ischemia associated with abnormalities of the coronary microcirculation. This is known as coronary microvascular disease (MVD), or "syndrome X." Prevention and treatment of MVD follow the same recommendations as for CAD.

Pathophysiology

Myocardial cells become hypoxic within the first 10 seconds of coronary occlusion. Anaerobic metabolism begins, and lactic acid accumulates. Lactic acid irritates myocardial nerve fibers and transmits a pain message to the cardiac nerves and upper thoracic posterior nerve roots. This accounts for referred cardiac pain to the shoulders, neck, lower jaw, and arms.

- Ischemic cardiac cells are viable for about 20 minutes. With restoration of blood flow, aerobic metabolism resumes and cellular repair begins.

Clinical Manifestations

When questioned, some patients may deny feeling pain but describe a pressure or ache in the chest. It is an unpleasant feeling, often described as a constrictive, squeezing, heavy, tight, or suffocating sensation (Table 10). Many people complain of severe indigestion or epigastric burning. Although most angina pain is substernal in location, the sensation may occur in the neck or radiate to locations including the jaw, neck, shoulders, and arms. Chronic angina pain usually does not change with position or breathing and is rarely described as sharp or stabbing.

- Some patients, especially women and older adults, report atypical symptoms of angina including dyspnea, nausea, and/or fatigue. This presentation is referred to as angina equivalent.

TABLE 10	**PQRST Assessment of Angina**	
Use the following memory aid to obtain information from the patient who has chest pain.		
	Factor	**Questions to Ask Patient**
P	Precipitating events	What events or activities precipitated the pain or discomfort (e.g., argument, exercise, resting)?
Q	Quality of pain	What does the pain or discomfort feel like (e.g., pressure, dull, aching, tight, squeezing, heaviness)?
R	Region (location) and radiation of pain	Can you point to where the pain or discomfort is located? Does the pain or discomfort radiate to other areas (e.g., back, neck, arms, jaw, shoulder, elbow)?
S	Severity of pain	On a scale of 0 to 10, with 0 indicating no pain and 10 being the most severe pain you could imagine, what number would you give the pain or discomfort?
T	Timing	When did the pain or discomfort begin? Has it changed since this time? Have you had pain/discomfort like this before?

- Often people will complain of pain between the shoulder blades and dismiss it as not being related to the heart.
- The pain usually lasts for only a few minutes (5 to 15 minutes) and commonly subsides with rest, calming down, and/or using sublingual nitroglycerin (e.g., Nitrostat).
- An ECG usually reveals ST-segment depression and/or T wave inversion, indicating ischemia. The ECG pattern returns to baseline when the pain is relieved.

Diagnostic Studies

Diagnostic studies used to evaluate angina are the same as those used to diagnose CAD (see Coronary Artery Disease, p. 153). For patients with known CAD and chronic stable angina, common diagnostic studies include 12-lead ECG, echocardiography, exercise stress testing, and pharmacologic nuclear imaging.

Interprofessional Care

The treatment of chronic stable angina is aimed at decreasing oxygen demand and/or increasing oxygen supply. The reduction of CAD risk factors is a priority. In addition to antiplatelet and cholesterol-lowering drug therapy, the most common interventions for chronic stable angina are nitrates, angiotensin-converting enzyme (ACE) inhibitors, β-blockers, and calcium channel blockers.

Emergency care of the patient with chest pain is presented in Table 33-12, Lewis et al, *Medical-Surgical Nursing,* ed 10, p. 723.

Drug Therapy

- Aspirin is given in the absence of contraindications.
- Short-acting nitrates are first-line therapy for the treatment of angina. Nitrates produce their principal effects by dilating peripheral blood vessels, coronary arteries, and collateral vessels. Sublingual nitroglycerin will usually relieve pain in approximately 3 minutes and lasts approximately 30 to 60 minutes. If symptoms are unchanged or worse after 5 minutes, the patient should activate the emergency response system. Sublingual nitroglycerin tablets can be used prophylactically before undertaking an activity that the patient knows may precipitate angina.
- Long-acting nitrates such as isosorbide dinitrate (Isordil) and isosorbide mononitrate can be used to reduce the frequency of anginal attacks. Longer-acting nitrates are available in oral preparations, ointments, and transdermal controlled-release patches.
- ACE inhibitors (e.g., captopril) are prescribed for patients with chronic stable angina who are at high risk for a cardiac event

(e.g., ejection fraction [EF] 40% or less, diabetes, hypertension, or chronic kidney disease). These drugs result in vasodilation and reduced blood volume. Most important, they can prevent or reverse ventricular remodeling.

- Patients with left ventricular dysfunction or elevated BP or those who have had a myocardial infarction (MI) take β-blockers such as carvedilol (Coreg), metoprolol (Lopressor, Toprol XL), and bisoprolol (Zebeta). These medications reduce myocardial oxygen demand by decreasing myocardial contractility, heart rate (HR), systemic vascular resistance (SVR), and BP.
- Calcium channel blockers, such as nifedipine (Procardia), verapamil (Calan), diltiazem (Cardizem), and nicardipine (Cardene), are used if β-adrenergic blocking agents are contraindicated, are poorly tolerated, or do not control symptoms. The two groups of calcium channel blockers are the dihydropyridines (e.g., amlodipine [Norvasc]), which have more vasodilatory effects, and the nondihydropyridines (e.g., verapamil [Calan], diltiazem [Cardizem]), which have more rate and contractility effects.

Cardiac Catheterization
Cardiac catheterization and coronary angiography provide images of the coronary circulation and identify the location and severity of any blockage. If a coronary blockage is amenable to intervention, coronary revascularization with an elective percutaneous coronary intervention (PCI) is done.

- During this procedure, which is called *balloon angioplasty,* a catheter equipped with a balloon tip is inserted into the appropriate coronary artery. When the blockage is located, the catheter is passed through the blockage, the balloon is inflated, and the atherosclerotic plaque is compressed, resulting in vessel dilation.

Intracoronary stents are usually inserted to prevent abrupt closure and restenosis after balloon angioplasty. A stent is an expandable, meshlike structure designed to keep the vessel open by supporting the arterial walls. Drugs commonly used during PCI are unfractionated heparin (UH) or low-molecular-weight heparin (LMWH), a direct thrombin inhibitor (e.g., bivalirudin [Angiomax]), and/or a glycoprotein IIb/IIIa inhibitor (e.g., eptifibatide [Integrilin]). After PCI, the patient is treated with dual antiplatelet drugs (e.g., aspirin [indefinitely] and clopidogrel) up to 12 months or longer, until the intimal lining can grow over the stent and provide a smooth vascular surface.

- Many stents are coated with a drug (e.g., paclitaxel, sirolimus) that prevents the overgrowth of new intima, which is the primary cause of stent restenosis.

- The most serious complications from stent placement are abrupt closure and vascular injury. Less common complications include acute MI, stent embolization, coronary spasm, contrast medium allergy, renal compromise, bleeding (e.g., retroperitoneal), infection, stroke, and emergent coronary artery bypass graft (CABG) surgery. The possibility of dysrhythmias during and after the procedure is always present.

Nursing Management
Goals and Nursing Diagnoses
Goals and nursing diagnoses for the patient with chronic stable angina are the same as those used for ACS (see Acute Coronary Syndrome, p. 5).
Nursing Interventions
If your patient experiences angina, perform the following measures: (1) position patient upright unless contraindicated and apply supplemental oxygen, (2) assess vital signs, (3) obtain a 12-lead ECG, (4) provide prompt pain relief first with nitroglycerin followed by an opioid analgesic if needed, and (5) assess heart and breath sounds.

- The patient is anxious and may have pale, cool, clammy skin. BP and HR may be elevated. Auscultation of the heart may reveal an atrial (S_4) or a ventricular (S_3) gallop.
- Ask the patient to describe the pain and to rate it on a scale of 0 to 10 before and after treatment, to evaluate the effectiveness of the interventions (Table 10).
- Assess for other manifestations of pain, such as restlessness; ECG changes; elevated HR, respiratory rate, or BP; clutching of the bed linens; or other nonverbal cues.
- Support and reassure the patient.

▼ Patient and Caregiver Teaching
Reassure the patient with a history of chronic stable angina that a long, productive life is possible.

- Teaching tools such as heart models and written information are important components of patient and caregiver teaching.
- Assist the patient to identify factors that precipitate angina and how to avoid or control these factors.
- Help the patient to identify personal risk factors for CAD. Discuss the ways modifiable risk factors can be reduced.
- Teach the patient and caregivers about diets low in sodium and saturated fats. Maintaining ideal body weight is important in controlling angina, because excess weight increases myocardial workload.
- Advise adhering to a regular, individualized exercise program that conditions rather than stresses the heart. For example,

patients can walk briskly on a flat surface at least 30 minutes a day, most days of the week, if not contraindicated.

- It is important to teach the patient and caregivers about the proper use of nitroglycerin.
- Patients with this condition may feel a threat to their roles, identity, and self-esteem. If needed, arrange for counseling to support psychologic adjustment of the patient and caregiver to the diagnosis of CAD and resulting angina.

ANKYLOSING SPONDYLITIS

Description
Ankylosing spondylitis (AS) is a chronic inflammatory disease that primarily affects the axial skeleton, including the sacroiliac joints, intervertebral spaces, and costovertebral articulations. The human leukocyte antigen HLA-B27 is found in 90% to 95% of people with AS. Onset of AS is usually in the third decade of life, but onset in adolescence is fairly common. Men are three times more likely to develop AS than women. The disease may go undetected in women because of a milder course.

Pathophysiology
Genetic predisposition appears to play a role in disease pathogenesis, but the precise cause is unknown. Inflammation in joints and adjacent tissue causes the formation of granulation tissue (pannus) and the development of dense fibrous scars that lead to joint fusion. Inflammation can affect the eyes, lungs, heart, kidneys, and peripheral nervous system.

Clinical Manifestations
Symptoms of inflammatory spine pain are the first clues to a diagnosis of AS. The patient typically reports lower back pain, stiffness, and limitation of motion that are worse during the night and in the morning but decrease with mild activity. Systemic manifestations such as fever, fatigue, anorexia, and weight loss are rare.

Uveitis (intraocular inflammation) is the most common nonskeletal manifestation. It can appear as an initial presentation of the disease years before joint symptoms develop. Patients may also experience chest pain and sternal/costal cartilage tenderness.

Severe postural abnormalities and deformity can cause significant disability. Aortic insufficiency and pulmonary fibrosis are frequent complications. Cauda equina syndrome can also result, contributing to lower extremity weakness and bladder dysfunction.

The patient is also at risk for spinal fracture because of associated osteoporosis.

Diagnostic Studies

- X-rays used to diagnose AS are limited in ability to detect early sacroiliitis or subtle changes in posterior vertebrae.
- MRI can be useful in assessing early cartilage abnormalities.
- Laboratory testing is not specific, but an elevated erythrocyte sedimentation rate (ESR) and mild anemia may be seen.
- Individuals with both the clinical signs of AS and the HLA-B27 antigen have an increased likelihood of being diagnosed with AS.

Interprofessional Care

Prevention of AS is not possible. However, families with other diagnosed HLA-B27–positive rheumatic diseases (e.g., acute anterior uveitis, juvenile spondyloarthritis) should be alert to signs of lower back pain and arthritis symptoms for early identification and treatment of AS.

Care of the patient is aimed at maintaining maximal skeletal mobility while decreasing pain and inflammation. Heat applications, nonsteroidal antiinflammatory drugs (NSAIDs) and salicylates, and disease-modifying antirheumatic drugs (DMARDs), such as sulfasalazine (Azulfidine) or methotrexate, can help in relieving symptoms. Etanercept (Enbrel), a biologic response modifier, inhibits the action of tumor necrosis factor (TNF) and has been shown to reduce active inflammation and improve spinal mobility. Additional anti-TNF agents (infliximab [Remicade], adalimumab [Humira], or golimumab [Simponi]) may also be effective.

Good posture and stretching exercises of the back, neck, and chest are important to minimize spinal deformity. Hydrotherapy may decrease pain and facilitate spinal extension. Surgery may be needed for severe deformity and mobility impairment. Spinal osteotomy and total joint replacement are the most commonly performed procedures.

Nursing Management

A key responsibility is to teach the patient about the nature of the disease and principles of therapy. The home management program consists of local moist heat, regular exercise, and knowledgeable use of drugs.

- Discourage excessive physical exertion during periods of active inflammation.
- Encourage smoking cessation to decrease the risk for lung complications in people with reduced chest expansion.

- Ongoing physical therapy should include gentle, graded stretching and strengthening exercises to preserve range of motion (ROM) and improve thoracolumbar flexion and extension.
- Proper positioning at rest is essential. Encourage the patient to use a firm mattress and sleep on the back with a flat pillow, avoiding positions that encourage flexion deformity.
- Postural training emphasizes avoiding spinal flexion (e.g., leaning over a desk), heavy lifting, and prolonged walking, standing, or sitting. Encourage sports that facilitate natural stretching, such as swimming and racquet games.
- Family counseling and vocational rehabilitation are important.

AORTIC DISSECTION

Description

Aortic dissection, often misnamed "dissecting aneurysm," is not a type of aneurysm. Rather, aortic dissection results from the creation of a false lumen between the intima (inner layer) and media (middle layer) of the arterial wall. Aortic dissection is classified according to the location of the dissection and duration of symptoms.

Type A dissection affects the ascending aorta and arch. Type B dissection begins in the descending aorta. Dissections are also classified as acute (first 14 days), subacute (14 to 90 days), or chronic (greater than 90 days) based on symptom onset.

- Approximately two thirds of dissections involve the ascending aorta and are acute in onset. Chronic dissections are almost always Type B.
- Aortic dissection affects men more often than women and occurs most frequently in the sixth and seventh decades of life. Predisposing factors include age, aortic diseases (e.g., aortitis, coarctation, arch hypoplasia), atherosclerosis, blunt or iatrogenic trauma, tobacco use, cocaine or methamphetamine use, congenital heart disease (e.g., bicuspid aortic valve), connective tissue disorders (e.g., Marfan's or Ehlers-Danlos syndrome), family history, history of heart surgery, male gender, pregnancy, and poorly controlled hypertension.

Pathophysiology

Most nontraumatic aortic dissections are attributed to degeneration of the elastic fibers in the medial layer. Chronic hypertension accelerates the degradation process. In aortic dissection, a tear develops in the inner wall of the aorta. Blood surges through this tear, causing the inner and middle layers to separate (dissect). If the blood-filled channel ruptures through the outside aortic wall, aortic dissection is often fatal.

As the heart contracts, each pulsation increases the pressure on the damaged area, which further increases dissection. Extension of the dissection may cut off blood supply to critical areas such as the brain, kidneys, spinal cord, and extremities. The false lumen may remain patent, become thrombosed (clotted), rejoin the true lumen by way of a distal tear, or rupture.

Clinical Manifestations and Complications

About 80% of patients with an acute Type A aortic dissection report an abrupt onset of excruciating anterior chest pain. Patients with acute Type B aortic dissection are more likely to report pain located in the back, abdomen, or legs. Pain location may overlap between Type A and B dissections. The pain is frequently described as "sharp" and "worst ever," or as "tearing," "ripping," or "stabbing." Dissection pain can be differentiated from myocardial infarction (MI) pain, which is more gradual in onset and has increasing intensity.

- Older patients are more likely to have hypotension and vague symptoms. In some cases, aortic dissection may be painless, emphasizing the importance of the physical examination.
- If the aortic arch is involved, the patient may exhibit neurologic deficits, including altered level of consciousness and dizziness, with weakened or absent carotid and temporal pulses.
- Type A aortic dissection usually produces some disruption of coronary artery blood flow and aortic valvular insufficiency.
- When either subclavian artery is involved, pulse quality and BP readings may differ between the left and right arms.
- As dissection progresses down the aorta, the abdominal organs and lower extremities demonstrate evidence of altered tissue perfusion.

A life-threatening complication of an acute ascending aortic dissection is cardiac tamponade, which occurs when blood from the dissection leaks into the pericardial sac. Clinical manifestations include hypotension, narrowed pulse pressure, distended neck veins, muffled heart sounds, and pulsus paradoxus.

- An aorta weakened by dissection may rupture. Hemorrhage may occur into the mediastinal, pleural, or abdominal cavity.
- Dissection can lead to occlusion of the blood supply to the spinal cord, kidneys, and abdominal structures. Spinal cord ischemia leads to weakness and decreased sensation. Renal ischemia can lead to renal failure. Signs of abdominal (mesenteric) ischemia include abdominal pain, decreased bowel sounds, and altered bowel elimination.

Diagnostic Studies

A

Studies to detect aortic dissection are similar to those performed for suspected aneurysms.

- Chest x-ray indicates widening of the mediastinum and pleural effusion.
- Three-dimensional (3-D) CT scanning, transesophageal echocardiography (TEE), or MRI may be used to diagnose acute aortic dissection.

Interprofessional Care

Reducing the HR, BP, and myocardial contractility limits extension of the acute dissection.

- An IV β-blocker (e.g., esmolol [Brevibloc]) is often titrated to a target HR of 60 beats/minute or less, or to a systolic BP between 100 and 110 mm Hg.
- Other antihypertensive agents, such as calcium channel blockers (e.g., diltiazem [Cardizem]) and angiotensin-converting enzyme (ACE) inhibitors (e.g., enalapril), may also be used.
- Morphine is the preferred analgesic because it decreases sympathetic nervous system stimulation and relieves pain.
- Supportive treatment for an acute aortic dissection serves as a bridge to surgery.

Endovascular repair of an acute descending aortic dissection with complications (e.g., hemodynamic instability) and of chronic descending aortic dissection with complications (e.g., peripheral ischemia) is a treatment option.

Patients with acute aortic dissection are managed in the intensive care unit (ICU). An acute ascending aortic dissection is considered a surgical emergency. Otherwise, surgery is indicated when conservative therapy is ineffective or when complications (e.g., heart failure) occur. Because the aorta is fragile after dissection, surgical intervention is delayed for as long as possible to allow time for edema to decrease and to permit clotting of the blood in the false lumen.

- Surgery involves resection of the aortic segment containing the intimal tear and replacement with a synthetic graft.

Even with prompt surgical intervention, the in-hospital mortality rate for acute aortic dissection is high. Causes of death include aortic rupture, mesenteric ischemia, MI, sepsis, and multiorgan failure.

The patient with an acute or chronic type B descending aortic dissection without complications can be managed nonsurgically. Such conservative treatment includes pain relief, heart rate (HR) and BP control, and cardiovascular disease (CVD) risk factor modification along with close surveillance imaging with CT or MRI.

Nursing Management

Preoperatively, nursing management includes keeping the patient in bed in a semi-Fowler's position and maintaining a quiet environment. These measures help to keep the HR and systolic BP at the lowest possible level that maintains vital organ perfusion (typically HR <60 beats/minute and systolic BP of 110 to 120 mm Hg). Give opioids and sedatives as ordered. To prevent extension of the dissection, manage pain and anxiety, which can cause elevations in the HR and systolic BP.

- Titrating IV administration of antihypertensive agents requires continuous ECG and intraarterial BP monitoring. Monitor vital signs frequently, sometimes as often as every 2 to 3 minutes, until target HR and BP are reached. Look for changes in peripheral pulses and signs of increasing pain, restlessness, and anxiety.

Postoperative care is similar to that after open aneurysm repair (see Aneurysm, Aortic, p. 45).

▼ **Patient and Caregiver Teaching**

- Instruct patients and caregivers about taking antihypertensive drugs daily for lifelong control of HR and BP.
- Tell the patient to discuss any side effects (e.g., dizziness, depression, fatigue, erectile dysfunction) with the HCP before discontinuing prescribed drugs.
- Follow-up monitoring with regularly scheduled MRI or CT evaluations is essential.
- Tell patients that if the pain or other symptoms return, they should contact emergency response system (ERS) for immediate care.

APPENDICITIS

Description

Appendicitis is an inflammation of the appendix, a narrow blind tube that extends from the inferior part of the cecum. It is most common in individuals 10 to 30 years of age. It is the most common reason for emergency abdominal surgery.

Pathophysiology

A common cause of appendicitis is obstruction of the lumen by a fecalith (accumulated feces). Obstruction results in distention,

A

venous engorgement, and the accumulation of mucus and bacteria, which can lead to gangrene, perforation, and peritonitis.

Clinical Manifestations and Complications

Appendicitis typically begins with dull periumbilical pain, followed by anorexia, nausea, and vomiting. The pain is persistent and continuous, eventually shifting to the right lower quadrant and localizing at McBurney's point (halfway between the umbilicus and right iliac crest).

- Further assessment reveals localized and rebound tenderness with muscle guarding. Coughing, sneezing, and deep inhalation magnify the pain.
- The patient usually prefers to lie still, often with the right leg flexed. A low-grade fever may develop.

If diagnosis and treatment are delayed, the appendix can rupture, and the resulting peritonitis can be fatal.

Diagnostic Studies

- White blood cell (WBC) count is usually elevated.
- Urinalysis is done to rule out genitourinary conditions that mimic manifestations of appendicitis.
- CT scan and ultrasound may be used.

Interprofessional Care

Treatment is immediate surgical removal of the appendix (appendectomy) if the inflammation is localized. If the appendix has ruptured and there is evidence of peritonitis or an abscess, antibiotic therapy and parenteral fluids are given for 6 to 8 hours before the appendectomy to prevent sepsis and dehydration.

Nursing Management

Encourage the patient with abdominal pain to see an HCP and to avoid self-treatment with laxatives and enemas. Increased peristalsis from these procedures may cause perforation.

- Nothing should be taken by mouth to ensure that the stomach will be empty if surgery is needed.
- Postoperative nursing management is similar to postoperative care of a patient after laparotomy (see Abdominal Pain, Acute, pp. 4-5).
- Patients are usually discharged within 24 hours after an uncomplicated laparoscopic appendectomy. Ambulation begins a few hours after surgery, and the diet is advanced as tolerated. Most patients resume normal activities 2 to 3 weeks after surgery.

ASTHMA

Description

Asthma is a lung disease that causes inflammation with variable episodes of airflow obstruction, which is usually reversible spontaneously or with treatment. Asthma is characterized by a combination of clinical manifestations along with reversible expiratory airflow limitation or bronchial hyperresponsiveness. Signs and symptoms can include episodes of wheezing, breathlessness, chest tightness, and cough, especially at night and in the early morning. The clinical course of asthma is unpredictable, ranging from periods of adequate control to exacerbations with poor control of symptoms.

- Asthma affects an estimated 18.8 million adult Americans. Among adults, women are 62% more likely to have asthma than men. Despite a decline in the number of deaths from asthma over the past 10 years, more than 3300 people die yearly from asthma.
- Risk factors for asthma and triggers of asthma attacks are listed in Table 11.

Pathophysiology

The primary pathophysiologic process in asthma is persistent but variable airway inflammation. The airflow is limited because the inflammation results in bronchoconstriction, airway hyperresponsiveness (hyperactivity), and airway edema. Exposure to allergens or irritants initiates the inflammatory cascade.

- As the inflammatory process begins, mast cells in the bronchial wall release multiple inflammatory mediators including leukotrienes, histamine, cytokines, prostaglandins, and nitric oxide.
- Inflammatory mediators have effects on the (1) blood vessels, causing vasodilation and increasing capillary permeability (runny nose); (2) nerve cells, causing itching; (3) smooth muscle cells, causing bronchial spasms and airway narrowing; and (4) goblet cells, causing mucus production.
- The *early-phase response* in asthma can occur within 30 to 60 minutes after exposure to a trigger or irritant.
- Symptoms can recur 4 to 6 hours after the early response because of the influx of many inflammatory cells and the further release of more inflammatory mediators. This *late-phase response* occurs in about 50% of people with asthma.
- Bronchoconstriction with symptoms persists for 24 hours or longer. Corticosteroids are effective in treating this inflammation.

Chronic inflammation may result in structural changes in the bronchial wall known as *remodeling*. A progressive loss of

TABLE 11 Triggers of Asthma Attacks	
Allergen Inhalation • Animal dander (e.g., cats, mice, guinea pigs) • House dust mites • Cockroaches • Pollens • Molds **Air Pollutants** • Exhaust fumes • Perfumes • Oxidants • Sulfur dioxides • Cigarette smoke • Aerosol sprays **Viral or Bacterial Infection** • Viral upper respiratory tract infection • Sinusitis, allergic rhinitis **Drugs** • Aspirin • Nonsteroidal antiinflammatory drugs • β-Adrenergic blockers	**Occupational Exposure** • Agriculture, farming • Paints, solvents • Laundry detergents • Metal salts • Wood and vegetable dusts • Industrial chemicals and plastics • Pharmaceutical agents **Food Additives** • Sulfites (bisulfites and metabisulfites) • Beer, wine, dried fruit, shrimp, processed potatoes • Monosodium glutamate • Tartrazine **Other Factors** • Exercise and cold, dry air • Stress • Hormones, menses • Gastroesophageal reflux disease (GERD)

lung function occurs that is not prevented or fully reversed by therapy.

During an asthma attack, decreased perfusion and ventilation of the alveoli and increased alveolar gas pressure lead to ventilation-perfusion abnormalities in the lungs.

- The patient is hypoxemic early on, with decreased partial pressure of CO_2 in arterial blood ($PaCO_2$) and increased pH caused by hyperventilation (respiratory alkalosis).
- As the airflow limitation worsens with air trapping, the $PaCO_2$ increases to produce respiratory acidosis, which is an ominous sign of respiratory failure.

Clinical Manifestations

Asthma signs and symptoms can differ for each patient. The most common manifestations include cough, shortness of breath (dyspnea), wheezing, chest tightness, and variable airflow obstruction. The presence of any of these (usually in combination) can indicate that an asthma episode or attack is occurring. Attacks may last for a few minutes to several hours.

- Characteristic manifestations are wheezing, cough, dyspnea, and chest tightness. Expiration may be prolonged, with an inspiratory/expiratory (I/E) ratio of 1:3 or 1:4.
- Wheezing is an unreliable sign to gauge the severity of an attack because many patients with minor attacks wheeze loudly, whereas others with severe attacks do not wheeze.
- In some patients with asthma, cough is the only symptom. The cough may be nonproductive because secretions may be so thick, tenacious, and gelatinous that their removal is difficult.
- During an acute attack, the patient usually sits upright or slightly bent forward, using accessory muscles of respiration. The more difficult the breathing becomes, the more anxious the patient feels.
- Signs of hypoxemia include restlessness, increased anxiety, inappropriate behavior, and increased pulse and BP.
- Percussion reveals hyperresonance of the lungs. Auscultation indicates inspiratory or expiratory wheezing.
- Diminished breath sounds may indicate a significant decrease in air movement. Severely diminished breath sounds or a "silent chest" is an ominous sign, indicating severe obstruction and impending respiratory failure.

Classification of Asthma

Asthma can be classified as intermittent, mild persistent, moderate persistent, or severe persistent (Table 12). The classification system is used to determine the treatment. Patients may have different asthma classifications over the course of the disease.

Complications

In severe asthma exacerbations, the patient is dyspneic at rest and speaks in single words because of the difficulty breathing.

- The patient is often agitated, sitting forward to maximize the diaphragmatic movement and using accessory muscles in the neck to lift the chest wall. Respiratory rate may be >30 breaths/minute and pulse >120 beats/minute. The peak flow (PEFR [peak expiratory flow rate]) is 40% of the patient's personal best, or <150 mL.
- Prominent wheezing may progress to no apparent wheezing if the airflow is exceptionally limited. The absence of a wheeze (i.e., silent chest) in a patient who is obviously struggling to

TABLE 12 Classification of Asthma Severity

Severity Component	Intermittent	ASTHMA SEVERITY Persistent Mild	Moderate	Severe
Impairment				
Symptoms	≤2 days/wk	>2 days/wk, not daily	Daily	Continuous
Nighttime awakenings	≤2/mo	3-4/mo	>1/wk, not nightly	Often 7/wk
SABA use for symptoms	≤2 days/wk	>2 days/wk, not daily	Daily	Several times per day
Interference with normal activity	None	Minor limitation	Some limitation	Extremely limited
Lung function*	Normal FEV_1 between exacerbations FEV_1 >80% FEV_1/FVC normal	FEV_1 >80% predicted FEV_1/FVC normal	FEV_1 60%-80% predicted FEV_1/FVC reduced by 5%	FEV_1 <60% predicted FEV_1/FVC reduced by 5%
Risk				
Exacerbations requiring oral corticosteroids	0-1/yr	≥2/yr even in the absence of impairment Consider severity and interval since last exacerbation. Frequency and severity may fluctuate over time. Relative annual risk of exacerbation may be related to FEV_1.		

Continued

A

TABLE 12 Classification of Asthma Severity—cont'd

Severity Component	Intermittent	Persistent		
		Mild	Moderate	Severe
Recommended Step for Initiating Treatment	Step 1	Step 2	Step 3†	Step 4 or 5†
	Reevaluate asthma control in 2-6 wk and adjust therapy accordingly.			

Guidelines for Using Table

- Patients should be assigned to the step of highest severity in which any feature occurs. Clinical features for individual patients may overlap across steps. Determine level of severity by assessment of both impairment and risk. Assess impairment by patient's recall of previous 2- to 4-week spirometry results.
- The individual patient's classification should change over time as treatment is initiated. After treatment, the focus switches to the level of control, not the classification of severity.
- Patients at any level of severity of chronic asthma can have mild, moderate, or severe exacerbations of asthma. Some patients with intermittent asthma experience severe and life-threatening exacerbations separated by long periods of normal lung function and no symptoms.

Source: Adapted from National Asthma Education and Prevention Program, National Heart, Lung, and Blood Institute: *Expert Panel Report 3: guidelines for the diagnosis and management of asthma*, NIH pub. no. 08-4051, Bethesda, Md, 2007, National Institutes of Health. Retrieved from www.nhlbi.nih.gov/guidelines.

FEV₁, Forced expiratory volume in 1 sec; FVC, forced vital capacity; SABA, short-acting β₂-adrenergic agonist.

*Percent predicted values for FEV_1 or ratio of FEV_1/FVC. Normal FEV_1/FVC: 8-19 yr, 85%; 20-39 yr, 80%; 40-59 yr, 75%; 60-80 yr, 70%.

†Consider short-term corticosteroid therapy.

breathe is a life-threatening situation that may require mechanical ventilation.

Diagnostic Studies

Underdiagnosis of asthma is common. In general, the HCP should consider a diagnosis of asthma if various indicators (i.e., clinical manifestations, health history, peak flow variability, or spirometry readings) are positive.

- Detailed history helps to identify asthma triggers.
- Spirometry determines the reversibility of bronchoconstriction and thus establishes the diagnosis of asthma.
- Sputum specimen can be used to rule out bacterial infection.
- Serum immunoglobulin E (IgE) levels and eosinophil count, when elevated, are highly suggestive of allergic tendency.
- Chest x-ray during an attack shows hyperinflation.
- Spirometry, oximetry, and arterial blood gases (ABGs) provide information about the severity of the attack and response to treatment.
- Allergy skin testing can be used to determine sensitivity to specific allergens.

Interprofessional Care

The goal of asthma treatment is to achieve and maintain control of the disease. At initial diagnosis, a patient may have severe asthma and require asthma medication. After treatment, the patient is assessed for level of asthma control. The HCP steps down the medication as the patient achieves control of the symptoms or steps it up as the symptoms worsen.

- Achieving rapid control of symptoms is the goal in order to return the patient to daily functioning at the best possible level. The level of control is determined by the patient's spirometry results and any exacerbations or adverse treatment effects.

Intermittent and Persistent Asthma

The classification of asthma severity (Table 12) at initial diagnosis helps determine which types of medications are best suited to control the symptoms.

- Patients in all classifications of asthma require a rescue medication for *short-term,* immediate control of symptoms. Short-acting β_2-adrenergic agonists (SABAs) (e.g., albuterol [ProAir HFA, Proventil HFA, Ventolin HFA]) are the most effective class of drugs used as rescue medications. Patients with persistent asthma must also be on a long-term or controller medication (see Table 28-6, Lewis et al, *Medical-Surgical Nursing,* ed 10, p. 546). Inhaled corticosteroids (ICSs) (e.g., fluticasone

[Flovent Diskus or HFA]) are the most effective class of drugs to treat the inflammation.

- For *long-term* control of moderate to severe persistent asthma, long-acting β_2-adrenergic agonists (LABAs) are added to daily ICSs (e.g., fluticasone [Flovent]). ICSs are the most effective class of drugs to treat the inflammation.

Acute Asthma Exacerbations

Asthma exacerbations may be mild to life-threatening. With mild exacerbations, patients have difficulty breathing only with activity and may feel that they "can't get enough air." Peak flow is >70% of personal best, and symptoms often are relieved at home promptly with an SABA such as albuterol delivered by a nebulizer or metered dose inhaler (MDI) with a spacer.

- With a moderate exacerbation, dyspnea interferes with usual activities and peak flow is 40% to 60% of personal best. In this situation, the patient usually comes to the ED or an HCP's office to get help. Relief is provided with the SABA and oral corticosteroids. Symptoms may persist for several days even after corticosteroids are started. Oxygen can be used with both mild and moderate exacerbations.

Severe and Life-Threatening Asthma Exacerbations

Management of the patient with severe and life-threatening asthma focuses on correcting hypoxemia and improving ventilation. The goal is to keep the O_2 saturation $\geq 90\%$. Continuous monitoring of the patient is critical.

- Many therapeutic measures are the same as those for acute asthma. Repetitive or continuous SABA administration is provided in the emergency department (ED). Initially, three treatments of SABA (spaced 20 to 30 minutes apart) are given. Then more SABA is given depending on the patient's airflow, improvement, and side effects from the SABA.
- In life-threatening asthma, IV corticosteroids are administered and are usually tapered rapidly. IV corticosteroids (methylprednisolone) are administered every 4 to 6 hours. Adjunctive medications such as IV magnesium sulfate may be administered for bronchodilation in patients with very low forced expiratory volume at 1 minute (FEV_1) or peak flow (<40% of predicted or personal best at presentation) or those who fail to respond to initial treatment.
- Supplemental O_2 is given by mask or nasal prongs to achieve a PaO_2 of at least 60 mm Hg or an O_2 saturation >90%.

Occasionally, asthma exacerbations are life-threatening, with impending respiratory arrest. The patient requires intubation and mechanical ventilation if there is no response to treatment. The patient is provided with 100% oxygen, hourly or continuously nebulized SABA, IV corticosteroids, and other adjunctive therapies as noted previously.

Drug Therapy

A stepwise approach to drug therapy is based initially on asthma severity and then on level of control. Persistent asthma requires daily long-term therapy in addition to appropriate medications to manage acute symptoms. Medications are divided into two general classifications:

- *Quick-relief or rescue medications* to treat symptoms and exacerbations, such as SABAs
- *Long-term control medications* to achieve and maintain control of persistent asthma such as ICS. Some of the controllers are used in combination to gain better asthma control (e.g., fluticasone/salmeterol [Advair]) (see Table 28-8, Lewis et al, *Medical-Surgical Nursing,* ed 10, pp. 548 to 549).

Patient teaching about medications should include the name, purpose, dosage, method of administration, and schedule, taking into consideration activities of daily living (ADLs) (e.g., bathing) that require energy expenditure and thus oxygen.

- Information should also include side effects, appropriate actions for side effects, and how to properly use and clean devices.

Nursing Management

Goals

The patient with asthma will have minimal symptoms during the day and night, acceptable activity levels (including exercise and other physical activity), greater than 80% of personal best PEFR, few or no adverse effects of therapy, no acute exacerbations, and adequate knowledge to participate in and carry out the plan of care.

Nursing Diagnoses

- Ineffective airway clearance
- Anxiety

Nursing Interventions

A goal in asthma care is to maximize the patient's ability to safely manage acute asthma exacerbations via an asthma action plan developed in conjunction with the HCP (see Fig. 28-8, Lewis et al, *Medical-Surgical Nursing,* ed 10, p. 555).

- The patient can take two to four puffs of an SABA every 20 minutes three times as a rescue plan. Depending on the response with alleviation of symptoms or improved peak flow, continued SABA use and/or oral corticosteroids may be a part of the home management plan. If symptoms persist or if the patient's peak flow is <50% of the personal best, the HCP or emergency medical services need to be immediately contacted.

- When the patient is in the health care facility with an acute exacerbation, it is important to monitor the respiratory and cardiovascular systems. This includes auscultating lung sounds and monitoring heart rate (HR) and respiratory rate, BP, pulse oximetry, and peak flow.
- An important nursing goal during an acute attack is to decrease the patient's sense of panic. Stay with the patient. A calm, quiet, reassuring attitude may help the patient relax. Position the patient comfortably (usually sitting) to maximize chest expansion.
- In a firm, calm voice, coach the patient to use pursed-lip breathing, which keeps the airways open by maintaining positive pressure, and abdominal breathing, which slows the respiratory rate and encourages deeper breaths.
- Also see eNursing Care Plan 28-1 on the website.

▼ **Patient and Caregiver Teaching**

A patient and caregiver teaching guide for the patient with asthma is presented in Table 13.

TABLE 13   Patient & Caregiver Teaching

Asthma

Include the following information in a teaching plan for the patient with asthma and the caregiver. It will help to improve the patient's quality of life and promote lifestyle changes that support successful living with asthma.

What Is Asthma?
- Basic anatomy and physiology of lung
- Pathophysiology of asthma
- Relationship of pathophysiology to signs and symptoms
- Measurement and correlation of spirometry and peak expiratory flow rate

What Is Good Asthma Control?
- Personal ideas of good control
- Use Asthma Control Test available at *www.asthmacontroltest.com.*

Hindrances to Asthma Treatment and Control
- Discuss possible hindrances (e.g., denial, poor perception of asthma severity) with patient and caregiver.

Environmental and Trigger Control
- Identification of possible triggers and possible preventive measures (use trigger diary)
- Avoidance of allergens and other triggers
- Need to maintain good hydration

TABLE 13 Patient & Caregiver Teaching

Asthma—cont'd

Medications
- Types (include mechanism of action)
  - β_2-Agonists
  - Corticosteroids
  - Methylxanthines
  - Anti-IgE
  - Leukotriene modifiers
  - Combination drugs
- Use of preventive and maintenance (e.g., antiinflammatory) agents
- Write out medication list and schedule.

Asthma Action Plan (Fig. 28-8 in Lewis et al, *Medical-Surgical Nursing,* ed 10, p. 555)

Correct Use of Inhalers, Spacer, and Nebulizer
- Demonstration–return demonstration with placebo devices (Figs. 28-5 to 28-7 and Tables 28-9 to 28-11 in Lewis et al, *Medical-Surgical Nursing,* ed. 10)

Breathing Techniques
- Pursed-lip breathing (Table 28-13 in Lewis et al, *Medical-Surgical Nursing,* ed 10, p. 554)

Correct Use of Peak Flow Meter (Table 28-14 in Lewis et al, *Medical-Surgical Nursing,* ed 10, p. 556)

IgE, Immunoglobulin E.

BELL'S PALSY

Description

Bell's palsy is the most common facial nerve disorder. It is characterized by inflammation of the facial nerve (cranial nerve [CN] VII) on one side of the face, with acute facial paresis.
- Most patients recover spontaneously within 3 weeks to 9 months.
- One third of patients may have residual effects of facial weakness, involuntary movements, and persistent tearing of the eye on the affected side.

Pathophysiology

It is believed that reactivation of a dormant viral infection such as viral meningitis, herpes simplex virus 1 (HSV1), herpes zoster virus

(HZV), or others may trigger Bell's palsy. The viral infection causes inflammation, edema, ischemia, and demyelination of the nerve, creating pain and alterations in motor and sensory function.

Clinical Manifestations

The onset of Bell's palsy is sudden, with a rapid onset of unilateral facial weakness over a few hours. Maximum facial weakness is seen within 2 days. Many patients have a history of a recent viral illness. Patients may complain of pain around and behind the ear. Additional manifestations include numbness of the face, tongue, and ear; tinnitus; headache; and hearing deficit.

Paralysis of the motor branches of the facial nerve typically results in a flaccidity of the affected side of the face, with drooping of the mouth accompanied by drooling. Inability to close the eyelid, with an upward movement of the eyeball when closure is attempted, is also evident.

- A widened palpebral fissure (opening between the eyelids); flattening of the nasolabial fold; unilateral loss of taste; and inability to smile, frown, or whistle are common.
- Decreased muscle movement may alter chewing ability, and some patients may experience a loss of tearing or excessive tearing.

Complications can include psychologic withdrawal because of changes in appearance, malnutrition, dehydration, mucous membrane trauma, corneal abrasions, and facial spasms and contractures.

Diagnosis of Bell's palsy is one of exclusion. Diagnosis and prognosis are indicated by observation of the pattern of onset and testing percutaneous nerve excitability by electromyography (EMG).

Interprofessional Care

Methods of treatment include moist heat, gentle massage, electrical stimulation of the nerve, and prescribed exercises. Stimulation may maintain muscle tone and prevent atrophy. Care is primarily focused on relief of symptoms, protection of the eye on the affected side, and prevention of complications.

- Corticosteroids (prednisone) are started immediately, with best results obtained if corticosteroids are initiated before paralysis is complete. When the patient improves to the point that corticosteroids are no longer necessary, they should be tapered off over 2 weeks.
- Treatment with antivirals has not been effective in the management of Bell's palsy.

Nursing Management

Mild analgesics can relieve pain. Hot, wet packs can reduce discomfort of herpetic lesions, aid circulation, and relieve pain. Tell the patient to protect the face from cold and drafts because extreme sensitivity to pain or touch may occur.

- Maintenance of good nutrition is important. Teach the patient to chew on the unaffected side of the mouth to avoid trapping food and improve taste. Thorough oral hygiene must be carried out after each meal to prevent development of parotitis, caries, and periodontal disease from residual food.
- Dark glasses may be worn for protective and cosmetic reasons. Artificial tears (methylcellulose) can be instilled frequently during the day to prevent corneal drying. Ointment and an impermeable eye shield can be used at night to retain moisture. Taping the eyelids closed at night may be necessary to provide protection.
- A facial sling may be fitted by an occupational or physical therapist to support affected muscles, improve lip alignment, and facilitate eating. When function begins to return, active facial exercises are performed several times per day.

The change in physical appearance as a result of Bell's palsy can be devastating. Reassure the patient that a stroke did not occur and that chances for a full recovery are good.

BENIGN PAROXYSMAL POSITIONAL VERTIGO

Benign paroxysmal positional vertigo (BPPV) is a condition in which free-floating debris in the semicircular canal causes vertigo with specific head movements, such as getting out of bed, rolling over in bed, and sitting up from lying down. BPPV causes about 50% of cases of vertigo. The debris ("ear rocks") is composed of small calcium carbonate crystals that may develop in the inner ear due to head trauma, infection, or the aging process, or from an unknown cause.

Symptoms are intermittent and include dizziness, vertigo, lightheadedness, loss of balance, and nausea. There is no hearing loss. The symptoms of BPPV may be confused with those of Ménière's disease. Diagnosis is based on auditory and vestibular testing results.

A person experiencing BPPV is at risk for falls. Repositioning maneuvers and procedures may provide symptom relief. (See Chapter 21 in Lewis et al, *Medical-Surgical Nursing,* ed 10, p. 387, for a description of these procedures.)

BENIGN PROSTATIC HYPERPLASIA

Description

Benign prostatic hyperplasia (BPH) is a condition in which the prostate gland increases in size, leading to disruption of the outflow of urine from the bladder through the urethra. Almost half of the men with BPH will have bothersome lower urinary tract symptoms (LUTS), such as difficulty starting a urine stream, a decreased flow of urine, or urinary frequency.

Pathophysiology

As men age, the amount of active testosterone in the blood decreases, leaving a higher proportion of estrogen. A higher amount of estrogen within the prostate gland increases the activity of substances, including dihydroxytestosterone (DHT), that promote prostate cell growth. BPH usually develops in the inner part of the prostate. As the prostate enlarges, it gradually compresses the urethra, leading to partial or complete obstruction.

- The location of the enlargement is most significant in the development of obstructive symptoms, so even mild prostate enlargement can cause severe symptoms.
- Risk factors for BPH include aging, obesity (in particular, increased waist circumference), lack of physical activity, alcohol consumption, erectile dysfunction, smoking, and diabetes. A family history of BPH in first-degree relatives may also be a risk factor.

Clinical Manifestations

Although early symptoms are often minimal, symptoms gradually worsen as the degree of urethral obstruction increases. Symptoms can be divided into two groups: obstructive and irritative.

- *Obstructive symptoms* of BPH due to urinary retention include a decrease in the caliber and force of the urinary stream, difficulty in initiating voiding, intermittency (stopping and starting stream several times while voiding), and dribbling at the end of urination.
- *Irritative symptoms,* including urinary frequency, urgency, dysuria, bladder pain, nocturia, and incontinence, are associated with inflammation and infection.

Complications

- Acute urinary retention is manifested as a sudden and painful inability to urinate. Treatment involves the insertion of a bladder catheter. Surgery may also be indicated.

- Urinary tract infections can result from incomplete bladder emptying, which provides a favorable environment for bacterial growth.
- Calculi may develop in the bladder because of alkalinization of the residual urine.
- Hydronephrosis and pyelonephritis caused by back pressure of urine in an obstructed system may lead to renal failure.

Diagnostic Studies
- Physical examination including a digital rectal examination (DRE) to determine prostate size, symmetry, and consistency
- Urinalysis with culture to determine the presence of infection
- Postvoid residual urine volume to assess the degree of urine flow obstruction
- Prostate-specific antigen (PSA) blood test to rule out prostate cancer
- Uroflowmetry studies and transrectal ultrasound scan of prostate
- Cystoscopy to visualize the urethra and bladder

Interprofessional Care
The goals of collaborative care are to restore bladder drainage, relieve the patient's symptoms, and prevent or treat the complications of BPH. Treatment is generally based on the degree to which the symptoms bother the patient or the presence of complications, rather than on the size of the prostate.
- Dietary changes (decreasing intake of caffeine and artificial sweeteners, limiting spicy or acidic foods), avoiding medications such as decongestants and anticholinergics, and restricting evening fluid intake may reduce symptoms.
- A timed voiding schedule may reduce or eliminate symptoms.

If the patient begins to have signs or symptoms that indicate an increase in obstruction, further treatment is indicated. Minimally invasive therapies are becoming more common as an alternative to watchful waiting or more invasive treatment. See Table 14 for descriptions of minimally invasive procedures and surgical treatment options.

Drug Therapy
Drugs are used to treat BPH with variable results.
- 5α-Reductase inhibitors reduce the size of the prostate gland. Finasteride (Proscar) blocks the enzyme needed to convert testosterone to DT, the principal intraprostatic androgen. This results in a regression of hyperplastic tissue. Dutasteride (Avodart) is a dual inhibitor of 5α-reductase type 1 and

TABLE 14 Treatment for Benign Prostatic Hyperplasia

Procedure/Description	Advantages	Disadvantages
Minimally Invasive		
Transurethral Microwave Thermotherapy (TUMT)		
Use of microwave radiating heat to produce coagulative necrosis of the prostate	• Outpatient procedure • Erectile dysfunction, urinary incontinence, and retrograde ejaculation are rare	• Potential for damage to surrounding tissue • Urinary catheter needed after procedure
Transurethral Needle Ablation (TUNA)		
Low-wave radiofrequency used to heat the prostate, causing necrosis	• Outpatient procedure • Erectile dysfunction, urinary incontinence, and retrograde ejaculation are rare • Precise delivery of heat to desired area • Very little pain experienced	• Urinary retention common • Irritative voiding symptoms • Hematuria

Laser Prostatectomy

Procedure uses a laser beam to cut or destroy part of the prostate.

Different techniques are available:
- Visual laser ablation of prostate (VLAP)
- Contact laser
- Photovaporization of prostate (PVP)
- Interstitial laser coagulation (ILC)

- Short procedure
- Comparable results to TURP
- Minimal bleeding
- Fast recovery time
- Rapid symptom improvement
- Very effective

- Catheter (up to 7 days) needed after procedure due to edema and urinary retention
- Delayed sloughing of tissue
- Takes several weeks to reach optimal effect
- Retrograde ejaculation

Transurethral Electrovaporization of Prostate (TUVP)

Electrosurgical vaporization and desiccation are used together to destroy prostatic tissue.

- Minimal risks
- Minimal bleeding and sloughing

- Retrograde ejaculation
- Intermittent hematuria

Invasive (Surgery)

Transurethral Resection of Prostate (TURP)

Use of excision and cauterization to remove prostate tissue via cystoscope

Remains the standard for treatment of BPH

- Erectile dysfunction unlikely

- Bleeding
- Retrograde ejaculation

Continued

B

TABLE 14   Treatment for Benign Prostatic Hyperplasia—cont'd

Procedure/Description	Advantages	Disadvantages
Transurethral Incision of Prostate (TUIP) Involves transurethral incisions into prostatic tissue to relieve obstruction Effective for men with small to moderate-sized prostates	• Outpatient procedure • Minimal complications • Low rate of occurrence of erectile dysfunction or retrograde ejaculation	• Urinary catheter needed after procedure
Open Prostatectomy Surgery of choice for men with large prostates, bladder damage, or other complicating factors Involves external incision with two possible approaches	• Complete visualization of prostate and surrounding tissue	• Erectile dysfunction • Bleeding • Postoperative pain • Risk of infection

2 isoenzymes. Serum PSA levels may decrease by almost 50% in patients taking finasteride.

- α-Adrenergic receptor blockers are used, including silodosin (Rapaflo), alfuzosin (Uroxatral), doxazosin (Cardura), prazosin (Minipress), terazosin, and tamsulosin (Flomax). These drugs offer BPH symptom relief by relaxing the smooth muscle of the prostate that surrounds the urethra, but these medications do not decrease the overall size of the prostate.
- The combination of a 5α-reductase inhibitor (dutasteride) and an α-adrenergic receptor blocker (tamsulosin) in a single oral medication (Jalyn) is available.
- Tadalafil (Cialis) has been used in men who have symptoms of BPH alone or in combination with erectile dysfunction (ED). The drug has shown to be effective in reducing symptoms for both of these conditions.
- Saw palmetto has been shown to have no benefit over a placebo in reducing BPH symptoms. Advise patients to discuss all herbal therapies being used with their HCP.

Nursing Management

The focus of nursing management is on health promotion for early detection and treatment, preoperative care, and postoperative care.

Goals

Overall preoperative goals for the patient having prostatic surgery are to have restoration of urinary drainage, treatment of any urinary tract infection, and understanding of the upcoming surgery. Overall postoperative goals are that the patient will have no complications, restoration of urinary control, complete bladder emptying, and satisfying sexual expression.

Nursing Diagnoses

Preoperative

- Acute pain
- Risk for infection

Postoperative

- Acute pain
- Impaired urinary elimination

Nursing Interventions

When symptoms of prostatic hyperplasia become evident, further diagnostic screening may be necessary.

- Ingestion of alcohol and caffeine may increase prostatic symptoms because of the diuretic effect that increases bladder distention.
- Advise patients with obstructive symptoms to urinate every 2 to 3 hours or when they first feel the urge, to minimize urinary stasis and acute urinary retention.

Preoperative Care. Urinary drainage must be restored before surgery; a urethral catheter such as a coudé (curved-tip) catheter may be needed.

- Any infection of the urinary tract must be treated before surgery. Restoring drainage and encouraging a high fluid intake (2 to 3 L/day) are helpful.
- Patients are often concerned about the impact of surgery on sexual function. Provide an opportunity for the patient and his partner to express concerns.

Postoperative Care.   Adjust the plan of care to the type of surgery, reasons for surgery, and patient response to surgery.

- Postoperatively, bladder irrigation is typically done to remove clotted blood from the bladder and ensure drainage of urine. The bladder is irrigated either manually on an intermittent basis or more commonly as continuous bladder irrigation (CBI) with sterile normal saline solution or another prescribed solution. Monitor the inflow and outflow of the irrigant. The infusion of the continuous bladder irrigation fluid should be at a rate to keep the urine drainage light pink without clots.
- The catheter should be connected to a closed drainage system and not disconnected unless it is being removed, changed, or irrigated. Blood clots are expected for the first 24 to 36 hours. However, large amounts of bright red blood in the urine can indicate hemorrhage.
- Painful bladder spasms occur as a result of irritation of the bladder mucosa. Instruct the patient not to urinate around the catheter because this increases the likelihood of spasm. If bladder spasms develop, check the catheter for clots. If present, remove the clots by irrigation so urine flows freely. Belladonna and opium suppositories, along with relaxation techniques, are used to relieve pain and decrease spasm.
- Sphincter tone may be poor immediately after catheter removal, resulting in urinary incontinence or dribbling. Sphincter tone can be strengthened by having the patient practice Kegel exercises (pelvic floor muscle technique). Continence can improve for up to 12 months.
- Observe the patient for signs of postoperative infection. If an external wound is present, the area should be observed for redness, heat, swelling, and purulent drainage. Rectal procedures, such as rectal temperatures and enemas (except insertion of well-lubricated belladonna and opium suppositories), should be avoided.
- Dietary intervention and stool softeners are important to prevent straining while having bowel movements. A diet high in fiber facilitates the passage of stool.

- Activities that increase abdominal pressure, such as sitting or walking for prolonged periods and straining to have a bowel movement (Valsalva maneuver), should be avoided.

▼ **Patient and Caregiver Teaching**

Discharge planning and home care issues are important aspects of care after prostate surgery.

B

- Instructions include (1) caring for an indwelling catheter, if one is in place; (2) managing urinary incontinence; (3) maintaining oral fluids between 2 and 3 L/day; (4) observing for signs and symptoms of urinary tract and wound infection; (5) preventing constipation; (6) avoiding heavy lifting (more than 10 lb [more than 4.5 kg]); and (7) refraining from driving or sexual intercourse as directed by the HCP.
- Many men experience retrograde ejaculation because of trauma to the internal sphincter. Semen is discharged into the bladder at orgasm and may produce cloudy urine when the patient urinates after orgasm. Discuss these changes with the patient and his partner and allow them to ask questions and express their concerns.
- Sexual counseling and treatment options may be necessary if ED becomes a chronic issue.
- The bladder may take up to 2 months to return to its normal capacity. The patient should be instructed to drink at least 2 to 3 L of fluid per day and to urinate every 2 to 3 hours to flush the urinary tract. Teach the patient to avoid or limit bladder irritants such as caffeine products, citrus juices, and alcohol.
- Advise the patient to discuss the need for a yearly DRE with his HCP if he has not had complete removal of the prostate. Hyperplasia or cancer can occur in the remaining prostatic tissue.

BLADDER CANCER

Description

Cancer of the bladder is most common between ages 60 and 70 years and is four times more common in men than in women. The most frequent malignant tumor of the urinary tract is transitional cell carcinoma of the bladder.

About one half of bladder cancers are related to cigarette smoking. Other risk factors include exposure to dyes used in the rubber and other industries. Also at increased risk for bladder cancer are women treated with radiation for cervical cancer, patients who received cyclophosphamide, and patients who take the diabetes drug pioglitazone (Actos).

Individuals with chronic, recurrent renal calculi (often bladder) and chronic lower urinary tract infections (UTIs) have an increased risk of squamous cell cancer of the bladder. Patients who have indwelling catheters for long periods are also at an increased risk for bladder cancer.

Clinical Manifestations

Microscopic or gross, painless hematuria (chronic or intermittent) is the most common clinical finding. Dysuria, frequency, and urgency may also occur because of bladder irritability.

Diagnostic Studies

- When cancer is suspected, obtain urine specimens to identify cancer or atypical cells.
- Ultrasound, CT, or MRI may be used to detect bladder cancer.
- Cystoscopy and biopsy are used to confirm a diagnosis of bladder cancer.

Pathologic grading systems are used to classify the malignant potential of tumor cells, indicating a scale ranging from well-differentiated to undifferentiated.

Nursing and Interprofessional Management

The majority of bladder cancers are diagnosed at an early stage when the cancer is treatable. Low-stage, low-grade, superficial bladder cancers are most common and most responsive to treatment.

Surgical therapies include a variety of procedures:

- *Transurethral resection of the bladder tumor* (TURBT) is used for superficial lesions of the bladder's inner lining. This procedure is also used to control bleeding in patients who are poor operative risks or who have advanced tumors.
- A *partial or radical cystectomy with urinary diversion* is the treatment of choice when the tumor is invasive or involves the trigone (area where ureters insert into the bladder) and the patient is free from metastases beyond the pelvic area.
- A *partial cystectomy* includes resection of that portion of the bladder wall containing the tumor, along with a margin of normal tissue.
- A *radical cystectomy* involves removal of the bladder, prostate, and seminal vesicles in men and the bladder, uterus, cervix, urethra, and ovaries in women.

Postoperative management for any of these surgical procedures includes instructions to drink large amounts of fluid each day for the first week after the procedure, avoid alcoholic beverages, use opioid analgesics and stool softeners if necessary, and take sitz baths to promote muscle relaxation and reduce urinary retention. Administer opioid analgesics for a brief period after the procedure, along with stool softeners.

Radiation therapy is used with cystectomy or as the primary therapy when the cancer is inoperable or when the patient refuses surgery. Chemotherapy drugs used in treating invasive cancer include cisplatin, vinblastine, doxorubicin, and methotrexate.

Chemotherapeutic or immune-stimulating agents can be delivered into the patient's bladder through a urethral catheter, usually at weekly intervals for 6 to 12 weeks. Intravesical agents are instilled directly into the bladder and retained for about 2 hours. The position of the patient may be changed every 15 minutes during the instillation for maximum contact in all areas of the bladder.

- Bacille Calmette-Guérin (BCG), a weakened strain of *Mycobacterium bovis,* is the treatment of choice for carcinoma in situ. When BCG fails, α-interferon, thiotepa, and valrubicin (Valstar) may be used.

After intravesical therapy, most patients have irritative voiding symptoms and hemorrhagic cystitis. Encourage patients to increase daily fluid intake and to quit smoking. Assess the patient for a secondary UTI and stress the need for routine urologic follow-up care. The patient may have fears or concerns about sexual activity or bladder function.

BONE TUMORS

Description

Primary *bone tumors,* both benign and malignant, are relatively rare in adults. They account for only about 3% of all tumors. Metastatic bone cancer in which the cancer has spread from another site is a more common problem.

- Benign bone tumors are more common than primary malignant tumors. These types of tumors, which include osteochondroma, osteoclastoma, and enchondroma, are often removed by surgery.
- Primary malignant bone cancer is called *sarcoma.* The more common types of primary bone cancer are osteosarcoma, chondrosarcoma, and Ewing's sarcoma. Primary malignant tumors occur most often during childhood and young adulthood. They are characterized by their rapid metastasis and bone destruction.

Osteochondroma

Osteochondroma is the most common primary benign bone tumor. It is characterized by an overgrowth of cartilage and bone near the end of the bone at the growth plate. It is more commonly found in the pelvis, scapula, or long bones of the leg.

- Clinical manifestations of osteochondroma include a painless, hard, and immobile mass; lower-than-normal-height for age; sore muscles near the tumor; one leg or arm longer than the other; and pressure or irritation with exercise. Patients may be asymptomatic.
- Diagnosis is confirmed using x-ray, CT scan, and MRI.
- No treatment is necessary for asymptomatic osteochondroma. If the tumor is causing pain or neurologic manifestations due to compression, surgical removal is usually done. Patients should have regular screening examinations for early detection of malignant transformation.

Osteosarcoma

- *Osteosarcoma* is an extremely aggressive primary malignant bone tumor that rapidly metastasizes. It usually occurs in the pelvis or metaphyseal region of long bones of the extremities, particularly in regions of the distal femur, proximal tibia, and proximal humerus. It is the most common malignant bone tumor affecting children and young adults, and is most often associated with Paget's disease and prior radiation.
- Clinical manifestations of osteosarcoma are usually associated with a gradual onset of pain and swelling, especially around the knee. A minor injury does not cause the tumor but rather serves to bring the preexisting condition to medical attention.
- Diagnosis is confirmed from tissue biopsy, elevation of serum alkaline phosphatase and calcium levels, and x-ray, CT or positron emission tomography (PET) scans, and MRI findings.
- Metastasis is present in 10% to 20% of individuals when they are diagnosed with osteosarcoma.

Preoperative chemotherapy may be used to decrease tumor size before surgery. Limb-salvage surgical procedures are usually considered if there is a clear (no cancer present) 6- to 7-cm margin surrounding the lesion. Adjunct chemotherapy after surgery has increased the 5-year survival rate to 70% in patients without metastasis.

Metastatic Bone Cancer

Metastatic bone cancer is the most common type of malignant bone tumor. It occurs as a result of metastasis from a primary tumor. Common sites for the primary tumor include the breast, prostate, lungs, kidney, and thyroid. Metastatic bone lesions are commonly found in the vertebrae, pelvis, femur, humerus, or ribs.

- Pathologic fractures at the site of metastasis are common because the bone has weakened. Serum calcium levels rise as calcium is released from damaged bones.
- Radionuclide bone scans may detect metastatic lesions before they are visible on x-ray. Metastatic bone lesions may occur at any time (even years later) after diagnosis and treatment of the primary tumor.
- Metastasis to the bone should be suspected in any patient who has local bone pain and a history of cancer.
- Treatment may be palliative and consists of radiation and pain management. Surgical stabilization of the fracture may be indicated if there is a fracture or impending fracture. Prognosis depends on the primary type of cancer and if other sites of metastasis are present.

Nursing Management: Bone Cancer

Nursing care of the patient with a malignant bone tumor is similar to care provided to the patient with cancer of any other body system. Use special care to reduce complications associated with prolonged bed rest and to prevent pathologic fractures by careful handling and support of the affected extremity and logrolling.

- Weakness caused by anemia and decreased mobility may be noted.
- Monitor the site of the tumor for swelling, changes in circulation, and decreased movement, sensation, or joint function.
- The pain caused by the tumor pressing against nerves and other organs near the bone can be very severe. Carefully monitor the patient's pain and ensure adequate pain medication. Sometimes radiation therapy is used as a palliative therapy to shrink the tumor and decrease the pain.
- The patient may be reluctant to participate in therapeutic activities because of weakness and fear of pain. Provide regular rest periods between activities.
- Assist the patient and family in adjusting to the guarded prognosis associated with bone cancer.
- Special attention is necessary for problems of pain and dysfunction, chemotherapy, and specific surgery, such as spinal cord decompression or amputation.

BRAIN TUMORS

Description

Brain tumors may be primary, arising from tissues within the brain, or secondary, resulting from a metastasis from a malignant neoplasm elsewhere in the body. Secondary brain tumors are the most common type.

Brain tumors are generally classified according to the tissue from which they arise. *Meningiomas* are the most common primary brain tumor. Other common brain tumors are gliomas (e.g., astrocytoma, glioblastoma [most common form of glioma]).

- More than half of brain tumors are malignant. They infiltrate the brain tissue and are not amenable to complete surgical removal. Other tumors may be histologically benign but are located such that complete removal is not possible.
- Brain tumors rarely metastasize outside the central nervous system (CNS) because they are contained by structural (meninges) and physiologic (blood-brain) barriers. (For a comparison of the most common brain tumors, see Table 56-12, Lewis et al, *Medical-Surgical Nursing,* ed 10, p. 1333.)
- Unless treated, all brain tumors eventually cause death from increasing tumor volume leading to increased intracranial pressure (ICP).

Clinical Manifestations

Manifestations depend on the location and size of the tumor. A wide range of clinical manifestations are associated with brain tumors.

- Headache is common. Tumor-related headaches tend to be worse at night and may awaken the patient. The headaches are usually dull and constant but occasionally are throbbing.
- Seizures are common in gliomas and brain metastases. Brain tumors can cause nausea and vomiting from increased ICP.
- Cognitive dysfunction, including memory problems and mood or personality changes, is common with brain metastases. Expanding tumors may produce signs of increased ICP, cerebral edema, or obstruction of cerebrospinal fluid (CSF) pathways.

Diagnostic Studies

- Extensive history and a comprehensive neurologic examination are essential in the diagnostic workup.
- MRI and positron emission tomography (PET) scans allow for detection of very small tumors.

- CT (with contrast) and brain scanning assist in tumor location.
- Other tests include angiography, magnetic resonance spectroscopy, functional MRI, PET scans, and single-photon emission computed tomography (SPECT).

Correct diagnosis of a brain tumor is made by obtaining tissue for histologic study. In most patients, tissue is obtained at time of surgery.

B

Interprofessional Care

Treatment goals are aimed at (1) identifying the tumor type and location, (2) removing or decreasing tumor mass, and (3) preventing or managing increased ICP.

Surgical removal is the preferred treatment for brain tumors (see section on cranial surgery in Chapter 56, Lewis et al, *Medical-Surgical Nursing,* ed 10, pp. 1334 to 1335). Surgical outcome depends on the type, size, and location of the tumor. Meningiomas and oligodendrogliomas can usually be completely removed, whereas more invasive gliomas and medulloblastomas can be only partially removed. Even if complete surgical removal of the tumor is not possible, surgery can reduce the tumor mass, which decreases ICP and provides relief of symptoms with an extension of survival time.

Radiation therapy is used as a follow-up measure after surgery. Radiation seeds can also be implanted into the brain. Cerebral edema and rapidly increasing ICP may be complications of radiation therapy, but they can be managed with high doses of corticosteroids (dexamethasone, prednisone, or methylprednisolone [Solu-Medrol]).

- Stereotactic radiosurgery delivers a highly concentrated dose of radiation precisely directed at a location within the brain. It may be used when conventional surgery has failed or is not an option because of the tumor location.

Normally the blood-brain barrier prohibits the entry of most drugs into brain tissue. The most malignant brain tumors cause a breakdown of the blood-brain barrier in the area, thus allowing chemotherapy drugs to reach the tumor. Chemotherapy drug–laden biodegradable wafers implanted during surgery can deliver chemotherapy directly to the tumor site. Intrathecal administration also allows direct delivery of chemotherapeutic drugs to the CNS.

Bevacizumab (Avastin) is used to treat patients with glioblastoma when this type of brain cancer continues to progress after standard therapy. Bevacizumab is a targeted therapy agent that inhibits the action of vascular endothelial growth factor (substance that helps form new blood vessels).

Nursing Management

Goals

The patient with a brain tumor will maintain normal ICP, maximize neurologic functioning, achieve control of pain and discomfort, and be aware of the long-term implications with respect to prognosis and cognitive and physical functioning.

Nursing Diagnoses/Collaborative Problems

- Risk for ineffective cerebral tissue perfusion
- Acute pain (headache)
- Anxiety
- Potential complication: seizures
- Potential complication: increased ICP

Nursing Interventions

Behavioral changes associated with a frontal lobe lesion, such as loss of emotional control, confusion, memory loss, and depression, are often not perceived by the patient but can be very disturbing and frightening to the family. Assist the caregiver and family in understanding what is happening.

- Care of the confused patient with behavioral instability can be a challenge. Close supervision of activity, use of padded side rails, and a calm, reassuring approach are all essential care techniques.
- Minimize environmental stimuli, create a routine, and use reality orientation for the confused patient.
- Seizures often occur with brain tumors. Seizure precautions should be instituted for the protection of the patient (see Seizure Disorders, p. 555).
- Motor and sensory dysfunctions are problems that interfere with the activities of daily living. Alterations in mobility must be managed, and encourage the patient to provide as much self-care as physically possible. Self-image often depends on the patient's ability to participate in care within the limitations of the physical deficits.
- Motor (expressive) or sensory (receptive) dysphasia may occur. Disturbances in communication can be frustrating for the patient and may interfere with your ability to meet patient needs. Make attempts to establish a communication system that can be used by both the patient and staff.
- Tumors in the temporal lobe can cause hallucinations, which may be confused with dementia or delirium in the patient.
- Nutritional intake may be decreased because of the patient's inability to eat, loss of appetite, or loss of desire to eat. Assessing the nutritional status of the patient and ensuring adequate nutritional intake are important aspects of care. The patient may

need encouragement to eat or, in some cases, may need enteral or parenteral nutrition (see Enteral Nutrition, p. 706, and Parenteral Nutrition, p. 731).

Social workers and home health nurses may be needed to assist the caregiver with discharge planning and to help the family adjust to role changes and psychosocial and socioeconomic factors. Issues related to palliative and end-of-life care need to be discussed with both the patient and family.

BREAST CANCER

Description

Breast cancer is the most common malignancy in women in the United States except for skin cancer and is second only to lung cancer as the leading cause of death from cancer in women. In the United States, over 231,000 new cases of invasive breast cancer and over 60,000 cases of in situ breast cancer are diagnosed annually. About 2200 new cases of breast cancer are diagnosed in men annually.

Pathophysiology

Although the etiology is not completely understood, a number of factors are related to breast cancer. Risk factors appear to be cumulative and interactive (Table 15). A breast cancer risk assessment tool for HCPs is available through the National Cancer Institute *(www.cancer.gov/bcrisk tool)*.

- The use of combined hormone therapy (estrogen plus progesterone) increases the risk of breast cancer and the risk of having a larger, more advanced breast cancer at diagnosis. The use of estrogen therapy alone for longer than 10 years (for women with a prior hysterectomy) increases a woman's long-term risk for breast cancer.
- About 5% to 10% of all breast cancers are hereditary and are associated with mutations in two genes: *BRCA1* and *BRCA2*.

In general, breast cancer arises from the epithelial lining of the ducts *(ductal carcinoma)* or from the epithelium of the lobules *(lobular carcinoma)*. Breast cancers may be *in situ* (within the duct) or invasive (arising from the duct and invading through the wall of the duct).

Breast cancer can be classified as noninvasive or invasive, and as ductal or lobular (Table 16).

- Factors that affect cancer prognosis are tumor size, axillary node involvement (the more nodes involved, the worse the prognosis), tumor differentiation (morphology of malignant

TABLE 15 Risk Factors for Breast Cancer

Risk Factor	Comments
Female	Women account for 99% of breast cancer cases.
Age ≥50 yr	Majority of breast cancers are found in postmenopausal women. After age 60, increase in incidence.
Hormone use	Use of estrogen and/or progesterone as hormone therapy, especially in postmenopausal women.
Family history	Breast cancer in a first-degree relative, particularly when premenopausal or bilateral, increases risk.
Genetic factors	Gene mutations *(BRCA1, BRCA2, P53, PTEN, PALB2)* play a role in 5%–10% of breast cancer cases.
Personal history of breast cancer, colon cancer, endometrial cancer, ovarian cancer	Personal history significantly increases risk of breast cancer, risk of cancer in other breast, and recurrence.
Early menarche (before age 12), late menopause (after age 55)	A long menstrual history increases the risk of breast cancer.
First full-term pregnancy after age 30, nulliparity	Prolonged exposure to unopposed estrogen increases risk for breast cancer.
Benign breast disease with atypical epithelial hyperplasia, lobular carcinoma in situ	Atypical changes in breast biopsy increase the risk of breast cancer.
Weight gain and obesity after menopause	Fat cells store estrogen, which increases the likelihood of developing breast cancer.
Exposure to ionizing radiation	Radiation damages DNA (e.g., prior treatment for Hodgkin's lymphoma).
Alcohol consumption	Women who drink ≥1 alcoholic beverage per day may have an increased risk of breast cancer.

TABLE 16 Classification of Breast Cancer

Based on Tissue Type
- Ductal carcinoma (affects milk ducts)
  - Medullary
  - Tubular
  - Colloid (mucinous)
- Lobular carcinoma (affects milk-producing glands)
- Other
  - Inflammatory
  - Paget's disease
  - Phyllodes tumor

Based on Invasiveness
Noninvasive (In Situ)
- Ductal carcinoma in situ (DCIS)
- Lobular carcinoma in situ (LCIS)

Invasive (Spreading to Other Locations)
- Invasive ductal carcinoma
- Invasive lobular carcinoma

Based on Hormone Receptor and Genetic Status
Estrogen and Progesterone Receptor Status
- Estrogen receptor–positive
- Estrogen receptor–negative
- Progesterone receptor–positive
- Progesterone receptor–negative

HER-2 Genetic Status
- HER-2–positive
- HER-2–negative

HER-2, Human epidermal growth factor receptor 2.

cells), estrogen and progesterone receptor status, and human epidermal growth factor receptor 2 (HER-2) status, which is a genetic marker.

Clinical Manifestations

Breast cancer is usually detected as a lump in the breast or mammographic abnormality. It occurs most often in the upper outer quadrant of the breast because that is the location of most of the glandular tissue.

- If palpable, breast cancer is characteristically hard and may be irregularly shaped, poorly delineated, nonmobile, and nontender.
- A small percentage of breast cancers cause nipple discharge. The discharge is usually unilateral and may be clear or bloody. Nipple retraction may occur.
- Plugging of the dermal lymphatics can cause skin thickening and exaggeration of the usual skin markings, giving skin the appearance of an orange peel (peau d'orange).
- In large cancers, infiltration, induration, and dimpling (pulling in) of the overlying skin may occur.

Recurrence may be local or regional (skin or soft tissue near mastectomy site, axillary lymph nodes) or distant (most commonly bone, brain, lung, and liver).

Diagnostic Studies
Screening
- Physical examination of breast and lymphatics
- Mammography and ultrasound
- Breast MRI
- Biopsy including fine-needle aspiration and stereotactic core biopsy

Post-Diagnosis
Axillary lymph node dissection is often performed. An examination of the nodes is often performed to determine if cancer has spread to the axilla on the side of the breast cancer. The more nodes involved, the greater the risk of recurrence.

Lymphatic mapping and *sentinel lymph node (SLN) biopsy* help the surgeon identify the lymph node(s) that drain from the tumor site (sentinel node). Assessment of this node can be used to determine the extent of tumor spread to axillary lymph nodes. If the SLNs are positive, a complete *axillary lymph node dissection* (ALND) may be done.

- Tumor size is a prognostic variable: the larger the tumor, the poorer the prognosis. In general, poorly differentiated tumors appear morphologically disorganized and are more aggressive.
- Estrogen and progesterone receptor status helps to determine treatment decisions and prognosis. Receptor-positive tumors commonly (1) show histologic evidence of being well differentiated, (2) have a lower chance for recurrence, and (3) are frequently responsive to hormonal therapy. Receptor-negative tumors (1) are often poorly differentiated histologically, (2) frequently recur, and (3) are usually unresponsive to hormonal therapy.

- DNA content (ploidy status) correlates with tumor aggressiveness. Diploid tumors have been shown to have a significantly lower risk of recurrence than aneuploid tumors.
- Overexpression of the HER-2 receptor has been associated with a greater risk for recurrence and a poorer prognosis in patients with breast cancer. About 10% to 20% of metastatic breast cancers produce excessive HER-2.
- Genomic assays (MammaPrint and Oncotype DX) are used to analyze the activity of a group of genes.

A patient whose breast cancer tests negative for all three receptors (estrogen, progesterone, and HER-2) has *triple-negative breast cancer,* an aggressive tumor with a poorer prognosis. The incidence of triple-negative breast cancer is higher in Hispanics, African Americans, women who are younger, and women with a *BRCA1* mutation.

Interprofessional Care

Prognostic factors are considered in treatment decisions, and tumor size (T), nodal involvement (N), and presence of metastasis (M) are used to stage breast cancer with the TNM system (see TNM Classification System, p. 781).

Surgical Therapy

The most common surgical options for resectable breast cancer are (1) breast-conserving surgery (lumpectomy, segmental mastectomy) and (2) mastectomy with or without reconstruction. Most women diagnosed with early-stage breast cancer (tumors smaller than 4 to 5 cm) are candidates for either treatment choice.

Breast-conserving surgery (lumpectomy) usually involves removal of the entire tumor along with a margin of normal tissue. Sentinel lymph node dissection (SLND) is the standard of care, with ALND reserved for patients when clinically indicated (evidence of disease in the axilla). After surgery, radiation therapy is delivered to the entire breast, ending with a boost to the tumor bed. If evidence exists that the risk for recurrence is high, chemotherapy may be administered before radiation therapy.

A *total* or *simple mastectomy* removes the entire breast. *Modified radical mastectomy* includes removal of the breast and axillary lymph nodes while preserving the pectoralis major muscle. See Table 51-7, Lewis et al, *Medical-Surgical Nursing,* ed 10, p. 1215, for treatment options, side effects, complications, and patient issues related to surgical procedures for breast cancer.

Radiation Therapy

Radiation therapy may be used for breast cancer as treatment to (1) prevent local tumor recurrences after breast-conserving surgery,

(2) prevent local and nodal recurrences after mastectomy, or (3) palliate pain caused by local, regional, and distant recurrence.
- The MammoSite system is a minimally invasive method of delivering internal radiation therapy. The technique uses a balloon catheter to insert radioactive seeds into the breast after the tumor is removed.

Chemotherapy
Many breast cancers are responsive to cytotoxic drugs. The use of a combination of drugs is most often superior to the use of a single drug. The incidence and severity of the side effects that accompany chemotherapy are influenced by the specific drug combinations, drug schedule, and dose of the drugs (see Chemotherapy, p. 694). In some patients, chemotherapy is given preoperatively.

Hormone Therapy
Estrogen can promote growth of breast cancer cells if cells are estrogen-receptor positive. Hormonal therapy can block the source of estrogen, thus promoting tumor regression. It may be used as an adjuvant to primary treatment or in patients with recurrent or metastatic cancer.

Hormone receptor assays can identify women who are likely to respond to hormone therapy. Hormonal therapy can block estrogen receptors or suppress estrogen synthesis through inhibiting aromatase, an enzyme needed for estrogen synthesis (Table 17).
- Antiestrogens include tamoxifen, toremifene (Fareston), and fulvestrant (Faslodex).
- Aromatase inhibitor drugs include anastrozole (Arimidex), letrozole (Femara), and exemestane (Aromasin) and are used in the treatment of breast cancer in postmenopausal women.

Immunotherapy and Targeted Therapy
Trastuzumab (Herceptin) is a monoclonal antibody to HER-2. After the antibody attaches to the antigen, it is taken into the cells and eventually kills them. It can be used alone or in combination with chemotherapy to treat patients with breast cancer whose tumors overexpress the HER-2 gene.

Lapatinib (Tykerb) may be used in combination with capecitabine (Xeloda) for patients with advanced, metastatic disease who are HER-2–positive. Pertuzumab (Perjeta) is a new anti–HER-2 therapy that is used for patients who have not received prior treatment for metastatic breast cancer with an anti–HER-2 therapy or chemotherapy. Pertuzumab is combined with trastuzumab and docetaxel.

Drugs in other classes used to treat breast cancer include everolimus (Afinitor) and palbociclib (Ibrance). Everolimus works by blocking mTOR, a protein that normally promotes cell growth and division. Palbociclib is a kinase inhibitor that prevents cells from dividing, thus slowing cancer growth.

TABLE 17 Drug Therapy

Breast Cancer

Drug Class/ Drug	Mechanism of Action	Indication(s)
Hormone Therapy		
Estrogen Receptor Blockers		
tamoxifen	Blocks estrogen receptors (ERs)	ER-positive breast cancer in premenopausal and postmenopausal women Used as a preventive measure in high-risk premenopausal and postmenopausal women
toremifene (Fareston)	Blocks ERs	ER-positive breast cancer in postmenopausal women only
fulvestrant (Faslodex)	Blocks ERs	ER-positive breast cancer in postmenopausal women only
Aromatase Inhibitors		
anastrozole (Arimidex) letrozole (Femara) exemestane (Aromasin)	Prevents production of estrogen by inhibiting aromatase	ER-positive breast cancer in postmenopausal women only
Estrogen Receptor Modulator		
raloxifene (Evista)	*In breast:* blocks the effect of estrogen *In bone:* promotes effect of estrogen and prevents bone loss	Postmenopausal women

Continued

B

TABLE 17   Drug Therapy
Breast Cancer—cont'd

Drug Class/ Drug	Mechanism of Action	Indication(s)
Immunotherapy and Targeted Therapy		
trastuzumab (Herceptin) pertuzumab (Perjeta)	Blocks HER-2 receptor	HER-2–positive breast cancer
lapatinib (Tykerb)	Inhibits HER-2 tyrosine kinase and EGFR tyrosine kinase	HER-2–positive breast cancer
ado-trastuzumab emtansine (Kadcyla)	Combination of trastuzumab and a chemotherapy drug called DM1	HER-2–positive breast cancer
everolimus (Afinitor)	Binds to mechanistic target of rapamycin (mTOR), thereby suppressing T cell activation and proliferation	ER-positive, HER-2–negative breast cancer in postmenopausal women
palbociclib (Ibrance)	Kinase inhibitor	ER-positive, HER-2–negative breast cancer in postmenopausal women

EGFR, Epidermal growth factor receptor; *HER-2,* human epidermal growth factor receptor 2.

Follow-up and Survivorship Care
After treatment for breast cancer, the patient will have ongoing survivorship care.

- Recommended follow-up examinations generally occur every 3 to 6 months for the first 5 years, and then annually thereafter.
- Advise women to perform monthly self-examinations of the breast and chest wall and report any changes to their HCP. The most common site of local recurrence of breast cancer is at the surgical site.

- The woman should have appropriate breast imaging at regular intervals (usually 6 months to 1 year) as determined by her risk of recurrence and breast cancer history.

Nursing Management
Goals

The patient with breast cancer will actively participate in the decision-making process related to treatment, adhere to the therapeutic plan, communicate about and manage the side effects of adjuvant therapy, and access and benefit from the support provided by significant others and the HCP.

Nursing Diagnoses
After a diagnosis of breast cancer and before a treatment plan has been selected, the following diagnoses apply:
- Decisional conflict
- Fear and/or anxiety
- Disturbed body image

If the patient undergoes a lumpectomy or modified radical mastectomy, nursing diagnoses may also include:
- Acute pain
- Impaired physical mobility

Nursing Interventions
The time between the diagnosis of breast cancer and the selection of a treatment plan is a difficult period for the woman and her family. Although the HCP discusses treatment options, the woman often relies on you to clarify and expand on these options.

- Appropriate nursing interventions are to explore the woman's usual decision-making processes, help her to evaluate the advantages and disadvantages of the options, provide information relevant to the decision(s), and support the patient and family once decisions are made.
- Regardless of the surgery planned, provide the patient with sufficient information to ensure informed consent. Teaching in the preoperative phase includes turning and deep breathing, a review of postoperative exercises, and an explanation of the recovery period from the time of surgery until the first postoperative visit.

The woman who has breast-conserving surgery usually has an uncomplicated postoperative course with variable pain intensity. After ALND or a mastectomy, patients are generally discharged home with drains in place. Teach the patient and family (including a return demonstration) how to manage the drains at home.

- Restoring arm function on the affected side after mastectomy and axillary lymph node dissection is a key nursing goal.

- Place the woman in a semi-Fowler's position with the arm on the affected side elevated on a pillow. Flexing and extending the fingers should begin in the recovery room, with progressive increases in activity.
- Postoperative arm and shoulder exercises are instituted gradually.
- Postoperative discomfort can be minimized by administering analgesics about 30 minutes before initiating exercises. When able to shower, the warm water on the affected shoulder often has a muscle-relaxing effect and reduces joint stiffness.

Lymphedema (accumulation of lymph in soft tissue) can occur as a result of excision or radiation of the lymph nodes. The patient may experience heaviness, pain, impaired motor function in the arm, and numbness and paresthesia of the fingers. Help the patient to understand that lymphedema can occur at any point after treatment. Teach measures to prevent or reduce lymphedema including:

- No BP readings, venipunctures, or injections on the affected arm.
- The affected arm should not be dependent for long periods of time, and caution should be used to prevent infection, burns, or compromised circulation on the affected side.
- If trauma to the arm occurs, the area should be washed thoroughly with soap and water and observed. A topical antibiotic ointment and a bandage or other sterile dressing may be applied.

Frequent and sustained elevation of the arm, regular use of a custom-fitted pressure sleeve, and treatment with an inflatable sleeve (pneumomassage) may also be helpful.

It is important to remain sensitive to the complex psychologic impact that a diagnosis of cancer and subsequent breast surgery can have on a woman and her family. Help to meet the woman's psychologic needs by the following:

- Help her identify sources of support and strength such as her partner, family, and spiritual practices.
- Provide a safe environment for the expression of the full range of feelings.
- Encourage the patient to identify and learn individual coping strengths.
- Promote communication between the patient and her family and/or friends.
- Provide accurate and complete answers to questions about the disease, treatment options, and reproductive or lactation issues (if appropriate).
- Make resources available for mental health counseling.

- Offer information about community resources, such as Reach to Recovery or local breast cancer organizations.

Breast reconstruction is discussed in Chapter 51, Lewis et al, *Medical-Surgical Nursing,* ed. 10.

▼ Patient and Caregiver Teaching

- Explain the specific follow-up plan to the patient, emphasizing the importance of ongoing monitoring and self-care.
- Immediately after surgery, advise the patient of symptoms to report to the HCP, including fever, inflammation at the surgical site, erythema, postoperative constipation, and unusual swelling.
- For women who have had a mastectomy without breast reconstruction, a variety of garment choice products are available, including camisoles with soft breast prosthetic inserts as well as a fitted prosthesis with bra.
- A preoperative sexual assessment provides baseline data that can be used to plan postoperative interventions.
- The spouse, sexual partner, or family members may need assistance in dealing with their emotional reactions to the diagnosis and surgery so that they can act as effective means of support for the patient.
- Depression and anxiety may occur with the continued stress and uncertainty of a cancer diagnosis. The support of family and friends and participation in a cancer support group are important aspects of care that are often helpful in improving quality of life and have a significant impact on survival.
- Additional information on expected outcomes for the patient after breast cancer surgery is presented in eNursing Care Plan 51-1 (available on the website).

BRONCHIECTASIS

Description

Bronchiectasis is characterized by permanent, abnormal dilation of medium-sized bronchi as a result of inflammatory changes that destroy elastic and muscular structures supporting the bronchial wall. Infection is the primary reason for the continuing cycle of inflammation, airway damage, and remodeling.

Stasis of thickened mucus occurs along with impaired movement by the cilia, resulting in a reduced ability to clear mucus from the lungs.

Cystic fibrosis is the main cause of bronchiectasis in children. In adults, the main cause is bacterial infections of the lungs that are either not treated or receive delayed treatment. Other causes include obstruction of an airway with mucus plugs, generalized impairment of pulmonary defenses, inflammatory bowel disease, rheumatoid arthritis, and immune disorders (e.g., acquired immunodeficiency syndrome [AIDS]).

Clinical Manifestations

The hallmark of bronchiectasis is persistent cough with consistent production of purulent, thick sputum. However, some patients with severe disease and upper lobe involvement may have no sputum production and little cough. Recurrent infections injure blood vessels, causing hemoptysis.

- Other manifestations are pleuritic chest pain, dyspnea, wheezing, clubbing of digits, weight loss, and anemia.
- Lung auscultation reveals a variety of adventitious sounds (e.g., crackles, wheezes).

Diagnostic Studies

An individual with a chronic productive cough with copious purulent sputum (which may be blood-streaked) should be suspected of having bronchiectasis.

- Chest x-ray shows nonspecific abnormalities.
- High-resolution CT (HRCT) scan of the chest is the preferred method for diagnosing bronchiectasis.
- Bronchoscopy may be used with localized bronchiectasis to diagnose obstruction.
- Sputum may provide additional information regarding severity of impairment and presence of active infection. Sputum samples are frequently found to contain *Haemophilus influenzae* or *Pseudomonas aeruginosa.*
- Spirometry usually shows an obstructive pattern, including a decrease in forced expiratory volume in 1 second (FEV_1) and in the ratio of FEV_1 to forced vital capacity (FVC).

Interprofessional Care

Bronchiectasis is difficult to treat. Therapy is aimed at treating acute flare-ups and preventing a decline in lung function. Antibiotics are the mainstay of treatment. Concurrent bronchodilator therapy or anticholinergics are given to prevent bronchospasm and stimulate mucociliary clearance.

- Maintaining good hydration is important to liquefy secretions. Chest physiotherapy and other airway clearance techniques facilitate expectoration of sputum.
- Teach the patient to reduce exposure to excessive air pollutants and irritants, avoid cigarette smoking, and obtain pneumococcal and influenza vaccinations.

- For selected patients who are disabled in spite of maximal therapy, lung transplantation is an option.

Nursing Management

Early detection and treatment of lower respiratory tract infections help prevent complications such as bronchiectasis. An important nursing goal is to promote drainage and removal of bronchial mucus. Various airway clearance techniques can be effectively used to facilitate secretion removal.

- The patient needs to understand the importance of taking the prescribed regimen of drugs to obtain maximum effectiveness.
- If hemoptysis occurs in the acute care setting, contact the HCP immediately. Elevate the head of the bed and place the patient in a side-lying position with the suspected bleeding side down.
- Good nutrition may be difficult to maintain because the patient is often anorexic. Oral hygiene to cleanse the mouth and remove dried sputum crusts may improve the patient's appetite.
- Unless there are contraindications, instruct the patient to drink at least 3 L of fluid daily.
- Direct hydration of the respiratory system may be beneficial in expectorating secretions. Often nebulized hypertonic saline may be ordered for a more aggressive effect. At home, a steamy shower can prove effective.
- Teach the patient and caregiver to recognize significant clinical manifestations to report to the HCP. These manifestations include increased sputum production, bloody sputum, increasing dyspnea, fever, chills, and chest pain.

BURNS

Description

Burns are tissue injuries caused by heat, chemicals, electric current, or radiation. An estimated 450,000 Americans seek medical care each year for burns. The highest fatality rates occur in children aged 4 years and younger and adults older than age 65.

Pathophysiology

Immediately after the burn injury occurs, there is increased blood flow to the area surrounding the wound. This is followed by the release of various vasoactive substances from burned tissue, which results in increased capillary permeability. Fluid then shifts from the intravascular compartment to the interstitial space, producing edema, hypovolemia, and (potentially) shock. After several days, diuresis from fluid mobilization occurs and healing begins.

Types of Burn Injury

Various types of burns may be seen alone or in combination with other burns.

- *Thermal burns* are caused by flame, flash, scald, or contact with hot objects. Severity depends on the temperature of the burning agent and duration of contact.
- *Chemical burns* are the result of tissue injury and destruction from acids, alkalis (e.g., cement, oven cleaner), and organic compounds such as petroleum products.
- *Smoke and inhalation injury* results from inhalation of hot air or noxious chemicals that damage the respiratory tract. These injuries include metabolic asphyxiation, upper airway injury, and lower airway injury.
- *Electrical burns* result from the intense heat of an electric current.

Classification of Burn Injury

The treatment of burns is related to the severity of injury. A variety of methods exist for determining burn severity.

1. Depth of burn is described according to the depth of skin destruction (epidermis, dermis, or subcutaneous tissue). Table 18 compares the various burn classifications according to the depth of injury.
2. Extent of the burn wound is calculated as percent of total body surface area (TBSA) affected. Two common methods for determining the extent of a burn include:
   - *Lund-Browder chart,* which is considered the most accurate because it takes into account patient age in proportion to relative body area size (Fig. 2, *A*).
   - *Rule of Nines chart,* which is often used for initial assessment because it is easy to remember (Fig. 2, *B*).
3. Severity of the burn injury is also determined by the location of the burn wound. For example, face and neck burns may inhibit respiratory function. Hands, feet, joint, and eye burns may limit self-care and functioning.
4. Preexisting disorders such as heart, lung, or kidney disease reduce the patient's ability to recover from the tremendous demands of burn injury. The patient with diabetes or peripheral vascular disease is at high risk for poor healing, especially with foot and leg burns.

The American Burn Association (ABA) has established referral criteria to determine which burn injuries should be treated in burn centers with specialized facilities (Table 19).

TABLE 18 Classification of Burn Injury Depth

Classification	Appearance	Possible Cause	Structures Involved
Partial-Thickness Skin Destruction			
• Superficial (first-degree) burn	Erythema, blanching on pressure, pain and mild swelling, no vesicles or blisters (although after 24 hr, skin may blister and peel).	Superficial sunburn Quick heat flash	Superficial epidermal damage with hyperemia. Tactile and pain sensation intact.
• Deep (second-degree) burn	Fluid-filled vesicles that are red, shiny, wet (if vesicles have ruptured). Severe pain caused by nerve injury. Mild to moderate edema.	Flame Flash Scald Contact burns Chemical Tar, cement Electric current	Epidermis and dermis involved to varying depths. Skin elements, from which epithelial regeneration occurs, remain viable.
Full-Thickness Skin Destruction			
• Third- and fourth-degree burns	Dry, waxy white, leathery, or hard skin. Visible thrombosed vessels. Insensitivity to pain because of nerve destruction. Possible involvement of muscles, tendons, and bones.	Flame Scald Chemical Tar, cement Electric current	All skin elements and local nerve endings destroyed. Coagulation necrosis present. Surgical intervention required for healing.

B

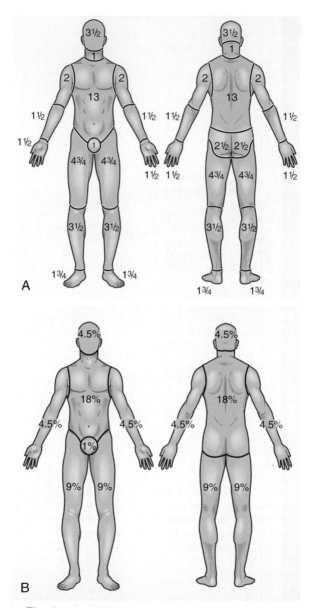

Fig. 2 A, Lund-Browder chart. **B,** Rule of Nines chart.

TABLE 19 Burn Center Referral Criteria

Burn injuries that should be referred to a burn center include the following:

1. Partial-thickness burns >10% of total body surface area (TBSA).
2. Burns that involve the face, hands, feet, genitalia, perineum, or major joints
3. Third-degree burns in any age group
4. Electrical burns, including lightning injury
5. Chemical burns
6. Inhalation injury
7. Burn injury in patients with preexisting medical disorders that could complicate management, prolong recovery, or affect mortality risk (e.g., heart or kidney disease)
8. Patients with burns and concomitant trauma (e.g., fractures) when the burn injury poses the greatest risk of morbidity or mortality. If the trauma poses the greater immediate risk, the patient may be initially stabilized in a trauma center before being transferred to a burn center. The HCP will need to use judgment, in consultation with the regional medical control plan and triage protocols.
9. Burn injury in children in hospitals without qualified personnel or equipment needed to care for them
10. Burn injury in patients who will require special social, emotional, or long-term rehabilitative intervention

Source: American Burn Association: Guidelines for the operation of burn centers. Retrieved from *http://www.ameriburn.org/Chapter14.pdf*.

Clinical Manifestations

Burns can be organized chronologically into three phases: emergent (resuscitative), acute (wound healing), and rehabilitative (restorative).

Emergent Phase

The greatest initial threat to a patient with a major burn is hypovolemic shock. Shivering (a result of heat loss or anxiety) and a paralytic ileus (if the burn area is large) may also be present. Full-thickness and deep partial-thickness burns are initially painless because nerve endings have been destroyed. Superficial to moderate partial-thickness burns are very painful. Blisters are common in partial-thickness burns. Unconsciousness or altered mental status is the result of smoke inhalation or head trauma. Complications may include respiratory distress, dysrhythmias, venous thromboembolism, and acute tubular necrosis.

Acute Phase

Partial-thickness wounds form eschar. After eschar is removed, reepithelialization begins at wound margins and appears as red or pink scar tissue. Wound closure and healing usually occur within 10 to 21 days. Separation of eschar from full-thickness wounds takes longer, and these wounds require surgical debridement and skin grafting for healing. Wound infection is a serious complication. Other possible complications include extreme disorientation and delirium, contractures, Curling's ulcer, and hyperglycemia.

Rehabilitative Phase

Mature healing occurs in about 12 months. New scar tissue shrinks, causing a contracture if not prevented with range-of-motion (ROM) exercises. The healing site, which is extremely sensitive to trauma, may itch. Complications are skin and joint contractures and hypertrophic scarring.

Diagnostic Studies

- Serum electrolytes, especially sodium (Na^+) and potassium (K^+), to monitor fluid and electrolyte shifts
- Chest x-ray, arterial blood gases (ABGs), and sputum for inhalation injury
- Urine output and specific gravity to evaluate fluid replacement and detect acute tubular necrosis and/or renal ischemia
- Complete blood count (CBC) to detect anemia and immunologic response to injury
- White blood cell (WBC) count and wound cultures if infection is suspected

Nursing and Interprofessional Management

Burn management can be classified into three phases: emergent, acute, and rehabilitative (Table 20).

Emergent Phase

Patient survival depends on rapid and thorough assessment and intervention.

- Assess adequacy of airway management and fluid therapy, provide pain medication and wound care, and offer support to patient and family. Begin feeding patient by most appropriate route as soon as possible.

Acute Phase

Predominant interventions are wound care, excision and grafting, pain management, physical and occupational therapy, nutritional therapy, and psychosocial care.

- Wound care consists of ongoing observation, assessment, cleansing, debridement, and dressing reapplication.
- Pain assessment and management are critical.

TABLE 20 Interprofessional Care

Burn Injury

Emergent Phase	Acute Phase	Rehabilitation Phase
Fluid Therapy	**Fluid Therapy**	• Continue to counsel and teach patient and caregiver about wound care.
• Assess fluid needs.	• Continue to replace fluids, depending on patient's clinical response.	• Continue to encourage and assist patient in resuming self-care.
• Begin IV fluid replacement (see Table 24-11, Lewis et al, *Medical-Surgical Nursing*, ed 10, p. 439).		• Continue to prevent or minimize contractures and assess likelihood for scarring (surgery, physical and occupational therapy, splinting, pressure garments).
• Insert urinary catheter.	**Wound Care**	• Discuss possible reconstructive surgery.
• Monitor urine output.	• Continue daily shower and wound care.	• Prepare for discharge home or transfer to rehabilitation hospital.
	• Continue debridement (if necessary).	• Discuss possible need for home care nursing.
Wound Care	• Assess wound daily and adjust dressing protocols as necessary.	
• Start daily shower and wound care.	• Observe for complications (e.g., infection).	
• Debride as necessary.		
• Assess extent and depth of burns.	**Early Excision and Grafting**	
• Administer tetanus toxoid or tetanus antitoxin.	• Provide temporary allografts.	
	• Provide permanent autografts.	
	• Care for donor sites.	

Continued

TABLE 20 Interprofessional Care

Burn Injury—cont'd

Emergent Phase	Acute Phase	Rehabilitation Phase
Pain and Anxiety • Assess and manage pain and anxiety.	**Pain and Anxiety** • Continue to assess for and treat pain and anxiety.	
Physical and Occupational Therapy • Place patient in position that prevents contracture formation and reduces edema. • Assess need for splints.	**Physical and Occupational Therapy** • Begin daily therapy program for maintenance of range of motion. • Assess need for splints and anticontracture positioning. • Encourage and assist patient with self-care as possible.	
Nutritional Therapy • Assess nutritional needs and begin feeding patient by most appropriate route as soon as possible.	**Nutritional Therapy** • Continue to assess diet to support wound healing.	

B

Respiratory Therapy

- Assess oxygenation needs.
- Provide supplemental O_2 as needed.
- Intubate if necessary.
- Monitor respiratory status.

Psychosocial Care

- Provide support to patient and caregiver during initial crisis phase.

Respiratory Therapy

- Continue to assess oxygenation needs.
- Continue to monitor respiratory status.
- Monitor for signs of complications (e.g., pneumonia).

Psychosocial Care

- Provide ongoing support, counseling, and teaching to patient and caregiver about physical and emotional aspects of care and recovery.
- Begin to anticipate discharge needs.

Drug Therapy

(see Table 24-13, Lewis et al, *Medical-Surgical Nursing*, ed 10, p. 441)

- Assess need for medications (e.g., antibiotics).
- Continue to monitor effectiveness and adjust dosage as needed.

Rehabilitative Phase

Encourage the patient and caregiver to actively participate in care.

- Continue to encourage patient to perform physical and occupational therapy routines.
- Apply water-based creams that penetrate the dermis on healed areas to keep skin supple and moisturized.
- Assist patients in adapting to a realistic, yet positive appraisal of the situation, emphasizing what they *can* do instead of what they *cannot* do.

▼ Patient and Caregiver Teaching

- Describe the burn injury process and the expected signs and symptoms related to phases of burn management.
- Explain therapeutic interventions, precautionary measures, gowning and hand washing, and visiting policy to elicit cooperation and decrease anxiety.
- Teach the patient to watch for injuries to new skin.
- Instruct about the signs and symptoms of infection so early treatment can be initiated.
- Teach caregivers how to perform dressing changes to ensure proper technique and increase their sense of control.
- Emphasize the importance of exercise and appropriate physical therapy. Plan a daily program with the patient and offer appropriate resources to provide a continuing activity program as needed.
- Help the patient and caregiver in setting realistic future expectations because anticipatory guidance decreases anxiety and inaccurate perceptions. In addition, they will need to know what to expect physiologically as well as psychologically during recovery.
- Assist the patient and caregivers to establish contact with family and patient support groups, such as the Phoenix Society (*www.phoenix-society.org*).

CARDIOMYOPATHY

Description

Cardiomyopathy (CMP) is a group of diseases that directly affect myocardial structure or function. CMP can be classified as primary or secondary:

- *Primary CMP* refers to those conditions in which the etiology of the heart disease is unknown. The heart muscle in this case is the only portion of the heart involved, and other cardiac structures are unaffected.

- In *secondary CMP,* the myocardial disease is the result of another disease process. Common causes of secondary CMP are coronary artery disease (CAD), myocarditis, hypertension, cardiotoxic agents (alcohol, cocaine), valve disease, and metabolic and autoimmune disorders.

Three major types of CMP are *dilated, hypertrophic,* and *restrictive.* Each type has its own pathogenesis, clinical presentation, and treatment (Table 21). CMP can lead to cardiomegaly and heart

C

TABLE 21 Types of Cardiomyopathy		
Dilated	**Hypertrophic**	**Restrictive**
Major Manifestations		
Fatigue, weakness, palpitations, dyspnea	Exertional dyspnea, fatigue, angina, syncope, palpitations	Dyspnea, fatigue
Cardiomegaly		
Moderate to severe	Mild to moderate	Mild
Contractility		
Decreased	Increased or decreased	Normal or decreased
Valvular Incompetence		
Atrioventricular (AV) valves, especially mitral	Mitral valve	AV valves
Dysrhythmias		
Sinus tachycardia, atrial and ventricular dysrhythmias	Atrial and ventricular dysrhythmias	Atrial and ventricular dysrhythmias
Cardiac Output		
Decreased	Normal or decreased	Normal or decreased
Outflow Tract Obstruction		
None	Increased	None

failure (HF). CMP is the primary reason for heart transplant procedures.

Dilated Cardiomyopathy

Pathophysiology

Dilated CMP is the most common type. It is characterized by diffuse inflammation and rapid degeneration of myocardial fibers that result in ventricular dilation, impairment of systolic function, atrial enlargement, and stasis of blood in the left ventricle. The ventricular walls do not hypertrophy.

- Dilated CMP often follows infectious myocarditis. Other common causes include alcohol, cocaine, hypertension, and CAD.

Clinical Manifestations

Signs and symptoms of dilated CMP may develop acutely after an infection or slowly over time. Most affected people eventually develop HF. Symptoms can include fatigue, dyspnea at rest, paroxysmal nocturnal dyspnea, and orthopnea. Dry cough, abdominal bloating, and anorexia may occur as the disease progresses. Signs can include an irregular heart rate with an abnormal S_3 and/or S_4, pulmonary crackles, edema, pallor, hepatomegaly, heart murmurs, dysrhythmias, and jugular venous distention.

Diagnostic Studies

A diagnosis is made on the basis of patient history and exclusion of other causes of HF.

- Doppler echocardiography is the basis for the diagnosis of dilated CMP.
- Chest x-ray may show cardiomegaly with pulmonary venous hypertension and pleural effusion.
- The electrocardiogram (ECG) may reveal tachycardia, bradycardia, and dysrhythmias with conduction disturbances.
- Serum levels of b-type natriuretic peptide (BNP) are elevated in the presence of HF.
- Heart catheterization confirms or excludes CAD, and multiple gated acquisition (MUGA) nuclear scan determines ejection fraction (EF).

Nursing and Interprofessional Management

Interventions focus on controlling HF by enhancing myocardial contractility and decreasing preload and afterload.

- Nitrates and loop diuretics decrease preload and angiotensin-converting enzyme (ACE) inhibitors reduce afterload.
- β-Adrenergic blockers (e.g., metoprolol [Lopressor]) and aldosterone antagonists (e.g., spironolactone [Aldactone]) control the neurohormonal stimulation that occurs in HF.

- Antidysrhythmics (e.g., amiodarone) and anticoagulants are used as indicated.
- Drug and nutritional therapy and cardiac rehabilitation may help alleviate symptoms of HF and improve cardiac output (CO) and quality of life.
- A patient with secondary dilated CMP must be treated for the underlying disease process. For example, the patient with alcohol-induced dilated CMP must abstain from alcohol.
- The use of statins (e.g., atorvastatin [Lipitor]) in ischemic and idiopathic dilated CMP improves survival and heart function while reducing inflammatory markers.
- Patients may also benefit from nondrug therapies. A ventricular assist device (VAD) allows the heart to rest and recover from acute HF. It may also serve as a bridge to heart transplantation. Cardiac resynchronization therapy and an implantable cardioverter-defibrillator are used in appropriate patients.
- The patient with terminal or end-stage CMP may consider heart transplantation. Currently, approximately 50% of heart transplantations that are performed are for treatment of CMP. Heart transplant recipients have a good prognosis.
- Observe for signs and symptoms of worsening HF, dysrhythmias, and embolus formation. Monitor for drug effectiveness. The goals of therapy are to keep the patient at an optimal level of functioning and out of the hospital.
- Encourage caregivers to learn cardiopulmonary resuscitation (CPR). Instruct them on when and how to activate emergency care.

Hypertrophic Cardiomyopathy
Pathophysiology
Hypertrophic cardiomyopathy (HCM) is asymmetric left ventricular hypertrophy without ventricular dilation. HCM occurs less commonly than dilated CMP and is more common in men than in women. It is usually diagnosed in young adulthood and is often seen in active, athletic individuals. HCM is the most common cause of sudden cardiac death (SCD) in otherwise healthy young people.
- The main characteristics of HCM result from massive ventricular hypertrophy: rapid, forceful contraction of the left ventricle; impaired relaxation (diastole); and obstruction to aortic outflow (not present in all patients). The primary defect is diastolic dysfunction from left ventricular stiffness. Decreased ventricular filling and obstruction to outflow result in decreased CO, especially during exertion.

Clinical Manifestations

Patients may be asymptomatic. The most common symptom is dyspnea, which is caused by an elevated left ventricular diastolic pressure. Other manifestations include fatigue, angina, syncope (especially during exertion), and dysrhythmias.

- Common dysrhythmias include atrial fibrillation, ventricular tachycardia, and ventricular fibrillation. Any of these dysrhythmias may lead to syncope or SCD.

Diagnostic Studies

Clinical findings on examination may be unremarkable. The following diagnostic studies may be used:

- Echocardiogram is the primary diagnostic tool to confirm HCM, which is hypertrophy of the left ventricle.
- Auscultation may reveal an S_4 and a systolic murmur between the apex and sternal border at the fourth intercostal space.
- Heart catheterization and nuclear stress testing may be helpful in diagnosing and guiding treatment.

Nursing and Interprofessional Management

Goals of care are to improve ventricular filling by reducing ventricular contractility and relieving left ventricular outflow obstruction. This can be done with the use of β-blockers (e.g., metoprolol) or calcium channel blockers (e.g., verapamil [Calan]).

- Amiodarone or sotalol (Betapace) are effective antidysrhythmic drugs. However, their use does not prevent SCD. For patients at risk for SCD, an implantable cardioverter-defibrillator is needed.
- Atrioventricular pacing can reduce the degree of outflow obstruction by causing the septum to move away from the left ventricular wall.
- Patients with severe symptoms unresponsive to therapy with marked obstruction to aortic outflow may be candidates for surgical treatment (ventriculomyotomy and myectomy) of their hypertrophied septum. Most patients have an improvement in symptoms and exercise tolerance after surgery.
- An alternative nonsurgical procedure to reduce symptoms is percutaneous transluminal septal myocardial ablation (PTSMA). Ablation of the septal wall decreases the obstruction to flow, and the patient's symptoms decrease.

Nursing interventions focus on relieving symptoms, observing for and preventing complications, and providing emotional support.

- Teaching should focus on helping the patients to adjust their lifestyle to avoid strenuous activity and dehydration. Any activity that causes an increase in systemic vascular resistance (thus increasing obstruction to forward blood flow) is dangerous and should be avoided.

- Rest and elevation of the feet to improve venous return to the heart can manage chest pain in these patients. Vasodilators such as nitroglycerin may worsen the chest pain by decreasing venous return and further increasing obstruction of blood flow from the heart.

Restrictive Cardiomyopathy

Pathophysiology

Restrictive cardiomyopathy is a disease of the heart muscle that impairs diastolic filling and stretch.

- A number of pathologic processes may be involved, including myocardial fibrosis, hypertrophy, and infiltration, which produce stiffness of the ventricular wall.
- The ventricles are resistant to filling and therefore demand high diastolic filling pressures to maintain CO.

Clinical Manifestations

Classic manifestations of restrictive CMP are fatigue, exercise intolerance, and dyspnea. Other manifestations may include angina, orthopnea, syncope, palpations, and signs of HF.

Diagnostic Studies

Chest x-ray may appear normal or show cardiomegaly with pleural effusions and pulmonary congestion.

- ECG may reveal mild tachycardia at rest. The most common dysrhythmias are atrial fibrillation and atrioventricular block.
- Echocardiography may reveal a left ventricle that is normal size with a thickened wall, a slightly dilated right ventricle, and dilated atria.
- Endomyocardial biopsy, CT scan, and nuclear imaging may help to determine a diagnosis.

Nursing and Interprofessional Management

Currently, no specific treatment for restrictive CMP exists. Interventions are aimed at improving diastolic filling and the underlying disease process. Treatment includes conventional therapy for HF and dysrhythmias. Heart transplantation may be a consideration.

Nursing care is similar to the care of a patient with HF. As with HCM, teach patients to avoid situations such as strenuous activity and dehydration that impair ventricular filling and increase systemic vascular resistance.

CARPAL TUNNEL SYNDROME

Description

Carpal tunnel syndrome (CTS) is a condition caused by compression of the median nerve, which enters the hand through the narrow

confines of the carpal tunnel. The carpal tunnel is formed by ligaments and bones. This condition is often caused by pressure from
trauma or edema from inflammation of a tendon (tenosynovitis),
cancer, rheumatoid arthritis, or soft tissue masses such as ganglion
cysts. It is the most common compression neuropathy in the upper
extremities.

- CTS is associated with hobbies or occupations that require
  continuous wrist movement (e.g., musicians, carpenters, computer users).
- Women are affected more often than men, possibly because of
  a smaller carpal tunnel.

Clinical Manifestations

Manifestations are weakness (especially of the thumb), pain and
numbness, impaired sensation in the distribution of the median
nerve, and clumsiness in performing fine hand movements. Numbness and tingling may awaken the patient at night. Shaking the
hands will often relieve these symptoms. Physical signs of CTS
include Tinel's sign and Phalen's sign.

- *Tinel's sign* can be elicited by tapping over the median nerve as
  it passes through the carpal tunnel in the wrist. A positive
  response is a sensation of tingling in the distribution of the
  median nerve over the hand.
- *Phalen's sign* can be elicited by allowing the wrists to fall freely
  into maximum flexion and maintain the position for more than
  60 seconds. A positive response is a sensation of tingling in the
  distribution of the median nerve over the hand.

In late stages, there is atrophy of the thenar muscles around the
base of the thumb, resulting in recurrent pain and eventual dysfunction of the hand.

Nursing and Interprofessional Management

Teach employees and employers about risk factors for CTS to
prevent its occurrence. Adaptive devices such as wrist splints may
be worn to relieve pressure on the median nerve. Special keyboard
pads and mice are available for computer users. Other ergonomic
changes include workstation modifications, change in body position, and frequent breaks from work-related activities.

Early symptoms of CTS can usually be relieved by stopping the
aggravating movement and by resting the hand and wrist by immo-
bilizing them in a hand splint. Splints worn at night help keep the
wrist in a neutral position and may reduce night pain and numbness. Injection of a corticosteroid drug directly into the carpal
tunnel may provide short-term relief.

If symptoms persist for more than 6 months, surgery is generally recommended, which involves severing the band of tissue around the wrist to reduce pressure on the median nerve. Surgery is done in an outpatient setting under local anesthesia. Endoscopic carpal tunnel release is performed through a small puncture incision(s) in the wrist and palm.

- After surgery, assess the neurovascular status of the hand regularly.
- Instruct the patient about wound care and the appropriate assessments to perform at home.

Although symptoms may be relieved immediately after surgery, full recovery may take months.

CATARACT

Description

A *cataract* is an opacity within the lens of one or both eyes, causing a gradual decline in vision. Cataract removal is the most common surgical procedure in the United States.

Pathophysiology

Although most cataracts are age-related (senile cataracts), they can be associated with other factors including trauma, congenital factors such as maternal rubella, radiation or ultraviolet (UV) light exposure, certain drugs such as systemic corticosteroids or long-term topical corticosteroids, and ocular inflammation. Patients with diabetes mellitus tend to develop cataracts at a younger age.

- In senile cataract formation, altered metabolic processes within the lens cause water accumulation and alterations in the lens fiber structure. These changes affect lens transparency, causing vision changes.

Clinical Manifestations

- Patients may complain of decreased vision, abnormal color perception, and glare.
- Visual decline is gradual, with the rate of cataract development varying from patient to patient.

Diagnostic Studies

- Lens opacity directly observable by ophthalmoscopic or slit lamp microscopic examination
- Visual acuity measurement
- Glare testing
- Keratometry and A-scan ultrasound if surgery is planned

Interprofessional Care

Currently no treatment is available to "cure" cataracts other than surgical removal.

- Helpful palliative measures include a change in eyeglass prescription, use of strong reading glasses or magnifiers, an increased amount of light for reading, and avoidance of nighttime driving if glare is worse at night.
- When palliative measures no longer provide an acceptable level of visual function, the patient is a candidate for surgery. Removal of the lens may also be medically necessary in patients with increased intraocular pressure and diabetic retinopathy, to allow visualization of the retina and adequate management.

Almost all patients have an intraocular lens (IOL) implanted at the time of cataract extraction surgery. Depending on the type of anesthesia, the patient's eye may be covered with a patch or protective shield, which is usually worn overnight and removed during the first postoperative visit. Most patients experience little visual impairment after surgery. IOL implants provide immediate visual rehabilitation, and many patients achieve a usable level of visual acuity within a few days after surgery.

Nursing Management

Goals

- Preoperatively, the patient will make an informed decision and experience minimal anxiety.
- Postoperatively, the patient will understand and comply with therapy, maintain an acceptable level of physical and emotional comfort, and remain free of infection and other complications.

Nursing Diagnoses

- Self-care deficits
- Anxiety

Nursing Interventions

For the patient who chooses not to have surgery, suggest vision enhancement techniques and a modification of activities and lifestyle to accommodate the visual deficit.

For the patient who elects surgery, provide information, support, and reassurance about the surgical and postoperative experience to reduce or alleviate anxiety. Postoperatively, offer mild analgesics for slight scratchiness or mild eye pain. The ophthalmologist needs to be notified if severe pain, increased or purulent drainage, increased redness, or decreased visual acuity is present.

TABLE 22 Patient & Caregiver Teaching
After Eye Surgery

Include the following information in the teaching plan for the patient and caregiver after eye surgery.

- Proper hygiene and eye care techniques to ensure that medications, dressings, and/or surgical wounds are not contaminated during eye care
- Signs and symptoms of infection and reporting these to allow for early recognition and treatment of possible infection
- Importance of complying with postoperative restrictions on head positioning, bending, coughing, and Valsalva maneuver to optimize visual outcomes and prevent increased intraocular pressure
- How to instill eye medications using aseptic techniques and adhere to prescribed eye medication routine to prevent infection
- How to monitor pain, take pain medication, and report pain not relieved by medication
- Importance of recommended follow-up to maximize visual outcomes

C

▼ Patient and Caregiver Teaching

- Written and verbal discharge teaching should include postoperative eye care, activity restrictions, medications, follow-up visit schedule, and signs of possible complications (Table 22).
- Include the patient's caregiver in your teaching. Some patients may have difficulty with self-care activities, especially if vision in the unoperated eye is poor. Provide an opportunity for the patient and caregiver to do return demonstrations of any self-care activities.
- Suggest ways of modifying activities and environment to maintain safe functioning. Suggestions may include getting assistance with stairs, removing area rugs and other obstacles, preparing meals for freezing before surgery, and obtaining audio books for diversion until visual acuity improves.

CELIAC DISEASE

Description

Celiac disease is an autoimmune disease characterized by damage to the small intestinal mucosa from the ingestion of wheat, barley, and rye in genetically susceptible individuals. It is a relatively common disease that occurs in all age groups with a wide variety of symptoms.

Celiac disease is not the same as the disease *tropical sprue,* a chronic disorder occurring primarily in tropical areas. Tropical sprue causes progressive disruption of jejunal and ileal tissue, resulting in malnutrition. It is treated with folic acid and tetracycline.

The incidence of celiac disease is thought to be about 1% of the U.S. population. High-risk groups include first- or second-degree relatives of someone with celiac disease and people with disorders associated with the disease, such as migraine and myocarditis. It is slightly more common in women, and symptoms often begin in childhood. Many people seek treatment for nonspecific complaints for years before celiac disease is diagnosed.

Pathophysiology

Three factors necessary for the development of celiac disease are a genetic predisposition, gluten ingestion, and an immune-mediated response.

- About 90% to 95% of patients with celiac disease have human leukocyte antigen (HLA) allele HLA-DQ2, and the other 5% to 10% have HLA-DQ8. However, not everyone with these genetic markers develops the disease.
- Tissue destruction that occurs with celiac disease is the result of chronic inflammation activated by the ingestion of gluten found in wheat, rye, and barley.
- Damage is most severe in the duodenum, probably because it is the site of the highest concentration of gluten. The inflammation lasts as long as gluten ingestion continues.

Clinical Manifestations

Classic manifestations of celiac disease include foul-smelling diarrhea, steatorrhea, flatulence, abdominal distention, and symptoms of malnutrition. Atypical signs and symptoms include decreased bone density and osteoporosis, dental enamel hypoplasia, iron and folate deficiencies, peripheral neuropathy, and reproductive problems.

- A pruritic, vesicular skin lesion called dermatitis herpetiformis may be present as a rash on the buttocks, scalp, face, elbows, and knees.
- Weight loss, muscle wasting, and other signs of malnutrition may be present. Patients may exhibit lactose intolerance.
- Iron-deficiency anemia is common.

- Celiac disease is associated with other autoimmune diseases, particularly rheumatoid arthritis, type 1 diabetes mellitus, and thyroid disease.

Diagnostic Studies

Celiac disease is confirmed by a combination of findings from the history and physical examination, serologic testing, and histologic analysis of small intestine biopsy specimens.

Nursing and Interprofessional Management

A gluten-free diet is the only effective treatment for celiac disease. Most patients recover completely within 3 to 6 months of treatment, but they need to maintain a gluten-free diet for life. If the condition is untreated, chronic inflammation and hyperplasia continue. Individuals with celiac disease have an increased risk for non-Hodgkin's lymphoma and gastrointestinal cancers.

- Dietary gluten comes from wheat, barley, rye, and oats (oats do not contain gluten but can become contaminated with gluten during milling). Gluten is also found in some medications, food additives, preservatives, and stabilizers.
- In patients with refractory celiac disease who do not respond to the gluten-free diet alone, corticosteroids may be used.

▼ **Patient and Caregiver Teaching**
- Refer all patients for a dietary consultation. Encourage patients to continue the gluten-free diet. Reinforce that continued gluten consumption will result in chronic inflammation, which can lead to complications such as anemia and osteoporosis.
- The Celiac Sprue Association website *(www.csaceliacs.info)* and the Celiac Disease Foundation *(www.celiac.org)* provide suggestions for maintaining a gluten-free diet and living with celiac disease.
- Many restaurants now indicate gluten-free menu options.

CERVICAL CANCER

Description

Cervical cancer was once the most frequent cause of cancer death in women. However, with early detection (using the Pap test), the mortality rate from cervical cancer has significantly declined. Approximately 12,900 women in the United States are diagnosed with cervical cancer and approximately 4100 die from the disease each year.

- Risk factors for cervical cancer include (1) infection with high-risk strains of human papillomavirus (HPV) 16 and 18,

(2) immunosuppression, (3) low socioeconomic status, (4) chlamydial infection, and (5) smoking.

Pathophysiology

The progression from normal cervical cells to dysplasia and on to cervical cancer occurs slowly over years. There is a strong relationship between sexual exposure to HPV and cervical dysplasia. A vaccine can protect against cervical cancer that is due to HPV types 16 and 18.

Clinical Manifestations

Early cervical cancer is generally asymptomatic, but leukorrhea and intermenstrual bleeding eventually occur.

- A vaginal discharge that is usually thin and watery becomes dark and foul-smelling as the disease advances.
- Vaginal bleeding is initially only spotting, but it becomes heavier and more frequent as the tumor enlarges.
- Pain is a late symptom and is followed by weight loss, anemia, and cachexia.

Diagnostic Studies

- Pap test, colposcopy, and biopsy

Interprofessional Care

Vaccination against HPV provides an opportunity for primary prevention of cervical cancer. Inform both parents and patients about the need to complete the HPV vaccination series before the first sexual contact.

Currently three vaccines are available to protect against HPV: (1) Gardasil protects against types 6, 11, 16, and 18; (2) Cervarix offers protection against HPV types 16 and 18; and (3) Gardasil 9 protects against HPV types 6, 11, 16, and 18 and five other HPV types. These vaccines are given in three IM doses over a 6-month period and have few side effects. The Centers for Disease Control and Prevention (CDC) recommends that all children, both male and female, be vaccinated at the age of 11 to 12 years. Vaccination can be started as early as age 9.

Treatment of cervical cancer is guided by the patient's age and general health and the stage of the tumor. Treatment options can include surgery or a combination of chemotherapy and irradiation.

- For patients with advanced disease, bevacizumab (Avastin), a targeted therapy drug, may be used in addition to cisplatin-based chemotherapy. Bevacizumab is an angiogenesis inhibitor and works by interfering with development of the blood vessels that fuel the development of cancer cells.

- Surgical procedures include hysterectomy, radical hysterectomy, and, rarely, pelvic exenteration (Table 23).

Nursing Management: Cervical Cancer and Other Cancers of the Female Reproductive System

In addition to cervical cancer, malignant tumors of the female reproductive system can be found in the endometrium, ovaries, vagina, and vulva. Management of the patient with any cancer of the female reproductive system includes many similar interventions.

Goals

The patient with a malignant tumor of the female reproductive system will actively participate in treatment decisions, achieve satisfactory pain and symptom management, recognize and report problems promptly, maintain preferred lifestyle as long as possible, and continue to practice cancer detection strategies.

Nursing Diagnoses

- Anxiety
- Acute pain
- Disturbed body image
- Ineffective sexuality patterns
- Grieving

Nursing Interventions

Teach women the importance of routine screening for cancers of the reproductive system. Cancer can be prevented when screening reveals precancerous conditions of the vulva, cervix, endometrium, and rarely the ovaries. Assist women to view routine cancer screening as an important self-care activity.

- Teaching women about risk factors for cancers of the reproductive system is important. Limiting sexual activity during adolescence, HPV vaccination against cervical cancer, using condoms, having fewer sexual partners, and not smoking reduce the risk of cervical cancer.

Hysterectomy. Preoperatively, the patient is prepared for surgery with the standard perineal or abdominal preparation. A vaginal douche and enema may be given according to surgeon preference. The bladder should be emptied before the patient is sent to the operating room. An indwelling catheter is often inserted.

- After a hysterectomy, abdominal distention may develop from the sudden release of pressure on the intestines when a large tumor is removed or from paralytic ileus secondary to anesthesia and pressure on the bowel. Food and fluids may be restricted

TABLE 23 Surgical Procedures Involving the Female Reproductive System

Type of Surgery	Description
Hysterectomy	
Total abdominal hysterectomy (TAH)	Uterus and cervix removed using abdominal incision (bikini cut)
Total abdominal hysterectomy and bilateral salpingo-oophorectomy (TAH-BSO)	Uterus, cervix, fallopian tubes, and ovaries removed using abdominal incision
Radical hysterectomy	Panhysterectomy, partial vaginectomy, and dissection of lymph nodes in pelvis
Vaginal hysterectomy	Uterus and cervix removed through a cut in the top of vagina
Laparoscopic hysterectomy	Laparoscope (video camera and small surgical instruments)
Laparoscopic-assisted vaginal hysterectomy (LAVH)	Incision made at top of vagina. Uterus and cervix removed through the vagina. Laparoscope inserted into abdomen to assist in the procedure.
Laparoscopic supracervical hysterectomy	Uterus removed using only laparoscopic instruments. Cervix is left intact.
Myomectomy	Surgical removal of fibroid from the uterus, leaving the uterus in place
Vulvectomy	Surgical procedure to remove part or all of the vulva
Skinning vulvectomy	Removal of top layer of vulvar skin where the cancer is found. Skin grafts from other parts of the body may be needed to cover the area.
Simple vulvectomy	Entire vulva is removed.
Radical vulvectomy	Entire vulva, including clitoris, labia majora and minora, and nearby tissue, is removed. Nearby lymph nodes may also be removed.
Vaginectomy	Removal of vagina
Pelvic exenteration	Radical hysterectomy, total vaginectomy, removal of bladder with diversion of urinary system and resection of colon and rectum with colostomy
Dilation and curettage	Dilation of cervix and scraping of endometrium

if the patient is nauseated. Ambulation will help relieve abdominal flatus.

- Take special care to prevent the development of deep vein thrombosis (DVT). Minimize stasis and pooling of blood with frequent changes of position, avoidance of the high Fowler's position, and avoidance of pressure under the knees. Pay special attention to patients with varicosities. Encourage leg exercises to promote circulation.

- Teach the patient what to expect after surgery (e.g., she will not menstruate). Instructions should include specific activity restrictions. Intercourse should be avoided until the wound is healed (about 4 to 6 weeks).

- If a vaginal hysterectomy is performed, inform the patient that she may have a temporary loss of vaginal sensation. Reassure her that the sensation will return in several months.

- Physical restrictions are limited for a short time. Heavy lifting should be avoided for 2 months. Teach the patient to avoid activities that may increase pelvic congestion, such as dancing and walking swiftly, for several months. However, activities such as swimming may be both physically and mentally helpful.

- See also eNursing Care Plan 53-1: Patient Having Abdominal Hysterectomy (on the website).

Salpingectomy and Oophorectomy. Postoperative care of the woman who has undergone removal of a fallopian tube (salpingectomy) or an ovary (oophorectomy) is similar to that for any patient having abdominal surgery. When both ovaries are removed (bilateral oophorectomy), surgical menopause results. Symptoms are similar to those of regular menopause but may be more severe because of the sudden withdrawal of hormones.

Pelvic Exenteration. When other forms of therapy are ineffective in controlling cancer spread and no metastases have been found outside the pelvis, pelvic exenteration may be performed. This radical surgery usually involves removal of the uterus, ovaries, fallopian tubes, vagina, bladder, urethra, and pelvic lymph nodes. In some situations the descending colon, rectum, and anal canal may also be removed. Postoperative care involves that of a patient who has had a radical hysterectomy, an abdominal perineal resection, and an ileostomy or colostomy. Physical, emotional, and social adjustments to life on the part of the woman and her family are great. Changes include urinary or fecal diversions in the abdominal wall, a reconstructed vagina, and the onset of menopausal symptoms.

- Much understanding and support are needed from the nursing staff during a long recovery period. Gently encourage the patient to regain independence.

CHLAMYDIAL INFECTIONS

Description

Chlamydia trachomatis infection is the most common sexually transmitted infection (STI) in the United States. *Chlamydia,* a gram-negative bacterium, is transmitted through exposure to sexual fluids during vaginal, anal, or oral sex. Numerous different strains of *C. trachomatis* cause urogenital infections (e.g., nongonococcal urethritis [NGU] in men and cervicitis in women), ocular trachoma, and lymphogranuloma venereum.

High-risk groups and risk factors include women and adolescents, new or multiple sexual partners, sexual partners who have had multiple partners, history of STIs and cervical ectopy, coexisting STIs, and inconsistent or incorrect use of a condom.

Clinical Manifestations

Symptoms may be absent or minor in most infected women and in many men.

- Men may experience pain with urination or a urethral discharge. Rarely, men can have pain or swelling of the testicles caused by infection of the epididymis.
- In women, manifestations of cervicitis include mucopurulent discharge (mucus with pus), bleeding, dysuria, and pain with intercourse.

Symptoms and signs of rectal chlamydial infection include rectal pain, discharge, and bleeding.

Complications

Complications often develop from poorly managed, inaccurately diagnosed, or undiagnosed chlamydial infections.

- In men, rare complications may result in epididymitis with possible infertility.
- In women, chlamydial infections may result in pelvic inflammatory disease, which damage fallopian tubes and increase the risk for an ectopic pregnancy (pregnancy outside of uterus), infertility, and chronic pelvic pain.

Diagnostic Studies

Chlamydial infections in men and women can be diagnosed by collecting urine or swab specimens from the endocervix or vagina (women), urethra (men), oropharynx, or rectum. The most common diagnostic test is the nucleic acid amplification test (NAAT).

Interprofessional Care

Because of the high prevalence of asymptomatic infections, regular screening for *Chlamydia* in high-risk populations is recommended.

Doxycycline (Vibramycin) or azithromycin (Zithromax) is used to treat patients and their partners. Treatment of pregnant women usually prevents transmission to the fetus.

- Patients treated for chlamydial infections should abstain from sexual intercourse for 7 days after treatment and until all sexual partners have completed a full course of treatment.
- Follow-up care includes advising the patient to return if symptoms persist or recur, treating sexual partners, and encouraging condom use during all sexual contacts.

Nursing Management

See Nursing Management: Sexually Transmitted Infections, pp. 564-565.

CHOLELITHIASIS/CHOLECYSTITIS

Description

The most common disorder of the biliary system is *cholelithiasis* (stones in the gallbladder). The stones may become lodged in the neck of the gallbladder or in the cystic duct. *Cholecystitis* (inflammation of the gallbladder) may be acute or chronic, and it is usually associated with cholelithiasis.

Gallbladder disease is a common health problem in the United States. Up to 10% of American adults have cholelithiasis.

- The incidence of cholelithiasis is higher in women, especially multiparous women and those older than 40 years of age. Postmenopausal women on estrogen replacement therapy and younger women on oral contraceptives are at an increased risk. Other factors that seem to increase the incidence of gallbladder disease are sedentary lifestyle, familial tendency, and obesity.
- The incidence of gallbladder disease is especially high in Native Americans, especially the Navajo and Pima tribes.

Pathophysiology

The cause of gallstones is unknown. Cholelithiasis develops when the balance that keeps cholesterol, bile salts, and calcium in solution is altered so that these substances precipitate. Conditions that upset this balance include infection and disturbances in the metabolism of cholesterol. Mixed cholesterol stones, which are predominantly cholesterol, are the most common gallstones.

The stones may remain in the gallbladder or migrate to the cystic duct or common bile duct. They cause pain as they pass through the ducts and may lodge in the ducts and cause obstruction. Stasis of bile in the gallbladder can lead to cholecystitis.

Cholecystitis is most commonly associated with obstruction resulting from gallstones or biliary sludge. Cholecystitis in the absence of obstruction occurs most frequently in older adults and patients who are critically ill. Bacteria reaching the gallbladder by the vascular or lymphatic route or chemical irritants in the bile can also produce cholecystitis. *Escherichia coli,* streptococci, and salmonellae are common causative bacteria. Other etiologic factors include adhesions, neoplasms, anesthesia, and opioids.

- During an acute attack of cholecystitis, the gallbladder is edematous and hyperemic and it may be distended with bile or pus. The cystic duct is also involved and may become occluded.
- The wall of the gallbladder becomes scarred after an acute attack. Decreased functioning occurs if large amounts of tissue are fibrosed.

Clinical Manifestations

Cholelithiasis may produce severe symptoms or none at all. Many patients have "silent cholelithiasis." Severity of symptoms depends on whether the stones are stationary or mobile and whether obstruction is present.

- When a stone is lodged in the ducts or when stones are moving through the ducts, spasms may result. This sometimes produces severe pain, which is termed *biliary colic*. The pain can be accompanied by tachycardia, diaphoresis, and prostration. The severe pain may last up to 1 hour, and when it subsides there is residual tenderness in the right upper quadrant.
- The attacks of pain frequently occur 3 to 6 hours after a high-fat meal or when the patient lies down.
- When total obstruction occurs, symptoms related to bile blockage are manifested. These include steatorrhea, pruritus, dark amber urine, bleeding tendencies, and jaundice.

Manifestations of cholecystitis vary from indigestion to moderate to severe pain, fever, and jaundice. Initial symptoms include indigestion and pain and tenderness in the right upper quadrant, which may be referred to the right shoulder and scapula. Pain may be acute and is accompanied by restlessness, diaphoresis, and nausea and vomiting.

- Symptoms of chronic cholecystitis include a history of fat intolerance, dyspepsia, heartburn, and flatulence.

Complications

Complications of cholecystitis include gangrenous cholecystitis, subphrenic abscess, pancreatitis, *cholangitis* (inflammation of biliary ducts), biliary cirrhosis, fistulas, and rupture of the gallbladder, which can produce bile peritonitis.

Diagnostic Studies

- Ultrasonography is used to diagnose gallstones.
- Endoscopic retrograde cholangiopancreatography (ERCP) allows for visualization of the gallbladder, cystic duct, common hepatic duct, and common bile duct. Bile taken during ERCP is sent for culture to identify any possible infecting organism.
- Percutaneous transhepatic cholangiography may be used to locate stones within the bile ducts.
- Laboratory tests reveal elevated serum enzymes and pancreatic enzymes, increased white blood cell (WBC) count, elevated direct and indirect bilirubin levels, and urinary bilirubin.

Interprofessional Care

The treatment of gallstones in cholelithiasis depends on the stage of disease. Bile acids (cholesterol solvents) such as ursodeoxycholic (ursodiol) and chenodeoxycholic (chenodiol) are used to dissolve stones. ERCP with sphincterotomy (papillotomy) may be used for stone removal. ERCP allows for visualization of the biliary system and placement of stents and sphincterotomy (if warranted).

Extracorporeal shock-wave lithotripsy (ESWL) may be used to treat cholelithiasis. In this procedure, a lithotriptor uses high-energy shock waves to disintegrate gallstones.

Drug therapy for gallbladder disease includes analgesics, anticholinergics (antispasmodics), fat-soluble vitamins, and bile salts. Morphine may be used initially for pain management. Cholestyramine, used to provide relief from pruritus, is a resin that binds bile salts in the intestine, increasing their excretion in the feces.

During an acute episode of cholecystitis, treatment focuses on pain control, control of possible infection with antibiotics, and maintenance of fluid and electrolyte balance. Treatment is mainly supportive and symptomatic. A cholecystostomy may be used to drain purulent material from the obstructed gallbladder.

- If nausea and vomiting are severe, nasogastric (NG) tube insertion and gastric decompression may be used to prevent further gallbladder stimulation.
- Anticholinergics may be administered to decrease secretions and counteract smooth muscle spasms.

Laparoscopic cholecystectomy is the preferred surgical procedure for symptomatic cholelithiasis. In this procedure, the gallbladder is removed through one of four small punctures in the abdomen. Most patients experience minimal postoperative pain and are discharged the day of surgery or the day after. In most cases they are able to resume normal activities and return to work within 1 week.

Nursing Management

Goals

The patient with gallbladder disease will have relief of pain and discomfort, no postoperative complications, and no recurrent attacks of cholecystitis or cholelithiasis.

Nursing Diagnoses

- Acute pain
- Ineffective health management

Nursing Interventions

Nursing goals for the patient undergoing conservative therapy include relieving pain, relieving nausea and vomiting, providing comfort and emotional support, maintaining fluid and electrolyte balance and nutrition, making accurate assessments to ensure effective treatment, and observing for complications.

The patient with acute cholecystitis or cholelithiasis is frequently experiencing severe pain. Medications ordered to relieve pain should be given as required before it becomes more severe. Assess what drugs relieve the pain and how much medication is required. Observe for signs of obstruction of the ducts by stones, including jaundice; clay-colored stools; dark, foamy urine; steatorrhea; fever; and increased white blood cell (WBC) count.

Postoperative nursing care after a laparoscopic cholecystectomy includes monitoring for complications such as bleeding, making the patient comfortable, and preparing the patient for discharge.

- A common postoperative problem is referred pain to the shoulder because of the CO_2 that was not released or absorbed by the body. CO_2 can irritate the phrenic nerve and diaphragm, causing some difficulty breathing. Placing the patient in Sims' position (left side with right knee flexed) helps move the gas pocket away from the diaphragm. Encourage deep breathing, movement, and ambulation.
- If the patient has a T tube, maintain bile drainage and observe for T tube functioning and drainage.

▼ Patient and Caregiver Teaching

- For the patient under conservative management, teach about a diet of smaller, more frequent meals with some fat at each meal to promote gallbladder emptying. If obesity is a problem, a reduced-calorie diet is indicated. The diet should be low in

TABLE 24 Patient & Caregiver Teaching

Postoperative Laparoscopic Cholecystectomy

Include the following instructions in the patient's postoperative teaching plan.

- Remove the bandages on the puncture site the day after surgery, and you can shower.
- Notify your surgeon if any of the following signs and symptoms occurs:
  - Redness, swelling, bile-colored drainage or pus from any incision
  - Severe abdominal pain, nausea, vomiting, fever, chills
- You can gradually resume normal activities.
- Return to work within 1 week of surgery.
- You can resume your usual diet, but a low-fat diet is usually better tolerated for several weeks after surgery.

saturated fats and high in fiber and calcium. The patient may need fat-soluble vitamin supplements.

- Instruct the patient on indications of biliary obstruction (stool and urine changes, jaundice, and pruritus).
- The patient who undergoes a laparoscopic cholecystectomy is discharged soon after the surgery, so home care and teaching are important (Table 24).

CHRONIC OBSTRUCTIVE PULMONARY DISEASE

Description

Chronic obstructive pulmonary disease (COPD) is a disease state characterized by persistent airflow limitation that is usually progressive. COPD is associated with an enhanced inflammatory response in the airways and lungs, primarily caused by cigarette smoking and other noxious particles or gases. Previous definitions of COPD encompassed two types of obstructive airway disease, emphysema and chronic bronchitis, but neither term is part of the current definition of COPD.

- *Emphysema* is the destruction of the alveoli and is a pathologic term that explains only one of several structural abnormalities in COPD.
- *Chronic bronchitis,* the presence of cough and sputum production for at least 3 months in each of 2 consecutive years, is an

independent disease that may precede or follow the development of airflow limitation.

- Patients with COPD may have a predominance of one of these conditions, but the conditions usually coexist, and COPD is considered one disease state in terms of pathophysiology and management.
- Patients with COPD may have asthma. Asthma may be a risk factor for the development of COPD. There is a considerable pathologic and functional overlap between these disorders, particularly among older adults, who may have components of both diseases. Recently this disorder has been called *asthma-COPD overlap syndrome*.

More than 12.7 million people have COPD in the United States, where it is the third leading cause of death.

Etiology

Cigarette smoking is the major risk factor for developing COPD. It affects about 15% of smokers.

- The irritating effect of cigarette smoke causes hyperplasia of cells, which subsequently results in increased mucus production. Hyperplasia reduces airway diameter and increases the difficulty in clearing secretions. Smoking reduces ciliary activity and produces abnormal dilation of the distal air space with destruction of alveolar walls.
- If a person has intense or prolonged exposure to various dusts, vapors, irritants, or fumes in the workplace, symptoms of lung impairment consistent with COPD can develop. If a person has occupational exposure and smokes, the risk of COPD increases.
- High levels of urban air pollution are harmful to people with existing lung disease. However, the effect of outdoor air pollution as a risk factor for the development of COPD is unclear.
- Passive smoking is the exposure of nonsmokers to cigarette smoke, also known as environmental tobacco smoke (ETS) or secondhand smoke.
- Severe recurring respiratory tract infections in childhood have been associated with reduced lung function and increased respiratory symptoms in adulthood. It is unclear whether the development of COPD can be related to recurrent infections in adults.
- Asthma may be a risk factor for COPD development.
- Genetic factors influence which smokers get the disease. α_1-*Antitrypsin (AAT) deficiency* is a genetic risk factor for COPD. The main function of AAT, an α_1-protease inhibitor, is to protect normal lung tissue from attack by proteases during inflammation related to cigarette smoking and infections.

Pathophysiology

COPD is characterized by chronic inflammation of the airways, lung parenchyma (respiratory bronchioles and alveoli), and pulmonary blood vessels. The pathogenesis of COPD is complex and involves many mechanisms. The defining features of COPD are irreversible airflow limitation during forced exhalation caused by loss of elastic recoil and airflow obstruction caused by mucus hypersecretion, mucosal edema, and bronchospasm.

The inflammatory process starts with inhalation of noxious particles (e.g., cigarette smoke) that causes the release of inflammatory mediators that damage lung tissue. This process causes tissue destruction and disrupts the normal defense mechanisms and repair process of the lung.

- The predominant inflammatory cells are neutrophils, macrophages, and lymphocytes. These cells attract other inflammatory mediators (e.g., leukotrienes) and proinflammatory cytokines (e.g., tumor necrosis factor). The end result of the inflammatory process is structural changes in the lungs.
- After the inhalation of oxidants in tobacco or air pollution, protease activity (which breaks down the connective tissue of the lungs) increases and antiproteases (which protect against the breakdown) are inhibited.
- Inability to expire air is the main characteristic of COPD. As the peripheral airways become obstructed, air is progressively trapped during expiration. The chest hyperexpands and becomes barrel shaped since the respiratory muscles are not able to function effectively.
- Gas exchange abnormalities result in hypoxemia and hypercapnia (increased CO_2). As air trapping increases and alveoli are destroyed, bullae (large air spaces in the parenchyma) and blebs (air spaces adjacent to pleurae) can form. There is a significant ventilation-perfusion (V/Q) mismatch, and hypoxemia results.
- Excess mucus production, resulting in a chronic productive cough, is due to an increased number of mucus-secreting goblet cells, enlarged submucosal glands, dysfunction of cilia, and stimulation from inflammatory mediators.
- Pulmonary vascular changes resulting in mild to moderate pulmonary hypertension may occur late in the course of COPD.

Cardiovascular diseases commonly occur along with COPD, because smoking is a primary risk factor for both.

Clinical Manifestations

COPD typically develops slowly, but COPD should be considered in a patient with chronic cough or sputum production, dyspnea, and a history of exposure to risk factors for the disease (e.g., tobacco smoke, occupational dusts and chemicals).

- A diagnosis of COPD should be considered for a patient who has symptoms of cough, sputum production, or dyspnea, and/or a history of exposure to risk factors for the disease.
- A chronic intermittent cough, often the first symptom to develop, may later be present every day.
- Dyspnea with exertion is often progressive. In the late stages of COPD, dyspnea may be present at rest. Wheezing and chest tightness may vary by time of the day or from day to day, especially in patients with more severe disease.
- The patient with advanced COPD experiences weight loss, even with adequate caloric intake. Fatigue is a prevalent symptom that affects activities of daily living.
- During physical examination, a prolonged expiratory phase of respiration, wheezes, or decreased breath sounds are noted in all lung fields. The anterior-posterior diameter of the chest is increased *(barrel chest)* from chronic air trapping. The patient may assume a tripod position and use pursed-lip breathing.
- Over time, hypoxemia may develop with hypercapnia. The bluish-red color of the skin results from polycythemia and cyanosis. Polycythemia develops as a result of increased production of red blood cells as the body attempts to compensate for chronic hypoxemia.

Complications

Cor pulmonale results from pulmonary hypertension. In COPD, pulmonary hypertension is caused primarily by constriction of pulmonary vessels in response to alveolar hypoxia, with acidosis further potentiating vasoconstriction. Chronic hypoxia also stimulates erythropoiesis, which causes polycythemia. This results in increased viscosity of the blood. When pulmonary hypertension develops, the pressure on the right side of the heart must increase to push blood into the lungs. Eventually right-sided heart failure develops (see Cor Pulmonale, p. 152).

A *COPD exacerbation* is an acute event characterized by a worsening of the patient's usual patterns of dyspnea, cough, and/or sputum production. The primary cause of exacerbation is bacterial or viral infection. Exacerbations are typical and increase in frequency (averaging one or two a year) as the disease progresses.

- Teach the patient and caregiver early recognition of the three cardinal symptoms of exacerbations (increase in dyspnea, sputum volume, or sputum purulence) to promote early treatment and thus prevent hospitalization and possible respiratory failure.

- Other complaints include malaise, insomnia, increased wheezing, fatigue, depression, confusion, and decreased exercise tolerance. Exacerbations are managed with short-acting bronchodilators, oral systemic corticosteroids, and antibiotics.

Acute respiratory failure may occur in patients with severe COPD who have exacerbations. Be alert for signs of increasing severity such as use of accessory muscles, central cyanosis, edema in the lower extremities, unstable BP, right-sided heart failure, and altered alertness. Frequently, patients with COPD wait too long to contact an HCP after first experiencing symptoms suggesting an exacerbation. Discontinuing bronchodilator or corticosteroid medication may also precipitate respiratory failure. (Respiratory failure is discussed in Chapter 67, Lewis et al, *Medical-Surgical Nursing,* ed 10, pp. 1609 to 1620.)

Diagnostic Studies

- A forced expiratory volume in 1 minute/forced vital capacity ratio (FEV_1/FVC) less than 70% along with the appropriate symptoms can help to diagnose COPD. A lower value of FEV_1 indicates more severe COPD.
- A history and physical examination are extremely important in the diagnostic workup.
- Chest x-rays are not diagnostic but may show a flat diaphragm due to hyperinflation of lungs.
- ECG can be used to determine right- and left-sided ventricular failure.
- Sputum culture and sensitivity are done if an acute exacerbation is present.
- Arterial blood gases (ABGs) in later stages usually indicate low PaO_2, elevated $PaCO_2$, decreased or low normal pH, and increased bicarbonate (HCO_3^-) levels.

Interprofessional Care

Most patients with COPD are treated as outpatients. They are hospitalized for complications such as acute exacerbations and acute respiratory failure.

Evaluate the patient's exposure to environmental or occupational irritants, and determine ways to control or avoid them. The patient with COPD and anyone who smokes should receive an influenza immunization yearly. The pneumococcal vaccine (see Table 27-5, Lewis et al, *Medical-Surgical Nursing,* ed 10, p. 504) is recommended for smokers 19 years of age or older and patients with COPD.

- Exacerbations of COPD should be treated as soon as possible, especially if the patient is in the severe stages.

- Cessation of cigarette smoking is the intervention that can have the biggest impact on reducing the risk of developing COPD, and on decreasing progression of the disease in any stage of COPD. Smoking cessation techniques are discussed in Lewis et al, *Medical-Surgical Nursing,* ed 10, pp. 146 to 148, 149, and 150, and in Tables 10-4 to 10-6, pp. 147, 149, and 150.

Medications for COPD can reduce symptoms, increase exercise capacity, improve overall health, and reduce the number and severity of exacerbations.

- Bronchodilator medications commonly used are β_2-adrenergic agonists, anticholinergic agents, and methylxanthines (see Table 28-8, Lewis et al, *Medical-Surgical Nursing,* ed 10, pp. 548 to 549). When the patient has mild COPD or intermittent symptoms, a short-acting bronchodilator is used as needed. In the moderate stage of COPD, a long-acting bronchodilator also is used.
- In patients with COPD associated with an FEV_1 less than 60%, regular treatment with inhaled corticosteroids (ICSs) is often prescribed, in addition to a long-acting β-agonist (LABA). Examples of combinations of ICSs with LABAs are fluticasone/salmeterol (Advair) and budesonide/formoterol (Symbicort).
- Roflumilast (Daliresp) is an oral medication used to decrease the frequency of exacerbations in patients with severe COPD and chronic bronchitis. This drug is a phosphodiesterase inhibitor, which is an antiinflammatory agent that suppresses the release of cytokines and other inflammatory mediators and inhibits the production of reactive oxygen radicals.

Long-term continuous (more than 15 hr/day) O_2 therapy (LTOT) increases survival and improves exercise capacity and mental status in hypoxemic patients with COPD (see Oxygen Therapy, p. 718).

The main types of breathing exercises commonly taught are pursed-lip breathing and diaphragmatic breathing. However, patients with moderate to severe COPD with marked hyperinflation may be poor candidates for diaphragmatic breathing.

Airway clearance techniques loosen mucus and secretions for clearance by coughing. A variety of treatments can be used to achieve airway clearance. Respiratory therapists, physical therapists, and nurses are involved in performing these techniques. See Lewis et al, *Medical-Surgical Nursing,* ed 10, pp. 569 to 570, for further information on airway clearance techniques.

- Weight loss and muscle wasting are common in the patient with severe COPD. To decrease dyspnea and conserve energy, the patient should rest at least 30 minutes before eating and use a bronchodilator before meals. A diet high in calories and protein, moderate in carbohydrates, and moderate to high in fat is recommended and can be divided into five or six small meals a day.

Surgical Therapy

Four different surgical procedures have been used in severe COPD. One type of surgery is *lung volume reduction surgery,* which is done to reduce the size of the lungs by removing the most diseased lung tissue so that the remaining healthy lung tissue can perform better. A second procedure, *bronchoscopic lung volume reduction surgery*, involves placing one-way valves in the airways. The valves let air out of diseased parts of the lung, but not in. Another surgical procedure is a *bullectomy*, which is used for patients with emphysematous COPD who have large bullae (>1 cm). The bullae are usually resected via thoracoscope. A fourth surgical procedure is *lung transplantation,* which benefits carefully selected patients with advanced COPD.

Nursing Management

Goals

The overall goals are that the patient with COPD will have prevention of disease progression, ability to perform activities of daily living (ADLs) and improved exercise tolerance, relief from symptoms, no complications related to COPD, knowledge and ability to implement a long-term treatment regimen, and overall improved quality of life.

See eNursing Care Plan 28-2 (available on the website) for specific goals related to the nursing diagnoses for the patient with COPD.

Nursing Diagnoses

- Ineffective airway clearance
- Ineffective breathing pattern
- Impaired gas exchange

Nursing Interventions

Counseling the patient regarding smoking cessation is vital, because it is the only way to slow the progression of COPD. Avoiding or controlling exposure to occupational and environmental pollutants and irritants is another preventive measure to maintain healthy lungs. Early diagnosis and treatment of respiratory tract infections and exacerbations of COPD help prevent progression of the disease.

- Patients with COPD should avoid people who are sick, practice good hand-washing techniques, take medications as prescribed, exercise regularly, and maintain a healthy weight. Influenza and pneumococcal vaccines are recommended for patients with COPD.

- The patient with COPD requires acute intervention for complications such as exacerbations of COPD, pneumonia, cor pulmonale, and acute respiratory failure.

▼ **Patient and Caregiver Teaching**

The most important aspect of long-term care of the patient with COPD is teaching (Table 25). In pulmonary rehabilitation (PR), an interprofessional team works to individualize the treatment plan for the patient with COPD.

- Components of PR vary but usually include exercise training, smoking cessation, nutrition counseling, and teaching.

TABLE 25 Patient & Caregiver Teaching

Chronic Obstructive Pulmonary Disease (COPD)

Include the following information in the teaching plan to assist the patient with COPD and the caregiver to improve quality of life through teaching and promotion of lifestyle practices that support successful living with COPD.

What Is COPD?
- Basic anatomy and physiology of lung
- Basic pathophysiology of COPD
- Signs and symptoms of COPD, exacerbation, cold, flu, pneumonia
- Tests to assess breathing

Breathing and Airway Clearance Exercises
- Pursed-lip breathing (see Table 28-13, Lewis et al, *Medical-Surgical Nursing,* ed 10, p. 554)
- Airway clearance technique—huff cough (see Table 28-23, Lewis et al, *Medical-Surgical Nursing,* ed 10, p. 569)

Energy Conservation Techniques
- Daily activities (e.g., bathing, grooming, shopping, traveling)
- Consultation with physical therapist and occupational therapist

Medications
Types (include mechanism of action and types of devices)
- Methylxanthines
- β_2-Adrenergic agonists
- Corticosteroids
- Anticholinergics
- Antibiotics
- Other medications
Establishing medication schedule

TABLE 25　Patient & Caregiver Teaching
Chronic Obstructive Pulmonary Disease (COPD)—cont'd

Correct Use of Inhalers, Spacer, and Nebulizer
- Demonstration–return demonstration with placebo devices (see Figs. 28-5 to 28-7 and Tables 28-9 to 28-11 in Lewis et al, *Medical-Surgical Nursing*, ed 10, pp. 547 to 552)

Home Oxygen
- Explanation of rationale for use
- Guide for home O_2 use and equipment

Psychosocial/Emotional Issues
Open discussion (sharing with patient, caregiver, and family)
- Concerns about interpersonal relationships (e.g., intimacy)
- Problems with emotions (e.g., depression, anxiety, panic)
- Dependency
Treatment decisions
- Support and rehabilitation groups
End-of-life issues

COPD Management Plan
Nurse and patient develop and write up COPD management plan that meets individual needs.
- Focus on self-management
- Need to report changes
- Cause of flare-ups or exacerbation
- Recognition of signs and symptoms of respiratory infection, heart failure
- Reduce risk factors, especially smoking cessation
- Exercise program of walking and arm strengthening
- Yearly follow-up evaluations

Healthy Nutrition (see Table 28-24 in Lewis et al, *Medical-Surgical Nursing*, ed 10, p. 571)
- Strategies to lose or gain weight, as appropriate
- Consultation with dietitian
For additional information, see American Lung Association at *www.lung.org/lung-disease/copd*.

- Other important topics include health promotion, psychologic counseling, and vocational rehabilitation. Smoking cessation is critical.

  Energy conservation is an important component in COPD rehabilitation. Exercise training of the upper extremities may improve muscle function and reduce dyspnea. Alternative energy-saving practices for ADLs and scheduled rest periods should be planned.

- Walking or other endurance exercises (e.g., cycling) combined with strength training are the best interventions to strengthen muscles and improve the patient's endurance. Teach the patient coordinated walking with slow, pursed-lip breathing. Encourage the patient to walk 15 to 20 minutes/day at least three times a week, with gradual increases.
- Modifying but not abstaining from sexual activity can also contribute to a healthy psychologic well-being. Using an inhaled bronchodilator before sexual activity can help ventilation.
- Adequate sleep is extremely important. The patient who is a restless sleeper, snores, stops breathing while asleep, and has a tendency to fall asleep during the day may need to be tested for sleep apnea.
- Healthy coping is a challenge for the patient and family. People with COPD frequently have to deal with many lifestyle changes that may involve decreased ability to care for themselves, decreased energy for social activities, and loss of a job. Support groups at local chapters of the American Lung Association, hospitals, and clinics may be helpful.

CIRRHOSIS

Description

Cirrhosis, the end stage of liver disease, is characterized by the extensive degeneration and destruction of liver cells. It is the eighth leading cause of death in the United States and is twice as common in men as in women. The most common causes of cirrhosis are chronic hepatitis C infection and alcohol-induced liver disease. Malnutrition, biliary obstruction, right-sided heart failure, and chronic liver diseases such as nonalcoholic fatty liver disease (NAFLD) also cause cirrhosis. NAFLD can be a complication of metabolic syndrome (see Metabolic Syndrome, p. 414).

Pathophysiology

Damaged liver cells attempt to regenerate, but a disorganized regenerative process results in abnormal blood vessel and bile duct architecture. The overgrowth of new and fibrous connective tissue distorts the liver's normal lobular structure, resulting in lobules of irregular size and shape with impeded blood flow and poor function.

Biliary causes of cirrhosis include primary biliary cirrhosis and primary sclerosing cholangitis. *Primary sclerosing cholangitis* is a chronic inflammatory condition affecting the liver and bile ducts. The etiology of primary sclerosing cholangitis is unknown. However, it is strongly associated with ulcerative colitis. The chronic inflammation can ultimately progress to cirrhosis and end-stage liver disease.

Clinical Manifestations

The onset of cirrhosis is usually insidious. Early symptoms may include fatigue or an enlarged liver. Later manifestations may be severe and result from liver failure and portal hypertension. Jaundice, peripheral edema, and ascites develop gradually. Other late signs and symptoms include skin lesions, hematologic disorders, endocrine disturbances, and peripheral neuropathies. In advanced stages, the liver becomes small and nodular. (See Fig. 3 for systemic clinical manifestations of cirrhosis.)

- *Jaundice* occurs as a result of the decreased ability of the liver to conjugate and excrete bilirubin.
- *Skin lesions* such as *spider angiomas* that occur on the nose, cheeks, upper trunk, and neck and a redness of the palms of the hands, known as *palmar erythema,* result from an increase in circulating estrogen because the liver cannot metabolize steroid hormones.
- *Hematologic disorders* such as anemia, leukopenia, and thrombocytopenia are thought to be caused by splenomegaly that results from backup of blood from the portal vein into the spleen (portal hypertension). Coagulation problems result from the liver's inability to produce prothrombin and other essential clotting factors.
- *Endocrine problems* result because adrenocortical hormones, estrogen, and testosterone cannot be metabolized by a damaged liver. Men lose masculine sex characteristics as a result of increased estrogen levels, and amenorrhea may occur in younger women. Sodium and water retention and potassium loss occur as a result of hyperaldosteronism.
- *Peripheral neuropathy* is probably caused by a dietary deficiency of thiamine, folic acid, and cobalamin.

Complications

Major complications of cirrhosis are portal hypertension with resultant esophageal and/or gastric varices, peripheral edema,

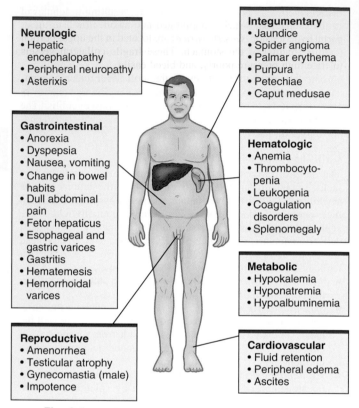

Fig. 3 Systemic clinical manifestations of liver cirrhosis.

abdominal ascites, hepatic encephalopathy (coma), and hepatorenal syndrome.

Portal hypertension, an increased pressure within the liver's circulatory system, and *esophageal* and *gastric varices* result when structural liver changes from cirrhosis obstruct blood flow in and out of the liver.

- Collateral channels commonly form in the lower esophagus, anterior abdominal wall, parietal peritoneum, and rectum.
- Varicosities may develop in areas where collateral and systemic circulations communicate, resulting in esophageal and gastric varices, *caput medusae* (ring of varices around the umbilicus), and hemorrhoids.

Esophageal varices are a complex of tortuous veins at the end of the esophagus, which are enlarged and swollen as a result of portal hypertension. *Gastric varices* are located in the upper portion (cardia, fundus) of the stomach. These fragile collateral vessels tolerate high pressure poorly, and bleed easily.

- Bleeding esophageal varices are the most life-threatening complication of cirrhosis. Patients may have melena or hematemesis. There may be slow oozing or massive bleeding, which is a medical emergency.

Peripheral edema results from decreased colloidal osmotic pressure from impaired liver synthesis of albumin and increased portacaval pressure from portal hypertension. Peripheral edema occurs in the lower extremities and presacral area.

Ascites is the accumulation of serous fluid in the peritoneal or abdominal cavity by three mechanisms. The first mechanism is portal hypertension which causes proteins to move from the blood vessels into the lymph space and then leak into the peritoneal cavity. A second mechanism is fluid shifting due to hypoalbuminemia and decreased colloidal oncotic pressure, which results from the liver's inability to synthesize albumin. A third mechanism is hyperaldosteronism, which results when aldosterone is not metabolized by damaged hepatocytes, causing increased renal reabsorption of sodium and water.

- Ascites is manifested by abdominal distention with weight gain. In severe ascites, the umbilicus may be everted. Abdominal striae with distended abdominal wall veins may be present.
- Patients may have signs of dehydration (e.g., dry tongue and skin, sunken eyeballs, muscle weakness) and decreased urinary output.
- Hypokalemia is common and is caused by an excessive loss of potassium from hyperaldosteronism and the use of diuretic therapy to treat ascites.

Hepatic encephalopathy is a neuropsychiatric manifestation of liver disease. When blood is shunted past the liver by way of collateral vessels or the liver is unable to convert ammonia to urea, the levels of ammonia in the systemic circulation rise. Ammonia crosses the blood-brain barrier and produces toxic neurologic manifestations.

- Factors that increase ammonia in the circulation include GI hemorrhage, constipation, infection, hypokalemia, hypovolemia, dehydration, and metabolic alkalosis.
- Hepatic encephalopathy is manifested by changes in neurologic and mental responsiveness, ranging from sleep disturbance to trouble concentrating to deep coma. A characteristic symptom is *asterixis* (flapping tremors), a rapid flexion and extension

movement of the hands when the arms and hands are held stretched out.

Hepatorenal syndrome is a type of renal failure with advancing azotemia, oliguria, and intractable ascites.

- There is no structural abnormality of the kidneys. The etiology is complex, but the final common pathway is usually portal hypertension along with liver decompensation that results in splanchnic and systemic vasodilation and decreased arterial blood volume. As a result, renal vasoconstriction occurs and renal failure follows.
- In the patient with cirrhosis, this syndrome frequently follows diuretic therapy, GI hemorrhage, or paracentesis.

Diagnostic Studies

- Liver function studies demonstrate an elevation in alkaline phosphatase, aspartate aminotransferase (AST), alanine aminotransferase (ALT), and γ-glutamyl transferase (GGT).
- Prothrombin time is prolonged.
- Serum albumin and protein levels are decreased and bilirubin and globulin levels are increased.
- Liver ultrasound and biopsy (percutaneous needle) can help determine severity of cirrhosis.
- Differential analysis of ascitic fluid may help to confirm the cause.

Interprofessional Care

The goal of treatment is to slow the progression of cirrhosis and prevent and treat any complications. Management of ascites focuses on sodium restriction (250 to 500 mg/day for severe ascites), diuretic therapy (e.g., a potassium-sparing diuretic combined with a loop diuretic), and fluid removal (paracentesis) for those patients with impaired respiration or abdominal pain. Transjugular intrahepatic portosystemic shunt (TIPS) is also used to alleviate ascites.

The main therapeutic goal related to esophageal varices is to prevent bleeding and hemorrhage. The patient who has esophageal varices should avoid ingesting alcohol, aspirin, and NSAIDs. Patients with varices at risk of bleeding are generally started on a nonselective β-adrenergic blocker (nadolol [Corgard] or propranolol [Inderal]) to decrease high portal pressure and reduce the incidence of hemorrhage.

- When variceal bleeding occurs, the first step is to stabilize the patient and manage the airway. IV therapy is initiated and may include administration of blood products. Management that involves a combination of drug therapy and endoscopic therapy is more successful than either approach alone. Drug therapy may include somatostatin analog octreotide (Sandostatin) or vasopressin (VP).

- At the time of endoscopy, band ligation or sclerotherapy may be used to prevent varices from rebleeding. Balloon tamponade may be used to control hemorrhage that cannot be controlled on initial endoscopy.

- Supportive measures during an acute variceal bleed include administration of fresh frozen plasma and packed red blood cells (RBCs), vitamin K, and proton pump inhibitors (e.g., pantoprazole [Protonix]). Lactulose and rifaximin (Xifaxan) may be administered to prevent hepatic encephalopathy from breakdown of blood and the release of ammonia in the intestine. Antibiotics are given to prevent bacterial infection.

- Nonsurgical (e.g., TIPS) and surgical methods of shunting blood away from the varices are available. Shunting procedures tend to be used more after a second major bleeding episode than during an initial bleeding episode.

The goal of management in hepatic encephalopathy is the reduction of ammonia formation. Lactulose discourages bacterial growth, traps ammonia in the gut, and expels ammonia from the colon. Antibiotics such as rifaximin may also be given, particularly in patients who do not respond to lactulose. Constipation should be prevented. Control of hepatic encephalopathy also involves treating GI bleeding and removing blood from the GI tract to decrease protein in the intestine.

A number of medications may be used to treat symptoms and complications of advanced liver disease (see Table 43-14, Lewis et al, *Medical-Surgical Nursing,* ed 10, p. 993). Specific nutritional therapy varies with the degree of liver damage and the danger of encephalopathy; generally, the diet is high in calories (3000 cal/day) and carbohydrates with sodium restricted. Protein restriction is rarely justified in patients with cirrhosis and persistent hepatic encephalopathy. Malnutrition is a more serious clinical problem than hepatic encephalopathy for many of these patients.

Nursing Management
Goals
The patient with cirrhosis will have relief of discomfort, have minimal to no complications (ascites, esophageal varices, hepatic encephalopathy), and return to as normal a lifestyle as possible.
Nursing Diagnoses
- Imbalanced nutrition: less than body requirement
- Excess fluid volume
- Impaired skin integrity

Nursing Interventions

Prevention and early treatment of cirrhosis focus on reducing or eliminating risk factors.

- Urge patients to abstain from alcohol and encourage those with history of alcohol abuse to enroll in Alcoholics Anonymous or other support groups.
- Adequate nutrition is essential to promote liver regeneration.
- Identify and treat acute hepatitis early so that it does not progress to chronic hepatitis and cirrhosis.

Nursing care for the patient with cirrhosis focuses on conserving the patient's strength while maintaining muscle strength and tone. Modify the activity and rest schedule according to signs of clinical improvement (e.g., decreasing jaundice, improvement in liver function studies).

- Anorexia, nausea and vomiting, pressure from ascites, and poor eating habits all interfere with adequate intake of nutrients. Make between-meal snacks available. Provide preferred foods whenever possible.
- Assess the patient for the presence and progression of jaundice and pruritus. Check urine and stool color.
- Accurate recordings of intake and output, daily weights, and measurements of extremities and abdominal girth help in the ongoing assessment of edema.
- A semi-Fowler's or Fowler's position allows for maximal respiratory efficiency when dyspnea is a problem. Use pillows to support arms and chest to increase patient comfort and ability to breathe.
- When the patient is taking diuretics, monitor serum electrolyte levels.
- Meticulous skin care is essential because edematous tissues are subject to breakdown. Use an alternating air pressure mattress or other special mattress. Adhere to a turning schedule (minimum of every 2 hours). Support the abdomen with pillows.
- Have the patient void immediately before a paracentesis to prevent puncture of the bladder. After the procedure, monitor for hypovolemia and electrolyte imbalances, and check the dressing for bleeding and leakage.
- Observe for signs of bleeding from esophageal or gastric varices, such as hematemesis and melena. If hematemesis occurs, assess the patient for hemorrhage, call the HCP, and be ready to assist with treatments to control bleeding.

▼ Patient and Caregiver Teaching

The patient and caregiver need to understand the importance of continuous health care and medical supervision. Teach the patient and caregiver about symptoms of complications and when to seek medical attention.

- Abstinence from alcohol is important and results in improvement in most patients. Provide information regarding community support programs such as Alcoholics Anonymous for help with alcohol abuse.
- Explain both verbally and in writing information about fluid or dietary recommendations.
- Instruct on the importance of adequate rest periods, skin care, drug therapy precautions, observation for bleeding, and protection from infection.
- Referral to a community or home health nurse may be helpful to ensure ongoing support and adequate adherence to prescribed therapy.

COLORECTAL CANCER

Description

Of cancers that affect both men and women, colorectal cancer (CRC) is the second leading cause of cancer-related deaths and is the third most common cancer in men and women. CRC is more common in men. Mortality rates are highest among African-American men and women. The risk of CRC increases with age, with about 90% of new cases detected in people older than 50 years of age.

Pathophysiology

No single risk factor accounts for most cases of CRC. The risk is highest in people with first-degree relatives with CRC and people with inflammatory bowel disease (IBD). About one third of cases of CRC occur in patients with a family history of CRC. Hereditary forms of CRC, including familial adenomatous polyposis (FAP) and hereditary nonpolyposis CRC (HNPCC) syndrome (Lynch syndrome), account for 5% to 10% of those cases.

About 30% to 50% of people with CRC have an abnormal *KRAS* gene. The *KRAS* gene, which is primarily involved in regulating cell division, belongs to a class of genes known as oncogenes. When mutated, oncogenes have the potential to cause normal cells to become cancerous.

- Physical exercise and a diet with large amounts of fruits, vegetables, and grains may decrease the risk. Long-term use of nonsteroidal antiinflammatory drugs (NSAIDs) (e.g., aspirin) is also associated with reduced risk.

Adenocarcinoma is the most common type of CRC. Typically it begins as adenomatous polyps. As the tumor grows, the cancer invades and penetrates the muscularis mucosae. Eventually tumor cells gain access to the regional lymph nodes and vascular system and spread to distant sites. Because venous blood leaving the colon and the rectum flows through the portal vein and the inferior rectal vein, the liver is a common site of metastasis. The cancer spreads from the liver to other sites (lungs, bones, and brain) or adjacent structures.

Clinical Manifestations and Complications

Manifestations are usually nonspecific or do not appear until the disease is advanced (Fig. 4). Signs and symptoms may include iron-deficiency anemia, rectal bleeding, abdominal pain, change in bowel habits, and intestinal obstruction or perforation.

- Additional findings in early disease may include fatigue, anorexia, and weight loss. In advanced disease, an abdominal mass, abdominal tenderness, abdominal distention, rectal pain, hepatomegaly, and ascites may be present.
- Right-sided lesions are more likely to bleed and cause diarrhea, whereas left-sided tumors are usually detected later and could present with bowel obstruction.

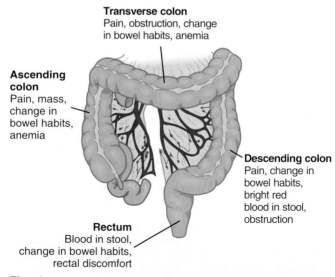

Transverse colon
Pain, obstruction, change in bowel habits, anemia

Ascending colon
Pain, mass, change in bowel habits, anemia

Descending colon
Pain, change in bowel habits, bright red blood in stool, obstruction

Rectum
Blood in stool, change in bowel habits, rectal discomfort

Fig. 4 Signs and symptoms of colorectal cancer by location of primary cancer.

- Complications include obstruction, bleeding, perforation, peritonitis, and fistula formation.

Diagnostic Studies

Because cancer symptoms do not become evident until the disease is advanced, regular screening is advocated to detect and remove polyps before they become cancerous. Beginning at age 50, both men and women at average risk for developing CRC should have screening tests to detect both polyps and cancer. African Americans should have their first colonoscopies at age 45.

- Colonoscopy is the screening procedure of choice to examine the entire colon, obtain biopsy specimens, and remove polyps.
- Fecal occult blood tests are done to detect blood.
- Complete blood count (CBC), coagulation studies, and liver function tests are done when the diagnosis is confirmed by colonoscopy and biopsy.
- CT scan or MRI of abdomen and pelvis is used to detect liver metastases.
- Carcinoembryonic antigen (CEA) serum test is used as a baseline to follow the progress of the patient after surgery or chemotherapy.

Interprofessional Care

Prognosis and treatment correlate with the pathologic staging of the disease. The TNM staging system is the most commonly used method to stage the tumor (see p. 781, Part Three). As with other cancers, prognosis worsens with greater size and depth of tumor, lymph node involvement, and metastasis.

Surgical Therapy

Surgical goals include complete resection of the tumor with adequate margins of healthy tissue, a thorough exploration of the abdomen to detect spread, removal of all lymph nodes that drain the cancer area, restoration of bowel continuity so that normal bowel function will return, and prevention of surgical complications.

- Polypectomy during colonoscopy can be used to resect CRC in situ.
- The site of the tumor determines the site of the resection (e.g., right hemicolectomy, left hemicolectomy).
- Surgery for stage I cancer includes removal of the tumor and at least 5 cm of intestine on either side of the tumor, plus removal of nearby lymph nodes. The remaining cancer-free ends are sewn back together. Laparoscopic surgery is sometimes used for stage I tumors, especially those in the left colon.

- Low-risk stage II tumors are treated with wide resection and reanastomosis, but chemotherapy is used in addition to surgery for high-risk stage II tumors.
- Stage III tumors are treated with surgery and chemotherapy.

In treating rectal cancer, the surgeon has three major options: (1) local excision, (2) abdominal-perineal resection (APR) with a permanent colostomy, and (3) low anterior resection (LAR) to preserve sphincter function. The surgical decision is based on the location and stage of the cancer and the likelihood of restoring normal bowel function and continence. Most patients with rectal cancer require APR or LAR.

Chemotherapy and Targeted Therapy

Chemotherapy can be used to shrink the tumor before surgery, as adjuvant therapy after colon resection, and as palliative treatment for nonresectable disease (see Chemotherapy, p. 694). Current chemotherapy protocols for CRC include 5-fluorouracil (5-FU) and folinic acid (leucovorin) alone or in combination with oxaliplatin (Eloxatin) or irinotecan (CPT-11). Oral regimens of a fluoropyrimidine (e.g., capecitabine [Xeloda]) in combination with oxaliplatin are an alternative to 5-FU/folinic acid therapy.

A variety of targeted therapies are used to treat metastatic disease. Angiogenesis inhibitors, which inhibit the blood supply to tumors, include bevacizumab (Avastin) and ziv-aflibercept (Zaltrap). Regorafenib (Stivarga) is a multikinase inhibitor that blocks several enzymes known to promote cancer growth. Cetuximab (Erbitux) and panitumumab (Vectibix) block the epidermal growth factor receptor.

Radiation Therapy

Radiation therapy may be used as an adjuvant to surgery and chemotherapy or as a palliative measure for patients with metastatic cancer. As a palliative measure, its primary objective is to reduce tumor size and provide symptomatic relief (see Radiation Therapy, p. 733).

Nursing Management

Goals

The patient with CRC will have normal bowel elimination patterns, quality of life appropriate to disease progression, relief of pain, and feelings of comfort and well-being.

Nursing Diagnoses

- Diarrhea or constipation
- Fear and anxiety
- Ineffective coping

Nursing Interventions

Encourage all patients older than 50 to have regular screening for CRC. Help identify those at high risk who need screening at an earlier age.

Preoperative Care.   Nursing care for patients with a colon resection is similar to care for patients undergoing a laparotomy (see Abdominal Pain, Acute, p. 3). Patients who have had an APR will have a permanent ostomy. Provide emotional support to cope with the diagnosis of cancer and the impending changes in body appearance and function.

Postoperative Care.   Many patients have immediate reanastomosis of bowel and require general postoperative care. Patients with more extensive surgery (e.g., APR) may have an open wound and drains (e.g., Jackson-Pratt, Hemovac) and a permanent stoma.

Postoperative care includes sterile dressing changes, care of drains, and patient and caregiver teaching about the stoma. Consult with a wound, ostomy, and continence nurse (WOCN) before surgery to select the ostomy site on the abdomen, and then provide follow-up care and teaching.

- A patient who has open and packed wounds requires meticulous postoperative care. Reinforce dressings and change them frequently during the first several hours postoperatively. Carefully assess all drainage for amount, color, and consistency. Examine the wound regularly and record bleeding, excessive drainage, and unusual odor.
- The patient may experience phantom rectal sensation because the sympathetic nerves responsible for rectal control are not severed during the surgery. Assess to distinguish phantom sensations from the pain of a developing perineal abscess.
- Sexual dysfunction is a possible complication of APR. Although the likelihood of sexual dysfunction depends on the surgical technique used, the surgeon should discuss the possibility with the patient.

▼ Patient and Caregiver Teaching

- The patient and caregiver should be aware of community resources and services available for assistance.
- Patients with colostomies need to know how to care for them.
- Patients and caregivers need to know about diet, incontinence products, and strategies for managing bloating, diarrhea, and bowel evacuation.
- Patients undergoing sphincter-sparing surgery may need antidiarrheal drugs or bulking agents to control diarrhea. A dietitian should help the patient choose foods that are less likely to cause diarrhea.

CONJUNCTIVITIS

Conjunctivitis is an inflammation or infection of the conjunctiva. Conjunctivitis may be caused by bacteria or viruses, and inflammation can result from exposure to allergens or chemical irritants. The tarsal conjunctiva (lining of the lid's interior surface) may become inflamed as a result of a long-term foreign body in the eye, such as a contact lens. See Table 26 for a comparison of clinical manifestations and management of the different types of conjunctivitis.

CONSTIPATION

Description

Constipation is a syndrome defined by difficult or infrequent stools; hard, dry stools that are difficult to pass; or a feeling of incomplete evacuation. Because individuals vary, it is important to compare the current symptoms with the patient's normal pattern of elimination.

Common causes of constipation include taking in insufficient dietary fiber or fluids, decreasing physical activity, and ignoring the defecation urge. Many drugs, especially opioids, cause constipation. Constipation occurs with diseases that slow GI transit and hamper neurologic function, such as diabetes mellitus, Parkinson's disease, and multiple sclerosis. Emotions, including anxiety, depression, and stress, affect the GI tract and can contribute to constipation.

Clinical Manifestations

Constipation may vary from a mild discomfort to a more severe acute event mimicking an "acute abdomen." Stools are absent or hard, dry, and difficult to pass. Abdominal distention, bloating, increased flatulence, and a sensation of increased rectal pressure may be present.

- Hemorrhoids are the most common complication of chronic constipation. They result from venous engorgement resulting from repeated Valsalva maneuvers (straining) and venous compression from hard impacted stool (see Hemorrhoids, p. 290).
- In the presence of obstipation (severe constipation with no passage of gas or stool) or fecal impaction secondary to constipation, colonic perforation may occur. Perforation, which is life-threatening, causes abdominal pain, nausea, vomiting, fever, and an elevated white blood cell (WBC) count.

C

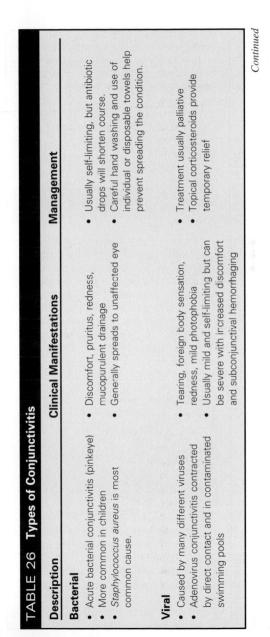

TABLE 26 Types of Conjunctivitis

Description	Clinical Manifestations	Management
Bacterial		
• Acute bacterial conjunctivitis (pinkeye) • More common in children • *Staphylococcus aureus* is most common cause.	• Discomfort, pruritus, redness, mucopurulent drainage • Generally spreads to unaffected eye	• Usually self-limiting, but antibiotic drops will shorten course. • Careful hand washing and use of individual or disposable towels help prevent spreading the condition.
Viral		
• Caused by many different viruses • Adenovirus conjunctivitis contracted by direct contact and in contaminated swimming pools	• Tearing, foreign body sensation, redness, mild photophobia • Usually mild and self-limiting but can be severe with increased discomfort and subconjunctival hemorrhaging	• Treatment usually palliative • Topical corticosteroids provide temporary relief

Continued

TABLE 26 Types of Conjunctivitis—cont'd

Description	Clinical Manifestations	Management
Chlamydial		
• *Chlamydia trachomatis* serotypes A-C cause trachoma, a chronic conjunctivitis that is a major cause of blindness worldwide. • Adult inclusion conjunctivitis (AIC) caused by *C. trachomatis* serotypes D-K is increasing with rise in chlamydial infections.	• Mucopurulent ocular discharge, irritation, redness, lid swelling • AIC does not lead to blindness as does trachoma.	• Antibiotic therapy usually effective for both trachoma and AIC • Patients with AIC have a high risk of concurrent chlamydial genital infection and other sexually transmitted infections.
Allergic		
• Conjunctivitis may develop in response to exposure to pollens, animal dander, ocular solutions, contact lenses, or other allergens.	• Itching (defining symptom), burning, redness, and tearing	• Artificial tears to dilute allergen and wash from eye • Topical antihistamines and corticosteroids • Teach to avoid known allergens.

Diagnostic Studies

Perform a thorough history and physical examination to identify the underlying cause.

- Diagnostic testing may include abdominal x-rays, barium enema, colonoscopy, sigmoidoscopy, rectal balloon expulsion test, anorectal manometry, defecography with barium or fluoroscopy, and colonic transit tests.

Interprofessional Care

Increasing dietary fiber, fluid intake, and exercise can prevent most cases of constipation. The diet should include fluid intake of at least 2 L/day unless contraindicated by cardiac or renal disease. Laxatives and enemas may be used to treat acute constipation but are used cautiously because overuse leads to chronic constipation.

- Methylnaltrexone (Relistor) and naloxegol (Movantik) are peripherally acting opioid receptor antagonists that reduce constipation caused by opioid use.
- Enemas are fast-acting and beneficial for immediate treatment of constipation but must be used cautiously. Soapsuds enemas produce inflammation of colon mucosa, tap water enemas can lead to water intoxication, and sodium phosphate (e.g., Fleet) enemas may cause electrolyte imbalances in some patients.
- Biofeedback therapy may benefit patients who are constipated as a result of anismus (uncoordinated contraction of the anal sphincter during straining).

A patient with severe constipation related to a motility or mechanical disorder may require more intensive treatment, including surgery

Nursing Management

Goals

The patient with constipation will increase dietary intake of fiber and fluids; increase physical activity; pass soft, formed stools; and not have any complications, such as bleeding hemorrhoids.

Nursing Diagnosis

- Constipation

Nursing Interventions

Interventions should be based on the patient's symptoms and assessment findings. Defecation is easiest when the person is sitting on a commode with the knees higher than the hips. The sitting position allows gravity to aid defecation, and flexing the hips straightens the angle between the anal canal and the rectum so that stool is expelled more easily.

Place a footstool in front of the toilet to promote flexion of the thighs. It is challenging to defecate while sitting on a bedpan. For a patient in bed, elevate the head of the bed as high as the patient can tolerate. Provide as much privacy as possible and offer an odor eliminator.

Encourage patients to exercise the abdominal muscles and contract the abdominal muscles several times each day. Sit-ups and straight-leg raises can also improve abdominal muscle tone.

▼ **Patient and Caregiver Teaching**
- Teach the patient and caregiver the importance of diet in the prevention of constipation. Emphasize the maintenance of a high-fiber diet, increased fluid intake, and a regular exercise program.
- Teach the patient to establish a regular time to defecate and not suppress the urge to defecate.
- Discourage the patient from using laxatives and enemas to achieve fecal elimination.

COR PULMONALE

Description

Cor pulmonale is enlargement of the right ventricle (RV) caused by a primary disorder of the respiratory system. Pulmonary hypertension is usually a preexisting condition in cor pulmonale. Cor pulmonale may be present with or without overt cardiac failure.
- The most common cause of cor pulmonale is chronic obstructive pulmonary disease (COPD) (see p. 127). Almost any disorder that affects the respiratory system can cause cor pulmonale.

Clinical Manifestations

- Manifestations are subtle and often masked by the symptoms of the pulmonary condition. Common signs and symptoms include exertional dyspnea, tachypnea, cough, and fatigue.
- Physical signs include evidence of right ventricular hypertrophy on the electrocardiogram (ECG) and increased intensity of the second heart sound. Chronic hypoxemia leads to polycythemia and increased total blood volume and viscosity of the blood.
- If heart failure accompanies cor pulmonale, additional manifestations include peripheral edema; weight gain; distended neck veins; full, bounding pulse; and enlarged liver.

Diagnostic tests may include arterial blood gases (ABGs), arterial O_2 saturation by pulse oximetry (SpO_2), b-type natriuretic peptide (BNP) level, ECG, chest x-ray, CT scan, MRI, and cardiac catheterization.

Nursing and Interprofessional Management

Early identification of cor pulmonale is essential before irreversible changes to the heart develop. Management is directed at treating the underlying pulmonary problem. Long-term, low-flow O_2 therapy to correct the hypoxemia reduces vasoconstriction and pulmonary hypertension.

- If fluid, electrolyte, and acid-base imbalances are present, they must be corrected. Diuretics and a low-sodium diet decrease the plasma volume and may reduce the workload on the heart. Diuretics must be used with extreme caution. In some cases, decreases in fluid volume from diuresis can worsen cardiac function.
- Bronchodilator therapy is indicated if the underlying respiratory problem is due to an obstructive disorder.
- Other treatments include those for pulmonary hypertension such as vasodilator therapy, calcium channel blockers, and anticoagulants.

Nursing management of cor pulmonale resulting from COPD is similar to that described for COPD (see pp. 133-136).

CORONARY ARTERY DISEASE

Description

Coronary artery disease (CAD) is a type of blood vessel disorder that is included in the general category of atherosclerosis. *Atherosclerosis* is derived from two Greek words: *athero,* meaning "fatty mush," and *skleros,* meaning "hard." Atherosclerosis is often referred to as "hardening of the arteries." Although this condition can occur in any artery in the body, the atheromas (fatty deposits) prefer the coronary arteries.

- Arteriosclerotic heart disease, cardiovascular heart disease, ischemic heart disease, coronary heart disease, and CAD all describe this disease process.
- Cardiovascular disease is the major cause of death in the United States. CAD is the most common type of cardiovascular disease and accounts for the majority of these deaths.
- Patients with CAD may be asymptomatic or develop *chronic stable angina (chest pain).*
- Unstable angina (UA) and myocardial infarction (MI) are more serious manifestations of CAD and are the defining disorders of *acute coronary syndrome* (ACS). (See Acute Coronary Syndrome, p. 5.)

Fig. 1 on p. 6 illustrates the relationship among the clinical manifestations of CAD.

TABLE 27   Risk Factors for Coronary Artery Disease

Nonmodifiable Risk Factors	Modifiable Risk Factors

• Increasing age
• Gender (more common in men than in women until the age of 75 years)
• Ethnicity (more common in white men than in African Americans)
• Genetic predisposition and family history of heart disease
	Major
	• Serum lipids:
	  • Total cholesterol >200 mg/dL
	  • Triglycerides ≥150 mg/dL*
	  • LDL cholesterol >160 mg/dL
	  • HDL cholesterol <40 mg/dL in men or <50 mg/dL in women*
	• BP ≥140/90 mm Hg*
	• Diabetes
	• Tobacco use
	• Physical inactivity
	• Obesity: Waist circumference ≥102 cm (≥40 in) in men and ≥88 cm (≥35 in) in women*
	
	Contributing
	• Fasting blood glucose ≥100 mg/dL*
	• Psychosocial risk factors (e.g., depression, hostility, anger, stress)
	• Elevated homocysteine levels

*Three or more of these risk factors meet the criteria for metabolic syndrome. Metabolic syndrome is discussed in Chapter 40 of Lewis et al, *Medical-Surgical Nursing*, ed 10, p. 890.
HDL, High-density lipoprotein; *LDL*, low-density lipoprotein.

Risk factors for CAD can be categorized as nonmodifiable and modifiable (Table 27).

Pathophysiology

Atherosclerosis is characterized by lipid deposits within the intima of the artery. Inflammation and endothelial injury play a central role in the development of atherosclerosis.

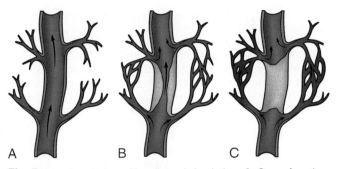

Fig. 5 Vessel occlusion with collateral circulation. **A,** Open, functioning coronary artery. **B,** Partial coronary artery closure, with collateral circulation being established. **C,** Total coronary artery occlusion with collateral circulation bypassing the occlusion to supply blood to the myocardium.

C

- The endothelial lining can be injured as a result of tobacco use, hyperlipidemia, hypertension, diabetes, hyperhomocystinemia, and infection causing a local inflammatory response.
- C-reactive protein (CRP), a protein produced by the liver, is a nonspecific marker of systemic inflammation. It is increased in many patients with CAD.
- CAD takes many years to develop. When it becomes symptomatic, the disease process is usually well advanced. Stages of development in atherosclerosis are (1) fatty streak, (2) fibrous plaque resulting from smooth muscle cell proliferation, and (3) complicated lesion.

   Normally some arterial anastomoses or connections, called *collateral circulation,* exist within the coronary circulation (Fig. 5).

- When blockages in coronary arteries occur slowly over a long period, there is a greater chance of collateral circulation developing, and the heart muscle may still receive an adequate amount of blood and oxygen.
- With rapid-onset CAD, time is inadequate for collateral development. Consequently, reduced blood flow results in more severe ischemia or infarction.

Clinical Manifestations

CAD is a progressive disease, and patients may be asymptomatic for many years or may develop chronic stable angina. When the demand for myocardial oxygen exceeds the ability of the coronary arteries to supply the heart with oxygen, myocardial ischemia occurs.

- *Angina,* or chest pain, is the clinical manifestation of reversible myocardial ischemia. The primary reason for insufficient blood flow is narrowing of coronary arteries by atherosclerosis.
- Chronic stable angina refers to chest pain that occurs intermittently over a long period with the same pattern of onset, duration, and intensity of symptoms (see Angina, Chronic Stable, p. 46).

When ischemia is prolonged and not immediately reversible, ACS develops and encompasses the spectrum of UA, non–ST-segment-elevation myocardial infarction (NSTEMI), and ST-segment-elevation myocardial infarction (STEMI) (see Fig. 1 on p. 6).

Diagnostic Studies

- Chest x-ray is used to detect cardiac enlargement, cardiac calcifications, and pulmonary congestion.
- The 12-lead ECG detects heart rhythm, pacemaker activity, conduction abnormalities, position of heart, size of atria and ventricles, and presence of ischemia/injury/infarction.
- Serum lipid levels are used to screen for risk factors.
- Exercise or stress testing is used to detect ST-segment and T wave changes that indicate ischemia with exercise.
- Ambulatory 24- to 48-hour ECG monitoring can help to identify silent ischemia.
- Nuclear imaging studies are used to determine myocardial perfusion, contractility, and ejection fraction.
- Positron emission tomography (PET) is used to identify and quantify ischemia and infarction.
- Angiography studies are used to visualize coronary arteries and help to determine treatment and prognosis.
- Echocardiography with exercise is used to diagnose coronary artery stenosis.

Interprofessional Care

People who have modifiable risk factors should be encouraged to make lifestyle changes to prevent, modify, or slow CAD progression. Lifestyle changes, including a low-saturated-fat, high-fiber diet; avoidance of tobacco; and increase in physical activity, can promote regression in the course of coronary atherosclerosis and a reduction in coronary events.

- A physical activity program should be designed to improve physical fitness by following the FITT formula: *f*requency (how often), *i*ntensity (how hard), *t*ype (isotonic), and *t*ime (how

long). Everyone should aim for at least 30 minutes of moderate
physical activity on most days of the week.

- Specific diet recommendations and plans are presented in
  Tables 33-3 and 33-4 in Lewis et al, *Medical-Surgical Nursing,*
  ed 10, p. 709.

Drug Therapy

People with serum cholesterol levels higher than 200 mg/dL are at
risk for CAD. Treatment usually begins with dietary caloric restriction (if overweight), decreased dietary fat and cholesterol intake,
and increased physical activity. Guidelines for the treatment of high
cholesterol recommend that the following groups of people receive
statin therapy: (1) patients with known cardiovascular disease
(CVD), (2) patients with primary elevations of low-density lipoprotein (LDL) cholesterol levels to 190 mg/dL or greater (e.g.,
familial hypercholesterolemia), (3) patients between 40 and 75
years of age with diabetes and LDL cholesterol levels between 70
and 189 mg/dL, and (4) patients between 40 and 75 years of age
with LDL cholesterol levels between 70 and 189 mg/dL and a
10-year risk for CVD of at least 7.5%. Serum lipid levels are reas-
sessed after 6 weeks of diet therapy. If they remain elevated, additional dietary options and drug therapy may be considered.

The statin drugs are the most widely used lipid-lowering drugs.
These drugs inhibit the synthesis of cholesterol in the liver by
blocking hydroxymethylglutaryl coenzyme A (HMG-CoA) reduc-
tase. Examples include lovastatin, pravastatin (Pravachol), simvastatin (Zocor), fluvastatin (Lescol), atorvastatin (Lipitor), and
rosuvastatin (Crestor). These drugs primarily lower LDL cholesterol and also cause an increase in high-density lipoprotein (HDL).
Niacin, a water-soluble B vitamin, also interferes with the synthesis
of LDL and triglyceride levels.

Fibric acid derivatives such as gemfibrozil (Lopid) are effective
in lowering very-low-density lipoprotein (VLDL) levels and triglycerides, while increasing HDL levels. Drugs that increase lipoprotein removal by increasing conversion of cholesterol to bile
acids include cholestyramine, colestipol (Colestid), and cole-
sevelam (Welchol) and are commonly used. Ezetimibe (Zetia)
inhibits the absorption of dietary and biliary cholesterol across the
intestinal wall and may be combined with a statin to promote
greater reductions in LDL.

- Drug therapy for hyperlipidemia often continues for a lifetime.
  Diet modification minimizes the need for drug therapy. The
  patient must fully understand the rationale and goals of treatment as well as drug safety and side effects.

Antiplatelet therapy with low-dose aspirin (e.g., 81 mg) is recommended for most people at risk for CAD unless contraindicated

(e.g., history of GI bleeding). For high-risk women who are aspirin-intolerant, clopidogrel (Plavix) can be considered.

Nursing Management

Regardless of the health care setting, it is extremely important to identify the person at risk for CAD. Risk screening involves obtaining a thorough health history. Question the patient about a family history of heart disease in parents and siblings. Note the presence of any cardiovascular symptoms.

Assess environmental factors, such as eating habits, type of diet, and level of exercise, to identify lifestyle patterns. Include a psychosocial history to determine tobacco use, alcohol intake, recent life-stressing events (e.g., loss of a spouse), and the presence of any negative psychologic states (e.g., anxiety, depression, anger). The place and type of employment provide important information on the kind of activity performed, exposure to pollutants or noxious chemicals, and the degree of stress associated with work.

- Identify patient attitudes and beliefs about health and illness. This information can give you insight into how disease and lifestyle changes may affect the patient and can reveal possible misconceptions about heart disease.
- Knowledge of the patient's educational background and health literacy is helpful in deciding on the level to begin teaching.
- If the patient takes prescribed drugs, it is important to know the names and dosages and if the patient adheres to the drug regimen.

CROHN'S DISEASE

Crohn's disease is an autoimmune disorder that, along with ulcerative colitis, is referred to as *inflammatory bowel disease* (IBD). See Inflammatory Bowel Disease, p. 348, for a discussion of the disorder.

CUSHING SYNDROME

Description

Cushing syndrome is a clinical condition that results from chronic exposure to excess corticosteroids, particularly glucocorticoids. The most common cause of Cushing syndrome is iatrogenic administration of *exogenous* corticosteroids (e.g., prednisone). About 85% of the cases of *endogenous* Cushing syndrome are caused by an adrenocorticotropic hormone (ACTH)–secreting pituitary tumor *(Cushing disease)*. Less common causes of Cushing syndrome include adrenal or other tumors.

Clinical Manifestations

Manifestations can be seen in most body systems and are related to excess levels of corticosteroids (see Table 49-13, Lewis et al, *Medical-Surgical Nursing,* ed 10, p. 1175). Although signs of glucocorticoid excess usually predominate, symptoms of mineralocorticoid and androgen excess can occur.

- Corticosteroid excess causes pronounced changes in physical appearance. Weight gain, the most common feature, results from an accumulation of adipose tissue in the trunk (centripetal obesity), face ("moon face"), and cervical areas ("buffalo hump").
- Hyperglycemia occurs because of glucose intolerance associated with cortisol-induced insulin resistance and increased gluconeogenesis by the liver.
- Muscle wasting leads to muscle weakness, especially in the extremities.
- Loss of bone protein matrix leads to osteoporosis with pathologic fractures (e.g., vertebral compression fractures) and bone and back pain.
- Loss of collagen makes the skin weaker, thinner, and easier to bruise. Purplish-red striae appear on the abdomen, breast, or buttocks.
- Mineralocorticoid excess may cause hypertension, whereas adrenal androgen excess may cause pronounced acne, with hirsutism and menstrual disorders in women.

Diagnostic Studies

- Plasma cortisol levels may be elevated with loss of diurnal variation.
- A 24-hour urine collection for free cortisol is done. Urine cortisol levels beyond the normal range of 80 to 120 mcg/24 hours in adults indicate Cushing syndrome. If these results are borderline, a low-dose dexamethasone suppression test is done.
- Plasma ACTH levels may be low, normal, or elevated depending on the underlying cause of Cushing syndrome.
- Other findings on diagnostic tests associated with, but not diagnostic of, Cushing syndrome include hyperglycemia, hypokalemia, glycosuria, hypercalciuria, and osteoporosis.
- CT scan and MRI of the pituitary and adrenal glands may be done.

Interprofessional Care

The primary goal is to normalize hormone secretion. The standard treatment for a pituitary adenoma is surgical removal of the pituitary tumor using the transsphenoidal approach. Radiation therapy may be used for patients who are not good surgical candidates. Adrenalectomy is indicated for adrenal tumors or hyperplasia. Patients with ectopic ACTH-secreting tumors (usually located in the lung or pancreas) are also treated surgically.

- When the patient is a poor candidate for surgery or prior surgery has failed, then drug therapy may be attempted. The goal of drug therapy is inhibition of adrenal function (*medical adrenalectomy*). Drug that inhibit corticosteroid synthesis include ketoconazole and mitotane (Lysodren).

If Cushing syndrome has developed during the course of prolonged administration of corticosteroids (e.g., prednisone), the following alternatives may be tried: (1) gradually discontinuing corticosteroid therapy, (2) reducing corticosteroid dose, or (3) converting to an alternate-day regimen.

Nursing Management

Goals

The patient with Cushing syndrome will experience relief of symptoms with no serious complications, maintain a positive self-image, and actively participate in the therapeutic plan.

Nursing Diagnoses

- Risk for infection
- Overweight
- Disturbed body image
- Impaired skin integrity

Nursing Interventions

Because the therapy for Cushing syndrome has many side effects, assessment focuses on signs and symptoms of hormone and drug toxicity and complicating conditions (e.g., cardiovascular disease, diabetes mellitus, infection).

- Monitor vital signs, glucose, and daily weights.
- Signs and symptoms of inflammation (e.g., fever, redness) may be absent, so assess for pain, loss of function, and purulent drainage.
- Monitor for signs of thromboembolic phenomena, such as sudden chest pain, dyspnea, and tachypnea.

Another important focus of nursing care is the provision of emotional support. Changes in appearance, such as truncal obesity, bruising, hirsutism in females, and gynecomastia in males, can be distressing. You can help by remaining sensitive to the patient's feelings and offering respect and unconditional acceptance. Reassure the patient that the physical changes and much of the emotional lability will resolve when hormone levels return to normal.

If treatment involves surgical removal of a pituitary adenoma, an adrenal tumor, or one or both adrenal glands, nursing care will include preoperative and postoperative care.

Preoperative Care. Before surgery, hypertension and hyperglycemia need to be controlled, with hypokalemia corrected by diet and potassium supplements. A high-protein meal plan helps correct protein depletion. Preoperative teaching should include information regarding the anticipated postoperative care.

Postoperative Care. Because of hormone fluctuations, the patient's BP, fluid balance, and electrolyte levels tend to be unstable after surgery. High doses of corticosteroids (hydrocortisone) are administered IV during surgery and for several days afterward to ensure adequate responses to the stress of the procedure.

- Report any rapid or significant changes in BP, respirations, or heart rate (HR).
- Carefully monitor fluid intake and output and assess for potential imbalance.
- If corticosteroid dosage is tapered too rapidly after surgery, acute adrenal insufficiency may develop. Vomiting, increased weakness, dehydration, and hypotension are signs of hypocortisolism. The patient may complain of painful joints, pruritus, or peeling skin and may experience severe emotional disturbances.
- After surgery the patient is usually maintained on bed rest until the BP stabilizes. Be alert for subtle signs of postoperative infections. Provide meticulous care when changing the dressing and during any other procedures that involve access to body cavities, circulation, or areas under skin.

▼ Patient and Caregiver Teaching

Discharge instructions are based on the patient's lack of endogenous cortisol and resulting inability to react physiologically to stressors.

- Instruct patients to wear a medical identification (Medic Alert) bracelet at all times and to carry documentation of the medical condition and instructions in a wallet or purse. Teach the patient to avoid exposure to extreme temperatures, infections, and emotional disturbances.
- Stress may produce or precipitate acute adrenal insufficiency because the remaining adrenal tissue cannot meet an increased hormonal demand. Teach patients to adjust their corticosteroid replacement therapy in accordance with stress levels.

- If the patient cannot adjust his or her own medication or if weakness, fainting, fever, or nausea and vomiting occur, the patient should contact the HCP.

Lifetime replacement therapy is required for many patients. It may take several months to satisfactorily adjust the hormone dose.

CYSTIC FIBROSIS

Description

Cystic fibrosis (CF) is an autosomal recessive, multisystem disease characterized by altered function of the exocrine glands involving primarily the lungs, pancreas, biliary tract, and reproductive tract.

Severity and progression of the disease vary. With early diagnosis and improvements in therapy, the prognosis has been significantly improved. The median predicted survival in 1970 was for 16 years but has currently increased to more than 41 years.

Pathophysiology

CF results from mutations in a gene located on chromosome 7 that produces a protein called CF transmembrane regulator (CFTR). CFTR regulates sodium and chloride channels in the epithelial surface of the airways, pancreatic ducts, and sweat gland ducts. Mutations in the *CFTR* gene alter this protein in such a way that the channel is blocked.

- Cells that line the passageways of the lungs, pancreas, and other organs produce abnormally thick, sticky mucus. This mucus plugs up the glands in these organs and causes the glands to atrophy, ultimately resulting in organ failure.
- The hallmark of respiratory involvement is its effect on the airways. The disease progresses from being a disease of the small airways *(chronic bronchiolitis)* to involvement of the larger airways, and finally causes destruction of lung tissue. CF is also characterized by chronic airway infection that cannot be eradicated. Lung disorders include chronic bronchiolitis and bronchitis that eventually lead to bronchiectasis, blebs, large cysts, and hemoptysis from erosion of pulmonary arteries.
- Pancreatic insufficiency is caused primarily by mucus plugging the pancreatic duct, which results in atrophy of the gland and progressive fibrotic cyst formation. Because the pancreatic digestive enzymes cannot reach the intestine, malabsorption of fat, protein, and fat-soluble vitamins occurs. Fat malabsorption results in steatorrhea, and protein malabsorption results in failure to grow and gain weight.

- CF-related diabetes mellitus results from fibrotic scarring of the pancreas.

Clinical Manifestations

Manifestations vary depending on the disease severity. Carriers are not affected by the gene mutation. Median age at diagnosis of CF is 5 months. An initial finding of meconium ileus in the newborn infant may prompt a diagnosis of CF. Other signs may include acute or persistent respiratory symptoms (wheezing, coughing, frequent pneumonia), failure to thrive or malnutrition, steatorrhea, and positive family history.

- In the adult, a common symptom is frequent cough that becomes persistent and produces viscous, purulent sputum.
- Over time exacerbations (increased cough and sputum, weight loss) become frequent, bronchiectasis worsens, and the recovery of lost lung function is less complete, which may ultimately lead to respiratory failure.
- Affected males and females both have delayed puberty, and some affected women are infertile.

Pneumothorax is an uncommon but serious complication caused by the formation of bullae and blebs. CF-related diabetes, bone disease, and liver disease are additional complications.

Diagnostic Studies

- Sweat chloride test (pilocarpine iontophoresis method) is the gold standard for diagnosing CF. Individuals with CF excrete four times the normal amount of sodium and chloride in their sweat.
- A genetic test is often used if the results from a sweat test are unclear.

Interprofessional Care

An interprofessional team should be involved in the care of a patient with CF, including a nurse, physician, respiratory and physical therapists, dietitian, and social worker.

- Management of pulmonary problems is focused on relieving airway obstruction and controlling infection. Drainage of thick bronchial mucus is assisted by aerosol and nebulization treatments that dilate the airways, liquefy mucus, and facilitate clearance.
- Airway clearance techniques include chest physiotherapy (CPT), positive expiratory pressure (PEP) devices, and breathing exercises.
- More than 95% of CF patients die of complications resulting from lung infection. Standard treatment includes antibiotics

for exacerbations and chronic suppressive therapy. The use of antibiotics should be carefully guided by sputum culture results.

Management of pancreatic insufficiency includes pancreatic enzyme replacement (e.g., pancrelipase [Pancreaze, Creon, Ultresa, Viokace, Zenpep]) administered before each meal and snack. Fat-soluble vitamins need to be supplemented. Added dietary salt is indicated whenever sweating is excessive, such as during hot weather, in the presence of fever, or from intense physical activity. Hyperglycemia may require treatment with insulin.

- Aerobic exercise also seems to be effective in clearing airways.
- More than 20% of adults with CF have depression because CF imposes a significant burden on the individual and family. Issues such as fertility, decreased life expectancy, costs of health care, and career choices may lead to depression.

Nursing Management
Goals
The patient with CF will have adequate airway clearance, reduced risk factors associated with respiratory infections, adequate nutritional support to maintain appropriate body mass index (BMI), ability to perform activities of daily living (ADLs), recognition and treatment of complications related to CF, and active participation in planning and implementing a therapeutic regimen.

Nursing Diagnoses
- Ineffective airway clearance
- Impaired gas exchange
- Imbalanced nutrition: less than body requirements
- Ineffective coping

Nursing Interventions
Acute intervention for the patient with CF includes relief of bronchoconstriction, airway obstruction, and airflow limitation. Interventions include aggressive CPT, antibiotics, and O_2 therapy in severe disease.

▼ Patient and Caregiver Teaching
- Sexuality is an important issue that should be discussed with the young adult. Delayed or irregular menstruation is not uncommon. There may also be delayed development of secondary sex characteristics, such as breasts in girls.
- With most individuals with CF now living to reproductive age, genetic counseling is important.
- The burden of living with a chronic disease can be emotionally overwhelming. Community resources and the Cystic Fibrosis Foundation may be helpful.

DEMENTIA

Description

Dementia is a neurocognitive disorder characterized by dysfunction or loss of memory, orientation, attention, language, judgment, and reasoning. Personality changes and behavioral problems such as agitation, delusions, and hallucinations may occur. Ultimately these problems result in alterations in the individual's ability to work, fulfill social and family responsibilities, and perform activities of daily living.

- Fifteen percent of older Americans have dementia. In the United States, about half of all patients in long-term care facilities have Alzheimer's disease (AD) or a related dementia.
- There are about 100 causes of dementia. About 60% to 80% of patients with dementia have a diagnosis of AD.

Pathophysiology

The two most common causes of dementia are neurodegenerative conditions (e.g., AD) and vascular disorders. Dementia is sometimes caused by treatable conditions that initially may be reversible, such as vitamin B_1 and B_{12} deficiencies, thyroid disorders, subarachnoid hemorrhage, prescribed drugs (e.g., anticholinergics, hypnotics, cocaine), alcoholism, and head injury. However, with prolonged exposure or disease, irreversible changes may occur.

Vascular dementia is loss of cognitive function resulting from ischemic or hemorrhagic brain lesions caused by cardiovascular disease. Vascular dementia may be caused by a single stroke (infarct) or by multiple strokes.

Clinical Manifestations

- Dementia associated with neurologic degeneration is often gradual and progressive. Vascular dementia often results in a more abrupt onset of manifestations or a stepwise pattern of progression.
- An acute (days to weeks) or subacute (weeks to months) pattern of change may indicate an infectious or metabolic cause of dementia, including encephalitis, meningitis, hypothyroidism, or drug-related dementia.

Other clinical manifestations of dementia are discussed with Alzheimer's Disease (pp. 22-25).

Diagnostic Studies

- Comprehensive medical, neurologic, and psychologic histories are important in determining the presence and cause of dementia.

- Physical examination and neuroimaging techniques (CT or MRI) may be performed to rule out some causes of dementia.
- Dementia is often diagnosed when two or more brain functions, such as memory loss or language skills, are significantly impaired.

Nursing and Interprofessional Management

Management of dementia is similar to management of the patient with AD (see Alzheimer's Disease, pp. 26-27). One form of dementia, vascular dementia, can often be prevented. Preventive measures include treatment of risk factors such as hypertension, diabetes, smoking, hypercholesterolemia, and cardiac dysrhythmias. Drugs that are used for patients with AD are also useful for patients with vascular dementia.

DIABETES INSIPIDUS

Description

Diabetes insipidus (DI) is caused by a deficiency of production or secretion of antidiuretic hormone (ADH) or a decreased renal response to ADH. The decrease in ADH results in fluid and electrolyte imbalances caused by increased urine output and increased plasma osmolality. Depending on the cause, DI may be transient or a lifelong condition.

There are several types of DI. *Central DI* (also known as *neurogenic DI*) results from an interference with ADH synthesis, transport, or release. Causes include brain tumor or surgery, central nervous system (CNS) infections, and head injury. It is the most common form of DI.

Nephrogenic DI occurs when there is adequate ADH, but there is a decreased response to ADH in the kidney. Causes include drug therapy (especially lithium), renal damage, and hereditary renal disease.

Psychogenic DI, a less common condition, is associated with excessive water intake. This can be caused by a structural lesion in the thirst center or a psychologic disorder.

Clinical Manifestations

The primary characteristic of DI is excretion of large quantities of urine (2 to 20 L/day) with a very low specific gravity (<1.005) and urine osmolality (100 mOsm/kg). Serum osmolality is elevated as a result of hypernatremia, which is caused by pure water loss in the kidney.

- Most patients compensate for fluid loss by drinking great amounts of water (polydipsia) so that serum osmolality is normal or only moderately elevated. The patient may be fatigued from nocturia and may experience generalized weakness.
- Central DI is usually acute and accompanied by excessive fluid loss.
- Although the clinical manifestations of nephrogenic DI are similar, the onset and amount of fluid losses are less dramatic than with central DI.
- Severe dehydration can result if oral fluid intake cannot keep up with urinary losses. This is manifested by poor tissue turgor, hypotension, tachycardia, and hypovolemic shock.
- The patient may also show CNS manifestations ranging from irritability and mental dullness to coma, which are related to rising serum osmolality and hypernatremia. Uncorrected hypernatremia can cause brain shrinkage and intracranial bleeding.

D

Diagnostic Studies
- Water deprivation test differentiates central DI from nephrogenic DI. Patients with central DI exhibit a dramatic increase in urine osmolality with this test, from 100 to 600 mOsm/kg, and a significant decrease in urine volume. The patient with nephrogenic DI will not be able to increase urine osmolality to >300 mOsm/kg.
- Measuring ADH levels after an analog of ADH (e.g., desmopressin) is given also differentiates central DI from nephrogenic DI. If the cause is central DI, the kidneys will respond to the hormone by concentrating urine. If the kidneys do not respond in this way, then the cause is nephrogenic.

Nursing and Interprofessional Management
Management of the patient with DI includes early detection, maintenance of adequate hydration, and patient teaching for long-term management. A therapeutic goal is the maintenance of fluid and electrolyte balance.

For central DI, fluid and hormone therapy is necessary. Fluids are replaced orally or IV, depending on the patient's condition and ability to drink. Monitor serum glucose levels because hyperglycemia and glucosuria can lead to osmotic diuresis, which increases the fluid volume deficit.

- Monitor level of consciousness, BP, heart rate, and urine output and specific gravity hourly in the acutely ill patient.
- Maintain an accurate record of intake and output and daily weights to determine fluid volume status.

- Desmopressin (DDAVP), a synthetic analog of ADH, is the hormone replacement of choice for central DI. Other ADH replacement drugs include aqueous vasopressin.

Treatment for nephrogenic DI revolves around dietary measures (low-sodium diet) and thiazide diuretics. Limiting sodium intake to no more than 3 g/day often helps decrease urine output. When a low-sodium diet and thiazide drugs are not effective, indomethacin may be prescribed. Indomethacin, a nonsteroidal antiinflammatory drug (NSAID), helps increase renal responsiveness to ADH.

DIABETES MELLITUS

Description

Diabetes mellitus (DM) is a chronic multisystem disease characterized by hyperglycemia related to abnormal insulin production, impaired insulin utilization, or both. Currently in the United States, an estimated 29.1 million people, or 9.3% of the population, have DM, and 86 million people have prediabetes. Approximately 8.1 million people with DM are unaware that they have the disease.

- Diabetes is the leading cause of adult blindness, end-stage renal disease, and nontraumatic lower limb amputations. It is also a major contributing factor to heart disease and stroke.
- The two most common types of diabetes are type 1 DM and type 2 DM (Table 28).

Type 1 Diabetes Mellitus

Type 1 DM, formerly known as "juvenile-onset" or "insulin-dependent" diabetes, accounts for approximately 5% to 10% of all cases of diabetes. This type generally affects people younger than 40 years of age, although it can occur at any age.

Pathophysiology. Type 1 diabetes is an autoimmune disorder in which the body develops antibodies against insulin and/or the pancreatic β-cells that produce insulin. This eventually results in insufficient insulin for survival. Autoantibodies to the islet cells cause a reduction of 80% to 90% of normal function before hyperglycemia and other manifestations occur.

- A genetic predisposition and exposure to a virus are factors that may contribute to the pathogenesis of immune-related type 1 diabetes.

Once the pancreas can no longer produce sufficient amounts of insulin to maintain normal glucose, the onset of symptoms is usually rapid.

TABLE 28 Comparison of Type 1 and Type 2 Diabetes Mellitus

Factor	Type 1 Diabetes Mellitus	Type 2 Diabetes Mellitus
Age at onset	More common in young people but can occur at any age	More common in adults, but can occur at any age Incidence is increasing in children
Type of onset	Signs and symptoms usually abrupt, but disease process may be present for several years.	Insidious, may go undiagnosed for years
Prevalence	Accounts for 5%-10% of all types of diabetes	Accounts for 90%-95% of all types of diabetes
Environmental factors	Virus, toxins	Obesity, lack of exercise
Primary defect	Absent or minimal insulin production	Insulin resistance, decreased insulin production over time, and alterations in production of adipokines
Islet cell antibodies	Often present at onset	Absent
Endogenous insulin	Absent	Initially increased in response to insulin resistance Secretion diminishes over time.
Nutritional status	Thin, normal, or obese	Frequently overweight or obese May be normal
Symptoms	Polydipsia, polyuria, polyphagia, fatigue, weight loss without trying	Frequently none Fatigue, recurrent infections May also experience polyuria, polydipsia, and polyphagia
Ketosis	Prone at onset or during insulin deficiency	Resistant except during infection or stress
Nutrition therapy	Essential	Essential
Insulin	Required for all	Required for some Disease is progressive and insulin treatment may need to be added to treatment regimen.
Vascular and neurologic complications	Frequent	Frequent

- The patient usually has a history of recent and sudden weight loss and the classic symptoms of *polydipsia* (excessive thirst), *polyuria* (frequent urination), and *polyphagia* (excessive hunger).
- The individual with type 1 diabetes requires a supply of insulin from an outside source *(exogenous insulin)* to sustain life. Without insulin, the patient develops *diabetic ketoacidosis* (DKA), a life-threatening condition resulting in metabolic acidosis.

Type 2 Diabetes Mellitus

Type 2 DM was formerly known as adult-onset diabetes mellitus (AODM) or non–insulin-dependent diabetes mellitus (NIDDM). This type is the most prevalent type of diabetes, accounting for greater than 90% of cases of diabetes.

Pathophysiology.   In type 2 diabetes, the pancreas usually continues to produce some endogenous (self-made) insulin. However, the body either does not produce enough insulin or does not use it effectively, or both. The presence of endogenous insulin is the major pathophysiologic distinction between type 1 and type 2 diabetes.

Genetic mutations that lead to insulin resistance and a higher risk for obesity have been found in many people with type 2 diabetes. Individuals with a first-degree relative with the disease are 10 times more likely to develop type 2 diabetes. Four major metabolic abnormalities play a role in the development of type 2 diabetes.

- The first factor is *insulin resistance,* which describes a condition in which body tissues do not respond to the action of insulin because insulin receptors are unresponsive, insufficient in number, or both. Entry of glucose into the cell is impeded, resulting in hyperglycemia.
- A second factor is a marked decrease in the ability of the pancreas to produce insulin as the β-cells become fatigued from the compensatory overproduction of insulin or when β-cell mass is lost.
- A third factor is inappropriate glucose production by the liver. Instead of properly regulating the release of glucose in response to blood levels, the liver does so in a haphazard way that does not correspond to the body's needs at the time.
- A fourth factor is alteration in the production of hormones and cytokines by adipose tissue (adipokines). Adipokines play a role in glucose and fat metabolism and likely contribute to the pathophysiology of type 2 diabetes.

Individuals with metabolic syndrome are at an increased risk for the development of type 2 diabetes. Overweight individuals with metabolic syndrome can reduce their risk for diabetes through a program of weight loss and regular physical activity (see Metabolic Syndrome, p. 414).

Disease onset in type 2 diabetes is usually gradual, with signs and symptoms of hyperglycemia developing when about 50% to 80% of β-cells no longer secrete insulin. Many people are diagnosed on routine laboratory testing or when they undergo treatment for other conditions and elevated glucose or glycosylated hemoglobin (A1C) levels are found.

Prediabetes

Individuals diagnosed with prediabetes are at increased risk for the development of type 2 diabetes. *Prediabetes,* an intermediate stage between normal glucose homeostasis and diabetes, is defined as impaired glucose tolerance (IGT), impaired fasting glucose (IFG), or both.

- A diagnosis of IGT is made if the 2-hour oral glucose tolerance test (OGTT) values are 140 to 199 mg/dL (7.8 to 11.0 mmol/L). IFG is diagnosed when fasting blood glucose levels are 100 to 125 mg/dL (5.56 to 6.9 mmol/L).

People with prediabetes usually do not have symptoms. However, long-term damage to the body, especially the heart and blood vessels, may already be occurring. It is important for patients to undergo screening and understand risk factors for diabetes.

- Encourage those with prediabetes to have their blood glucose and A1C tested regularly and to self-monitor for symptoms of diabetes, such as polyuria, polyphagia, and polydipsia.
- Maintaining a healthy weight, exercising regularly, and eating a healthy diet reduce the risk of developing overt diabetes in people with prediabetes.

Clinical Manifestations

Type 1 Diabetes

Because the onset of type 1 DM is rapid, the initial manifestations are usually acute. The osmotic effect of glucose produces polydipsia and polyuria. Polyphagia is a consequence of cellular malnourishment when insulin deficiency prevents use of glucose for energy. Weight loss, weakness, and fatigue may also occur.

Type 2 Diabetes

Manifestations of type 2 DM are often nonspecific, including fatigue, recurrent infections, prolonged wound healing, and visual changes. Polydipsia, polyuria, and polyphagia may also occur.

Acute Complications

Acute complications arise from events associated with hyperglycemia and hypoglycemia (also referred to as *insulin reaction*). It is important for the HCP to distinguish between hyperglycemia and hypoglycemia because hypoglycemia worsens rapidly and constitutes a serious threat if action is not immediately taken. Table 29 compares hyperglycemia and hypoglycemia.

Diabetic Ketoacidosis

Diabetic ketoacidosis (DKA) is caused by a profound deficiency of insulin and is characterized by hyperglycemia, ketosis, acidosis, and dehydration. Precipitating factors include illness and infection, inadequate insulin dosage, undiagnosed type 1 diabetes, poor self-management, and neglect.

- DKA is most likely to occur in type 1 diabetes but may be seen in type 2 during severe illness or stress when the pancreas cannot meet the extra demand for insulin. If it is left untreated, death is inevitable.
- Manifestations of DKA include dehydration signs (e.g., poor skin turgor, dry mucous membranes), tachycardia, orthostatic hypotension with a weak and rapid pulse, vomiting, Kussmaul respirations, and a sweet fruity odor of acetone on the breath.
- Laboratory findings include a blood glucose level of 250 mg/dL (13.9 mmol/L) or greater, arterial blood pH less than 7.30, serum bicarbonate level less than 16 mEq/L (16 mmol/L), and moderate to large amount of ketones in the urine or serum.

TABLE 29   Comparison of Hyperglycemia and Hypoglycemia

Hyperglycemia	Hypoglycemia
Manifestations*	
• Elevated blood glucose†	• Blood glucose <70 mg/dL
• Increase in urination	(3.9 mmol/L)
• Increase in appetite followed by lack of appetite	• Cold, clammy skin
• Weakness, fatigue	• Numbness of fingers, toes, mouth
• Blurred vision	• Rapid heartbeat
• Headache	• Emotional changes
• Glycosuria	• Headache
• Nausea and vomiting	• Nervousness, tremors
• Abdominal cramps	• Faintness, dizziness
• Progression to DKA or HHS	• Unsteady gait, slurred speech
	• Hunger
	• Changes in vision
	• Seizures, coma

TABLE 29 Comparison of Hyperglycemia and Hypoglycemia—cont'd

Hyperglycemia	Hypoglycemia
Causes	
• Illness, infection • Corticosteroids • Too much food • Too little or no diabetes medication • Inactivity • Emotional, physical stress • Poor absorption of insulin	• Alcohol intake without food • Too little food—delayed, omitted, inadequate intake • Too much diabetes medication • Too much exercise without adequate food intake • Diabetes medication or food taken at wrong time • Loss of weight without change in medication • Use of β-adrenergic blockers interfering with recognition of symptoms
Treatment	
• Get medical care. • Continue diabetes medication as prescribed. • Check blood glucose frequently and check urine for ketones; record results. • Drink fluids at least on an hourly basis. • Contact HCP regarding ketonuria.	• *Conscious person*: Give 15 g of a simple (fast-acting) carbohydrate (fruit juice or regular soft drink). Recheck the blood glucose 15 minutes later. If the value is still below 70 mg/dL, have the patient ingest 15 g more of carbohydrate and recheck the blood glucose in 15 minutes. Have the patient ingest a complex carbohydrate after recovery to prevent a rebound hypoglycemic attack. If no significant improvement occurs after two or three doses of 15 g of simple carbohydrate, contact the health care provider. • *Worsening symptoms or unconscious patient*: Subcutaneous or IM injection of 1 mg glucagon, or IV administration of 25-50 mL of 50% glucose.

D

Continued

TABLE 29   Comparison of Hyperglycemia and Hypoglycemia—cont'd

Hyperglycemia	Hypoglycemia
Preventive Measures	
• Take prescribed dose of medication at proper time.	• Take prescribed dose of medication at proper time.
• Accurately administer insulin, noninsulin injectables, and/or OAs.	• Accurately administer insulin, noninsulin injectables, OAs.
• Make healthy food choices.	• Coordinate eating with medications.
• Follow sick-day rules when ill.	• Eat adequate food intake needed for calories for exercise.
• Check blood glucose routinely.	• Be able to recognize and know symptoms and treat them immediately.
• Wear or carry diabetes identification.	• Carry simple carbohydrates.
	• Educate family and caregiver about symptoms and treatment.
	• Check blood glucose routinely.
	• Wear or carry diabetes identification.

DKA, Diabetic ketoacidosis; *HHS,* hyperosmolar hyperglycemic syndrome; *OAs,* oral agents.

*There is usually a gradual onset of symptoms in hyperglycemia and a more rapid onset in hypoglycemia. Many signs and symptoms of hyper- and hypoglycemia overlap. Signs and symptoms of hypoglycemia often change over time.

†Specific clinical manifestations related to elevated levels of blood glucose vary according to the patient.

Hyperosmolar Hyperglycemic Syndrome

Hyperosmolar hyperglycemic syndrome (HHS) is a life-threatening syndrome that can occur in the patient with DM who is able to produce enough insulin to prevent DKA but not enough to prevent severe hyperglycemia, osmotic diuresis, and extracellular fluid depletion.

- The main difference between HHS and DKA is that the patient with HHS usually has enough circulating insulin so that keto-acidosis does not occur. Because HHS produces fewer symptoms in the earlier stages, blood glucose levels can climb quite high before the problem is recognized. The higher blood glucose levels increase serum osmolality and produce more severe neurologic manifestations, such as somnolence, coma, seizures, hemiparesis, and aphasia.

- HHS is less common than DKA. It often occurs in patients greater than 60 years of age with type 2 diabetes. Common causes of HHS are urinary tract infections, pneumonia, sepsis, and any acute illness. HHS is more common among patients with newly diagnosed type 2 diabetes.
- Laboratory values include a blood glucose level above 600 mg/dL (33.33 mmol/L) and a marked increase in serum osmolality. Ketone bodies are absent or minimal in both blood and urine.

Hypoglycemia

Hypoglycemia, or low blood glucose, occurs when there is too much insulin in proportion to available glucose in the blood. This causes the blood glucose level to drop below 70 mg/dL. Manifestations include shakiness, palpitations, nervousness, diaphoresis, anxiety, hunger, and pallor. Untreated hypoglycemia can progress to loss of consciousness, seizures, coma, and death.

Chronic Complications

Chronic complications are primarily those of end-organ disease arising from damage to the blood vessels from chronic hyperglycemia. *Angiopathy,* or blood vessel disease, is one of the leading causes of diabetes-related deaths. These chronic blood vessel problems are divided into two categories: macrovascular complications and microvascular complications.

Macrovascular Complications

Macrovascular complications are diseases of the large and medium-sized blood vessels that occur with greater frequency and an earlier onset in people with diabetes. Risk factors associated with macrovascular complications, such as obesity, smoking, hypertension, high fat intake, and sedentary lifestyle, can be reduced. Insulin resistance appears to play a role in the development of cardiovascular disease and is implicated in the pathogenesis of essential hypertension and dyslipidemia.

Microvascular Complications

Microvascular complications result from thickening of the vessel membranes in the capillaries and arterioles in response to chronic hyperglycemia. Although microangiopathy can be found throughout the body, the areas most noticeably affected are the eyes (retinopathy), kidneys (nephropathy), and nerves (neuropathy).

Diabetic retinopathy is estimated to be the most common cause of new cases of adult blindness.

- In *nonproliferative retinopathy,* the most common form, partial occlusion of the small blood vessels in the retina causes microaneurysms to develop in the capillary walls. Capillary fluid leaks out, causing retinal edema and eventually hard exudates or intraretinal hemorrhages. Vision may be affected if the macula is involved.

- *Proliferative retinopathy* is more severe and involves the retina and vitreous. When retinal capillaries become occluded, new, fragile blood vessels are formed. Eventually light does not reach the retina as vessels tear and bleed. A tear or retinal detachment may then occur. If the macula is involved, vision is lost. Treatment involves laser photocoagulation.

Diabetic nephropathy is a microvascular complication associated with damage to the small blood vessels that supply the glomeruli of the kidney. It is the leading cause of end-stage renal disease in the United States. Tight blood glucose control is critical in the prevention and delay of diabetic nephropathy. Hypertension significantly accelerates the progression of nephropathy. Therefore aggressive BP management is indicated for all patients with diabetes. See Hypertension, p. 323.

- Patients with diabetes are screened for nephropathy annually with a random spot urine collection to assess for albuminuria and measure the albumin-to-creatinine ratio. Serum creatinine is also measured to provide an estimation of the glomerular filtration rate and thus the degree of kidney function.

Neuropathy is nerve damage that occurs because of the metabolic alterations associated with diabetes. About 60% to 70% of patients with diabetes have some degree of neuropathy. More than 60% of nontraumatic amputations in the United States are done for people with diabetes. Screening for neuropathy should begin at the time of diagnosis in patients with type 2 diabetes and 5 years after diagnosis in patients with type 1 diabetes.

Two major categories of diabetes-related neuropathy are *sensory neuropathy,* which affects the peripheral nervous system and is the more common type of neuropathy, and *autonomic neuropathy,* which can affect nearly all body systems.

- The most common form of sensory neuropathy is distal symmetric neuropathy, which affects the hands or feet bilaterally. Characteristics include loss of sensation, abnormal sensations, pain, and paresthesias. The pain, which is often described as burning, cramping, crushing, or tearing, is usually worse at night. The paresthesias may be associated with tingling, burning, and itching sensations.

- Autonomic neuropathy can lead to hypoglycemia unawareness, bowel incontinence and diarrhea, and urinary retention. Delayed gastric emptying *(gastroparesis),* a complication of autonomic neuropathy, can produce nausea, vomiting, gastroesophageal reflux, and persistent feelings of fullness. Cardiovascular abnormalities, such as postural hypotension, painless myocardial infarction, and resting tachycardia, can occur.

Control of blood glucose is the only treatment for diabetic neuropathy. It is effective in many but not all cases. Drug therapy may be used to treat neuropathic symptoms, particularly pain.

Diagnostic Studies

The diagnosis of diabetes can be made through one of the following four methods. In the absence of unequivocal hyperglycemia, criteria 1 to 3 should be confirmed by repeat testing.

1. A1C level of 6.5% or greater
2. Fasting plasma glucose (FPG) level at or above 126 mg/dL (7.0 mmol/L). *Fasting* is defined as no caloric intake for at least 8 hours.
3. Two-hour plasma glucose level at or above 200 mg/dL (11.1 mmol/L) during an OGTT, using a glucose load of 75 g
4. In a patient with classic symptoms of hyperglycemia (polyuria, polydipsia, unexplained weight loss) or hyperglycemic crisis, a random plasma glucose of at least 200 mg/dL (11.1 mmol/L)

Interprofessional Care

The goals of diabetes management are to reduce symptoms, promote well-being, prevent acute complications related to hypo- or hyperglycemia, and prevent or delay the onset and progression of long-term complications. Nutritional therapy, drug therapy, exercise, and self-monitoring of blood glucose are the tools used in the management of diabetes. The major types of glucose-lowering agents (GLAs) used in the treatment of diabetes are insulin and oral and noninsulin injectable agents. For a majority of patients, drug therapy is necessary.

Drug Therapy: Insulin

Exogenous (injected) insulin is needed when the patient has inadequate insulin to meet specific metabolic needs. People with type 1 diabetes require exogenous insulin to survive. People with type 2 diabetes usually controlled with diet, exercise, and/or OAs may require exogenous insulin during periods of severe stress, such as illness or surgery. When patients with type 2 diabetes cannot maintain satisfactory blood glucose levels, exogenous insulin is added to the management plan.

Human insulin is prepared using genetic engineering. The insulin is derived from common bacteria (e.g., *Escherichia coli*) or yeast cells using recombinant DNA technology. Insulins differ in their onset, peak action, and duration of effect and are categorized as rapid-acting, short-acting, intermediate-acting, and long-acting insulin.

Examples of insulin regimens ranging from one to four injections per day are presented in Table 48-4 in Lewis et al, *Medical-Surgical Nursing,* ed 10, p. 1127.

- The insulin regimen that most closely mimics endogenous insulin production is a basal-bolus regimen that uses rapid- and short-acting (bolus) insulin before meals and long-acting (basal) background insulin once or twice per day.

- In addition to mealtime insulin, people with type 1 diabetes must also use a long- or intermediate-acting (background) insulin to control blood glucose levels between meals and overnight.

- Combination insulin therapy involves the mixing of short- or rapid-acting insulin with intermediate-acting insulin to provide both mealtime and basal coverage with one injection. Premixed formulas are available for this regimen, but optimal blood glucose control is not as likely because there is less flexibility in dosing.

The steps in administering a subcutaneous insulin injection are outlined in Table 48-5 in Lewis et al, *Medical-Surgical Nursing,* ed 10, p. 1128.

Continuous subcutaneous insulin infusion can be administered through an insulin pump, a small battery-operated device that resembles a standard pager in size and appearance. Every 2 or 3 days the insertion site is changed. A major advantage of the pump is the potential for tight glucose control.

A rapid-acting inhaled insulin (Afrezza) is administered at the beginning of each meal or within 20 minutes after starting a meal. It is not a substitute for long-acting insulin.

Nursing Care Related to Insulin Therapy. Nursing responsibilities for the patient receiving insulin include proper administration, assessment of patient's response to insulin therapy, and teaching the patient about administration of, adjustment to, and side effects of insulin.

- Assess the patient who is new to insulin and evaluate his or her ability to manage insulin therapy safely. This includes the ability to understand the interaction of insulin, diet, and activity and to recognize and appropriately treat the symptoms of hypoglycemia.

- The patient or the caregiver also must be able to prepare and inject the insulin (see Table 48-5, Lewis et al, *Medical-Surgical Nursing,* ed 10, p. 1128). If the patient or caregiver lacks this ability, additional resources will be needed.

- Follow-up assessment of the patient who has been using insulin therapy includes inspection of insulin sites for *lipodystrophy* (atrophy of subcutaneous tissue) and other reactions, a review of the insulin preparation and injection technique, a history pertaining to the occurrence of hypoglycemic episodes, and assessment of the patient's method for handling hypoglycemic episodes.

Drug Therapy: Oral and Noninsulin Injectable Agents

Oral agents (OAs) and noninsulin injectable agents work to improve the mechanisms by which the body produces and uses insulin and glucose (Fig. 6). These drugs work on the three defects of type 2 diabetes: insulin resistance, decreased insulin production, and increased hepatic glucose production. These drugs may be used

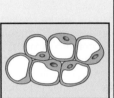
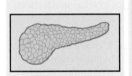

Pancreas

Sulfonylureas, meglitinides, DPP-4 inhibitors, and GLP-1 receptor agonists
↑ Insulin production

Adipose tissue   Muscle

Biguanides and thiazolidinediones
↑ Uptake and use of glucose
↓ Insulin resistance

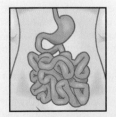
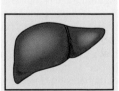
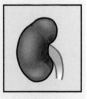

Stomach and small intestine

α-Glucosidase inhibitors
Delay absorption of starches
DPP-4 inhibitors
↑ Activity of incretins
GLP-1 receptor agonists and amylin
↓ Gastric emptying

Liver

Biguanides, thiazolidinediones, and DPP-4 inhibitors
↓ Hepatic glucose production

Kidney

SGLT inhibitors
↓ Glucose reabsorption

Fig. 6 Sites and methods of action of type 2 diabetes drugs. *DPP-4*, Dipeptidyl peptidase-4; *GLP-1*, glucagon-like peptide-1; *SGLT*, sodium-glucose co-transporter.

in combination with agents from other classes or with insulin to achieve blood glucose targets.

Many types of OAs and noninsulin injectable agents (Table 30) are used in the treatment of type 2 diabetes:

- *Biguanides* primarily reduce glucose production by the liver, but they also enhance insulin sensitivity and improve glucose transport into cells. Metformin is the most effective first-line treatment for type 2 diabetes. Forms of metformin include Glucophage (immediate-release), Glucophage XR (extended-release), Fortamet (extended-release), and Riomet (liquid form of metformin).

- *Sulfonylureas* increase insulin production by the pancreas and include glipizide (Glucotrol, Glucotrol XL), glyburide (DiaBeta, Glynase), and glimepiride (Amaryl).

- *Meglitinides* also increase insulin production from the pancreas, but they are more rapidly absorbed and eliminated than the sulfonylureas, decreasing the potential for hypoglycemia. Meglitinides include repaglinide (Prandin) and nateglinide (Starlix).

- *α-Glucosidase inhibitors* slow down the absorption of carbohydrate in the small intestine. Acarbose (Precose) and miglitol (Glyset) are the drugs in this class.

- *Thiazolidinediones* improve insulin sensitivity, transport, and utilization at target tissues. These agents include pioglitazone (Actos) and rosiglitazone (Avandia).

- *Dipeptidyl peptidase-4 (DDP) inhibitors* slow the inactivation of incretin hormones. Incretin hormones are released by the intestines throughout the day, but levels increase in response to a meal. This class of drugs includes sitagliptin (Januvia), linagliptin (Tradjenta), saxagliptin (Onglyza), and alogliptin (Nesina).

- The amylin analog class of drugs, synthetic analogs of human amylin (a hormone secreted by the β-cells of the pancreas), work to control diabetes by slowing gastric emptying, reducing postprandial glucagon secretion, and increasing satiety. The available drug in this class is pramlintide (Symlin), which must be administered subcutaneously and cannot be mixed in the same syringe as for insulin.

- *Glucagon-like peptide (GLP-1) receptor agonists* stimulate GLP-1 (one of the incretin hormones), which is decreased in type 2 diabetes. These drugs increase insulin synthesis and release from the pancreas, inhibit glucagon secretion, decrease gastric emptying, and reduce food intake by increasing satiety. These drugs are administered subcutaneously and may be used as monotherapy or adjunct therapy for patients with type 2 diabetes who have not achieved optimal glucose control on

TABLE 30 Drug Therapy

Oral Agents and Noninsulin Injectable Agents

Type/Agent	Mechanism of Action
Oral Agents	
Biguanides	
metformin (Glucophage, Glucophage XR, Riomet, Fortamet, Glumetza)	Decreases rate of hepatic glucose production Augments glucose uptake by tissues, especially muscles
Sulfonylureas	
glipizide (Glucotrol, Glucotrol XL) glyburide (DiaBeta, Glynase PresTab) glimepiride (Amaryl)	Stimulate release of insulin from pancreatic islets Decrease glycogenolysis and gluconeogenesis Enhance cellular sensitivity to insulin
Meglitinides	
nateglinide (Starlix) repaglinide (Prandin)	Stimulate a rapid and short-lived release of insulin from the pancreas
α-Glucosidase Inhibitors	
acarbose (Precose) miglitol (Glyset)	Delay absorption of complex carbohydrates (starches) from gastrointestinal tract
Thiazolidinediones	
pioglitazone (Actos) rosiglitazone (Avandia)	Increase glucose uptake in muscle Decrease endogenous glucose production
Dipeptidyl Peptidase-4 (DPP-4) Inhibitors	
linagliptin (Tradjenta) saxagliptin (Onglyza) sitagliptin (Januvia) alogliptin (Nesina)	Enhance activity of incretins Stimulate release of insulin from pancreatic β-cells Decrease hepatic glucose production

D

Continued

TABLE 30   Drug Therapy

Oral Agents and Noninsulin Injectable Agents—cont'd

Type/Agent	Mechanism of Action
Dopamine Receptor Agonists	
bromocriptine (Cycloset)	Activates dopamine receptors in central nervous system
	Unknown how it improves glycemic control
Sodium-Glucose Cotransporter 2 (SGLT2) Inhibitors	
canagliflozin (Invokana)	Decrease renal glucose reabsorption and increase urinary glucose excretion
dapagliflozin (Farxiga)	
empagliflozin (Jardiance)	
Combination Oral Therapy	
Glucovance	metformin and glyburide
Duetact	pioglitazone and glimepiride
Actoplus Met, Actoplus Met XR	metformin and pioglitazone
Janumet, Janumet XR	metformin and sitagliptin
Jentadueto	linagliptin and metformin
PrandiMet	metformin and repaglinide
Kombiglyze	saxagliptin and metformin
Kazano	alogliptin and metformin
Oseni	alogliptin and pioglitazone
Glyxambi	empagliflozin and linagliptin
Xigduo	dapagliflozin and metformin
Noninsulin Injectable Agents	
Glucagon-Like Peptide-1 (GLP-1) Receptor Agonists*	
exenatide (Byetta)	Stimulate release of insulin, decrease glucagon secretion, and slow gastric emptying
exenatide extended-release (Bydureon)	
liraglutide (Victoza)	
albiglutide (Tanzeum)	Increase satiety
dulaglutide (Trulicity)	
Amylin Analogs†	
pramlintide (Symlin)	Slows gastric emptying, decreases glucagon secretion and endogenous glucose output from liver
	Increases satiety

*Administered subcutaneously.
†Administered subcutaneously only in abdomen or thigh.

OAs. Drugs in this class include exenatide (Byetta), exenatide extended-release (Bydureon), liraglutide (Victoza), albiglutide (Tanzeum), and dulaglutide (Trulicity).

- *Sodium-glucose co-transporter 2 (SGLT2) inhibitors* work by blocking the reabsorption of glucose by the kidney, increasing glucose excretion, and lowering blood glucose levels. Drugs in this class include canagliflozin (Invokana),dapagliflozin (Farxiga), and empagliflozin (Jardiance).

Nursing Care Related to Oral and Noninsulin Injectable Agents. Your responsibilities for the patient taking oral and noninsulin injectable agents are similar to those for the patient taking insulin. Proper administration, assessment of the patient's use of and response to these drugs, and teaching the patient and family are all essential nursing actions.

- Your assessment is valuable in determining the most appropriate drug for a patient. This includes assessing the patient's mental status, eating habits, home environment, attitude toward diabetes, and medication history.
- Teach the importance of diet and activity plans.

Nutritional Therapy

Nutritional therapy is a cornerstone of diabetes care. Guidelines from the American Diabetes Association (ADA) indicate that within the context of an overall healthy eating plan, a person with DM can eat the same foods as a person who does not have diabetes. This means that the same principles of good nutrition that apply to the general population also apply to people with diabetes. See Table 48-8, which describes nutritional therapy for patients with diabetes, Lewis et al, *Medical-Surgical Nursing*, ed 10, p. 1133.

- *Type 1 diabetes:* People with type 1 diabetes base their meal planning on usual food intake and preferences balanced with insulin and exercise patterns. Day-to-day consistency in timing and amount of food eaten makes it much easier to manage blood glucose levels, especially for those individuals using conventional, fixed insulin regimens. Rapid-acting insulin doses can be adjusted before the meal depending on current blood glucose level and the carbohydrate content of the meal. Multiple daily injections or the use of an insulin pump allows considerable flexibility in food selection, and regimens can be adjusted for variations in eating and exercise habits.
- *Type 2 diabetes:* Nutritional therapy in type 2 diabetes should emphasize achieving glucose, lipid, and BP goals. Modest weight loss has been associated with improved insulin resistance and blood glucose control.

Most often, a dietitian initially teaches the principles of the nutritional therapy regimen as part of an interprofessional diabetes care team. When patients do not have access to a dietitian, you may need to assume responsibility for teaching basic dietary management to patients with diabetes.

Exercise

Regular, consistent exercise is an essential part of diabetes and prediabetes management. The ADA recommends that people with diabetes engage in at least 150 minutes weekly (30 minutes, 5 days/wk) of a moderate-intensity aerobic physical activity. Encourage people with type 2 diabetes to perform resistance training three times a week in the absence of contraindications.

Exercise decreases insulin resistance and can have a direct effect on lowering blood glucose levels. It also contributes to weight loss, which further decreases insulin resistance, and in addition it may help reduce triglyceride and low-density lipoprotein (LDL) cholesterol levels, increase high-density lipoprotein (HDL), reduce BP, and improve circulation. Additional information is provided in the patient and caregiver teaching guide (see Table 48-10, Lewis et al, *Medical-Surgical Nursing,* ed 10, p. 1134).

Blood Glucose Monitoring

Self-monitoring of blood glucose is a critical part of diabetes management. By providing a current blood glucose reading, self-monitoring enables the patient to make decisions regarding food intake, activity patterns, and medication dosages.

Because incorrect monitoring technique can cause errors in management strategies, comprehensive patient teaching is essential. Initial instruction should be followed up with regular reassessment. Table 48-11 in Lewis et al, *Medical-Surgical Nursing,* ed 10, p. 1136, presents instructions for teaching the patient to perform self-monitoring of blood glucose.

Management of Acute Complications

Diabetic Ketoacidosis

DKA may be managed on an outpatient basis if fluid and electrolyte imbalances are not severe and blood glucose levels can be safely monitored at home. Emergency management of the DKA is needed when fluid imbalance is potentially life-threatening. The initial goal of therapy is to establish IV access and begin fluid and electrolyte replacement. The aim of fluid and electrolyte therapy is to replace extracellular and intracellular water and to correct deficits of sodium, chloride, bicarbonate, potassium, phosphate, magnesium, and nitrogen.

- IV insulin administration is directed toward correcting hyperglycemia and hyperketonemia. Insulin is immediately started by a continuous infusion.

Hyperosmolar Hyperglycemic Syndrome
HHS constitutes a medical emergency with a high mortality rate. Therapy is similar to that for DKA except that HHS requires more fluid replacement.
- Insulin is given immediately by IV infusion.
- Electrolytes are monitored and replaced as needed. Assess vital signs, intake and output, tissue turgor, laboratory values, and cardiac monitoring to monitor the efficacy of fluid and electrolyte replacement.

Hypoglycemia
At the first sign of hypoglycemia, check the blood glucose if possible. If it is below 70 mg/dL (3.9 mmol/L), immediately begin treatment for hypoglycemia. If the patient has manifestations of hypoglycemia and monitoring equipment is not available, or if the patient has a history of chronic poor glucose control, hypoglycemia should be assumed and treatment initiated.
- Hypoglycemia is treated by ingesting 15 g of a simple (fast-acting) carbohydrate, such as 4 to 6 ounces of fruit juice or regular soft drink. Avoid overtreatment with large quantities of quick-acting carbohydrates, such as candy bars, so that a rapid fluctuation to hyperglycemia does not occur.
- Recheck the blood glucose 15 minutes later. If the value is still below 70 mg/dL, have the patient ingest 15 g more of carbohydrate and recheck the blood glucose in 15 minutes. Because of the potential for rebound hypoglycemia after an acute episode, have the patient ingest a complex carbohydrate after recovery to prevent another hypoglycemic attack.
- If no significant improvement occurs after two or three doses of 15 g of simple carbohydrate, contact the health care provider.

Once acute hypoglycemia has been reversed, you should explore with the patient the reasons for why the situation developed. This assessment may indicate a need for additional teaching of the patient and caregiver to avoid future episodes of hypoglycemia.

Nursing Management
Goals
The patient with diabetes will engage in self-care behaviors to actively manage his or her diabetes, experience few or no episodes of acute hyperglycemic or hypoglycemic emergencies, maintain blood glucose levels at normal or near-normal levels, prevent or minimize chronic complications of diabetes, and adjust lifestyle to accommodate the diabetes regimen with a minimum of stress.

Nursing Diagnoses
- Ineffective health management
- Risk for unstable blood glucose levels

- Risk for injury
- Risk for peripheral neurovascular dysfunction

Nursing Interventions

Your role in health promotion is to identify, monitor, and teach the patient at risk for diabetes.

Management of Acute Illness and Surgery. Emotional and physical stress can increase blood glucose levels and result in hyperglycemia. Acute illness, injury, and surgery are situations that may evoke a counterregulatory hormone response resulting in hyperglycemia. When patients with diabetes are ill, they should check blood glucose at least every 4 hours. An acutely ill patient with type 1 diabetes with a blood glucose level above 240 mg/dL (13.3 mmol/L) should test the urine for ketones every 3 to 4 hours.

- Patients should report to the HCP when glucose levels are above 300 mg/dL for two tests in a row or urine ketone levels are moderate to high.
- If patients are able to eat normally, they should continue with the regular meal plan while increasing the intake of noncaloric fluids, such as broth, water, dietary gelatin, and other decaffeinated beverages, and continue taking oral agents and insulin as prescribed.
- If illness causes the patient to eat less than normal, drug therapy should be continued as prescribed while supplementing food intake with carbohydrate-containing fluids. Notify the HCP if the patient is unable to keep down fluid or food.
- Adjustments in the diabetes regimen during the intraoperative period can be planned to ensure glycemic control. The patient is given IV fluids and insulin (if needed) immediately before, during, and after surgery when there is no oral intake.
- When caring for an unconscious surgical patient receiving insulin, be alert for hypoglycemic signs, such as sweating, tachycardia, and tremors.

Ambulatory Care. Successful management of diabetes requires ongoing interaction among the patient, family, and interprofessional health care team. It is important that a certified diabetes educator be involved in the care of the patient and family.

Individuals with diabetes must continually face lifestyle choices that affect the food they eat, their activities, and demands on their time and energy. In addition, they face the challenge of preventing or dealing with the devastating complications of diabetes. Careful assessment of what it means to have diabetes is the starting point of patient teaching.

The potential for infection requires diligent skin care and dental hygiene. Routine care includes toothbrushing and flossing and regular bathing, with particular emphasis on foot care. Skin injuries should be treated promptly and monitored carefully. If the injury does not begin to heal within 24 hours or signs of infection develop, the HCP should be notified immediately.

▼ **Patient and Caregiver Teaching**

The goals of diabetes self-management education are to match the level of self-management to the patient's individual ability so that he or she can become the most active participant possible. Patients who actively manage their diabetes care have better outcomes than those who do not. Guidelines for patient and caregiver teaching for management of diabetes are listed in Table 31.

Assess the patient's knowledge base frequently so that gaps in knowledge or incorrect or inaccurate ideas can be quickly corrected.

- Instruct the patient to carry medical identification at all times indicating that he or she has diabetes. An identification card can supply valuable information, such as the name of the health care provider and the type and dose of insulin or other drug therapy.

D

TABLE 31	Patient & Caregiver Teaching

Management of Diabetes Mellitus

Include the following instructions when teaching the patient and caregiver how to manage diabetes mellitus.

Component	What to Teach
Disease process	• Include an introduction about the pancreas and the islets of Langerhans. • Describe how insulin is made and what affects its production. • Discuss the relationship of insulin and glucose. • Explain the differences between type 1 and type 2 diabetes.
Physical activity	• Discuss the effect of regular exercise on the management of blood glucose, improvement of cardiovascular function, and general health.
Menu planning	• Stress the importance of a well-balanced diet as part of a diabetes management plan. • Explain the impact of carbohydrates on blood glucose levels.

Continued

TABLE 31 Patient & Caregiver Teaching

Management of Diabetes Mellitus—cont'd

Medication	• Ensure that the patient understands the proper use of prescribed medication (e.g., insulin [Table 48-4, Lewis et al, *Medical-Surgical Nursing*, ed 10, p. 1127], OAs, and noninsulin injectables [Table 30, pp. 181-182]). • Account for a patient's physical limitations or inabilities for self-medication. If necessary, involve the family or the caregiver in proper use of medication. • Discuss all side effects and safety issues regarding medication.
Monitoring blood glucose	• Teach correct blood glucose monitoring. • Include when to check blood glucose levels, how to record them, and how to adjust insulin levels if necessary.
Risk reduction	• Ensure that the patient understands and appropriately responds to the signs and symptoms of hypoglycemia and hyperglycemia (see Table 48-16, Lewis et al, *Medical-Surgical Nursing*, ed 10, p. 1143). • Stress the importance of proper foot care (see Table 48-21, Lewis et al, *Medical-Surgical Nursing*, ed 10, p. 1151), regular eye examinations, and consistent glucose monitoring. • Inform the patient about the effect that stress can have on blood glucose.
Psychosocial	• Help the patient identify resources that are available to facilitate the adjustment and answer questions about living with a chronic condition such as diabetes.

OAs, Oral agents.

DIARRHEA

Description

Diarrhea is the passage of at least three loose or liquid stools per day. It may be acute, or it may be considered chronic if it lasts longer than 30 days.

Pathophysiology

The primary cause of acute diarrhea is ingesting infectious organisms. Viruses cause most cases of infectious diarrhea in the United States. Bacterial infections are also common. *Escherichia coli* O157:H7 is the most common cause of bloody diarrhea in the United States. It is transmitted by undercooked beef or chicken contaminated with the bacteria or by fruits and vegetables exposed to contaminated manure. *Giardia lamblia* is the most common intestinal parasite that causes diarrhea in the United States.

Infectious organisms attack the intestines in different ways. Some organisms (e.g., *Rotavirus, Norovirus, G. lamblia*) alter secretion and/or absorption of the enterocytes of the small intestine without causing inflammation. Other organisms (e.g., *Clostridium difficile*) impair absorption by destroying cells and producing inflammation in the colon.

Patients receiving broad-spectrum antibiotics (e.g., clindamycin [Cleocin], cephalosporins, or fluoroquinolones) are susceptible to infections with pathogenic strains of *C. difficile*. Probiotics—in particular, *Saccharomyces boulardii* and *Lactobacillus*—may be helpful in preventing antibiotic-induced diarrhea in some patients.

Diarrhea is not always due to infection. Drugs and specific food intolerances can also cause diarrhea.

Clinical Manifestations

Infections that attack the upper GI tract (e.g., *Norovirus* organisms, *G. lamblia*) usually produce large-volume, watery stools; cramping; and periumbilical pain. Patients have either a low-grade or no fever and often experience nausea and vomiting before the diarrhea begins.

Infections of the colon and distal small bowel (e.g., *Shigella* or *Salmonella* organisms or *C. difficile*) produce fever and frequent bloody diarrhea with a small volume. Leukocytes, blood, and mucus may be present in the stool.

Severe diarrhea produces life-threatening dehydration, electrolyte disturbances (e.g., hypokalemia), and acid-base imbalances (metabolic acidosis). *C. difficile* infection (CDI) can progress to fulminant colitis and intestinal perforation.

Diagnostic Studies

Because most cases of diarrhea resolve quickly, stool cultures are only indicated for patients who are very ill, have a significant fever, or have had diarrhea longer than 3 days.

- Stools are examined for blood, mucus, white blood cells (WBCs), and parasites, and cultures are done to identify infectious organisms.

- CDI is detected by enzyme immunoassay (EIA).
- In a patient with chronic diarrhea, measurement of stool electrolytes, pH, and osmolality may help determine whether diarrhea is related to decreased fluid absorption or increased fluid secretion.
- Measurement of stool fat and undigested muscle fibers may indicate fat and protein malabsorption conditions, including pancreatic insufficiency.

Interprofessional Care

Treatment depends on the cause. Foods and drugs that cause diarrhea should be avoided. Acute infectious diarrhea is usually self-limiting. The major concerns are preventing transmission, replacing fluid and electrolytes, and protecting the skin. Oral solutions containing glucose and electrolytes (e.g., Gatorade, Pedialyte) may be sufficient to replace losses from mild diarrhea. In severe diarrhea, parenteral administration of fluids, electrolytes, vitamins, and nutrition may be necessary.

Antidiarrheal agents may be given to coat and protect mucous membranes, absorb irritating substances, inhibit GI motility, decrease intestinal secretions, or decrease central nervous system (CNS) stimulation to the GI tract. Antidiarrheal agents are contraindicated in the treatment of infectious diarrhea because they potentially prolong exposure to the organism.

- Antidiarrheal agents are contraindicated in the treatment of some infectious diarrheas because they potentially prolong exposure to the infectious agent. They are used cautiously in inflammatory bowel disease because of the danger of *toxic megacolon* (colonic dilation to greater than 5 cm).
- Regardless of the cause, antidiarrheal medications should be given only for a short period. Antibiotics are rarely used to treat infectious diarrhea.

CDI is a particularly hazardous health care–associated infection (HAI). Its spores can survive for up to 70 days on objects including commodes, telephones, thermometers, bedside tables, and floors. CDI can be transmitted from patient to patient by health care workers who do not adhere to infection control precautions.

- The infection is usually treated by stopping nonessential antibiotics and administering metronidazole (Flagyl) or vancomycin (Vancocin).

Nursing Management: Acute Infectious Diarrhea

Goals

The patient with infectious diarrhea will have no transmission of the microorganism causing the diarrhea, cessation of diarrhea and resumption of normal bowel patterns, normal fluid and electrolyte and acid-base balance, normal nutritional status, and no perianal skin breakdown.

Nursing Diagnoses
- Diarrhea
- Deficient fluid volume

Nursing Interventions
Consider all cases of acute diarrhea to be infectious until the cause is known.
- Strict infection control precautions are necessary to prevent the illness from spreading to others. Wash your hands before and after contact with each patient and when handling any body fluids.
- Provide private rooms for patients with CDI and ensure that visitors and HCPs wear gloves and gowns.

▼ **Patient and Caregiver Teaching**
- Teach the patient and caregiver the principles of hygiene, infection control precautions, and potential dangers of an illness that is infectious to themselves and others.
- Discuss proper food handling, cooking, and storage.

DISSEMINATED INTRAVASCULAR COAGULATION

Description
Disseminated intravascular coagulation (DIC) is a serious bleeding and thrombotic disorder that results from abnormally initiated and accelerated clotting. Subsequent decreases in clotting factors and platelets may lead to uncontrollable hemorrhage. The term *DIC* can be misleading because it only suggests that blood is clotting. However, DIC is characterized by profuse bleeding resulting from depletion of platelets and clotting factors.

Pathophysiology
DIC is an abnormal response of the normal clotting cascade stimulated by a disease process or disorder. The diseases and disorders known to predispose patients to acute DIC are major physiologic assaults and include shock, septicemia, abruptio placentae, malignancies, severe head injury, heatstroke, and pulmonary emboli. The underlying disease must be treated for DIC to resolve.
- DIC can occur as an acute, catastrophic condition, or it may exist at a subacute or chronic level. Each condition may have one or multiple triggering mechanisms to start the clotting cascade.

Tissue factor is released at the site of tissue injury and by some malignancies, such as leukemia, and enhances normal coagulation mechanisms. Abundant intravascular thrombin, the most powerful coagulant, is produced. It catalyzes the conversion of fibrinogen to fibrin and enhances platelet aggregation. There is widespread fibrin and platelet deposition in capillaries and arterioles, resulting in thrombosis. Excessive clotting activates the fibrinolytic system, which in turn breaks down newly formed clots, creating fibrin-split (fibrin-degradation) products (FSPs), which inhibit normal blood clotting. Ultimately the blood loses its ability to form a stable clot at injury sites, which predisposes the patient to hemorrhage.

- Chronic and subacute DIC is most commonly seen in patients with long-standing illnesses such as malignant disorders or autoimmune diseases. Occasionally these patients have subclinical disease manifested only by laboratory abnormalities.

Clinical Manifestations

Bleeding in a person with no previous history or obvious cause should be investigated further because it may be one of the first manifestations of acute DIC. Other nonspecific manifestations include weakness, malaise, and fever. There are both bleeding and thrombotic manifestations in DIC (Fig. 7).

- *Bleeding manifestations* include petechiae, oozing blood, tachypnea, hemoptysis, tachycardia, hypotension, bloody stools, hematuria, dizziness, headache, changes in mental status, and bone and joint pain.
- *Thrombotic manifestations* are a result of fibrin or platelet deposition in the microvasculature. Manifestations include ischemic tissue necrosis (e.g., gangrene), acute respiratory distress syndrome (ARDS), cardiovascular and ECG changes, kidney damage, and paralytic ileus.

Diagnostic Studies

For comparison of laboratory results in DIC with other types of thrombocytopenia, see Table 30-12, Lewis et al, *Medical-Surgical Nursing,* ed 10, p. 623.

Diagnostic findings include:

- Prolonged prothrombin time and partial thromboplastin time
- Prolonged activated partial thromboplastin time and thrombin time
- Reduced fibrinogen, antithrombin III (AT III), and platelets
- Elevated FSPs and elevated D-dimers (cross-linked fibrin fragments)
- Reduced levels of factors V, VII, VIII, X, and XIII

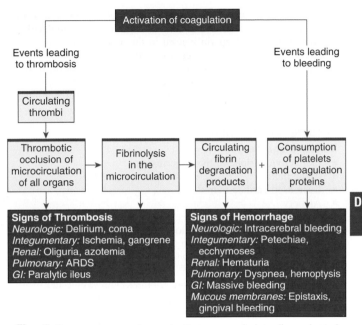

Fig. 7 The sequence of events that occur during disseminated intravascular coagulation (DIC).

Interprofessional Care

It is important to diagnose DIC quickly, stabilize the patient if needed (e.g., with oxygenation or volume replacement), treat the underlying causative disease or problem, and control the ongoing thrombosis and bleeding. Depending on its severity, a variety of different methods are used to manage DIC.

- If chronic DIC is diagnosed in a patient who is not bleeding, no therapy for DIC is necessary. Treatment of the underlying disease may be sufficient to reverse DIC (e.g., chemotherapy when DIC is caused by malignancy).
- When the patient with DIC is bleeding, therapy is directed toward providing support with necessary blood products while treating the primary disorder. Blood product support is usually reserved to stabilize the patient with life-threatening hemorrhage. Platelets are given to correct thrombocytopenia, and cryoprecipitate replaces factor VIII and fibrinogen. Fresh frozen plasma (FFP) replaces all clotting factors except platelets and provides a source of antithrombin.

- A patient with manifestations of thrombosis is often treated by anticoagulation with unfractionated heparin or low-molecular-weight heparin. Heparin is used in the treatment of DIC only when the benefit (reducing clotting) outweighs the risk of bleeding. Antithrombin III (AT III) (ATnativ) may be useful in fulminant DIC, although it increases the risk of bleeding.
- Chronic DIC does not respond to oral anticoagulants, but it can be controlled with long-term use of heparin.

Nursing Management

Nursing Diagnoses
- Ineffective peripheral tissue perfusion
- Acute pain
- Decreased cardiac output
- Anxiety

Nursing Interventions
Be alert to the possible development of DIC. Remember that because DIC is secondary to an underlying disease, the causative problem needs to be managed while providing supportive care for the manifestations of DIC.
- Early detection of bleeding and clotting, both occult and overt, must be a primary goal. Assess for signs of external bleeding (e.g., petechiae, oozing at IV or injection sites) and internal bleeding (e.g., changes in mental status, increasing abdominal girth, pain) and any indications that microthrombi may be causing clinically significant organ damage (e.g., decreased renal output).
- Minimize tissue damage and protect the patient from additional bleeding.
- Administer blood products and medications correctly.

DIVERTICULOSIS/DIVERTICULITIS

Description
Diverticula are saccular dilations or outpouchings of the mucosa that develop in the colon. Diverticulosis is the presence of multiple noninflamed diverticula. Diverticulitis is inflammation of one or more diverticula, resulting in perforation into the peritoneum. Clinically, diverticular disease covers a spectrum from asymptomatic, uncomplicated diverticulosis to diverticulitis with complications such as perforation, abscess, fistula, and bleeding.
- Diverticula are common, especially in older adults, but they seldom progress to diverticulitis.
- The disease is more prevalent in populations with diets low in fiber and high in refined carbohydrates. Diverticula are uncommon in vegetarians.

- Other risk factors for development of diverticula are obesity, inactivity, smoking, excessive alcohol use, and immunosuppression.

Pathophysiology

Diverticula may occur anywhere in the gastrointestinal (GI) tract but are most commonly found in the left (descending, sigmoid) colon. The etiology of diverticulosis of the sigmoid colon is thought to be associated with high intraluminal pressures from a deficiency in dietary fiber intake.

Inadequate dietary fiber slows transit time, allowing more water to be absorbed from the stool. Decreased stool size increases intraluminal pressure, thereby promoting diverticula formation.

Clinical Manifestations and Complications

Most patients with diverticulosis have no symptoms. Those with symptoms typically have abdominal pain, bloating, flatulence, or changes in bowel habits but no symptoms of inflammation.

The most common signs and symptoms of diverticulitis include acute pain in the left lower quadrant (location of sigmoid colon), a palpable abdominal mass, nausea, vomiting, and evidence of systemic infection (fever, increased C-reactive protein, and leukocytosis with a shift to the left). Older patients with diverticulitis may be afebrile, with a normal WBC count and little, if any, abdominal tenderness.

The diverticula may bleed, or diverticulitis can develop. Diverticulitis is characterized by inflamed diverticula and increased luminal pressures that cause erosion of the bowel wall and perforation into the peritoneum. A localized abscess develops when the body is able to wall off the area of perforation. Peritonitis develops if it cannot be contained. Bleeding can be extensive but usually stops spontaneously.

Diagnostic Studies

- History and physical examination
- Abdominal and chest x-rays to rule out other causes of acute abdominal pain
- CT scan with contrast to confirm the diagnosis

Interprofessional Care

A high-fiber diet, mainly from fruits and vegetables, and decreased intake of fat and red meat are the best ways to prevent diverticular disease. High levels of physical activity may decrease the risk. A high-fiber diet is also recommended once diverticular disease is present. Weight reduction is important for the obese person.

In acute diverticulitis, the goal of treatment is to allow the colon to rest and the inflammation to subside. Some patients can be managed at home with oral antibiotics and a clear liquid diet. Hospitalization is necessary if symptoms are severe, the patient is unable to tolerate oral fluids, or the patient has comorbid diseases.

Surgery is reserved for patients with frequently recurring diverticulitis or complications, such as an abscess or obstruction that cannot be managed medically. The usual surgical procedures involve resection of the involved colon, with a primary anastomosis if adequate bowel cleansing is feasible or a temporary diverting colostomy with later reanastomosis of the colon.

Nursing Management

Teach patients with diverticular disease to avoid increased intraabdominal pressure because it may precipitate an attack.

- Factors that increase intraabdominal pressure are straining at stool, vomiting, bending, lifting, and wearing tight, restrictive clothing.
- When the acute attack subsides, give oral fluids first and then progress the diet to semisolids. Ambulation is allowed.
- Provide the patient with a full explanation of the condition. Patients who understand the disease process well and adhere to the prescribed regimen are less likely to experience an exacerbation of the disease and its complications.
- Weight reduction is important for the obese person with diverticular disease.

DYSMENORRHEA

Description

Dysmenorrhea is painful menses with abdominal cramping. The degree of pain and discomfort varies. The two types of dysmenorrhea are primary (no pathologic condition exists) and secondary (pelvic disease is the underlying cause). Dysmenorrhea is one of the most common gynecologic problems.

Pathophysiology

Primary dysmenorrhea begins in the first few years after menarche, typically with the onset of regular menstrual cycles. It is usually related to elevated levels of prostaglandin, a hormone that is found in the endometrium.

- Stimulation of the endometrium by estrogen and progesterone increases prostaglandin production. Prostaglandin stimulates the uterus to contract. Uterine contractions and constriction of small endometrial blood vessels cause tissue ischemia and sensitize pain receptors, resulting in painful menstrual cramps. As menstruation continues, prostaglandin levels decrease each day and cramping lessens.

Secondary dysmenorrhea usually occurs after adolescence, most commonly at 30 to 40 years of age, and worsens as the woman ages. Common pelvic conditions that cause secondary dysmenorrhea include endometriosis, chronic pelvic inflammatory disease, and uterine leiomyomas (fibroids).

Clinical Manifestations

In *primary dysmenorrhea,* symptoms start 12 to 24 hours before the onset of menses. The pain is most severe the first day of menses and rarely lasts more than 2 days.

- Characteristic manifestations include lower abdominal cramping pain that is colicky in nature, frequently radiating to the lower back and upper thighs. The abdominal pain is often accompanied by nausea, diarrhea, loose stools, fatigue, and headache.

In *secondary dysmenorrhea,* usually the woman previously had little to no pain during the menstrual cycle. The pain, which may be unilateral, is generally more constant in nature and continues for a longer time than with primary dysmenorrhea.

- Depending on the cause, signs and symptoms such as *dyspareunia* (painful intercourse), painful defecation, or irregular bleeding may occur at times other than menstruation.

Diagnostic Studies

Evaluation begins with a complete health history and a pelvic examination.

- If the pelvic examination is normal and the history reveals an onset shortly after menarche with symptoms only associated with menses, the probable diagnosis is primary dysmenorrhea.
- If a specific cause is evident, the diagnosis is secondary dysmenorrhea.

Interprofessional Care

Treatment for primary dysmenorrhea includes heat applied to the lower abdomen or back, exercise, and drug therapy. Regular exercise may reduce endometrial hyperplasia and subsequent prostaglandin production. Nonsteroidal antiinflammatory drugs (NSAIDs) (e.g., naproxen [Naprosyn]) inhibit prostaglandins. Oral contraceptives may also be used to decrease estrogen and progesterone, lower prostaglandin levels, decrease monthly endometrial lining proliferation, and decrease menstrual flow.

Nursing Management
- Teach the patient that applying heat to the abdomen or back and taking NSAIDs may relieve acute pain.
- Suggest noninvasive pain-relieving practices such as relaxation breathing, guided imagery, and yoga.
- Other measures to reduce the discomfort of dysmenorrhea include regular exercise and good nutrition.

DYSRHYTHMIAS

Description
Dysrhythmias are abnormal cardiac rhythms. Prompt assessment of abnormal cardiac rhythms and the patient's response to the rhythm is critical. Dysrhythmias result from disorders of impulse formation, conduction of impulses, or both.

A pacemaker from a site other than the sinoatrial (SA) node may be fired in two ways.
- If the SA node fires more slowly than a secondary pacemaker, electrical discharges from the secondary pacemaker may passively "escape" and fire automatically at its intrinsic rate. Secondary pacemakers can also originate when they fire more rapidly than the normal pacemaker of the SA node.
- *Triggered beats* (early or late) may come from an *ectopic focus* (area outside the normal conduction pathway) in the atria, atrioventricular (AV) node, or ventricles. This results in a dysrhythmia, which replaces the normal sinus rhythm.

Dysrhythmias occur as the result of various abnormalities and disease states. The cause of a dysrhythmia influences the patient's treatment. Common causes of dysrhythmias are presented in Table 32. Table 33 presents a systematic approach to assessing a cardiac rhythm.

Types of Dysrhythmias
The characteristics of common dysrhythmias are described in Part Three (Reference Appendix) on pp. 761-762. Examples of ECG tracings of common dysrhythmias are presented in Figs. 35-11 to 35-19, Lewis et al, *Medical-Surgical Nursing,* ed 10, pp. 763 to 770.

Sinus Bradycardia
Sinus bradycardia occurs when the SA node discharges at a rate less than 60 beats/minute. It may be a normal rhythm in aerobically trained athletes or in some people during sleep. It also occurs in response to carotid sinus massage, Valsalva maneuver, hypothermia, increased intraocular pressure, vagal stimulation, and the administration of certain drugs (e.g., β-adrenergic blockers,

TABLE 32   Common Causes of Dysrhythmias*

Heart Conditions
- Accessory pathways
- Cardiomyopathy
- Conduction defects
- Heart failure
- Myocardial ischemia, infarction
- Valve disease

Other Conditions
- Acid-base imbalances
- Alcohol
- Caffeine, tobacco
- Connective tissue disorders
- Drug effects (e.g., antidysrhythmia drugs, stimulants, β-adrenergic blockers) or toxicity
- Electric shock
- Electrolyte imbalances (e.g., hyperkalemia, hypocalcemia)
- Emotional crisis
- Herbal supplements (e.g., areca nut, wahoo root bark, yerba maté)
- Hypoxia
- Metabolic conditions (e.g., thyroid dysfunction)
- Near-drowning
- Sepsis, shock
- Toxins

*List is not all-inclusive.

calcium channel blockers). Disease states associated with sinus bradycardia are hypothyroidism, increased intracranial pressure, hypoglycemia, and inferior wall myocardial infarction (MI).

- Clinical significance depends on how the patient tolerates the dysrhythmia. Signs of symptomatic bradycardia include pale, cool skin; hypotension; weakness; angina; dizziness or syncope, confusion, or disorientation; and shortness of breath.
- Treatment consists of administration of atropine for patients with symptoms. Pacemaker therapy may be required. If caused by drugs, these may need to be held or discontinued, or given in reduced dosages.

Sinus Tachycardia

Sinus tachycardia involves a heart rate (HR) of 101 to 200 beats/minute from the SA node, occurring as a result of vagal inhibition or sympathetic stimulation. This dysrhythmia is associated with physiologic and psychologic stressors, such as exercise, fever, pain,

---

TABLE 33 Approach to Assessing Heart Rhythm

When assessing a heart rhythm, use a consistent and systematic approach. One such approach includes the following:

1. Look for the P wave. Is it upright or inverted? Is there one for every QRS complex or more than one? Are atrial fibrillatory or flutter waves present?
2. Evaluate the atrial rhythm. Is it regular or irregular?
3. Calculate the atrial rate.
4. Measure the duration of the PR interval. Is it normal duration or prolonged? Is it consistent in its duration before each QRS?
5. Evaluate the ventricular rhythm. Is it regular or irregular?
6. Calculate the ventricular rate.
7. Measure the duration of the QRS complex. Is it of normal duration or prolonged?
8. Assess the ST segment. Is it isoelectric (flat), elevated, or depressed?
9. Measure the duration of the QT interval. Correct for heart rate (cQT) to determine if it is normal or prolonged.*
10. Note the T wave. Is it upright or inverted?

Additional questions to consider include the following:

1. What is the dominant or underlying rhythm and/or dysrhythmia?
2. What is the clinical significance of your findings?
3. What is the treatment for the particular rhythm?

A website for calculating the cQT interval for heart rate is available (www.mdcalc.com/corrected-qt-interval-qtc).

hypotension, hypovolemia, anemia, hypoglycemia, myocardial ischemia, heart failure (HF), hyperthyroidism, and anxiety. It can also be an effect of drugs such as epinephrine, norepinephrine, caffeine, theophylline, nifedipine (Procardia), or hydralazine. Pseudoephedrine (Sudafed), which is found in many over-the-counter cold remedies, can also cause tachycardia.

- Clinical significance depends on the patient's tolerance of the increased HR. The patient may experience dizziness, dyspnea, and hypotension. Angina or an increase in infarct size may accompany sinus tachycardia in the patient with an acute MI.
- Treatment is based on the underlying cause. For example, if the patient is experiencing tachycardia from pain, effective pain management is important to treat the tachycardia. In patients who are clinically stable, vagal maneuvers can be attempted. In addition, IV β- blockers (e.g., metoprolol [Lopressor]), adenosine (Adenocard), or calcium channel blockers (e.g., diltiazem [Cardizem]) can be given to reduce HR and decrease

myocardial oxygen consumption. In clinically unstable patients, synchronized cardioversion is used.

Premature Atrial Contraction

Premature atrial contraction (PAC) is a contraction starting from an ectopic focus in the atrium (in a location other than the SA node) sooner than the next expected sinus beat. The ectopic focus starts in the left or right atrium and travels across the atria by an abnormal pathway, creating a distorted P wave. At the AV node it may be stopped (nonconducted PAC), delayed (lengthened PR interval), or conducted normally. If the impulse moves through the AV node, in most cases it is conducted normally through the ventricles.

In a normal heart, a PAC can result from emotional stress or physical fatigue or from the use of caffeine, tobacco, or alcohol. PACs can also result from hypoxia, electrolyte imbalances, and disease states such as hyperthyroidism, chronic obstructive pulmonary disease (COPD), and heart disease, including coronary artery disease (CAD) and valvular heart disease.

- HR varies with the underlying rate and frequency of PACs, and the rhythm is irregular.
- Isolated PACs are not significant in people with healthy hearts. In people with heart disease, PACs may warn of or start more serious dysrhythmias (e.g., supraventricular tachycardia).
- Treatment depends on patient symptoms. Withdrawal of sources of stimulation such as caffeine or sympathomimetic drugs may be warranted. β-Blockers may also be used to decrease PACs.

Paroxysmal Supraventricular Tachycardia

Paroxysmal supraventricular tachycardia (PSVT) is a dysrhythmia originating in an ectopic focus anywhere above the bifurcation of the bundle of His. Identification of the ectopic focus is often difficult even with a 12-lead ECG, because it requires recording the dysrhythmia as it starts. *Paroxysmal* refers to an abrupt onset and termination. In the normal heart, PSVT is associated with overexertion, emotional stress, deep inspiration, and stimulants such as caffeine and tobacco. PSVT is also associated with rheumatic heart disease, *Wolff-Parkinson-White (WPW) syndrome* (conduction by way of accessory pathways), digitalis intoxication, CAD, and cor pulmonale.

- HR is 150 to 220 beats/minute and rhythm is regular. Some degree of AV block may be present.
- Clinical significance depends on the associated symptoms. A prolonged episode and HR above 180 beats/minute decreases cardiac output (CO), resulting in hypotension, dyspnea, and angina.
- Treatment includes vagal stimulation and drug therapy. Common vagal maneuvers include Valsalva, carotid massage, and

coughing. IV adenosine (Adenocard) is the drug of choice to convert PSVT to a normal sinus rhythm. IV β-blockers (e.g., sotalol [Betapace]), calcium channel blockers (e.g., diltiazem [Cardizem]), and amiodarone can also be used. If vagal stimulation and drug therapy are ineffective and the patient becomes hemodynamically unstable, synchronized cardioversion is used.

Atrial Flutter

Atrial flutter is an atrial tachydysrhythmia identified on the ECG by recurring, regular, sawtooth-shaped flutter waves that originate from a single ectopic focus in the right atrium. Atrial flutter is associated with CAD, hypertension, mitral valve disorders, pulmonary embolus, chronic lung disease, cor pulmonale, cardiomyopathy, hyperthyroidism, and the use of drugs such as digoxin, quinidine, and epinephrine.

- The atrial rate is 250 to 350 beats/minute. The ventricular rate varies depending on the conduction ratio. In 2:1 conduction, the ventricular rate is typically about 150 beats/minute. Atrial and ventricular rhythms are usually regular.
- High ventricular rates (>100 beats/minute) can decrease CO and cause serious consequences, such as HF.
- The primary treatment goal is to slow ventricular response by increasing AV block. Drugs used to control the ventricular rate include calcium channel blockers and β-blockers.
- Antidysrhythmic drugs used to convert atrial flutter to sinus rhythm or maintain sinus rhythm include amiodarone, ibutilide (Corvert), dronedarone (Multaq), and flecainide.
- Electrical cardioversion may be used to convert atrial flutter to sinus rhythm in an emergency situation. Radiofrequency catheter ablation of the ectopic focus is the treatment of choice for atrial flutter.

Atrial Fibrillation

Atrial fibrillation is a consequence of total disorganization of atrial electrical activity associated with multiple ectopic foci, resulting in loss of effective atrial contraction. The dysrhythmia may be paroxysmal (i.e., beginning and ending spontaneously) or persistent (lasting longer than 7 days).

Atrial fibrillation is the most common, clinically significant dysrhythmia with respect to morbidity, mortality, and economic impact. Its prevalence increases with age. Atrial fibrillation usually occurs with underlying heart disease. It often develops acutely with thyrotoxicosis, alcohol intoxication, caffeine use, electrolyte disturbances, stress, or heart surgery.

- The atrial rate may be as high as 350 to 600 beats/minute. The ventricular rate varies, and the rhythm is usually irregular.

- Atrial fibrillation results in a decrease in CO secondary to ineffective atrial contractions and/or rapid ventricular response. Thrombi form in the atria because of blood stasis. An embolized clot may develop and pass to the brain, causing a stroke.

The goals of treatment include a decrease in ventricular response to <100 beats/minute, prevention of cerebral embolic events, and conversion to sinus rhythm, if possible. Drugs used for rate control include calcium channel blockers (e.g., diltiazem), β-blockers (e.g., metoprolol), dronedarone, and digoxin (Lanoxin). Antidysrhythmic drugs used for maintenance of sinus rhythm after cardioversion include amiodarone and ibutilide.

Electrical cardioversion may convert atrial fibrillation to normal sinus rhythm.

- If a patient is in atrial fibrillation for longer than 48 hours, anticoagulation therapy is needed for 3 to 4 weeks before the cardioversion and for several weeks after successful cardioversion.
- For patients with drug-refractory atrial fibrillation or those who do not respond to electrical conversion, radiofrequency catheter ablation (similar to the procedure for atrial flutter) and the Maze procedure (surgical intervention that interrupts ectopic electrical signals) may be used.

First-Degree Atrioventricular Block

In first-degree AV block, every impulse from the atria is conducted to the ventricles, but the time of AV conduction is prolonged. After the impulse moves through the AV node, the ventricles usually respond normally. First-degree AV block is associated with MI, CAD, rheumatic fever, hyperthyroidism, vagal stimulation, and drugs such as digoxin, β-blockers, calcium channel blockers, and flecainide.

- HR is normal and rhythm is regular.
- First-degree AV block may be a precursor of higher degrees of AV block.
- Patients with first-degree AV block are asymptomatic.
- There is no treatment for first-degree AV block.

Second-Degree Atrioventricular Block, Type I
(Mobitz I, Wenckebach)

A type I second-degree AV block is characterized by gradual lengthening of the PR interval. It occurs because of an AV conduction time that is prolonged until an atrial impulse is nonconducted and a QRS complex is blocked (missing). Type I AV block may result from use of digoxin or β-blockers. It may be associated with CAD. It is usually the result of myocardial ischemia or inferior MI. It is generally transient and well tolerated. However, it may be a warning signal of a more serious AV conduction disturbance (e.g., complete heart block).

- The rhythm appears on the ECG in a pattern of grouped beats.
- If the patient is symptomatic, atropine is used to increase HR, or a temporary pacemaker may be needed, especially if the patient has experienced an MI.

Second-Degree Atrioventricular Block, Type II (Mobitz II)

In type II second-degree AV block, the P wave is nonconducted without progressive PR lengthening. This usually occurs when a bundle branch block is present. On conducted beats, the PR interval is constant. In a second-degree heart block, a certain number of impulses from the SA node are not conducted to the ventricles. This occurs in ratios of 2:1, 3:1, and so on when there are two P waves to one QRS complex, three P waves to one QRS complex, and so on. It may occur with varying ratios. Type II AV block is associated with rheumatic heart disease, CAD, anterior MI, and drug toxicity.

- The atrial rate is usually normal. The ventricular rate depends on the intrinsic rate and degree of AV block. The atrial rhythm is regular, but the ventricular rhythm may be irregular.
- Type II AV block often progresses to third-degree AV block and is associated with a poor prognosis.
- Reduced HR frequently results in decreased CO with subsequent hypotension and myocardial ischemia.
- Transcutaneous pacing or the insertion of a temporary pacemaker may be necessary before the insertion of a permanent pacemaker if the patient becomes symptomatic (e.g., hypotension, angina) (see Pacemakers, p. 727). Atropine is not an effective drug for this dysrhythmia.

Third-Degree Atrioventricular Block (Complete Heart Block)

Third-degree AV block constitutes a form of AV dissociation in which no impulses from the atria are conducted to the ventricles. The atria are stimulated and contract independently of the ventricles. Ventricular rhythm is an escape rhythm from above or below the bifurcation of the bundle of His. This rhythm is associated with severe heart disease, including CAD, MI, myocarditis, cardiomyopathy, and some systemic diseases such as amyloidosis and scleroderma. Some drugs can also cause third-degree AV block, such as digoxin, β-blockers, and calcium channel blockers.

- Atrial rate is usually a sinus rate of 60 to 100 beats/minute. Ventricular rate depends on the site of the block. If it is in the AV node, the rate is 40 to 60 beats/minute, and if it is in the Purkinje system, it is 20 to 40 beats/minute. Atrial and ventricular rhythms are regular but unrelated to each other.
- Third-degree AV block almost always results in reduced CO with subsequent ischemia and heart failure.

- For symptomatic patients, a temporary transcutaneous pacemaker is used until a permanent pacemaker can be inserted. Atropine is not an effective drug for this dysrhythmia. Drugs such as epinephrine and dopamine are temporary measures to increase HR and support BP before pacemaker insertion (see Pacemakers, p. 727).

Premature Ventricular Contractions

Premature ventricular contractions (PVCs) originate in an ectopic focus in the ventricles. PVCs are a premature occurrence of the QRS complex, which is wide and distorted in shape. PVCs that are initiated from different foci appear different in shape from each other and are termed *multifocal PVCs*. When every other beat is a PVC, the condition is called *ventricular bigeminy*. When every third beat is a PVC, the condition is called *ventricular trigeminy*. Two consecutive PVCs are called *couplets*. *Ventricular tachycardia* (VT) appears as three or more consecutive PVCs. A PVC falling on the T wave of a preceding beat is termed the R-on-T phenomenon and is considered to be dangerous because it may precipitate VT or ventricular fibrillation (VF).

PVCs are associated with stimulants such as caffeine, alcohol, nicotine, epinephrine, and digoxin. They are also associated with electrolyte imbalances, hypoxia, fever, exercise, and emotional stress. Disease states associated with PVCs include MI, cardiomyopathy, mitral valve prolapse, HF, and CAD.

- HR varies depending on the intrinsic rate and number of PVCs. Rhythm is irregular because of premature beats.
- PVCs are usually not harmful in the patient with a normal heart. In heart disease, PVCs may reduce CO and precipitate angina and HF. PVCs in a patient with CAD or acute MI represent ventricular irritability.
- Treatment relates to the cause of the PVCs (e.g., oxygen therapy for hypoxia, electrolyte replacement). Assessing the patient's hemodynamic status is important to determine if drug therapy is indicated. Drug therapy includes β-blockers, procainamide, or amiodarone.

Ventricular Tachycardia

VT is seen on the ECG as a run of three or more PVCs that occurs when an ectopic focus or foci fire repetitively. VT is a life-threatening dysrhythmia because of the associated decrease in CO and the possibility of the development of VF, which is a lethal dysrhythmia. VT is associated with MI, CAD, significant electrolyte imbalances, hypoxemia, cardiomyopathy, mitral valve prolapse, long QT syndrome, digitalis toxicity, and central nervous system disorders. The dysrhythmia can be seen in patients who have no evidence of cardiac disease.

D

- The ventricular rate is 150 to 250 beats/minute.
- VT can be stable (patient has a pulse) or unstable (patient is pulseless). Sustained VT causes a severe decrease in CO because of decreased ventricular diastolic filling times and loss of atrial contraction. This results in hypotension, pulmonary edema, decreased cerebral blood flow, and cardiopulmonary arrest.
- The dysrhythmia must be treated quickly, even if it occurs only briefly and stops abruptly. Episodes may recur if prophylactic treatment is not started.

  Different forms of VT exist:
- If the patient is hemodynamically stable and has *monomorphic VT* (QRS complexes have same shape, size, and direction) with preserved left ventricular function, then IV procainamide, sotalol, amiodarone, or lidocaine is used. These drugs can also be used if the VT is polymorphic with a normal baseline QT interval.
- *Polymorphic VT* with a prolonged baseline QT interval is treated with IV magnesium, isoproterenol, phenytoin, or antitachycardia pacing. Drugs that prolong the QT interval (e.g., dofetilide [Tikosyn]) should be discontinued. Cardioversion is used when drug therapy is ineffective.
- VT without a pulse is a lethal dysrhythmia and is treated in the same manner as for VF.

Ventricular Fibrillation

VF is a severe derangement of the heart rhythm characterized on the ECG by irregular waveforms of various shapes and amplitudes. This pattern represents the firing of multiple ectopic foci in the ventricle. Mechanically, the ventricle is simply "quivering," and no effective contraction or CO occurs. This dysrhythmia is lethal. VF occurs in acute MI and myocardial ischemia and in chronic diseases such as CAD and cardiomyopathy. It may occur during cardiac pacing or cardiac catheterization procedures because of catheter stimulation of the ventricle. It may also occur with coronary reperfusion after thrombolytic therapy. Other clinical associations are accidental electrical shock, hyperkalemia, hypoxemia, acidosis, and drug toxicity.

- HR is not measurable. Rhythm is irregular and chaotic.
- VF results in an unresponsive, pulseless, and apneic state. If it is not rapidly treated, the patient will die.
- Treatment consists of immediate initiation of cardiopulmonary resuscitation (CPR) and advanced cardiac life support (ACLS) with the use of defibrillation and definitive drug therapy (e.g., epinephrine, vasopressin). There should be no delay in using a defibrillator once available.

EATING DISORDERS

Description

Eating disorders are psychiatric conditions associated with physiologic alterations. Patients with eating disorders may be hospitalized for fluid and electrolyte alterations; cardiac dysrhythmias; and nutritional, endocrine, and metabolic disorders. Menstrual problems may be reported in women of childbearing age.

The three most common types of eating disorders are *anorexia nervosa, bulimia nervosa, and binge-eating disorder*. Binge-eating disorder is less severe than bulimia nervosa and anorexia nervosa. Individuals with binge-eating disorder do not have a distorted body image and are often overweight or obese.

Anorexia Nervosa

Anorexia nervosa is characterized by self-starvation, an intense fear of being fat, and disturbed self-image. Anorexia nervosa clinically manifests as extreme thinness, unwillingness to maintain a healthy weight, distorted body image, lanugo (soft, downy hair covering the body except the palms and soles), refusal to eat, continuous dieting, hair loss, sensitivity to cold, compulsive exercise, dry and yellowish skin, constipation, and absent or irregular menstruation in women of childbearing age. Signs of malnutrition are noted during the physical examination.

Diagnostic studies often show osteopenia or osteoporosis, iron-deficiency anemia, and an elevated blood urea nitrogen level from marked intravascular volume depletion and abnormal renal function.

- Lack of potassium in the diet and loss of potassium in the urine lead to potassium deficiency. Manifestations of potassium deficiency include muscle weakness, cardiac dysrhythmias, and renal failure.
- Leukopenia, hypoglycemia, hyponatremia, hypomagnesemia, and hypophosphatemia may also be present.

Interprofessional care must involve a combination of nutritional support and psychiatric care. Nutritional care focuses on reaching and maintaining a healthy weight, normal eating patterns, and perception of hunger and satiety.

Hospitalization may be necessary if the patient has medical complications that cannot be managed in an outpatient therapy program. Nutritional repletion must be closely supervised to ensure consistent and ongoing weight gain. Refeeding syndrome is a rare but serious complication of behavioral refeeding programs. The use of enteral or parenteral nutrition may be necessary (see Enteral Nutrition, p. 706, and Parenteral Nutrition, p. 731).

Improved nutrition is not a cure for anorexia nervosa. The underlying psychiatric problem must be addressed by identifying disturbed patterns of personal and family interactions, followed by personal and family counseling.

Bulimia Nervosa

Bulimia nervosa is a disorder characterized by episodes of frequent binge eating and inappropriate behaviors to avoid weight gain (vomiting, laxative abuse, overexercise), associated with loss of control related to eating and a persistent concern with body image. Individuals with bulimia nervosa may have normal weight for height, or their weight may fluctuate with bingeing and purging. They may abuse laxatives, diuretics, exercise, or "diet drugs." They may exhibit signs of frequent self-induced vomiting, such as macerated knuckles, swollen salivary glands, broken blood vessels in the eyes, and dental problems.

- The person with bulimia nervosa goes to great lengths to conceal abnormal eating habits. Abnormal laboratory parameters, including hypokalemia, metabolic alkalosis, and elevated serum amylase, may be seen with frequent vomiting.

The cause of bulimia remains unclear but is thought to be similar to that of anorexia nervosa. Substance abuse, anxiety, affective disorders, and personality disturbances have been reported among people with bulimia.

- Combination treatment with psychologic counseling and nutritional therapy is essential.
- Fluoxetine (Prozac) is the only FDA-approved antidepressant for treating bulimia nervosa. Antidepressants are not helpful for all patients with bulimia.
- Education and emotional support for the patient and the family are vital. Support groups such as the National Association of Anorexia Nervosa and Associated Disorders (ANAD) *(www.anad.org)* may be helpful.

ENCEPHALITIS

Description

Encephalitis is a serious, sometimes fatal, acute inflammation of the brain. It is usually caused by a virus. Many different viruses have been implicated in encephalitis; some of them are associated with certain seasons of the year and are endemic to certain geographic areas. Ticks and mosquitoes transmit epidemic encephalitis, whereas nonepidemic encephalitis may occur as a complication of measles, chickenpox, or mumps.

- Herpes simplex virus (HSV) encephalitis is the most common form of nonepidemic viral encephalitis.
- Cytomegalovirus encephalitis is a common complication in patients with acquired immunodeficiency syndrome (AIDS).

Clinical Manifestations and Diagnostic Studies

The onset of infection is typically nonspecific, with fever, headache, nausea, and vomiting. Infection can be acute or subacute. Signs of encephalitis appear on day 2 or 3 and may range from minimal alterations in mental status to coma.

- Almost any central nervous system (CNS) abnormality can occur, including hemiparesis, tremors, seizures, dysphasia, cranial nerve palsies, personality changes, memory impairment, and amnesia.
- Diagnostic findings related to viral encephalitis are shown in Table 34.
- Brain imaging techniques include CT, MRI, and positron emission tomography (PET).
- Polymerase chain reaction (PCR) tests can be used to detect herpes simplex virus (HSV) and West Nile encephalitis.

West Nile virus infection should be strongly considered in adults older than 50 years who develop encephalitis or meningitis in summer or early fall. The best diagnostic test to identify West Nile virus is a blood test that detects viral ribonucleic acid (RNA).

Nursing and Interprofessional Management

To prevent encephalitis, mosquito control should be practiced, including cleaning rain gutters, removing old tires, draining bird baths, and removing water where mosquitoes can breed. In addition, insect repellant should be used outdoors during mosquito season.

Management of encephalitis, including West Nile virus infection, is symptomatic and supportive. Initially many patients require intensive care. Acyclovir is used to treat HSV encephalitis. For maximal benefit, antiviral agents must be started before the onset of coma.

- Prophylactic treatment with antiseizure drugs may be used in severe cases of encephalitis.

E

TABLE 34 Comparison of Cerebral Inflammatory Conditions

Feature	Meningitis	Encephalitis	Brain Abscess
Cause	Bacteria* (*Streptococcus pneumoniae*, *Neisseria meningitidis*, group B streptococci), viruses, fungi	Bacteria, fungi, parasites, herpes simplex virus (HSV), other viruses (e.g., West Nile virus)	Streptococci, staphylococci (acquired through bloodstream)
CSF (reference interval)			
• Pressure (70-150 mm H_2O)	Increased *Bacterial:* 200-500 mm H_2O *Viral:* ≤250 mm H_2O	Normal to slight increase	Increased
• WBC count (0-5 cells/μL)	*Bacterial:* >1000/μL (mainly neutrophils) *Viral:* 25-500/μL (mainly lymphocytes)	500/μL, neutrophils (early), lymphocytes (later)	25-300/μL (neutrophils)
• Protein (15-45 mg/dL [0.15-0.45 g/L])	*Bacterial:* >500 mg/dL *Viral:* 50-500 mg/dL	Slight increase	Normal
• Glucose (40-70 mg/dL [2.2-3.9 mmol/L])	*Bacterial:* Decreased at 5-40 mg/dL *Viral:* Normal or low at >40 mg/dL	Normal	Low or absent
• Appearance	*Bacterial:* Turbid, cloudy *Viral:* Clear or cloudy	Clear	Clear
Diagnostic studies	CT scan, Gram stain, smear, culture, PCR assay†	CT scan, EEG, MRI, PET, PCR, IgM antibodies to virus in serum or CSF	CT scan
Treatment	Antibiotics, dexamethasone, supportive care, prevention of ↑ ICP	Supportive care, prevention of ↑ ICP, acyclovir (Zovirax) for HSV infection	Antibiotics, incision and drainage Supportive care

CSF, Cerebrospinal fluid; *EEG,* electroencephalography; *ICP,* intracranial pressure; *PCR,* polymerase chain reaction; *PET,* positron emission tomography.
*See also Meningitis, Bacterial on p. 410.
†PCR testing is used to detect viral RNA or DNA.

ENDOCARDITIS, INFECTIVE

Description

Infective endocarditis (IE) is an infection of the endocardial (innermost) surface of the heart. Therefore IE affects the valves. An estimated 10,000 to 15,000 new cases of IE are diagnosed in the United States each year.

Classification

IE is most often classified by cause (e.g., IV drug abuse, fungal endocarditis) or site of involvement (e.g., prosthetic valve endocarditis).

- IE was traditionally classified as *subacute* (typically affecting preexisting valve disease and extending over months) or *acute* (typically affecting healthy valves and manifesting as a rapidly progressive illness).

Pathophysiology

The most common causative agents, *Staphylococcus aureus* and *Streptococcus viridans,* are bacterial. Other pathogens include fungi and viruses.

IE occurs when blood flow within the heart allows the causative organism to infect previously damaged valves or other endothelial surfaces. IE can occur in individuals with a variety of underlying cardiac conditions, including prior endocarditis, prosthetic valves, acquired valve disease, and cardiac lesions. A variety of invasive procedures (e.g., IV drug abuse, renal dialysis) can also allow large numbers of organisms to enter the bloodstream and trigger the infectious process.

Vegetations, the primary lesions of IE, consist of fibrin, leukocytes, platelets, and microbes, which adhere to the valve surface or endocardium. The loss of portions of this vegetation into the circulation results in embolization. Many persons with IE will develop systemic embolization. This occurs when left-sided heart vegetations move to various organs (e.g., kidney, spleen, brain) and extremities. Right-sided heart lesions embolize to the lungs, resulting in pulmonary emboli.

The infection may spread locally to cause damage to valves or their supporting structures. This results in dysrhythmias, valve dysfunction, and eventual invasion of the myocardium, leading to heart failure (HF), sepsis, and heart block.

At one time rheumatic heart disease was the most common cause of IE. However, now it accounts for less than 20% of cases. The main contributing factors in the development of IE are (1) aging (more than 50% of older people have calcified aortic stenosis), (2) IV drug abuse, (3) use of prosthetic valves, (4) use of intravascular devices resulting in health care–associated infections (HAIs) (e.g., methicillin-resistant *S. aureus* [MRSA]), and (5) renal dialysis.

Clinical Manifestations

The clinical manifestations are nonspecific and can involve multiple organ systems. Symptoms include fever, chills, weakness, malaise, fatigue, and anorexia. Arthralgias, myalgias, abdominal discomfort, back pain, weight loss, headache, and clubbing of fingers may occur in subacute forms of endocarditis. Fever may be absent in older adults or those who are immunocompromised.

Vascular signs may include splinter hemorrhages (black longitudinal streaks) in the nail beds. Petechiae, which may result from fragmentation and microembolization of vegetative lesions, are common on the conjunctivae, lips, buccal mucosa, and palate and over the ankles, feet, and antecubital and popliteal areas. *Osler's nodes* (painful, tender, red or purple, pea-size lesions) may be found on the fingertips or toes. *Janeway lesions* (flat, painless, small, red spots) may be found on the palms and soles. Funduscopic examination may reveal hemorrhagic retinal lesions called *Roth's spots*. A new-onset or changing murmur is frequently noted, with the aortic and mitral valves most commonly affected.

Clinical signs and symptoms secondary to embolization in various body organs may also be present. These include:

- Embolization to the spleen may result in sharp, left upper quadrant pain and splenomegaly, local tenderness, and abdominal rigidity.
- Embolization to the kidneys may cause pain in the flank, hematuria, and renal failure.
- Emboli may lodge in the small peripheral blood vessels of the arms and legs, causing ischemia and gangrene.
- Embolization to the brain may result in hemiplegia, ataxia, aphasia, visual changes, and change in mental status.
- Pulmonary emboli may occur in right-sided endocarditis.

Diagnostic Studies

A health history should be obtained with inquiry made regarding any recent dental, urologic, surgical, or gynecologic procedures including normal or abnormal obstetric delivery. Document previous history of heart disease, IV drug abuse, recent cardiac catheterization, cardiac surgery, intravascular device placement, renal dialysis, and infection (e.g., skin, respiratory, urinary tract).

- Blood culture of two samples drawn 1 hour apart from two different sites will be positive in more than 90% of patients.

- A mild leukocytosis occurs in acute endocarditis.
- Erythrocyte sedimentation rate (ESR) and C-reactive protein (CRP) levels may be elevated.
- Chest x-ray is used to detect an enlarged heart.
- ECG may show first- or second-degree heart block because the valves lie in close proximity to the atrioventricular (AV) node.
- Cardiac catheterization may be used to evaluate valve functioning.

Major criteria to diagnose IE include at least two of the following: two positive blood cultures 12 hours apart, nonvalvular regurgitation, or intracardiac mass or vegetation noted on echocardiography.

Interprofessional Care
Prophylactic Treatment
Antibiotic prophylaxis is recommended for high cardiac risk conditions including prosthetic heart valves, history of endocarditis, surgically constructed systemic-pulmonary shunts, congenital heart disease, and heart valve disease after heart transplantation. Specific antibiotic regimens are recommended for dental, respiratory, GI and genitourinary (GU) procedures (see Table 36-2, Lewis et al, *Medical-Surgical Nursing,* ed 10, p. 783).

Drug Therapy
Accurate identification of the causative organism is the key to successful treatment. Complete removal of the organisms generally takes weeks, and relapses are common. Patients are hospitalized and IV antibiotic therapy is started based on blood cultures.

- Blood cultures that remain positive indicate inadequate or inappropriate antibiotic administration, aortic root or myocardial abscess, or the wrong diagnosis (e.g., an infection elsewhere).
- Fever may persist for several days after treatment has been started and is treated with aspirin, acetaminophen, fluids, and rest.
- Complete bed rest is usually not needed unless the temperature remains elevated or there are signs of heart failure.
- Endocarditis coupled with heart failure responds poorly to antibiotic therapy and valve replacement and is often life-threatening.

Nursing Management
Goals
The patient with IE will have normal or baseline cardiac function, perform activities of daily living without fatigue, and know the therapeutic regimen to prevent recurrence of endocarditis.

Nursing Diagnoses
- Decreased cardiac output
- Activity intolerance

Nursing Interventions

The incidence of IE can be decreased by identifying individuals who are at risk for development of the disease. Assessment of the patient's history and an understanding of the disease process is important for planning and implementing appropriate health maintenance strategies.

IE generally requires treatment with antibiotics for 4 to 6 weeks. After initial treatment in the hospital, the patient may continue treatment in the home setting if hemodynamically stable and adherent.

- Patients who receive outpatient IV antibiotics require vigilant home nursing care. Instruct the patient or caregiver about the importance of monitoring body temperature because persistent, prolonged temperature elevations may indicate that the drug therapy is ineffective. Teach patients and caregivers to recognize signs and symptoms of these complications (e.g., change in mental status, dyspnea, chest pain).
- The patient needs adequate periods of physical and emotional rest. Bed rest may be necessary when fever is present or there are complications (e.g., heart damage). Otherwise the patient may walk and perform moderate activity.
- Monitor laboratory data to determine the effectiveness of the antibiotic therapy. Assess IV lines for patency and any signs of complications (e.g., phlebitis). Administer antibiotics as scheduled and monitor the patient for adverse drug reactions.
- To prevent problems related to decreased mobility, teach the patient to wear elastic compression gradient stockings, perform range-of-motion (ROM) exercises, and cough and deep breathe every 2 hours.
- Recognize that the patient may experience anxiety and fear associated with the illness. Implement strategies to help the patient cope.

▼ Patient and Caregiver Teaching
- Instruct the patient about symptoms that may indicate another infection, such as fever, fatigue, malaise, and chills, and the importance of notifying the HCP if they occur.
- Tell the patient about the importance of prophylactic antibiotic therapy before certain invasive procedures.
- Explain to the patient and caregiver the relationship of follow-up care, good nutrition, and early treatment of common infections (e.g., colds) to maintaining good health.

ENDOMETRIAL CANCER

Description

Endometrial cancer is the most common gynecologic malignancy. If endometrial cancer is diagnosed in the early stage, it has a relatively low mortality rate, with survival rates over 95%.

- The major risk factor for endometrial cancer is exposure to estrogen, especially unopposed estrogen. Obesity is a risk factor because adipose cells store estrogen, thus increasing the amount of circulating estrogen. Additional risk factors include increasing age, never being pregnant, early menarche, late menopause, smoking, diabetes mellitus, and a patient or family history of hereditary nonpolyposis colorectal cancer
- Pregnancy, use of oral contraceptives and intrauterine devices (IUDs), and physical exercise are associated with reduced risk.

Pathophysiology

Endometrial cancer arises from the endometrial lining and most tumors are adenocarcinomas. If endometrial cancer is not diagnosed in early stages, it can invade the myometrium (muscle of the uterus) and the regional lymph nodes.

If metastasis occurs, the common sites include the lung, liver, bone, and brain. Prognosis depends on the tumor size, cell type, degree of invasion into the myometrium, and metastasis.

Clinical Manifestations

- Early clinical manifestations include abnormal uterine bleeding, especially in postmenopausal women.
- Later symptoms can include pain during urination or intercourse or in the pelvic area.

Diagnostic Studies

Endometrial biopsy is the primary diagnostic procedure for endometrial cancer.

Interprofessional Care

Treatment of endometrial cancer in the early stage is a total hysterectomy and bilateral salpingo-oophorectomy with lymph node biopsies. Surgery may be followed by external irradiation either to the pelvis or abdomen or internal radiation (brachytherapy) intravaginally if there is local or distant metastasis. If the woman has advanced or recurrent disease, chemotherapy and hormonal therapy may be indicated.

Nursing Management: Cancers of the Female Reproductive Tract

See Cervical Cancer, p. 117.

ENDOMETRIOSIS

Description

Endometriosis is a common benign gynecologic condition in which endometrial tissue accumulates outside the endometrial cavity. The most frequent sites are in or near the ovaries, uterosacral ligaments, and uterovesical peritoneum (Fig. 8). The endometrial tissue responds to the hormones of the ovarian cycle and undergoes a "mini-menstrual cycle" similar to that of the uterine endometrium. Endometriosis can cause considerable pain.

■ Endometriosis is a common cause of infertility and increases the risk of ovarian cancer. The etiology of endometriosis is unknown.

Clinical Manifestations

A wide range of manifestations and severity exists. The magnitude of a woman's symptoms does not necessarily correlate with the clinical extent of her endometriosis.

■ The most common signs and symptoms are secondary dysmenorrhea, infertility, pelvic pain, dyspareunia, and irregular bleeding.

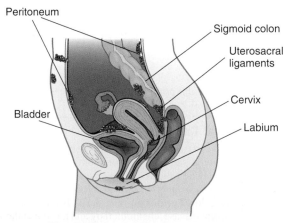

Fig. 8 Common sites of endometriosis.

- Less common symptoms include backache, painful bowel movements, and dysuria.
- With menopause, estrogen is no longer produced in the ovaries, which may lead to the disappearance of symptoms.

Diagnostic Studies

Diagnosis is frequently confirmed by patient history and the palpation of firm nodular lumps in the adnexa on bimanual examination. Laparoscopic examination is necessary for a definitive diagnosis.

Interprofessional Care

Treatment is influenced by the patient's age, desire for pregnancy, symptom severity, and the extent and location of the disease. When symptoms are not disruptive, a "watch and wait" approach is used.

Drug Therapy

Drugs are often used to reduce symptoms. Pain may be relieved with nonsteroidal antiinflammatory drugs such as ibuprofen and diclofenac. Drugs to inhibit estrogen production by the ovary may shrink the endometrial tissue. These drugs produce changes that imitate a state of pregnancy or menopause.

- Continuous use (for 9 months) of combined oral contraceptives causes regression of endometrial tissue. Ovulation is suppressed by progestin agents such as medroxyprogesterone (Depo-Provera).
- Another class of drugs used is gonadotropin-releasing hormone (GnRH) agonists, such as leuprolide acetate (Lupron) and nafarelin (Synarel). These drugs result in amenorrhea.

Surgical Therapy

The only cure for endometriosis is surgical removal of all endometrial tissue by means of laparoscopic laser surgery or laparotomy. Definitive surgery involves removal of the uterus, fallopian tubes, ovaries, and as many endometrial implants as possible. GnRH agonist therapy can be given for 4 to 6 months to reduce the size of the lesions before surgery.

- For women wishing to get pregnant, conservative surgical therapy is used to remove implants that may block the fallopian tube. Adhesions are removed from the tubes, ovaries, and pelvic structures.

Nursing Management

Teach and reassure the patient that endometriosis is not a life-threatening situation, which may permit her to accept a progressive treatment approach.

- When the symptoms are less severe, teach about nondrug comfort measures.
- Assist the patient to understand the drugs ordered to treat the condition.
- Psychologic support may be needed for the patient experiencing severe disabling pain, sexual difficulties secondary to dyspareunia, and infertility.
- Each woman should be actively involved in making the decision about preserving part or all of her ovaries if surgically possible. Help her to explore her feelings about maintaining her cyclic ovarian function.
- If conservative surgery is the treatment selected, nursing care is similar to general preoperative and postoperative care of a patient undergoing laparotomy (see Abdominal Pain, Acute, p. 3).
- If definitive surgery is planned, nursing care is similar to care of the patient undergoing an abdominal hysterectomy.

ESOPHAGEAL CANCER

Description

Esophageal cancer is uncommon although the incidence is increasing. Approximately 17,000 new cases of esophageal cancer are diagnosed annually in the United States. The 5-year survival rate is 37% for localized cancer and 18% for regional cancer.

Risk factors include Barrett's esophagus, smoking, excessive alcohol intake, and obesity. Patients with occupational exposure to asbestos and cement dust are at greater risk.

Pathophysiology

Most esophageal cancers are adenocarcinomas, with the remainder being squamous cell tumors. Adenocarcinomas arise from the glands lining the esophagus and resemble cancers of the stomach and small intestine.

- Most tumors are located in the middle and lower portions of the esophagus. The tumor may penetrate the muscular layer and extend outside the esophageal wall.
- The malignant tumor usually appears as an ulcerated lesion and has often advanced by the time the patient notices symptoms.
- Obstruction of the esophagus occurs in the later stages.
- Achalasia, a condition in which there is delayed emptying of the lower esophagus, is associated with squamous cell cancer.

Clinical Manifestations

The onset of symptoms is usually late relative to tumor growth.

- Progressive dysphagia is the most common symptom and may be expressed as a substernal feeling that food is not passing. Initially dysphagia occurs only with meat, then with soft foods, and eventually with liquids.
- Pain develops late and is described as occurring in the substernal, epigastric, or back areas and usually increases with swallowing. The pain may radiate to the neck, jaw, ears, and shoulders.
- If the tumor is in the upper third of the esophagus, symptoms such as sore throat, choking, and hoarseness may occur. Weight loss is common.
- When esophageal stenosis (narrowing) is severe, regurgitation of blood-flecked esophageal contents is common.

Complications may include hemorrhage from cancer eroding through the esophagus and into the aorta. Esophageal perforation into the lung or trachea may also develop. The liver and lung are common metastatic sites.

Diagnostic Studies

- Barium swallow with fluoroscopy may detect esophageal narrowing at the tumor site.
- Endoscopic biopsy is used to make a definitive diagnosis.
- Endoscopic ultrasonography, bronchoscopy, CT scan, and MRI assess the extent of disease.

Interprofessional Care

Treatment depends on the tumor location and whether metastasis has occurred. The best results may be obtained with a combination of surgery, endoscopic ablation, chemotherapy, and radiation therapy.

- The surgical approaches may be open (thoracic or abdominal incision) or minimally invasive (e.g., laparoscopic vagal nerve–sparing surgery).
- Endoscopic approaches using photodynamic therapy, endoscopic mucosal resection (EMR), and radiofrequency ablation are also used.

Concurrent radiation therapy and chemotherapy are used for palliation of symptoms, especially dysphagia, as well as to increase survival. Palliative therapy consists of restoration of the swallowing function and maintenance of nutrition and hydration. Dilation, stent placement, or both can relieve obstruction.

Nutritional Therapy

After esophageal surgery, parenteral fluids are given. A swallowing study is often done before the patient is allowed to have oral fluids. When fluids are permitted, water (30 to 60 mL) is given hourly, with gradual progression to small, frequent, bland meals. The patient should be in an upright position to prevent regurgitation. Observe the patient for signs of intolerance to the feeding or leakage of the feeding into the mediastinum. Symptoms indicating leakage are pain, increased temperature, and dyspnea. A jejunostomy, gastrostomy, or esophagostomy feeding tube may be placed for the purpose of feeding the patient.

Nursing Management

Goals

The patient with esophageal cancer will have relief of symptoms, including pain and dysphagia, achieve optimal nutritional intake, understand the prognosis of the disease, and experience a quality of life appropriate to disease progression.

Nursing Diagnoses

- Chronic pain
- Imbalanced nutrition: less than body requirements
- Risk for aspiration
- Anxiety and grieving

Nursing Interventions

In addition to general preoperative teaching and preparation, pay particular attention to the patient's nutritional needs. Many patients are poorly nourished because of the inability to ingest adequate food and fluids. Teaching should include information about chest tubes (if a thoracic approach is used), IV lines, nasogastric (NG) tube, gastrostomy or jejunostomy feeding, turning, coughing, and deep breathing. Meticulous oral care is essential.

Postoperative care should include assessment of drainage; maintenance of the NG tube; oral and nasal care; and prevention of respiratory complications by turning, coughing, and deep breathing, with incentive spirometry every 2 hours, and placing the patient in a semi-Fowler's position to prevent gastric reflux and aspiration.

▼ Patient and Caregiver Teaching

- Know what the interprofessional team has told the patient regarding the prognosis in order to provide appropriate and consistent counseling.
- Provide emotional and physical support, provide information, clarify test results, and maintain a positive attitude with respect to the patient's immediate recovery and long-term survival.

- Referral to a home health nurse may be needed for continued care of the patient (e.g., gastrostomy teaching and follow-up wound care).

FIBROCYSTIC BREAST CHANGES

Description

Fibrocystic breast changes include the development of excess fibrous tissue, hyperplasia of the epithelial lining of the mammary ducts, proliferation of mammary ducts, and cyst formation. These benign changes are the most frequently occurring breast disorder. Fibrocystic changes occur most frequently in women between 35 and 50 years old but often begin as early as the age of 20 years. They are not associated alone with increased breast cancer risk.

Fibrocystic changes most commonly occur in women with premenstrual abnormalities, nulliparous women, women with a history of spontaneous abortion, nonusers of oral contraceptives, and women with early menarche and late menopause.

Pathophysiology

Fibrocystic changes are thought to be heightened responsiveness of breast tissue to circulating estrogen and progesterone. These changes produce pain from nerve irritation due to connective tissue edema and fibrosis from nerve pinching.

- Masses or nodules are often found in the upper, outer quadrants. They usually occur bilaterally.
- Symptoms of fibrocystic changes often worsen in the premenstrual phase and subside after menstruation.

Clinical Manifestations

Manifestations of fibrocystic breast changes include one or more palpable lumps that are usually round, well delineated, and freely movable within the breast. Discomfort ranging from tenderness to pain may also occur.

- The lump usually increases in size and perhaps in tenderness before menstruation. Cysts may enlarge or shrink rapidly.
- Nipple discharge associated with fibrocystic breasts is often milky, watery-milky, yellow, or green.
- Pain and nodularity often increase over time but tend to subside after menopause unless high doses of estrogen replacement are used.

Mammography may be helpful in distinguishing fibrocystic changes from breast cancer. However, in some women the breast tissue is so dense that it is difficult to obtain a mammogram. In these situations, ultrasound may be more useful in differentiating a cystic mass from a solid mass.

Nursing and Interprofessional Management

With the initial discovery of a discrete breast mass, aspiration or surgical biopsy may be indicated. If the nodularity is recurrent, a wait of 7 to 10 days may be planned to note any changes related to the menstrual cycle.

- An excisional biopsy should be done if no fluid is found on aspiration, the fluid that is found is hemorrhagic, or a residual mass remains after fluid aspiration.

Many types of treatment have been suggested for a fibrocystic condition. Some relief for cyclic pain may occur by reducing intake of caffeine and dietary fat; taking vitamins E, A, B complex, gamma-linolenic acid (evening primrose oil); and continually wearing a supportive bra. Compresses, ice, analgesics, and antiinflammatory drugs may also help. Prescription medication such as oral contraceptives and danazol may also be used. However, the androgenic side effects of danazol (acne, edema, hirsutism) may make this therapy unacceptable.

▼ **Patient and Caregiver Teaching**

Your role in the care of the patient with fibrocystic breast changes is primarily one of teaching.

- Teach the patient that she may expect recurrences of the cysts in one or both breasts until menopause, and that cysts may enlarge or become painful just before menstruation. In addition, offer reassurance that cysts do not "turn into" cancer.
- Encourage the woman with cystic changes to get regular follow-up care. Also teach her breast self-examination (BSE) to self-monitor changes. Severe fibrocystic changes may make palpation of the breast more difficult. Teach her to report any changes in symptoms or changes found during the BSE so they can be evaluated.

FIBROMYALGIA

Description

Fibromyalgia is a chronic central pain syndrome marked by widespread, nonarticular musculoskeletal pain and fatigue with multiple tender points. People with fibromyalgia may also experience nonrestorative sleep, morning stiffness, irritable bowel syndrome, and anxiety. Fibromyalgia affects an estimated 2% of the general U.S. population. The disease is 4 to 10 times more common in women than in men.

Fibromyalgia and systemic exertion intolerance disease (SEID), formerly called chronic fatigue syndrome, share many common features (see Table 82, p. 616).

Pathophysiology

Fibromyalgia is a disorder involving abnormal central processing of nociceptive pain input. The increased pain experienced by the patient is due to abnormal sensory processing in the CNS.

Multiple physiologic abnormalities have been found, including increased levels of substance P in the spinal fluid, low blood flow to the thalamus, dysfunction of the hypothalamic-pituitary-adrenal (HPA) axis, low levels of serotonin and tryptophan, and abnormalities in cytokine function.

- Serotonin and substance P play a role in mood regulation, sleep, and pain perception. Changes in the HPA axis can lead to depression and a decreased response to stress.
- Genetic factors contribute to the etiology of fibromyalgia, as a familial tendency exists. Recent illness or trauma may be a trigger.

Clinical Manifestations

Widespread burning pain worsens and subsides through the course of a day. The patient often has difficulty discriminating whether pain occurs in the muscles, joints, or soft tissues.

- Head or facial pain often results from stiff or painful neck and shoulder muscles. This pain can accompany temporomandibular joint dysfunction. Physical examination characteristically reveals point tenderness at 11 or more of 18 identified sites (Fig. 9).
- Cognitive effects range from difficulty concentrating to memory lapses and a feeling of being overwhelmed when dealing with multiple tasks. Many individuals report migraine headaches, depression, and anxiety.
- Numbness or tingling in the hands or feet (paresthesia) often accompanies fibromyalgia. Restless legs syndrome is common.
- Women with fibromyalgia may experience more difficult menstruation, with a worsening of disease symptoms during this time.
- Irritable bowel syndrome with manifestations of diarrhea or constipation, abdominal pain, and bloating can occur. In addition, increased urinary frequency and urgency may occur.

Diagnostic Studies

A definitive diagnosis is often difficult to establish. Laboratory results may serve to rule out other suspected disorders.

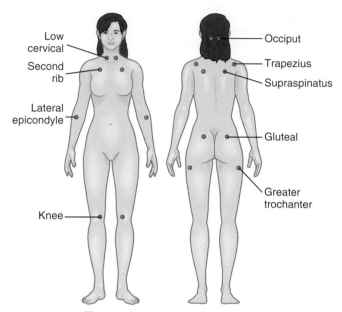

Fig. 9 Tender points in fibromyalgia.

- Muscle biopsy may reveal a nonspecific moth-eaten appearance or fiber atrophy.

The American College of Rheumatology classifies an individual as having fibromyalgia if two criteria are met: (1) pain in 11 of the 18 tender points on palpation and (2) a history of widespread pain for at least 3 months.

Interprofessional Care

Treatment is symptomatic and requires a high level of patient motivation. Teach the patient to be an active participant in the therapeutic regimen. Rest can help the pain, aching, and tenderness.

Drug therapy for the chronic widespread pain associated with fibromyalgia includes pregabalin (Lyrica), duloxetine (Cymbalta), and milnacipran (Savella). Low-dose tricyclic antidepressants (TCAs), selective serotonin reuptake inhibitors (SSRIs), or benzodiazepines (e.g., diazepam ([Valium]) may be prescribed. If the TCA is not well tolerated, similar drugs can be substituted, such as doxepin, imipramine (Tofranil), or trazodone.

- SSRI antidepressants (e.g., sertraline [Zoloft] or paroxetine [Paxil]) tend to be reserved for patients who also have depression. Both antidepressants and muscle relaxants (e.g., baclofen) have sedative effects that can help in improving nighttime rest for the patient with fibromyalgia.
- Long-acting opioids generally are not recommended unless fibromyalgia is refractory to other therapies.
- In some patients, pain may be managed with over-the-counter (OTC) analgesics such as acetaminophen (Tylenol), ibuprofen, or naproxen (Aleve) used in combination with a TCA. Nonopioids, such as tramadol (Ultram), may also be used. In addition, zolpidem (Ambien) or trazodone is sometimes prescribed for short-term intervention in the patient with severe sleep problems.

Because of the chronic nature of fibromyalgia and the need to maintain an ongoing rehabilitation program, the patient needs information and consistent support from the interprofessional team. Massage combined with ultrasound or the application of alternating heat and cold packs soothes tense, sore muscles and increases blood circulation.

- Gentle stretching can be performed by a physical therapist and practiced by the patient at home to relieve muscle tension and spasm.
- Limit consumption of muscle irritants such as sugar, caffeine, and alcohol.
- Pain and the related symptoms of fibromyalgia can cause significant stress. Effective relaxation strategies include biofeedback, guided imagery, and autogenic training. Counseling and a support group may prove beneficial.

F

FLAIL CHEST

Description

Flail chest results from the fracture of several consecutive ribs in two or more separate locations that cause an unstable segment.

Pathophysiology

The affected (flail) area moves in the opposite direction with respect to the intact portion of the chest. During inspiration, the affected portion is sucked in, and during expiration it bulges out. This paradoxical chest movement prevents adequate ventilation of the lung in the injured area and increases the work of breathing.

Clinical Manifestations and Diagnostic Studies

A flail chest is usually apparent on visual examination of the unconscious patient.

- The patient manifests rapid, shallow respirations and tachycardia.
- A flail chest may not be initially apparent in the conscious patient as a result of splinting of the chest wall. The patient moves air poorly. Movement of the thorax is asymmetric and uncoordinated.
- Palpation of abnormal respiratory movements, evaluation for crepitus near the rib fractures, chest x-ray, and arterial blood gases (ABGs) all assist in the diagnosis.

Interprofessional Care

Initial therapy consists of airway management, adequate ventilation, supplemental oxygen therapy, careful administration of IV solutions to support circulation, and pain control. Definitive therapy is to facilitate lung expansion. Intubation and ventilation may be necessary. Surgical fixation of the flail segment may be done. Lung parenchyma and fractured ribs will heal with time.

FRACTURE

Description

A *fracture* is a disruption or break in the continuity of the structure of bone. Traumatic injuries account for the majority of fractures, although some fractures are secondary to a disease process (pathologic fractures from cancer or osteoporosis).

Fractures can be classified as *open* or *closed* depending on communication with the external environment. In an open fracture, the skin is broken, exposing the bone and causing soft tissue injury. In a closed fracture, the skin has not been ruptured and remains intact.

- Fractures can also be classified as complete or incomplete. Fractures are termed *complete* if the break goes completely through the bone and *incomplete* if the break occurs partly across a bone shaft but the bone is still intact. An incomplete fracture is often the result of bending or crushing forces applied to a bone.
- Fractures are also described and classified according to the direction of the fracture line. Types include linear, oblique, transverse, longitudinal, and spiral fractures.

- Fractures can also be classified as *displaced* or *nondisplaced.* In a displaced fracture the two ends of the broken bone are separated from one another and out of their normal positions.
- Displaced fractures are often comminuted (more than two fragments) or oblique. In a nondisplaced fracture the periosteum is intact across the fracture and the bone is still in alignment. Nondisplaced fractures are usually transverse, spiral, or greenstick.

Illustrations of the various classifications of fractures can be found in Figs. 62-6 and 62-7 in Lewis et al, *Medical-Surgical Nursing,* ed 10, pp. 1468 to 1469.

Clinical Manifestations

Manifestations include immediate localized pain, decreased function, and inability to bear weight on or use the affected part.

- The patient guards the extremity (protects it against movement). Obvious bone deformity may not be visible.
- If a fracture is suspected, the extremity is immobilized in the position in which it is found. Unnecessary movement increases soft tissue damage and may convert a closed fracture to an open fracture or create further injury to adjacent nerves and blood vessels.

Complications

The majority of fractures heal without complications. If death occurs after a fracture, it is usually the result of damage to underlying organs and vascular structures or from complications of the fracture or immobility.

- Direct complications include problems with bone union, avascular necrosis, and bone infection.
- Indirect complications are associated with blood vessel and nerve damage resulting in conditions such as compartment syndrome, venous thromboembolism, rhabdomyolysis, fat embolism, and traumatic or hypovolemic shock. A discussion of these complications is in Lewis et al, *Medical-Surgical Nursing,* ed 10, pp. 1478 to 1480. Hypovolemic shock may also occur (see Shock, p. 565).
- Most musculoskeletal injuries are not life-threatening. However, open fractures or fractures accompanied by severe blood loss and fractures that damage vital organs (e.g., lung, heart) are medical emergencies requiring immediate attention.

Open fractures and soft tissue injuries have a high risk of infection. Devitalized and contaminated tissue is an ideal medium for many common pathogens, including gas-forming (anaerobic) bacilli.

Diagnostic Studies
- History and physical examination
- X-ray examination
- CT scan and MRI

Interprofessional Care

The goals of treatment are anatomic realignment of bone fragments through reduction of the fracture, immobilization to maintain realignment, and restoration of function of the injured part.

Fracture Reduction

Closed reduction is a nonsurgical, manual realignment of bones to their previous anatomic position. Traction and countertraction are manually applied to bone fragments to restore position, length, and alignment.

- Closed reduction is usually performed with the patient under local or general anesthesia. After reduction, the injured part is immobilized by casting, traction, external fixation, splints, or orthoses (braces) to maintain alignment until healing occurs.

Open reduction is correction of bone alignment through a surgical incision. It usually includes internal fixation of the fracture with the use of wires, screws, pins, plates, intramedullary rods, or nails.

- Open reduction with internal fixation (ORIF) facilitates early ambulation, which decreases the risk of complications related to prolonged immobility.

Traction devices apply a pulling force on the fractured extremity while countertraction pulls in the opposite direction. The two most common types of traction are skin traction and skeletal traction.

- *Skin traction* is generally used for short-term treatment (48 to 72 hours) until skeletal traction or surgery is possible. Tape, boots, or slings are applied directly to the skin to help diminish muscle spasms in the injured extremity. A *Buck's traction* boot is a type of skin traction device that is used preoperatively for the patient with a hip fracture.
- *Skeletal traction,* generally in place for longer periods, is used to align injured bones and joints or treat joint contractures and congenital hip dysplasia. It provides a long-term pull that keeps injured bones and joints aligned. Skeletal traction requires the insertion of a pin or wire into the bone to align and immobilize the injured body part. Fracture alignment depends on correct positioning and alignment of the patient while the traction forces remain constant. For extremity traction to be effective, forces must be pulling in the opposite direction *(countertraction).*

- Countertraction is commonly supplied by the patient's body weight or may be augmented by elevating the end of the bed.

Fracture Immobilization

Casting may occur after closed reduction has been performed. It allows the patient to perform many normal activities of daily living (ADLs) while providing sufficient immobilization to ensure stability. Synthetic casting materials are commonly used because they are light in weight and dry more quickly than plaster of Paris.

Immobilization of an acute fracture or soft tissue injury of the upper extremity is often accomplished by use of the (1) sugar-tong splint, (2) posterior splint, (3) short arm cast, or (4) long arm cast. A discussion of these casts is in Lewis et al, *Medical-Surgical Nursing,* ed 10, pp. 1471 to 1473.

An *external fixator* is a metal device composed of metal pins that are inserted into the bone and attached to external rods to stabilize the fracture while it heals. It can be used to apply traction or to immobilize reduced fragments when the use of a cast or traction is not appropriate. The external fixator is attached directly to the bones by percutaneous pins or wires. Ongoing assessment for pin loosening and infection is critical. Infection signaled by exudate, redness, tenderness, and pain may require removal of the device.

Internal fixation devices (pins, plates, intramedullary rods, and metal and bioabsorbable screws) are surgically inserted to realign and maintain bony fragments. These metal devices are biologically inert and made from stainless steel, vitallium, or titanium. Proper alignment is evaluated by x-ray studies at regular intervals.

Other Therapy

Electrical bone growth stimulation may be used to facilitate the healing process for certain types of fractures, especially when there is nonunion or delayed healing.

Central and peripheral muscle relaxants, such as carisoprodol (Soma), cyclobenzaprine, or methocarbamol (Robaxin), may be prescribed for management of pain associated with muscle spasms.

The threat of tetanus from an open fracture can be reduced by administering tetanus and diphtheria toxoid or tetanus immunoglobulin for the patient who has not been previously immunized or whose immunization has expired.

Proper nutrition is an essential component of the reparative process in injured tissue. The patient's diet must include ample protein (e.g., 1 g/kg body weight daily), vitamins (especially B, C, and D), and calcium, phosphorus, and magnesium.

Nursing Management

Goals
The patient with a fracture will have healing with no associated complications, obtain satisfactory pain relief, and achieve maximal rehabilitation potential.

Nursing Diagnoses
- Impaired physical mobility
- Risk for peripheral neurovascular dysfunction
- Acute pain
- Readiness for enhanced health management

Nursing Interventions
Patients with fractures may be treated in an emergency department or a physician's office and released to home care, or they may require hospitalization. Specific nursing measures depend on the type of treatment used and setting in which patients are placed.

Preoperative Management. If surgical intervention is required to treat the fracture, patients will need preoperative preparation. In addition to the usual preoperative nursing measures, inform patients of the type of immobilization and assistive devices that will be used and the expected activity limitations after surgery.

- Assure patients that nursing staff will help meet personal needs until they can resume self-care. Remind patients that pain medication will be available if needed.

Postoperative Management. Frequent neurovascular assessments of the affected extremity are necessary to detect early and subtle changes. Closely monitor any limitations of movement or activity related to turning, positioning, and extremity support.

- Pain and discomfort can be minimized through proper alignment and positioning.
- Carefully observe dressings or casts for any overt signs of bleeding or drainage. Report a significant increase in the size of the drainage area.
- If a wound drainage system is in place, regularly assess the patency of the system and the volume and characteristics of drainage. Whenever the contents of a drainage system are measured or emptied, use sterile technique to avoid contamination.

Plan care to prevent complications of immobility if the patient is immobilized as a result of the fracture. Prevent constipation by increasing activity, maintaining a high fluid intake, and providing a diet high in bulk and roughage. Maintain a regular time for elimination. If these measures are not effective in maintaining the patient's normal bowel pattern, administer stool softeners, laxatives, or suppositories as necessary.

■ Renal calculi can develop as a result of bone demineralization related to reduced mobility. Unless contraindicated, a fluid intake of 2500 mL/day is recommended.

■ Rapid deconditioning of the cardiovascular system can occur as a result of prolonged bed rest, resulting in orthostatic hypotension and decreased lung capacity. Unless activity is contraindicated, these effects can be diminished by having the patient sit on the side of the bed, allowing the lower limbs to dangle over the bedside, and having the patient perform standing transfers.

■ When the patient is allowed to increase activity, assess for orthostatic hypotension. Also assess patients for deep vein thrombosis (DVT) and pulmonary emboli.

When slings are used with traction, inspect exposed skin areas regularly. Observe skeletal traction pin sites for signs of infection. Pin site care may vary but often includes regularly cleansing with chlorhexidine, rinsing pin sites with sterile saline, and drying of area with sterile gauze.

▼ **Patient and Caregiver Teaching**

Teaching is important to prevent complications. In addition to specific instructions for cast care and recognition of complications, encourage the patient to contact the HCP if questions arise. Validate patient and caregiver understanding of instructions before discharge.

For further information on rehabilitation management of fractures, including the use of assistive devices such as walkers and crutches, see Lewis et al, *Medical-Surgical Nursing*, ed 10, pp. 1477 to 1478, and see the specific types of fractures discussed in this *Companion*.

FRACTURE, HIP

Description

Hip fractures are common in older adults, with 95% of these due to a fall. By age 90, approximately 33% of all women and 17% of all men will have sustained a hip fracture. In adults more than 65 years old, hip fracture occurs more frequently in women than in men because of osteoporosis. Many older adults with a hip fracture develop disabilities that require long-term care.

A fracture of the hip refers to a fracture of the proximal (upper) third of the femur, which extends up to 5 cm below the lesser trochanter.

■ Fractures that occur within the hip joint capsule are called *intracapsular fractures*. Intracapsular fractures (femoral neck) are further identified by their specific locations: capital, sub-capital, and transcervical. These fractures are associated with osteoporosis and minor trauma.

- *Extracapsular fractures* occur outside the joint capsule. They are termed intertrochanteric if they occur in a region between the greater and lesser trochanter or subtrochanteric if they occur in the region below the lesser trochanter. Extracap-sular fractures are usually caused by severe direct trauma or a fall.

Clinical Manifestations

Manifestations of a hip fracture are external rotation, muscle spasm, shortening of the affected extremity, and severe pain and tenderness in the region of the fracture site. Displaced femoral neck fractures may cause serious disruption of the blood supply to the femoral head, which can result in avascular necrosis.

Interprofessional Care

Initially the affected extremity may be temporarily immobilized by Buck's traction until the patient's physical condition is stabilized and surgery can be performed. Buck's traction relieves painful muscle spasms and can be used for 24 to 48 hours.

Surgical treatment permits early mobilization of the patient and decreases the risk of major complications. The type of surgery depends on the location of the fracture, severity of the fracture, and person's age. Better outcomes are associated with surgery per-formed within 24 hours of injury.

- Surgical options include (1) repair with internal fixation devices (e.g., hip compression screw, intramedullary devices), (2) re-placement of part of the femoral head with a prosthesis (partial hip replacement), and (3) total hip replacement (involves both the femur and acetabulum).

These types of surgical repair are shown in Figs. 62-18 and 62-19 in Lewis et al, *Medical-Surgical Nursing,* ed 10 p. 1482.

Nursing Management

Preoperative Management

Before surgery, severe muscle spasms can increase pain. Appropri-ate analgesics or muscle relaxants, comfortable positioning unless contraindicated, and properly adjusted traction can help manage spasms.

- When possible, teach patient the method and frequency for exercising the unaffected leg and both arms. Encourage the patient to use the overhead trapeze bar and opposite side rail to assist in changing positions. A physical therapist can begin to teach out-of-bed and chair transfers.

■ Inform the caregiver about the patient's weight-bearing status after surgery. Plans for discharge begin as the patient enters the hospital because the length of postoperative stay is only a few days.

Postoperative Management

The principles of patient care for any of the surgical procedures for hip fractures are similar. In the initial postoperative period, assess vital signs and intake and output, monitor respiratory activities such as deep breathing and coughing, administer pain medication, and observe the dressing and incision for signs of bleeding and infection.

In the early postoperative period there is potential for neurovascular impairment. Assess the patient's extremity for motor function, temperature and color, sensation, distal pulses, capillary refill, edema, and pain.

■ Edema is alleviated by elevation of the leg whenever the patient is in a chair.

■ Pain resulting from surgical repair of the affected extremity can be reduced by maintaining limb alignment with pillows between the knees when turning the patient to the nonoperative side. Avoid turning patient to the affected side unless approved by the surgeon.

■ Encourage patient to use overhead trapeze bar and the opposite side rail to assist in changing positions. A physical therapist can teach the patient how to perform out-of-bed and chair transfers.

■ If the hip fracture has been treated by insertion of a prosthesis with a *posterior approach* (accessing the hip joint from the back), measures to prevent dislocation must be used.

■ Patient and caregiver must be fully aware of positions and activities that predispose the patient to dislocation (>90 degrees of flexion, abduction, or internal rotation). Many daily activities may reproduce these positions, including putting on shoes and socks, crossing legs or feet while seated, assuming the side-lying position incorrectly, standing up or sitting down while the body is flexed more than 90 degrees relative to the chair, and sitting on low seats, especially low toilet seats.

■ Until the soft tissue capsule surrounding the hip has healed sufficiently to stabilize the prosthesis, teach the patient to avoid these activities, usually for at least 6 weeks.

In addition to teaching patient and caregiver how to prevent prosthesis dislocation, you should also place a large pillow between

F

the patient's legs when turning, avoid extreme hip flexion, and avoid turning the patient on the affected side until it is approved by the surgeon. Some HCPs prefer that patients keep leg abductor splints on except when bathing.

When the hip fracture is accessed during surgery with an *anterior approach* (joint reached from front of body), the hip muscles are left intact. This approach generally results in a more stable hip in the postoperative period with a lower rate of complications. Patient precautions related to motion and weight bearing are few and may include instructions to avoid hyperextension.

The patient is usually out of bed on the first postoperative day. In collaboration with the physical therapist, monitor the patient's ambulation status for proper crutch walking or use of the walker. For the patient to be discharged home, have the patient demonstrate the proper use of crutches or a walker, the ability to transfer into and from a chair and bed, and the ability to ascend and descend stairs.

Weight bearing on the involved extremity varies. Weight bearing after open reduction and internal fixation (ORIF) surgery is generally restricted until x-ray examination indicates adequate healing, usually 6 to 12 weeks. Limited weight bearing is typically the only restriction for the patient who had ORIF of the hip fracture. Inform caregiver about the patient's weight-bearing status after surgery.

- Sudden severe pain, a lump in the buttock, limb shortening, or extreme external rotation indicate prosthesis dislocation. This requires a closed reduction or open reduction to realign the femoral head in the acetabulum.

Assist both the patient and caregiver in adjusting to the restrictions and dependence imposed by the hip fracture. Depression can easily occur, but creative nursing care and awareness of the problem can do much to prevent it.

- Inform the patient and caregivers about community referral services that can assist in the postdischarge rehabilitation phase.
- Hospitalization averages 3 or 4 days. Patients frequently require care in a subacute unit, skilled nursing facility, or rehabilitation facility before returning home.

Home care considerations include ongoing assessment of pain management, monitoring for infection, and prevention of venous thromboembolism.

▼ Patient and Caregiver Teaching

Teach patient the following:
- Use an elevated toilet seat.
- Place chair inside shower or tub and remain seated while washing.

- Use pillow between legs for first 6 weeks after surgery when lying on nonoperative side or when supine.
- Keep hip in neutral, straight position when sitting, walking, or lying.
- Notify surgeon immediately if severe pain, deformity, or loss of function occurs.
- Discuss risk factors for prosthetic joint infection with surgeon and dentist before dental work.

FRACTURE, HUMERUS

Fractures involving the shaft of the humerus are common among young and middle-aged adults. Clinical manifestations are an obvious displacement of the humeral shaft, shortened extremity, abnormal mobility, and pain.
- Major complications are radial nerve injury and vascular injury to the brachial artery as a result of laceration, transection, or muscle spasm.

Treatment for a fracture of the humerus depends on the location and displacement of the fracture.
- Nonoperative treatment may include use of a hanging arm cast, shoulder immobilizer, or the sling and swathe, which is a type of immobilization that prevents glenohumeral movement.

When these devices are used, elevate the head of the bed to assist gravity in reducing the fracture. Allow the arm to hang freely when the patient is sitting and standing.

Include measures in your care to protect the axilla and prevent skin maceration. Carefully place lightly powdered absorption pads in the axilla and change them twice daily or as needed.
- Skin or skeletal traction may be used for purposes of reduction and immobilization.
- During the rehabilitative phase, an exercise program geared toward improving strength and motion of the injured extremity is extremely important. This program should include assisted motion of the hands and fingers. If the fracture is stable, the shoulder can be exercised to prevent stiffness secondary to "frozen shoulder" or fibrosis of the shoulder capsule.

FRACTURE, PELVIS

Pelvic fractures may be relatively minor or life-threatening, depending on the mechanism of injury and associated vascular damage. Although only a small percentage of all fractures are pelvic fractures, this type of injury is associated with a high mortality rate. Preoccupation with more obvious injuries at the time of a traumatic event may result in pelvic injuries being overlooked.

- Pelvic fractures may cause serious intraabdominal injury, such as paralytic ileus, hemorrhage, and laceration of the urethra, bladder, or colon. Patients may survive the initial pelvic injury, only to die from complications such as sepsis, fat embolism syndrome, or thromboembolism.
- Pelvic fractures are diagnosed by x-ray and CT.
- Physical examination of the abdomen demonstrates local swelling, tenderness, deformity, unusual pelvic movement, and ecchymosis.

Treatment of pelvic fractures depends on the severity of the injury.

- Stable, nondisplaced fractures require limited intervention. Bed rest, sometimes with the use of a pelvic sling, is typically maintained for a few days. Progressive ambulation with guarded weight bearing is then encouraged.
- Complex or displaced fractures (e.g., open book fracture) are often performed emergently with external fixation alone or combined with open reduction and internal fixation (ORIF) surgery. Use extreme care in handling or moving the patient to prevent additional injury. Only turn the patient when approved by the HCP. Because a pelvic fracture can damage other organs, assess bowel and urinary tract function, as well as distal neurovascular status.
- Provide back care while the patient is raised from the bed, with either independent use of the trapeze or adequate assistance.

GASTRITIS

Description

Gastritis, an inflammation of the gastric mucosa, is one of the most common problems affecting the stomach. Gastritis may be acute or chronic and diffuse or localized.

Pathophysiology

Gastritis occurs as the result of a breakdown in the normal gastric mucosal barrier. When the barrier is broken, HCl acid and pepsin can diffuse back into the mucosa. This back diffusion results in stomach tissue edema, disruption of capillary walls with plasma lost into the gastric lumen, and possible hemorrhage.

Drugs contribute to the development of acute and chronic gastritis. Nonsteroidal antiinflammatory drugs (NSAIDs), including aspirin, and corticosteroids inhibit the synthesis of prostaglandins that are protective to the gastric mucosa, making the mucosa more susceptible to injury. Risk factors for NSAID-induced gastritis include being female; age older than 60 years; a history of ulcer disease; taking anticoagulants, other NSAIDs (including low-dose aspirin), or other ulcerogenic drugs (including corticosteroids); and presence of a chronic debilitating disorder such as cardiovascular disease.

Repeated alcohol abuse results in chronic gastritis. Eating large quantities of spicy, irritating food and metabolic conditions such as renal failure can cause acute gastritis.

Another cause of chronic gastritis is *Helicobacter pylori* infection, which is highest in underdeveloped countries and among people of low socioeconomic status.

Autoimmune metaplastic atrophic gastritis (also called autoimmune atrophic gastritis) is an inherited condition in which there is an immune response directed against parietal cells. Atrophic gastritis is associated with an increased risk of stomach cancer.

Clinical Manifestations

- *Acute gastritis* symptoms include anorexia, nausea and vomiting, epigastric tenderness, and a feeling of fullness. Hemorrhage is commonly associated with alcohol abuse and may be the only symptom. Acute gastritis is self-limiting, lasting from a few hours to a few days.
- *Chronic gastritis* symptoms are similar to those of acute gastritis. Some patients are asymptomatic. However, when parietal cells are lost as a result of atrophy, the source of intrinsic factor is lost, and cobalamin (vitamin B_{12}) cannot be absorbed in the ileum, resulting in pernicious anemia and neurologic complications.

Diagnostic Studies

Diagnosis of acute gastritis is most often based on the patient's symptoms and history.

- Endoscopic examination with biopsy is used to obtain a definitive diagnosis.
- Breath, urine, serum, stool, and gastric tissue biopsy tests are available for determination of *H. pylori* infection.
- CBC may demonstrate anemia from blood loss or lack of intrinsic factor.
- Stools are tested for occult blood.

- Serum tests for antibodies to parietal cells and intrinsic factor are done.

Interprofessional Care

Treatment of acute gastritis focuses on eliminating the cause and preventing or avoiding it in the future. The plan of care is supportive (see Nausea and Vomiting, p. 429).

- If vomiting accompanies acute gastritis, rest, nothing by mouth (NPO) status, and IV fluids may be prescribed. Antiemetics are given for nausea and vomiting. In severe cases, a nasogastric (NG) tube may be used to monitor for bleeding, lavage the precipitating agent from the stomach, or keep the stomach empty and free of noxious stimuli.
- Monitor for dehydration. It can occur rapidly in acute gastritis with vomiting.
- Clear liquids are resumed when acute symptoms have subsided, with gradual reintroduction of solid, bland foods.
- Management strategies discussed in the section on upper GI bleeding apply to the patient with severe gastritis (see Gastrointestinal Bleeding, Upper, p. 242).
- Drug therapy focuses on reducing irritation of the gastric mucosa and providing symptomatic relief. Histamine (H_2)-receptor blockers (e.g., ranitidine, cimetidine) or proton pump inhibitors (PPIs) (e.g., omeprazole, lansoprazole) reduce gastric HCl acid secretion.

Treatment of chronic gastritis focuses on evaluating and eliminating the specific cause.

- Antibiotic combinations are used to eradicate *H. pylori.*
- The patient with pernicious anemia needs lifelong administration of cobalamin.

The patient undergoing treatment for chronic gastritis may have to adapt to lifestyle changes and strictly adhere to a drug regimen. An interprofessional team approach in which the HCP, nurse, dietitian, and pharmacist provide consistent information and support may increase patient success in making these alterations.

GASTROESOPHAGEAL REFLUX DISEASE

Description

Gastroesophageal reflux disease (GERD) results from mucosal damage caused by reflux of stomach acid into the lower esophagus. GERD is not a disease but a syndrome. GERD is the most common

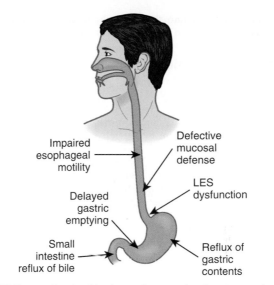

Fig. 10 Factors involved in the pathogenesis of gastroesophageal reflux disease. *LES,* Lower esophageal sphincter.

upper GI problem. Approximately 10% to 20% of the U.S. population experience GERD symptoms (heartburn or regurgitation) at least once a week.

Pathophysiology

GERD has no single cause (Fig. 10). GERD results when the defenses of the esophagus are overwhelmed by the reflux of acidic gastric contents into the esophagus. One of the primary etiologic factors in GERD is an incompetent lower esophageal sphincter (LES). Under normal conditions, the LES acts as an antireflux barrier. An incompetent LES lets gastric contents move from the stomach to the esophagus when the patient is supine or has an increase in intraabdominal pressure.

Gastric HCl acid and pepsin secretions that reflux cause esophageal irritation and inflammation *(esophagitis).* The degree of inflammation depends on the amount and composition of the gastric reflux and on the esophagus's mucosal defense mechanisms.

Predisposing conditions include hiatal hernia, incompetent LES, decreased esophageal clearance (ability to clear liquids or food

G

from the esophagus into the stomach) resulting from impaired esophageal motility, and decreased gastric emptying.

Clinical Manifestations

Symptoms vary, but symptoms that persistently occur more than twice a week indicate GERD.

- Heartburn (*pyrosis*), caused by irritation of the esophagus by secretions, is the most common manifestation. Heartburn is a burning, tight sensation that is felt intermittently beneath the lower sternum and spreads upward to the throat or jaw.
- Patients may complain of dyspepsia, which is pain or discomfort centered in the upper abdomen (mainly in or around the midline, as opposed to the right or left hypochondrium).
- Regurgitation is common and often described as a hot, bitter, or sour liquid in the throat or mouth.
- GERD-related chest pain can mimic angina. It is described as burning, squeezing, or radiating to the back, neck, jaw, or arms. Unlike angina, GERD-related chest pain is relieved with antacids.

Complications

Complications are related to the effects of gastric acid secretion on the esophageal mucosa. Esophagitis (inflammation of the esophagus) is a common complication of GERD. Repeated esophagitis may cause scar tissue formation, stricture, and ultimately dysphagia. *Barrett's esophagus,* a precancerous lesion, increases the patient's risk for esophageal cancer.

- Respiratory complications due to irritation of the upper airway by gastric secretions include cough, bronchospasm, laryngospasm, asthma, and chronic bronchitis.
- Dental erosion may result from acid reflux into the mouth.

Diagnostic Studies

Diagnostic studies help determine the cause of the GERD.

- Barium swallow determines if there is protrusion of the upper part of the stomach into the esophagus.
- Endoscopy is useful in assessing LES competence and extent of inflammation (if present), potential scarring, and strictures.
- Biopsy and cytologic specimens can differentiate stomach and esophageal cancer from Barrett's esophagus (see Esophageal Cancer, p. 218).
- Radionuclide tests can detect gastric reflux and the rate of esophageal clearance.

Interprofessional Care

Most patients with GERD can successfully manage the condition through lifestyle modifications and drug therapy. Give particular attention to diet and other medications that may affect the LES, acid secretion, or gastric emptying. Encourage patients who smoke to stop.

No specific diet is necessary. Teach patients to avoid foods that aggravate their symptoms such as chocolate, peppermint, tomatoes, fatty foods, coffee, and tea. Small, frequent meals help prevent overdistention of the stomach. Late evening meals and nocturnal snacking should be avoided. Weight reduction is recommended if the patient is obese.

Drug Therapy

Drug therapy focuses on improving LES function, increasing esophageal clearance, decreasing volume and acidity of reflux, and protecting esophageal mucosa. Proton pump inhibitors (PPIs) and H_2-receptor blockers are effective treatments for symptomatic GERD. The goal of HCl acid suppression treatment is to reduce the acidity of the gastric refluxate. Patients who are symptomatic with GERD but do not have evidence of esophagitis achieve symptom relief with PPIs and H_2-receptor agents. The PPIs are more effective in healing esophagitis than are H_2-receptor blockers.

- PPIs include omeprazole (Prilosec), esomeprazole (Nexium), lansoprazole (Prevacid), and rabeprazole (Aciphex).
- H_2-receptor blockers such as cimetidine, ranitidine (Zantac), famotidine (Pepcid), and nizatidine (Axid) reduce symptoms and promote esophageal healing in 50% of patients.

Antacids with or without alginic acid (e.g., Gaviscon) may be useful in patients with mild, intermittent heartburn.

Surgical Therapy

Surgical therapy is reserved for patients with complications of reflux, including esophagitis, intolerance of medications, stricture, Barrett's esophagus, and persistence of severe symptoms. Most surgical procedures are performed laparoscopically.

Nursing Management

Nursing care for the patient with acute symptoms consists of encouraging the patient to follow the necessary regimen (Table 35).

TABLE 35 Patient & Caregiver Teaching
Gastroesophageal Reflux Disease (GERD)

Include the following instructions when teaching the patient and caregivers about management of GERD.

1. Explain the reason for a low-fat diet.
2. Encourage the patient to eat small, frequent meals to prevent gastric distention.
3. Explain the reason for avoiding alcohol, smoking (causes an almost immediate, marked decrease in lower esophageal sphincter pressure), and beverages that contain caffeine.
4. Advise the patient to not lie down for 2 to 3 hours after eating, wear tight clothing around the waist, or bend over (especially after eating).
5. Have the patient avoid eating within 3 hours of bedtime.
6. Encourage the patient to sleep with head of bed elevated on 4- to 6-inch blocks or 30-degree angle (gravity fosters esophageal emptying).
7. Provide information about drugs, including reasons for their use and common side effects.
8. Discuss strategies for weight reduction if appropriate.
9. Encourage patient and caregiver to share concerns about lifestyle changes and living with a chronic problem.

GASTROINTESTINAL BLEEDING, UPPER

Description

In the United States, approximately 300,000 hospital admissions occur each year for upper GI bleeding. Approximately 60% of these are adults older than 65 years of age. Despite advances in the drug management of predisposing conditions and identification of risk factors, the mortality rate for upper GI bleeding has remained at approximately 6% to 13% for many years.

Pathophysiology

Although the most serious loss of blood from the upper GI tract is characterized by a sudden onset, insidious occult bleeding can be a major problem. Bleeding severity depends on whether the origin is venous, capillary, or arterial. Bleeding from an arterial source is profuse, and the blood is bright red. By contrast, "coffee ground" vomitus indicates that the blood has been in the stomach for some time. *Melena* (black, tarry stools) indicates slow bleeding from an upper GI source.

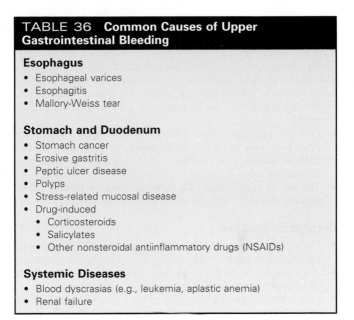

TABLE 36 Common Causes of Upper Gastrointestinal Bleeding

Esophagus
- Esophageal varices
- Esophagitis
- Mallory-Weiss tear

Stomach and Duodenum
- Stomach cancer
- Erosive gastritis
- Peptic ulcer disease
- Polyps
- Stress-related mucosal disease
- Drug-induced
  - Corticosteroids
  - Salicylates
  - Other nonsteroidal antiinflammatory drugs (NSAIDs)

Systemic Diseases
- Blood dyscrasias (e.g., leukemia, aplastic anemia)
- Renal failure

A variety of areas in the GI tract may be involved. Table 36 lists common causes of upper GI bleeding. The most common sites are the esophagus, stomach, and duodenum.

- Bleeding from the esophagus is most likely caused by chronic esophagitis, Mallory-Weiss tear, or esophageal varices. Chronic esophagitis can be caused by GERD, smoking, alcohol use, and the ingestion of drugs irritating to the mucosa. Esophageal varices most often occur from cirrhosis of the liver (see Cirrhosis, p. 136).
- Bleeding peptic ulcers account for 40% of the cases of upper GI bleeding. Drugs are a major cause of upper GI bleeding. Aspirin and other NSAIDs and corticosteroids can cause irritation and disruption of the gastroduodenal mucosa.
- Stress-related mucosal disease (SRMD), also called physiologic stress ulcers, is a continuum of conditions ranging from stress-related injury (superficial mucosal damage) to stress ulcers (focal deep mucosal damage). SRMD is most commonly seen in critically ill patients who have had severe burns, trauma, or major surgery.

Complications

To facilitate early intervention, the physical examination should focus on identifying signs and symptoms of shock such as tachycardia, weak pulse, hypotension, cool extremities, prolonged capillary refill, and apprehension. Monitor vital signs every 15 to 30 minutes. The patient is at risk for gut perforation and peritonitis, which may be indicated by a tense, rigid, boardlike abdomen.

- IV lines, preferably two, with a 16- or 18-gauge needle are placed for fluid and blood replacement. An indwelling urinary catheter may also be inserted so that output can be accurately assessed hourly.
- The use of supplemental O_2 delivered by face mask or nasal cannula may help increase blood oxygen saturation.

Diagnostic Studies

- Endoscopy is the primary tool for diagnosing the source (e.g., esophageal or gastric varices, gastritis) of upper GI bleeding.
- Angiography is used to diagnose upper GI bleeding when endoscopy cannot be done or when bleeding persists.
- Laboratory studies include CBC, blood urea nitrogen (BUN), serum electrolytes, prothrombin time, partial thromboplastin time, liver enzymes, and arterial blood gases (ABGs).

Interprofessional Care

The first-line management of upper GI bleeding is endoscopy. Endoscopy performed within the first 24 hours of bleeding is important for diagnosis, determining the need for surgical intervention, and providing treatment. Injection therapy with epinephrine (1 : 10,000 dilution) during endoscopy is effective for acute hemostasis. The goal of endoscopic hemostasis is to coagulate or thrombose the bleeding vessel.

Surgical intervention is indicated when bleeding continues from an identified site. The site of the hemorrhage determines the choice of operation.

During the acute phase, drugs are used to decrease bleeding, decrease HCl acid secretion, and neutralize the HCl acid that is present.

- Efforts are made to reduce acid secretion because the acidic environment can alter platelet function, as well as interfere with clot stabilization. Proton pump inhibitors (PPIs) (e.g., pantoprazole [Protonix]) or H_2-receptor blockers (e.g., cimetidine) are administered IV to decrease acid secretion (see

Table 41-10 in Lewis et al, *Medical-Surgical Nursing,* ed 10, p. 903).

Octreotide (Sandostatin) or vasopressin may be given when upper GI bleeding is from esophageal or gastric varices.

Nursing Management

Goals

The patient with upper GI bleeding will have no further GI bleeding, have the cause of the bleeding identified and treated, experience a return to a normal hemodynamic state, and have minimal or no symptoms of pain or anxiety.

Nursing Diagnoses

- Decreased cardiac output
- Deficient fluid volume
- Ineffective peripheral tissue perfusion
- Anxiety

Nursing Interventions

The patient with a history of chronic gastritis or peptic ulcer disease is at high risk for upper GI bleeding. Teach the at-risk patient to avoid known gastric irritants such as alcohol and smoking, and to take only prescribed medications. OTC drugs can be harmful because they may contain ingredients (e.g., aspirin) that increase the risk of bleeding.

Once an infusion has been started, maintain the IV line for fluid or blood replacement. An accurate intake and output record is essential so that the patient's hydration status can be assessed.

Although room-temperature, cool, or iced gastric lavage is used in some institutions, its effectiveness as a treatment for upper GI bleeding is questionable. When lavage is used, approximately 50 to 100 mL of fluid is instilled at a time into the stomach.

- Monitor vital signs, especially in patients with cardiovascular disease, because dysrhythmias may occur.
- Keep the head of the bed elevated to provide comfort and prevent aspiration.
- Assess stools for blood. Black, tarry stools indicate prolonged upper GI bleeding.
- Monitor the patient's laboratory studies. The hemoglobin and hematocrit are usually evaluated about every 4 to 6 hours if the patient is actively bleeding.
- When oral nourishment is begun, observe the patient for symptoms of nausea and vomiting and a recurrence of bleeding. Feedings initially consist of hourly clear fluids until tolerance is determined. Gradual introduction of foods follows if the patient has no discomfort.

- When hemorrhage is the result of chronic alcohol abuse, closely observe the patient for delirium tremens as alcohol withdrawal takes place.

▼ **Patient and Caregiver Teaching**

- Teach the patient and caregivers how to avoid future bleeding episodes, emphasizing adherence to prescribed drug therapy and avoiding aspirin and other NSAIDs.
- Smoking and alcohol should be eliminated because they are sources of gastric irritation.
- Instruct the patient and family on what to do if an acute hemorrhage occurs in the future.

GLAUCOMA

Description

Glaucoma is a group of disorders characterized by increased intraocular pressure (IOP) and the consequences of elevated pressure, optic nerve atrophy, and peripheral visual field loss. Many people with glaucoma are unaware of their condition.

- Glaucoma is the second leading cause of permanent blindness in the United States and the leading cause of blindness among African Americans.
- Blindness from glaucoma is largely preventable with early detection and appropriate treatment.

Pathophysiology

Increased IOP results when the rate of aqueous production (inflow) is greater than aqueous reabsorption (outflow). If the pressure remains elevated, permanent vision loss may occur.

- *Primary open-angle glaucoma* (POAG) is the most common type of primary glaucoma. In POAG, the aqueous outflow is decreased in the trabecular meshwork. The drainage channels become clogged, like a clogged kitchen sink. Damage to the optic nerve can result.
- *Primary angle-closure glaucoma* (PACG) is due to a reduction in the outflow of aqueous humor that results from angle closure. Usually this is caused by the lens bulging forward as a result of the aging process. Angle closure may also occur as a result of pupil dilation in the patient with anatomically narrow angles. An acute attack may occur because of drug-induced mydriasis, emotional excitement, or darkness. Check the medical record before administering medications to the patient with angle-closure glaucoma and instruct the patient not to take any mydriatic medications.

Clinical Manifestations

- POAG develops slowly without symptoms of pain or pressure. The patient usually does not notice gradual visual field loss until peripheral vision is severely compromised (tunnel vision).
- Acute angle-closure glaucoma causes symptoms of sudden, excruciating pain in or around the eye that is often accompanied by nausea and vomiting. Visual symptoms include seeing colored halos around lights, blurred vision, and ocular redness.
- Manifestations of subacute or chronic angle-closure glaucoma appear gradually. The patient who has had a previous unrecognized episode of subacute angle-closure glaucoma may report a history of blurred vision, colored halos around lights, ocular redness, or eye or brow pain.

Diagnostic Studies

- IOP measurement with tonometry
- Visual acuity measurement and visual field perimetry
- Slit-lamp microscopy
- Ophthalmoscopy (direct and indirect)

Interprofessional Care

The primary focus of therapy is to keep the IOP low enough to prevent the patient from developing optic nerve damage. Therapy varies with the type of glaucoma.

- In chronic open-angle glaucoma, initial drug therapy can include β-adrenergic receptor blocking agents, α-adrenergic agents, cholinergic agents (miotics), and carbonic anhydrase inhibitors (hyperosmotic agents).
- When prescribed medications are not effective or are not used as recommended, surgical options include argon laser trabeculoplasty (ALT) and trabeculectomy.
- Acute angle-closure glaucoma is an ocular emergency that requires immediate interventions, including miotics and oral or IV hyperosmotic agents. Laser peripheral iridotomy or surgical iridectomy is necessary for definitive treatment and prevention of subsequent episodes.

Nursing Management

Because glaucoma is a chronic condition requiring long-term management, assess the patient's ability to understand the rationale and adhere to the regimen of the prescribed therapy. Also assess the patient's reaction to the diagnosis of a potentially sight-threatening chronic disorder.

Goals

The patient with glaucoma will have no progression of visual impairment, understand the disease process and rationale for therapy, comply with all aspects of therapy (including drug administration and follow-up care), and have no postoperative complications.

Nursing Diagnoses

- Acute pain
- Self-care deficits
- Risk for injury
- Noncompliance

Nursing Interventions

- Encourage adherence by helping the patient identify the most convenient and appropriate times for drug administration or advocating a change in therapy if the patient reports unacceptable side effects.

▼ **Patient and Caregiver Teaching**

See Table 22, Patient and Caregiver Teaching: After Eye Surgery, p. 115.

Provide accurate information about the disease process and treatment options, including the rationale underlying each option. In addition, the patient needs information about the purpose, frequency, and technique for administration of antiglaucoma drugs.

GLOMERULONEPHRITIS

Glomerulonephritis is an inflammation of renal glomeruli caused by immunologic processes. It affects both kidneys equally and is the third leading cause of end-stage renal disease (ESRD) in the United States. Although the glomerulus is the primary site of inflammation, tubular, interstitial, and vascular changes also occur.

- A variety of conditions can cause glomerulonephritis, ranging from kidney infections to systemic diseases. Glomerulonephritis can be acute or chronic. In *acute glomerulonephritis* symptoms come on suddenly and may be temporary or reversible. By contrast, *chronic glomerulonephritis* is slowly progressive and generally leads to irreversible renal failure.

Acute Poststreptococcal Glomerulonephritis

Acute poststreptococcal glomerulonephritis (APSGN) is most common in children and young adults. It develops 1 to 2 weeks after an infection of the tonsils, pharynx, or skin (e.g., streptococcal sore throat, impetigo) by nephrotoxic strains of group A β-hemolytic streptococci. Antibodies are produced to the streptococcal antigen, and tissue injury occurs as the antigen-antibody complexes are deposited in the glomeruli and complement is activated.

- More than 95% of patients with APSGN recover completely or improve rapidly with conservative management. Accurate recognition and assessment are critical because chronic glomerulonephritis can develop if the patient is not treated appropriately. Clinical manifestations of APSGN include generalized body edema, hypertension, oliguria, hematuria with a smoky or rusty appearance, and proteinuria. Fluid retention occurs as a result of decreased glomerular filtration.
- Edema initially appears in low-pressure tissues, such as the eyes *(periorbital edema),* but later progresses to involve the total body as ascites or peripheral edema in the legs.
- Smoky urine indicates bleeding in the upper urinary tract. The degree of proteinuria varies with the severity of the glomerulonephropathy.
- Hypertension mainly results from increased extracellular fluid volume.
- The patient may have abdominal or flank pain. In other cases, the patient may be asymptomatic and the problem is found on routine urinalysis.

An immune response to the streptococci is often demonstrated by assessment of antistreptolysin-O (ASO) titers. Decreased complement levels indicate an immune-mediated response. Renal biopsy may be done to confirm the disease. Urinalysis reveals significant numbers of erythrocytes. Erythrocyte casts are highly suggestive of acute glomerulonephritis. Proteinuria may be mild to severe. Blood tests include blood urea nitrogen (BUN) and serum creatinine to assess the extent of renal impairment.

Nursing and Interprofessional Management

Management of APSGN focuses on symptomatic relief. Rest is recommended until the signs of glomerular inflammation (proteinuria, hematuria) and hypertension subside. Edema is treated by restricting sodium and fluid intake and administering diuretics.

- Severe hypertension is treated with antihypertensive drugs.
- Dietary protein intake may be restricted if there is evidence of an increase in nitrogenous wastes (e.g., elevated BUN).
- Antibiotics are given if streptococcal infection is still present. Corticosteroids and cytotoxic drugs have not been shown to be of value.

One of the most important ways to prevent APSGN is to encourage early diagnosis and treatment of sore throats and skin lesions.

G

If streptococci are found in the culture, encourage the patient to take the full course of antibiotics to ensure that the bacteria have been eradicated.

- Good personal hygiene is an important factor in preventing the spread of cutaneous streptococcal infections.

Chronic Glomerulonephritis

Chronic glomerulonephritis is a syndrome that reflects the end stage of glomerular inflammatory disease. Most types of glomerulonephritis and nephrotic syndrome can eventually lead to chronic glomerulonephritis.

- Some people who develop chronic glomerulonephritis have no history of kidney disease. Frequently the cause of chronic glomerulonephritis is not found.
- The syndrome is characterized by proteinuria, hematuria, and the slow development of the uremic syndrome as a result of decreasing renal function.

Chronic glomerulonephritis is often found coincidentally with an abnormality on a urinalysis or elevated BP. It is common that the patient has no recollection or history of renal problems. Ultrasound and CT scan are the preferred diagnostic studies. A renal biopsy may be performed to determine the exact cause of the glomerulonephritis. Treatment is supportive and symptomatic (see Kidney Disease, Chronic, p. 370).

GONORRHEA

Description

Gonorrhea is the second most frequently occurring sexually transmitted infection (STI) in the United States.

Pathophysiology

Gonorrhea is caused by *Neisseria gonorrhoeae,* a gram-negative diplococcus bacterium. Gonorrhea can be transmitted by exposure to sexual fluids during vaginal, anal, or oral sex. The most common site of infection for men is the urethra and for women, the cervix. Both men and women can get gonorrheal infections of the rectum from anal sex or of the oropharynx from oral sex.

- Gonococcal infection elicits an inflammatory response, which, if left untreated, leads to formation of fibrous tissue and adhesions. This fibrous scarring is subsequently responsible for many complications such as strictures and tubal abnormalities, which can lead to tubal pregnancy, chronic pelvic pain, and infertility.

Clinical Manifestations

- Many men with gonorrhea are asymptomatic, whereas others do report symptoms. The most common symptoms of gonococcal urethritis among men are dysuria, purulent urethral discharge, and epididymitis.
- Most women who contract gonorrhea are asymptomatic or have symptoms that are overlooked. For women, common symptoms are increased vaginal discharge, dysuria, frequency of urination, and bleeding after sex. Redness and swelling can occur at the cervix or urethra along with a purulent exudate.
- Symptoms and signs of rectal gonorrhea may include mucopurulent rectal discharge, bleeding, pain, pruritus, and painful bowel movements.
- Most patients with gonorrheal infections in the throat have few if any symptoms. Some may complain of a sore throat.

Complications

Because men often seek treatment early in the course of the infection, they are less likely to develop complications. Complications that do occur in men are prostatitis, urethral strictures, and sterility from orchitis or epididymitis.

Because women who are asymptomatic seldom seek treatment, complications are more common and usually are the reason for seeking medical attention. In women, pelvic inflammatory disease (PID), Bartholin's abscess, ectopic pregnancy, and infertility are the main complications.

Neonates can develop *gonococcal conjunctivitis* (ophthalmia neonatorum) from exposure to an infected mother during delivery, which can result in permanent blindness. Almost all states have a law or a health department regulation requiring the use of a prophylactic treatment in the eyes of all newborns to prevent such infections.

G

Diagnostic Studies

- For men, a presumptive diagnosis of gonorrhea is made if there is a history of sexual contact with a new or infected partner followed within a few days by a urethral discharge. Typical clinical manifestations combined with a positive finding in a Gram-stained smear of discharge from the penis give an almost certain diagnosis.
- The nucleic acid amplification test (NAAT) is a nonculture test with sensitivity similar to that of culture tests for *N. gonorrhoeae*. It can be done on a wide variety of samples, including vaginal, endocervical, urethral, and urine specimens.

- For women, making a diagnosis of gonorrhea on the basis of symptoms is difficult. Most women are asymptomatic or have complaints that may be confused with other conditions, such as chlamydial infection or a urinary tract infection. A culture must be performed to confirm the diagnosis.

Interprofessional Care

Because of a short incubation period and high infectivity, treatment is generally instituted without waiting for culture results. The first-line treatment for gonorrhea is dual therapy with IM ceftriaxone (Rocephin) and oral azithromycin. Because of the increasing rate of drug resistance, all patients with gonococcal infection must receive treatment with at least two antibiotics.

- All sexual contacts of patients with gonorrhea must be treated to prevent reinfection after resumption of sexual relations. The "ping-pong" effect of reexposure, treatment, and reinfection can cease only when infected partners are treated simultaneously.

Nursing Management

See Nursing Management: Sexually Transmitted Infections, pp. 564-565.

GOUT

Description

Gout is a type of acute arthritis characterized by elevation of uric acid (hyperuricemia) and the deposit of uric acid crystals in one or more joints. Sodium urate crystals may be found in articular, periarticular, and subcutaneous tissues. Unlike chronic forms of arthritis, gout is marked by painful flares lasting days to weeks followed by long periods without symptoms. More than 8 million Americans are affected by gout, with men affected three times as often as women. The incidence in African American men is nearly twice that in white men.

Hyperuricemia may be classified as primary or secondary. In *primary hyperuricemia* a hereditary error of purine metabolism leads to the overproduction or retention of uric acid. *Secondary hyperuricemia* may be related to another acquired disorder or may be caused by drugs known to inhibit uric acid excretion (e.g., thiazide diuretics, β-adrenergic blockers, angiotensin-converting enzyme inhibitors). Postmenopausal women and organ transplant recipients taking immunosuppressive agents are also at risk for hyperuricemia.

Pathophysiology

Uric acid is the major end product of purine catabolism and is primarily excreted by the kidneys. Gout is caused by an increase in uric acid production, reduced excretion of uric acid by the kidneys (the most common cause), or increased intake of foods containing purines (e.g., red and organ meat, shellfish, fructose drinks), which are metabolized to uric acid by the body. Increased uric acid production is most commonly linked to obesity. Excessive alcohol consumption is also a risk factor.

- High dietary intake of purine alone has relatively little effect on uric acid levels. Hyperuricemia may result from prolonged fasting or excessive alcohol drinking because of the increased production of keto acids, which then inhibit uric acid excretion. Reduced uric acid excretion can occur with chronic kidney disease or metabolic syndrome.

Clinical Manifestations

Gouty arthritis may occur acutely in one or more joints. Affected joints may appear dusky or cyanotic and are extremely tender. Inflammation of the great toe *(podagra)* is the most common initial problem. Other joints affected may include the midfoot, ankle, knee, wrist, and olecranon bursa.

- Acute gouty arthritis is usually triggered by events such as trauma, surgery, alcohol ingestion, or systemic infection. Symptom onset is usually rapid as swelling and pain peak within several hours, often accompanied by a low-grade fever.
- Individual attacks usually subside in 2 to 10 days with or without treatment. The affected joint returns to normal and patients have no symptoms between attacks.

Chronic gout is characterized by multiple joint involvement and visible deposits of sodium urate crystals *(tophi)*. These are typically seen in the synovium, subchondral bone, olecranon bursa, and vertebrae; along tendons; and in the skin and cartilage. Tophi are generally noted many years after the onset of the disease.

Chronic inflammation may cause joint deformity, and cartilage destruction may predispose the joint to secondary osteoarthritis. Large urate crystal deposits may pierce overlying skin, producing draining sinuses that often become infected. Excessive uric acid excretion may lead to urinary tract stone formation. Pyelonephritis related to intrarenal sodium urate deposits and obstruction may contribute to kidney disease.

The severity of gouty arthritis is variable. The clinical course may consist of infrequent mild attacks or multiple severe episodes and slowly progressive disability.

G

Diagnostic Studies

- Serum uric acid levels are usually elevated above 6 mg/dL.
- Specimens may be obtained for 24-hour urine uric acid levels to determine if the disease is caused by decreased renal excretion or overproduction of uric acid.
- X-rays appear normal in the early stages of gout, with tophi, an indicator of chronic disease, appearing as eroded areas in the bone.
- Synovial fluid aspiration helps distinguish gout from septic arthritis and *pseudogout* (in which calcium phosphate crystals are formed). Affected fluid characteristically contains needle-like crystals of sodium urate.

Interprofessional Care

Goals for care include ending an acute attack with an antiinflammatory agent such as colchicine. Drug therapy is the primary way to treat acute and chronic gout. Weight reduction (as needed) and possible avoidance of alcohol and foods high in purine (red and organ meats) are recommended.

Drug Therapy

Acute gouty arthritis is treated with colchicine and nonsteroidal antiinflammatory drugs (NSAIDs). Because colchicine has antiinflammatory effects but is not an analgesic, an NSAID is added to the treatment regimen for pain management. Future attacks are prevented in part by combining colchicine with a xanthine oxidase inhibitor (allopurinol [Zyloprim]), or a drug that increases the excretion of uric acid in the urine (uricosuric) (probenecid [Probalan]). Febuxostat (Uloric), a selective inhibitor of xanthine oxidase, is used for long-term management of hyperuricemia in people with chronic gout.

- Aspirin inactivates the effect of uricosurics, resulting in urate retention, and should be avoided while patients are taking uricosuric drugs (e.g., probenecid). Acetaminophen can be used safely if analgesia is required.

Patients who cannot take or do not respond to drugs that lower uric acid in the blood may be given pegloticase (Krystexxa). This drug metabolizes uric acid into a harmless chemical excreted in the urine.

- Corticosteroids, either orally or by intraarticular injection, can be helpful in treating acute attacks.
- Adequate urine volume with normal renal function (2 to 3 L/day) must be maintained to prevent precipitation of uric acid in the renal tubules. Allopurinol, which blocks production of uric acid, is particularly useful in patients with uric acid stones or

renal impairment, in whom uricosuric drugs may be ineffective or dangerous.

Regardless of which drugs are used to treat gout, serum uric acid levels must be checked regularly to monitor treatment effectiveness.

Nutritional Therapy

Dietary restrictions that limit alcohol and foods high in purine help minimize uric acid production. Instruct obese patients in a carefully planned weight-reduction program.

Nursing Management

Nursing intervention is directed at supportive care of the inflamed joints.

- Bed rest may be appropriate, with affected joints properly immobilized. Use a bed cradle or footboard to protect a painful lower extremity from the weight of bed clothes.
- Assess the limitation of motion and degree of pain. Document treatment response.

▼ **Patient and Caregiver Teaching**

Hyperuricemia and gouty arthritis are chronic problems that can be controlled with careful adherence to a treatment program.

- Explain the importance of drug therapy and the need for periodic determination of serum uric acid levels.
- Teach the patient about triggers for an attack, including overindulgence in purine-containing foods and alcohol, starvation (fasting), medication use (e.g., diuretics), and major medical events (e.g., surgery, myocardial infarction).

G

GUILLAIN-BARRÉ SYNDROME

Description

Guillain-Barré syndrome (GBS) is a collection of clinical syndromes that manifest as acute inflammatory polyneuropathy. GBS is characterized by an autoimmune process that occurs a few days or weeks after a viral or bacterial infection. The most common type of GBS diagnosed in the United States is acute inflammatory demyelinating polyneuropathy (AIDP). GBS is rare, affecting approximately 1 person in every 100,000.

The main features of GBS include acute, ascending, rapidly progressive, symmetric weakness of the limbs. Maximal weakness is reached in 4 weeks. Reflexes in the affected limbs are weak or absent. Respiratory muscles may also be affected and some patients require mechanical ventilation.

- Although 80% of patients almost completely recover, the process may take months or years.

Pathophysiology

The etiology is unknown. Both cellular and humoral immune mechanisms play a role in the immune reaction directed at the nerves. The result is a loss of myelin (a segmental demyelination) and edema and inflammation of the affected nerves. As demyelination occurs, the transmission of nerve impulses is stopped or slowed. Muscles innervated by the damaged peripheral nerves undergo denervation and atrophy. In the recovery phase, remyelination occurs slowly and function returns in a proximal-to-distal pattern.

- Most cases of GBS follow a viral or bacterial infection of the gastrointestinal or upper respiratory tract. Cytomegalovirus is the most common viral cause. *Campylobacter jejuni* gastroenteritis is the most common bacterial cause.

Clinical Manifestations

GBS is a heterogeneous condition, with symptoms ranging from mild to severe.

- The first symptoms are pain, paresthesia (numbness and tingling), and hypotonia (reduced muscle tone) of the limbs.
- Areflexia (lack of reflexes) and weakness or paralysis of the limbs usually peak within 4 weeks.
- Autonomic nervous system dysfunction manifests with orthostatic hypotension, hypertension, and abnormal vagal responses (bradycardia, heart block, asystole). Other autonomic dysfunctions include bowel and bladder dysfunction, facial flushing, and diaphoresis.
- Cranial nerve involvement is manifested as facial weakness and paresthesia, extraocular eye movement difficulties, and dysphagia.
- Pain is a common symptom including paresthesias, muscular aches and cramps, and hyperesthesias. Pain appears to be worse at night. Pain may lead to a decrease in appetite and interfere with sleep.

The most serious complication of GBS is respiratory failure, which occurs as paralysis progresses to the nerves that innervate the thoracic area.

Diagnostic Studies

Diagnosis is based primarily on patient history and clinical signs. Clinical features required for the diagnosis include progressive weakness of more than one limb and diminished or absent reflexes.

- Cerebrospinal fluid (CSF) analysis is helpful in excluding other causes. In GBS, the CSF has more protein than normal.
- Results of EMG and nerve conduction studies are used to confirm the diagnosis.

Nursing and Interprofessional Management

Management of GBS is supportive. Ventilator support is critical during the acute phase, as 30% of GBS cases progress to respiratory failure. Immunomodulating treatments such as plasma exchange (plasmapheresis) or high-dose IV immunoglobulin (IVIG) are most effective if administered within the first 2 weeks of symptom onset.

- Plasmapheresis removes antibodies and other immune factors. It is used 5 times either daily or every other day in the first 2 weeks.
- IVIG interferes with antigen presentation and is given over 5 days. Because it is more readily available, IVIG therapy has replaced plasmapheresis as the preferred treatment in many centers. Assessment of the patient is the most important aspect of nursing care during the acute phase.
- Assess the respiratory system frequently by checking respiratory rate and depth to determine the need for immediate intervention, including intubation and mechanical ventilation (see Tracheostomy, p. 735, and Artificial Airways: Endotracheal Tubes, p. 683). Monitor arterial blood gases (ABGs) and vital capacity.
- Evaluate motor and sensory function. Report changes in motor function (e.g., ascending paralysis), deep tendon reflexes, cranial nerve functions (e.g, swallowing, gag reflex, corneal reflex), and level of consciousness.
- Monitor BP and cardiac rate and rhythm during the acute phase because dysrhythmias may occur. Autonomic dysfunction usually takes the form of bradycardia and dysrhythmias. Orthostatic hypotension secondary to muscle atony may occur in severe cases. Vasopressor agents and volume expanders may be needed.
- If fever develops, obtain sputum cultures to identify the pathogen. Appropriate antibiotic therapy is then initiated.
- Respiratory infection or urinary tract infection (UTI) may occur. Immobility from paralysis can cause paralytic ileus, muscle atrophy, venous thromboembolism (VTE), pressure ulcers, orthostatic hypotension, and nutritional deficiencies.

Nutritional needs must be met in spite of possible problems associated with gastric dilation, paralytic ileus, and aspiration potential if the gag reflex is lost.

- Note drooling and other difficulties with secretions, which may indicate an inadequate gag reflex.
- Initially, enteral feedings or parenteral nutrition may be used to ensure adequate caloric intake. Monitor fluid and electrolyte therapy to prevent electrolyte imbalances.

HEAD AND NECK CANCER

Description

Most head and neck cancers arise from squamous cells that line the mucosal surfaces of the head and neck. These cancers may involve the nasal cavity and paranasal sinuses, nasopharynx, oropharynx, larynx, oral cavity, and/or salivary glands. Most patients present with locally advanced disease. Disability from the disease and treatment is great because of the potential loss of voice, disfigurement, and social consequences.

- Head and neck cancer occurs most frequently in patients 50 to 60 years of age. Men are affected twice as often as women.
- Most head and neck cancers are caused by tobacco use. Excessive alcohol consumption is also a major risk factor.
- Cancers in patients younger than 50 have been associated with human papillomavirus (HPV) infection. Other risk factors include sun exposure (oral cavity), radiation therapy to the head and neck, exposure to asbestos and other industrial carcinogens, and poor oral hygiene.

Clinical Manifestations

Early signs of head and neck cancer vary with tumor location.

- Cancer of the oral cavity may initially be seen as a red or white patch in the mouth, an ulcer that does not heal, or a change in the fit of dentures.
- Hoarseness that lasts more than 2 weeks may be a symptom of early laryngeal cancer. Some patients experience what feels like a lump in the throat or a change in voice quality.
- Other clinical manifestations include sore throat that does not get better with treatment, unilateral sore throat or otalgia (ear pain), swelling or lumps in the neck, and coughing up blood.
- Difficulties with chewing, swallowing, moving the tongue, and breathing are typically late symptoms.

Diagnostic Studies

- If lesions are suspected, upper airways may be examined by indirect laryngoscopy or using a flexible nasopharyngoscope.

The larynx and vocal cords are visually inspected for lesions and tissue mobility.

- A CT scan or MRI may be performed to detect local and regional spread.
- Multiple biopsy specimens are obtained to determine the extent of the disease.

Interprofessional Care

The stage of the disease is determined on the basis of tumor size (T), number and location of involved nodes (N), and extent of metastasis (M). TNM classifies disease as stage I to stage IV (see p. 781, Part Three).

- Stage I and II cancers are potentially curable with radiation therapy or larynx-sparing surgery.
- Patients with advanced disease (stages III and IV) are treated with various combinations of surgery, radiation, chemotherapy, and targeted therapy. Radiation can be delivered by either external-beam therapy or internal implants (brachytherapy).
- Advanced lesions of the larynx are treated by a total laryngectomy, in which the entire larynx and preepiglottic region are removed and a permanent tracheostomy is created (see Tracheostomy, p. 735, in Part Two). Radical neck dissection frequently accompanies total laryngectomy. Depending on the extent of involvement, extensive dissection and reconstruction may be performed.
- Changes after a total laryngectomy include loss of speech, loss of the ability to taste and smell, inability to produce audible sounds (including laughing and crying), and a permanent tracheal stoma.
- Some patients refuse surgical intervention for advanced lesions because of the extent of the procedure and the potential risk. In this situation, external radiation therapy is used as the sole treatment or in combination with chemotherapy.
- Chemotherapy (e.g., cisplatin and targeted therapy (cetuximab [Erbitux]) are used in combination with radiation therapy for patients with stage III or IV cancers.

Nutritional Therapy

After radical neck surgery, the patient may be unable to take in nutrients through the normal route of ingestion. Parenteral fluids are given for the first 24 to 48 hours.

- Because of swelling and difficulty swallowing postoperatively, tube feedings are usually given through a nasogastric, nasointestinal, or gastrostomy tube that was placed during surgery.

H

When the patient can successfully swallow with low or no risk of aspiration, small amounts of thickened liquids or pureed foods may be given with the patient in high Fowler's position. Avoid thin, watery fluids because they are difficult to swallow, increasing the risk of aspiration. Closely observe for choking. Suctioning may be necessary to prevent aspiration.

Nursing Management

Goals

The patient with head or neck cancer will have a patent airway, no complications related to therapy, adequate nutritional intake, minimal to no pain, the ability to communicate, and an acceptable body image.

Nursing Diagnoses

- Ineffective airway clearance
- Risk for aspiration
- Anxiety
- Impaired verbal communication
- Acute pain

Nursing Interventions

Include information about risk factors in health teaching. Encourage good oral hygiene. Teach patients about safe sex practices to prevent HPV infection. Tobacco and alcohol cessation is still important after a cancer has been diagnosed because continued use of those substances diminishes the likelihood of a cure.

- Interventions to reduce side effects of radiation therapy include teaching the patient oral care measures to reduce dry mouth and encouraging regular exercise to reduce fatigue.

For procedures that involve a laryngectomy, teaching should include information about expected changes in speech. Establish a means of communication for the immediate postoperative period.

After surgery, maintenance of a patent airway is essential, and a laryngectomy (tracheostomy) tube will be in place. Keep the patient in semi-Fowler's position to decrease edema and tension on the suture lines. Monitor vital signs frequently because of the risk of hemorrhage and respiratory compromise. Immediately after surgery, the postlaryngectomy patient requires frequent suctioning via the tracheostomy tube.

- Encourage deep breathing and coughing and provide tracheostomy care as needed.
- Depression and changes in sexuality patterns because of altered body image are common in the patient who has had radical neck dissection. Help the patient regain an acceptable self-concept.

- A speech therapist should meet with the patient who had a total laryngectomy to discuss voice restoration options.

▼ **Patient and Caregiver Teaching**
- Monitor patency of any wound drainage tubes every 4 hours to ensure proper functioning. After drainage tubes are removed, closely monitor the area for swelling. If fluid accumulates, aspiration may be necessary.
- Instruct the patient and caregivers on how to manage tubes and whom to call if there are problems.
- Provide pictorial instructions for tracheostomy care, suctioning, stoma care, and tube feedings as appropriate.
- Teach the patient to cover the stoma before performing activities such as shaving and applying makeup to avoid inhalation of foreign materials.
- Address measures to provide adequate humidity at home using a bedside humidifier and high oral fluid intake.
- Encourage preparation of food that is colorful, attractive, and nutritious, because taste may also be diminished with loss of the sense of smell after surgery or radiation therapy.

HEAD INJURY

Description

Head injury includes any trauma to the scalp, skull, or brain. A serious form of head injury is *traumatic brain injury* (TBI). In U.S. hospital emergency departments, an estimated 1.7 million people are treated and released with TBI.
- Falls and motor vehicle crashes are the most common causes of head injury. Other causes of head injury include firearms, assaults, sports-related trauma, recreational injuries, and war-related injuries.
- Males are twice as likely to sustain a TBI as females.

Deaths from head trauma occur at three time points after injury: immediately after injury, within 2 hours of injury, and approximately 3 weeks after injury.
- The majority of deaths occur immediately after the injury, either from the direct head trauma or massive hemorrhage and shock.
- Deaths occurring within a few hours of the trauma are caused by progressive worsening of the head injury or internal bleeding. Immediately recognizing changes in neurologic status and rapid surgical intervention are critical in the prevention of deaths.
- Deaths occurring 3 weeks or more after the injury result from multisystem failure.

H

Types of Head Injuries

Scalp Laceration

Because the scalp contains many blood vessels with poor constrictive abilities, even relatively small wounds can bleed profusely. The major complications of scalp lesions are blood loss and infection.

Skull Fracture

Fractures frequently occur with head trauma. Fractures may be closed or open, depending on the presence of a scalp laceration or extension of the fracture into the air sinuses or dura.

- The type and severity of a skull fracture depend on the velocity, momentum, and direction of the injuring agent, and the site of impact. Specific manifestations of a skull fracture are generally associated with the location of the injury (see Table 56-7, Lewis et al, *Medical-Surgical Nursing,* ed 10, p. 1327).

Major potential complications of skull fracture are intracranial infections and hematoma, as well as meningeal and brain tissue damage.

Head Trauma

Brain injuries are categorized as *diffuse* (generalized) or *focal* (localized). In *diffuse injury* (i.e., concussion, diffuse axonal), damage to the brain cannot be localized to one particular area of the brain, whereas a *focal injury* (e.g., contusion, hematoma) can be localized to a specific area of the brain.

Diffuse Injury. *Concussion* is a minor, sudden, transient, and diffuse head injury associated with a disruption in neural activity and a change in the level of consciousness (LOC). The patient may not lose total consciousness. Manifestations such as a brief disruption in LOC, amnesia for the event (retrograde amnesia), and headache are generally of short duration.

- Postconcussion syndrome may develop in some patients and is usually seen from 2 weeks to 2 months after the injury. Manifestations include persistent headache, lethargy, behavior changes, decreased short-term memory, and changes in intellectual ability.

Although concussion is generally considered benign and usually resolves spontaneously, the signs and symptoms may be the beginning of a more serious, progressive problem. At the time of discharge it is important to give the patient and caregiver instructions for observation and accurate reporting of symptoms or changes in neurologic status.

Diffuse axonal injury (DAI) is widespread axonal damage occurring after a mild, moderate, or severe TBI.

- Clinical signs of DAI include decreased LOC, increased intracranial pressure (ICP), decortication or decerebration, and global cerebral edema. Approximately 90% of patients with DAI remain in a persistent vegetative state.
- Patients are rapidly triaged to an intensive care unit (ICU), where they will be vigilantly watched for signs of increased ICP and treated for increased ICP (see Increased Intracranial Pressure, p. 342).

Focal Injury. Focal injury can be minor to severe and can be localized to an area of injury. Focal injury consists of lacerations, contusions, hematomas, and cranial nerve injuries.

Lacerations involve actual tearing of brain tissue and often occur with compound fractures and penetrating injuries. Tissue damage is severe, and surgical repair of the laceration is impossible because of the nature of brain tissue. If bleeding is deep into the brain parenchyma, focal and generalized signs develop. Prognosis is generally poor for the patient with a large intracerebral hemorrhage.

A *contusion* is the bruising of brain tissue within a focal area. It is usually associated with a closed head injury. A contusion may contain areas of hemorrhage, infarction, necrosis, and edema and frequently occurs at a fracture site.

- Contusions or lacerations may occur both at the site of the direct impact of the brain on the skull *(coup)* and at a secondary area of damage on the opposite side away from injury *(contrecoup),* leading to multiple contused areas.
- Neurologic assessment may reveal focal as well as generalized findings, depending on the size and location of the contusion. Seizures are a common complication.

Complications

Epidural Hematoma

An *epidural hematoma* results from bleeding between the dura and inner surface of the skull. An epidural hematoma is a neurologic emergency and is usually associated with a linear fracture crossing a major artery in the dura, causing a tear. It can have a venous or an arterial origin.

- Venous epidural hematomas are associated with a tear of the dural venous sinus and develop slowly.
- With arterial hematomas, the middle meningeal artery lying under the temporal bone is often torn. Because this is an arterial hemorrhage, the hematoma develops rapidly.

Manifestations typically include an initial period of unconsciousness at the scene, with a brief lucid interval followed by a

H

decrease in LOC. Other symptoms may be headache, nausea and vomiting, or focal manifestations. Rapid surgical intervention to evacuate the hematoma and prevent cerebral herniation, along with medical management for increasing ICP, can dramatically improve outcomes.

Subdural Hematoma

A *subdural hematoma* occurs from bleeding between the dura mater and arachnoid layer of the meninges. The hematoma usually results from injury to the brain tissue and its blood vessels. A subdural hematoma is usually venous in origin and develops slowly, but development can occur rapidly if the hematoma is of arterial origin. Subdural hematomas may be acute, subacute, or chronic (Table 37).

TABLE 37 Types of Subdural Hematomas

Occurrence After Injury	Progression of Symptoms	Treatment
Acute		
24-48 hr after severe trauma	Immediate deterioration	Craniotomy, evacuation and decompression
Subacute		
48 hr–2 wk after severe trauma	Alteration in mental status as hematoma develops Progression dependent on size and location of hematoma	Evacuation and decompression
Chronic		
Weeks or months, usually >20 days after injury Often injury seemed trivial or was forgotten by patient	Nonspecific, nonlocalizing progression Progressive alteration in LOC	Evacuation and decompression, membranectomy

LOC, Level of consciousness.

- An *acute subdural hematoma* manifests within 24 to 48 hours of the injury. Manifestations are similar to those associated with brain tissue compression in increased ICP (see Increased Intracranial Pressure, p. 342). The patient may be drowsy, confused, or unconscious. The ipsilateral pupil dilates and becomes fixed if ICP is significantly elevated.

- A *subacute subdural hematoma* usually occurs within 2 to 14 days of the injury. After the initial bleeding, a subdural hematoma may appear to enlarge over time as the breakdown products of the blood draw fluid into the subdural space.

- A *chronic subdural hematoma* develops over weeks or months after a seemingly minor head injury. Chronic subdural hematomas are more common in older adults because of a potentially larger subdural space secondary to brain atrophy. The presenting complaints are focal symptoms rather than signs of increased ICP.

Intracerebral Hematoma

An *intracerebral hematoma* occurs from bleeding within the brain tissue. It usually occurs within the frontal and temporal lobes, possibly from the rupture of intracerebral vessels at the time of injury.

Diagnostic Studies

- CT scan is the best diagnostic test to evaluate for craniocerebral trauma.
- MRI, positron emission tomography (PET), and evoked potential studies assist in diagnosis and differentiation of head injuries.
- Transcranial Doppler studies are used to measure cerebral blood flow velocity.
- Cervical spine x-ray series, CT scan, or MRI of the spine may be done.

Interprofessional Care

Emergency management of the patient with head injury includes measures to prevent secondary injury by treating cerebral edema and managing increased ICP (see Table 56-9, Lewis et al, *Medical-Surgical Nursing,* ed 10, p. 1330). The principal treatment of head injuries is timely diagnosis and surgery if necessary. For the patient with a concussion or contusion, observation for and management of increased ICP are primary management strategies.

- The treatment of skull fractures is usually conservative. For depressed fractures and fractures with loose fragments, a craniotomy is necessary to elevate depressed bone and remove free fragments. If large amounts of bone are destroyed, the bone may be removed (craniectomy) and a cranioplasty will be needed at a later time (see the section on cranial surgery in Lewis et al, *Medical-Surgical Nursing,* ed 10, pp. 1336 to 1338).

- In cases of large acute subdural and epidural hematomas or those associated with significant neurologic impairment, the blood must be removed. A craniotomy is generally performed to visualize and allow control of the bleeding vessels. Burr-hole openings may be used in an extreme emergency for more rapid decompression, followed by a craniotomy. A drain may be placed postoperatively for several days to prevent reaccumulation of blood.

Nursing Management

Goals

The patient with an acute head injury will maintain adequate cerebral oxygenation and perfusion; remain normothermic; achieve control of pain and discomfort; be free from infection; have adequate nutrition; and attain maximal cognitive, motor, and sensory function.

Nursing Diagnoses/Collaborative Problem

- Risk for ineffective cerebral tissue perfusion
- Hyperthermia
- Impaired physical mobility
- Anxiety
- Potential complication: increased ICP

Nursing Interventions

One of the best ways to prevent head injuries is to prevent car and motorcycle crashes.

- Be active in campaigns that promote driving safety, and speak to driver education classes regarding the dangers of unsafe driving and driving after drinking alcohol and using drugs.
- Teach community members that using seat belts in cars and helmets for riding on motorcycles are the most effective measures for increasing survival after crashes.
- Protective helmets should also be worn by lumberjacks, construction workers, athletes who play contact sports, miners, horseback riders, bicycle riders, snowboarders, skiers, and skydivers.

Acute Care. The general goal of nursing management of the head-injured patient is to maintain cerebral oxygenation and perfusion and prevent secondary cerebral ischemia. Surveillance or monitoring for changes in neurologic status is critically important because the patient's condition may deteriorate rapidly, necessitating emergency surgery.

- Explain the need for frequent neurologic assessments to both patient and caregiver.
- Behavioral manifestations associated with head injury can result in a frightened, disoriented patient who is combative and resists help.

The Glasgow Coma Scale (GCS) is useful in assessing the LOC (see Glasgow Coma Scale, p. 767). Indications of a deteriorating neurologic state, such as a decreasing LOC or lessening of motor strength, should be reported to the HCP, and the patient's condition should be closely monitored.

The major focus of nursing care for the brain-injured patient relates to increased ICP (see Increased Intracranial Pressure: Nursing Management, p. 346).

- Loss of the corneal reflex may necessitate administering lubricating eye drops or taping the eyes shut to prevent abrasion.
- Periorbital ecchymosis and edema disappear spontaneously, but cold and, later, warm compresses provide comfort and hasten the process.
- Diplopia can be relieved by use of an eye patch.
- Hyperthermia can result in increased metabolism, cerebral blood flow, cerebral blood volume, and ICP. Increased metabolic waste also produces further cerebral vasodilation. Avoid hyperthermia, with a goal of maintaining a body temperature of 36° to 37°C.
- If cerebrospinal fluid (CSF) rhinorrhea or otorrhea occurs, inform the HCP immediately. The head of the bed may be elevated to decrease the CSF pressure. A loose collection pad may be placed under the nose or over the ear. Instruct the patient not to sneeze or blow the nose. Do not insert a gastric tube or suction catheter through the nose.
- Nausea and vomiting may be a problem and can be alleviated by antiemetic drugs.
- Headache can usually be controlled with acetaminophen or small doses of codeine.

If the patient's condition deteriorates, intracranial surgery may be necessary. A burr-hole opening or craniotomy may be indicated, depending on the underlying injury. The patient is often unconscious before surgery, making it necessary for a family member to sign the consent form for surgery. This is a difficult and frightening time for the patient's caregiver and family and requires sensitive nursing management. The suddenness of the situation makes it especially difficult for the family to cope.

Rehabilitation.   Once the condition has stabilized, the patient is usually transferred for acute rehabilitation management. There may

H

be chronic problems related to motor and sensory deficits, communication, memory, and intellectual functioning.

- The patient's outward appearance is not a good indicator of how well the patient will function in the home or work environment, given recovery time and rehabilitation.
- The mental and emotional sequelae of brain trauma are often the most incapacitating problems. Many of the patients with head injuries who have been comatose for more than 6 hours undergo some personality change. The patient's behavior may indicate a loss of social restraint, judgment, tact, and emotional control.

Progressive recovery may continue for 6 months or more before a plateau is reached and a prognosis for recovery can be made. Nursing management depends on specific residual deficits. The family needs to understand what is happening and be taught appropriate interaction patterns.

- The family often has unrealistic expectations for the patient's full return to pretrauma status as the coma begins to recede. In reality, the patient usually experiences a reduced awareness and ability to interpret environmental stimuli.
- Prepare the family for the emergence of the patient from coma and explain that the process of awakening often takes several weeks. Arrange for social work and chaplain consultations for the family, in addition to providing open visitation and frequent status updates.
- Family members, particularly spouses, go through role transition from that of spouse to that of caregiver.

HEADACHE

Description

Headache is probably the most common type of pain experienced by humans. The majority of people have functional headaches, such as migraine or tension-type, whereas others have organic headaches caused by intracranial or extracranial disease.

- *Primary headaches* are those not caused by a disease or another medical condition. They include tension-type, migraine, and cluster headaches. Characteristics and management of tension-type, migraine, and cluster headaches are shown in Table 38.
- *Secondary headaches* are caused by another condition or disorder, such as sinus infection, neck injury, or brain tumor.

The examination findings of a person with a headache are often normal. Unexplained abnormal findings require additional

Text continued on p. 273

TABLE 38 Interprofessional Care

Headaches

	Tension-Type Headache	Migraine Headache	Cluster Headache
Location	Bilateral, bandlike pressure at base of skull	Unilateral (in 60%), may switch sides, commonly anterior location	Unilateral, radiating up or down from one eye
Quality	Constant, squeezing tightness	Throbbing, synchronous with pulse	Severe—"bone crushing"
Frequency	Cycles for many years	Periodic, cycles of several months and years	May have months or years between attacks. Attacks occur in clusters over a period of 2-12 wk
Duration	30 min–7 days	4-72 hr	5 min–3 hr

Continued

H

TABLE 38 Interprofessional Care
Headaches—cont'd

Tension-Type Headache	Migraine Headache	Cluster Headache
Time and Mode of Onset		
Not related to time	May be preceded by premonitory symptoms or aura Onset after awakening Improves with sleep	Nocturnal, commonly awakens person from sleep
Associated Symptoms		
Palpable neck and shoulder muscle tension, stiff neck, tenderness	Irritability, sweating Nausea, vomiting Photophobia Phonophobia Premonitory symptoms: sensory, motor, or psychic phenomena Family history (in 65%)	Facial flushing or pallor Unilateral lacrimation, ptosis, rhinitis

Treatment: Abortive and Symptomatic Drugs

Nonopioid analgesics: aspirin, acetaminophen, NSAIDs

Analgesic combinations
- butalbital/aspirin/caffeine (Fiorinal)
- butalbital/acetaminophen/caffeine (Fioricet)
- dichloralphenazone/acetaminophen/isomethepetene (Midrin)

Muscle relaxants

Nonopioid analgesics: aspirin, NSAIDs

Serotonin receptor agonists
- almotriptan (Axert)
- eletriptan (Relpax)
- frovatriptan (Frova)
- naratriptan (Amerge)
- rizatriptan (Maxalt)
- sumatriptan (Imitrex)
- zolmitriptan (Zomig)
- sumatriptan transdermal system (Zecuity)

Combination
- sumatriptan/naproxen (Treximet)

α-Adrenergic blockers
- ergotamine tartrate (Ergomar)
- dihydroergotamine nasal spray (Migranal)

Analgesic combinations
- acetaminophen/caffeine/aspirin
- acetaminophen/isometheptene/dichloralphenazone

Corticosteroids
- dexamethasone

α-Adrenergic blockers
- ergotamine tartrate (Ergomar)
- O_2 100% inhalation via mask

Serotonin receptor agonists
- almotriptan
- eletriptan
- frovatriptan
- naratriptan
- rizatriptan
- sumatriptan
- zolmitriptan

Continued

H

TABLE 38   Interprofessional Care

Headaches—cont'd

Tension-Type Headache	Migraine Headache	Cluster Headache
Treatment: Preventive		
Tricyclic antidepressants	β-Adrenergic blocker:	α-Adrenergic blockers
• amitriptyline	• propranolol	• ergotamine tartrate (Ergomar)
• nortriptyline (Pamelor)	Antidepressants	Corticosteroid
• doxepin	• amitriptyline	• prednisone
Selective serotonin reuptake inhibitors	• imipramine (Tofranil)	Calcium channel blocker
• fluoxetine (Prozac)	Antiseizure drugs	• verapamil
• paroxetine (Paxil)	• valproic acid (Depakene)	Lithium
β-Adrenergic blocker	• divalproex	Biofeedback
• propranolol (Inderal)	• topiramate (Topamax)	
Antiseizure drugs	• gabapentin (Neurontin)	
• topiramate (Topamax)	Calcium channel blockers	
• divalproex (Depakote)	• verapamil (Calan)	
Other drugs	Botulinum toxin A (Botox)	
• mirtazapine (Remeron)	Biofeedback	
Biofeedback	Relaxation therapy	
Psychotherapy	Cognitive-behavioral therapy	
Muscle relaxation training		

diagnostic studies to identify underlying causes and additional risk factors.

Nursing Management

Goals
The patient with a headache will have reduced or no pain, experience increased comfort and decreased anxiety, demonstrate understanding of triggering events and treatment strategies, use positive coping strategies to deal with pain, and experience increased quality of life and decreased disability.

Nursing Diagnoses
- Acute pain
- Ineffective health management

Nursing Interventions
Headaches may result from an inability to cope with daily stresses. An effective therapy may be to help patients examine their daily routine, recognize stressful situations, and learn to use effective coping strategies. Help the patient identify precipitating factors and develop ways to avoid them. Encourage daily exercise, relaxation periods, and socializing to decrease the recurrence of headache.

- Suggest alternative ways of handling the pain of headache through techniques such as relaxation, meditation, yoga, and self-hypnosis. Massage and moist hot packs to the neck and head can help a patient with tension-type headaches.
- The patient should learn about drugs prescribed for prophylactic and symptomatic treatment of headache and should be able to describe the purpose, action, dosage, and side effects.
- For the patient whose headaches are triggered by food, provide dietary counseling. The patient needs to be encouraged to eliminate foods and substances that may provoke headaches (e.g., chocolate, alcohol, excessive caffeine, cheese, fermented foods, monosodium glutamate).
- Cluster headache attacks may occur at high altitudes with low O_2 levels during air travel. Ergotamine, taken before the plane takes off, may decrease the likelihood of these attacks.

▼ Patient and Caregiver Teaching
A teaching guide for the patient with a headache is provided in Table 39.

H

TABLE 39 Patient & Caregiver Teaching

Headaches

Include the following instructions when teaching the patient with a headache and the patient's caregiver.

1. Keep a diary or calendar of headaches and possible precipitating events.
2. Avoid possible triggers for a headache:
   * Foods containing amines (cheese, chocolate), nitrites (meats such as hot dogs), vinegar, onions, monosodium glutamate
   * Fermented or marinated foods
   * Caffeine
   * Oranges
   * Tomatoes
   * Aspartame
   * Nicotine
   * Ice cream
   * Alcohol (particularly red wine)
   * Emotional stress
   * Fatigue
   * Drugs such as ergot-containing preparations (ergotamine tartrate [Ergomar]) and monoamine oxidase inhibitors (e.g., rasagiline [Azilect])
3. Learn the purpose, action, dosage, and side effects of drugs taken.
4. Self-administer sumatriptan (Imitrex) subcutaneously if prescribed.
5. Self-administer sumatriptan transdermal patch (Zecuity) (if prescribed), and describe appropriate disposal method for used patch.
6. Use stress management techniques.
7. Participate in regular exercise.
8. Contact HCP if any of the following occurs:
   * Symptoms become more severe, last longer than usual, or are resistant to medication.
   * Nausea and vomiting (if severe or not typical), change in vision, or fever occurs with the headache.
   * Problems occur with any drugs.

HEART FAILURE

Description

Heart failure (HF) is a complex clinical syndrome that results in the inability of the heart to provide sufficient blood to meet the O_2

needs of tissues and organs. A defect in either ventricular filling (diastolic dysfunction) or ventricular ejection (systolic dysfunction) is the key manifestation of HF.

The amount of blood pumped by the left ventricle with each heartbeat is called the ejection fraction (EF). The American Academy of Cardiology Foundation (ACCF) has adopted the terms *heart failure with reduced EF* (HFrEF) and *heart failure with preserved EF* (HFpEF) to describe systolic and diastolic HF.

HF is associated with numerous types of cardiovascular diseases, particularly long-standing hypertension, coronary artery disease (CAD), and myocardial infarction (MI).

- HF is a major health problem in the United States. In contrast with other cardiovascular diseases, HF is increasing in incidence and prevalence because of improved survival after cardiovascular events and the increasing population of older adults. HF is a common reason for hospital admission in older adults.
- CAD and hypertension are the primary risk factors for HF. Other factors including diabetes, metabolic syndrome, advanced age, tobacco use, and vascular disease contribute to the development of HF.

Pathophysiology

HF may be caused by any interference with the normal mechanisms regulating cardiac output (CO). CO depends on (1) preload, (2) afterload, (3) myocardial contractility, and (4) heart rate (HR). Any changes in these factors can lead to decreased ventricular function with subsequent HF.

- Major causes of HF may be divided into two subgroups: (1) *primary causes,* consisting of underlying cardiac diseases, such as CAD and cardiomyopathy, and (2) *precipitating causes,* such as anemia, pulmonary disease, and hypervolemia (see the complete listing of causes in Tables 34-1 and 34-2, Lewis et al, *Medical-Surgical Nursing,* ed. 10, p. 738).

HF is classified as systolic or diastolic failure. *Systolic failure,* or HFrEF, results from an inability of the heart to pump effectively. It is caused by impaired contractile function (e.g., MI), increased afterload (e.g., hypertension), cardiomyopathy, or a mechanical abnormality (e.g., valvular heart disease). The hallmark of systolic dysfunction is a decrease in the left ventricular EF.

Diastolic failure, or HFpEF, is the inability of the ventricles to relax and fill during diastole. Decreased filling results in decreased stroke volume and CO and venous engorgement in both the pulmonary and systemic vascular systems. The diagnosis of diastolic failure is based on the presence of HF symptoms with a normal EF. Diastolic failure is usually the result of left ventricular hypertrophy from chronic hypertension, aortic stenosis, or hypertrophic cardiomyopathy.

Mixed systolic and diastolic failure is seen in disease states such as dilated cardiomyopathy, in which poor systolic function (weakened muscle function) is further compromised by dilated left ventricular walls that are unable to relax.

The patient with ventricular failure of any type has low systemic arterial BP, low CO, and poor renal perfusion. Whether the patient arrives at this point acutely (from an MI) or chronically (from worsening cardiomyopathy or hypertension), the body's response to this low CO is to mobilize compensatory mechanisms to maintain CO and BP. The main compensatory mechanisms are (1) sympathetic nervous system activation, (2) neurohormonal responses, (3) ventricular dilation, and (4) ventricular hypertrophy.

HF is usually manifested as biventricular failure, although one ventricle may precede the other in dysfunction.

- *Left-sided failure* is the most common form of initial HF. Left-sided failure causes blood to back up into the left atrium and pulmonary veins. The increased pulmonary pressure causes fluid leakage from the pulmonary capillary bed into the interstitium and then the alveoli, which is manifested as pulmonary congestion and edema.
- *Right-sided failure* causes a backup of blood into the right atrium and venous circulation. Venous congestion in the systemic circulation results in peripheral edema, hepatomegaly, and jugular venous distention. The primary cause of right-sided failure is left-sided failure. In this situation, left-sided HF results in pulmonary congestion and increased pressure in the blood vessels of the lung (pulmonary hypertension). Eventually, chronic pulmonary hypertension (increased right ventricular afterload) results in right-sided hypertrophy and HF. *Cor pulmonale* (right ventricular dilation and hypertrophy caused by pulmonary pathologic conditions) can also cause right-sided failure (see Cor Pulmonale, p. 152).

Clinical Manifestations
Acute Decompensated Heart Failure
In acute decompensated HF (ADHF), an increase in the pulmonary venous pressure is caused by failure of the left ventricle (LV). This results in engorgement of the pulmonary vascular system. This early stage is clinically associated with a mild increase in the respiratory rate and a decrease in partial pressure of O_2 in arterial blood (PaO_2).

ADHF can manifest as *pulmonary edema*. This is an acute, life-threatening situation in which the lung alveoli become filled with serosanguineous fluid. The most common cause of pulmonary edema is acute LV failure secondary to CAD.

- Manifestations of pulmonary edema are distinct. The patient is usually anxious, pale, and possibly cyanotic, with clammy and cold skin.
- The patient has dyspnea, respiratory rate greater than 30 breaths/min, and orthopnea. Wheezing and coughing with production of frothy, blood-tinged sputum may also occur.
- Auscultation of the lungs may reveal bubbling, crackles, and wheezes. The patient's HR is rapid, and BP may be elevated or decreased depending on the severity of the HF.

Chronic Heart Failure

Manifestations of chronic HF depend on the patient's age, underlying type and extent of heart disease, and which ventricle is failing to pump effectively. Table 40 lists manifestations of left-sided and right-sided failure. The patient with chronic HF usually has manifestations of biventricular failure.

- Fatigue after usual activities is one of the earliest symptoms.
- Dyspnea is common. Shortness of breath occurs in the recumbent position (orthopnea).
- Paroxysmal nocturnal dyspnea (PND) occurs when the patient is asleep. The patient awakens in a panic, has feelings of suffocation, and has a strong desire to sit or stand up.
- A cough is often associated with HF and may be the first clinical symptom. It begins as a dry, nonproductive cough that is not relieved by position change or over-the-counter cough medicine.
- Other common signs include tachycardia; edema in the legs, liver, abdominal cavity, and lungs; nocturia; dusky skin; restlessness and confusion; angina; and weight changes.

Complications

Pleural effusion results from increasing pressure in the pleural capillaries. Enlargement of the heart chambers in chronic HF can cause atrial fibrillation. Patients also are at risk for ventricular dysrhythmias.

Left ventricular thrombus may occur with ADHF or chronic HF, in which the enlarged LV and decreased CO combine to increase the chance of thrombus formation within the LV. This places the patient at risk for stroke.

Hepatomegaly may result as the liver becomes congested with venous blood. Hepatic congestion leads to impaired liver function; eventually liver cells die, and cirrhosis can develop. The decreased CO that accompanies chronic HF also results in decreased perfusion to the kidneys and can lead to renal insufficiency or failure.

H

TABLE 40	**Manifestations of Heart Failure**	
	Right-Sided Failure	**Left-Sided Failure**
Signs	• RV heaves • Murmurs • Jugular venous distention • Edema (e.g., pedal, scrotum, sacrum) • Weight gain • ↑ HR • Ascites • Anasarca (massive generalized body edema) • Hepatomegaly (liver enlargement)	• LV heaves • Pulsus alternans (alternating pulses: strong, weak) • ↑ HR • PMI displaced inferiorly and posteriorly (LV hypertrophy) • ↓ PaO_2, slight ↑ $PaCO_2$ (poor O_2 exchange) • Crackles (pulmonary edema) • S_3 and S_4 heart sounds • Pleural effusion • Changes in mental status • Restlessness, confusion
Symptoms	• Fatigue • Anxiety, depression • Dependent, bilateral edema • Right upper quadrant pain • Anorexia and GI bloating • Nausea	• Weakness, fatigue • Anxiety, depression • Dyspnea • Shallow, rapid respirations • Paroxysmal nocturnal dyspnea • Orthopnea • Dry, hacking cough • Nocturia • Frothy, pink-tinged sputum (advanced pulmonary edema)

GI, gastrointestinal; *HR*, heart rate; *LV*, left ventricular; *PaCO₂*, partial pressure of CO_2 in arterial blood; *PaO₂*, partial pressure of O_2 in arterial blood; *PMI*, point of maximal impulse; *RV*, right ventricular.

Diagnostic Studies

Diagnosing HF is often difficult because signs and symptoms are not highly specific and may mimic those of many other medical conditions (e.g., anemia, lung disease). Diagnostic tests for ADHF and chronic HF are presented in Table 41.

TABLE 41 Interprofessional Care

Heart Failure

Both ADHF and Chronic HF	ADHF	Chronic HF
Diagnostic Assessment		
• History and physical examination • Determination of underlying cause • Serum chemistry panel, cardiac markers, BNP or NT-proBNP level (see Table 31-6 in Lewis et al, *Medical-Surgical Nursing*, ed 10, pp. 673 to 677), liver function tests, thyroid function tests, CBC, lipid profile, kidney function tests, urinalysis • Chest x-ray • 12-lead ECG • Two-dimensional echocardiogram • Nuclear imaging studies (see Table 31-6 in Lewis et al, *Medical-Surgical Nursing*, ed 10, pp. 673 to 677) • Cardiac catheterization	• Measurement of LV function • Hemodynamic monitoring • Endomyocardial biopsy in select patients	• Cardiopulmonary exercise stress test • 6-minute walk test • Sleep studies in select patients

Continued

H

TABLE 41 Interprofessional Care

Heart Failure—cont'd

Both ADHF and Chronic HF	ADHF	Chronic HF
Management		
• Treatment of underlying cause	• High Fowler's position	• O₂ therapy by nasal cannula if indicated
• Circulatory assist devices (e.g., ventricular assist device)	• O₂ by mask or nasal cannula	• Drug therapy (Table 34-7)
• Daily weights	• Noninvasive positive pressure ventilation	• Cardiac resynchronization therapy with biventricular pacing and implantable cardioverter-defibrillator (ICD)
• Sodium- and possibly fluid-restricted diet	• Circulatory assist device: intraaortic balloon pump	• LVAD
	• Endotracheal intubation and mechanical ventilation	• Heart transplantation
	• Vital signs, urine output at least q1hr	• Rest-activity periods
	• Continuous ECG and pulse oximetry monitoring	• Dietitian consult
	• Hemodynamic monitoring (e.g., intraarterial BP, PAWP, CO)	• Physical/occupational therapy consult
	• Drug therapy (Table 34-7 in Lewis et al., *Medical-Surgical Nursing,* ed 10, p. 745)	• Cardiac rehabilitation
	• Possible cardioversion (e.g., atrial fibrillation)	• Home health nursing care (e.g., telehealth monitoring)
	• Ultrafiltration	• Palliative and end-of-life care

ADHF, Acute decompensated heart failure; *BNP,* b-type natriuretic peptide; *BP,* blood pressure; *CBC,* complete blood count; *CO,* cardiac output; *ECG,* electrocardiogram; *HF,* heart failure; *LV,* left ventricular; *LVAD,* LV assist device; *NT-proBNP,* N-terminal prohormone of BNP; *PAWP,* pulmonary artery wedge pressure.

A primary diagnostic goal is to determine the underlying etiology. An endomyocardial biopsy (EMB) may be done in patients who develop unexplained, new-onset HF that is unresponsive to usual care. An echocardiogram provides information on the EF, which helps to differentiate between HFpEF and HFrEF. In general, b-type natriuretic peptide (BNP) levels correlate positively with the degree of left ventricular dysfunction.

Nursing and Interprofessional Management: Acute Decompensated Heart Failure

With the addition of new drugs and device therapies, the management of HF has dramatically changed in the past few years. Table 41 summarizes interprofessional care of the patient with ADHF.

Patients with ADHF need continuous monitoring and assessment, which may be done in an intensive care unit (ICU) setting. Monitor ECG and O_2 saturation. The patient may have continuous hemodynamic monitoring. Supplemental O_2 helps increase the percentage of O_2 in inspired air. In severe pulmonary edema, the patient may need noninvasive ventilatory support or intubation and mechanical ventilation.

- If the patient is dyspneic, place in a high Fowler's position with the legs horizontal in the bed or dangling at the bedside. This position helps decrease venous return through pooling of blood in the extremities.
- Ultrafiltration is an option for the patient with volume overload. It can rapidly remove intravascular fluid volume while maintaining hemodynamic stability.
- Circulatory assist devices are used to manage patients with worsening HF. The intraaortic balloon pump (IABP) increases coronary blood flow to the heart muscle and decreases the heart's workload. Ventricular assist devices (VADs) can be used to maintain the pumping action of the heart.
- Assess patients with HF for depression and anxiety, and treatment plans should be initiated if appropriate.

Drug Therapy

Drug therapy is essential in treating acute HF.

- *Diuretics:* Diuretics are the mainstay of treatment in patients with volume overload. These agents act to decrease sodium reabsorption in the nephrons, thereby enhancing sodium and water loss. Decreasing venous return (preload) reduces the amount of volume returned to the LV during diastole. Decreasing intravascular volume with the use of loop diuretics (e.g., furosemide [Lasix], bumetanide [Bumex]) reduces venous return.
- *Vasodilators:* IV nitroglycerin reduces preload, slightly reduces afterload (in high doses), and increases myocardial oxygen

H

supply. Sodium nitroprusside reduces both preload and after-load, thereby improving myocardial contraction, increasing CO, and reducing pulmonary congestion. IV nesiritide (Natre-cor), a recombinant form of BNP, causes both arterial and venous dilation.

- *Morphine:* Morphine sulfate reduces preload and afterload and is used in the treatment of ADHF and pulmonary edema. It dilates the pulmonary and systemic blood vessels, thereby decreasing pulmonary pressures and improving gas exchange.
- *Positive inotropics:* Inotropic therapy increases myocardial contractility. Drugs include β-adrenergic agonists (e.g., dopamine, dobutamine, epinephrine, norepinephrine [Levophed]), phos-phodiesterase inhibitors (inamrinone, milrinone), and digitalis.

Digitalis is a positive inotrope that improves LV function but also increases myocardial oxygen consumption. Inotropic therapy is recommended for use only in the short-term management of patients with ADHF who have not responded to conventional phar-macotherapy (e.g., diuretics, vasodilators, morphine).

Interprofessional Care: Chronic Heart Failure

The main goals in the treatment of chronic HF are to treat the underlying cause and contributing factors, maximize CO, reduce symptoms, improve ventricular function, improve quality of life, preserve target organ function, and improve mortality and morbid-ity. The treatment of causes such as dysrhythmias, hypertension, valvular disorders, and CAD is discussed elsewhere in this book.

Nondrug Therapy

- Administration of O_2 improves O_2 saturation and assists in meeting tissue oxygen needs, thereby helping to relieve dyspnea and fatigue.
- Physical and emotional rest conserves energy and decreases the need for additional O_2. A patient with severe HF may be on bed rest with limited activity. A patient with mild to moder-ate HF can be ambulatory with a restriction of strenuous activity.

Cardiac resynchronization therapy (CRT), unlike traditional pacing, coordinates right and left ventricular contractility through biventricular pacing. The ability to have normal simultaneous elec-trical conduction (synchrony) within the right and left ventricles increases left ventricular function and CO.

Mechanical options such as the IABP and VADs are available for patients with deteriorating clinical condition, especially those awaiting cardiac transplantation. Limitations of bed rest, risk of infection, and vascular complications preclude long-term use of

IABPs. VADs provide highly effective long-term support and have become standard care in many heart transplant centers.

Drug Therapy

- *Diuretics:* Diuretics reduce edema, pulmonary venous pressure, and preload. Thiazide diuretics (e.g., hydrochlorothiazide) inhibit sodium reabsorption in the distal tubule, thus promoting excretion of sodium and water. Loop diuretics such as furosemide (Lasix), bumetanide (Bumex), and torsemide (Demadex) are potent but can cause hypokalemia and ototoxicity. In chronic HF, the lowest effective dose of diuretic should be used.
- *Angiotensin-converting enzyme (ACE) inhibitors:* ACE inhibitors (e.g., captopril, enalapril [Vasotec]) are the primary drugs of choice for blocking the renin-angiotensin-aldosterone system in patients with systolic HF. A reduction in systemic vascular resistance (SVR) with the use of ACE inhibitors causes a significant increase in CO. Although BP decreases, tissue perfusion is maintained or increased as a result of improved CO, and diuresis is enhanced by the suppression of aldosterone.
- *Nitrates:* Nitrates (e.g., nitroglycerin) cause vasodilation by acting directly on the smooth muscle of the vessel wall. Nitrates are of particular benefit in the management of myocardial ischemia related to HF because they promote vasodilation of the coronary arteries.
- *BiDil:* A combination drug containing isosorbide dinitrate and hydralazine (BiDil) is used for the treatment of HF in African Americans who are already being treated with standard therapy.
- *β-Adrenergic blockers:* β-Adrenergic blockers, including carvedilol (Coreg), metoprolol (Toprol-XL), and bisoprolol (Zebeta), directly block the negative effects of the sympathetic nervous system on the failing heart.
- *Positive inotropes:* Positive inotropes are used to improve cardiac contractility. Digitalis preparations (e.g., digoxin [Lanoxin]) increase the force of cardiac contraction *(inotropic action)*. They also decrease conduction speed within the myocardium and slow the HR *(chronotropic action)*. The slower heart rate allows for more complete emptying of the ventricles, reducing the volume remaining in the ventricles during diastole. CO increases because of increased stroke volume from improved contractility.

Nutritional Therapy

Diet teaching and weight management are essential to the patient's control of chronic HF. You or a dietitian should obtain a detailed diet history to determine not only what foods the patient eats but also when, where, and how often the person dines out.

H

The edema associated with chronic HF is often treated by dietary restriction of sodium. Teach the patient what foods are low and high in sodium and ways to enhance food flavors without the use of salt (e.g., substituting lemon juice, various spices). The degree of sodium restriction depends on the severity of the HF and effectiveness of diuretic therapy.

- A commonly prescribed diet for a patient with mild HF is a 2-g sodium diet. All foods high in sodium should be eliminated. (For sample menu plans for sodium-restricted diets, see Table 34-8, Lewis et al, *Medical-Surgical Nursing,* ed 10, p. 749.)

Fluid restrictions are not commonly prescribed for mild to moderate HF. However, for moderate to severe HF, fluid restrictions are usually implemented.

- Instruct patients to weigh themselves at the same time each day, preferably before breakfast, while wearing the same type of clothing. For a weight gain of 3 lb (1.4 kg) over 2 days or a 5-lb (2.3-kg) gain over 1 week, the HCP should be contacted.

Nursing Management: Chronic Heart Failure
Goals
The patient with HF will have a decrease in symptoms (e.g., shortness of breath, fatigue), decreased peripheral edema, increased exercise tolerance, adherence with medical regimen, and no complications related to HF.

See care of the patient with HF in the eNursing Care Plan 34-1 on the website.

Nursing Diagnoses
- Activity intolerance
- Excess fluid volume
- Decreased cardiac output
- Impaired gas exchange

Nursing Interventions
Help to aggressively identify and treat risk factors for HF to prevent or slow the progression of the disease. For example, teach the patient with hypertension or hyperlipidemia measures to manage BP or cholesterol with medication, diet, and exercise. Patients with valvular disease should have valve replacement planned before lung congestion develops.

Acute Care.   Many people with HF will experience one or more episodes of ADHF. Such episodes are usually managed in an ICU, an intermediate care unit with continuous cardiac monitoring capability, or a specialized HF unit.

- Successful HF management depends on several important principles: (1) HF is a progressive disease, and treatment plans are established along with quality-of-life goals; (2) symptoms are controlled by the patient with self-management tools (e.g., daily weights, drug regimens, diet and exercise plans); (3) salt and, at times, water must be restricted; (4) energy must be conserved; and (5) support systems are essential to the success of the entire treatment plan.

- Reduction of anxiety is an important nursing function, because anxiety may increase the sympathetic nervous system (SNS) response and further increase myocardial workload. Reducing anxiety may be facilitated by a variety of nursing interventions and the use of sedatives (e.g., benzodiazepines, morphine sulfate).

Ambulatory Care.   HF is a chronic illness for most people. Important nursing responsibilities are to (1) teach the patient about physiologic changes that have occurred, (2) help the patient adapt to both physiologic and psychologic changes, and (3) integrate patient and caregiver preferences into the overall care plan.

A patient and caregiver teaching guide for HF is presented in Table 42.

TABLE 42   Patient & Caregiver Teaching

Heart Failure

Include the following instructions when teaching the patient and caregiver about the management of heart failure.

Dietary Therapy
- Consult the diet plan and list of permitted and restricted foods.
- Examine labels to determine sodium content. Also examine the labels of over-the-counter drugs such as laxatives, cough medicines, and antacids for sodium content.
- Avoid using salt when preparing foods or adding salt to foods.
- Weigh yourself at the same time each day, preferably in the morning, using the same scale and wearing similar clothes.
- Eat small, frequent meals.

Activity Program
- Increase walking and other activities gradually, provided that they do not cause fatigue or dyspnea.
- Consider a cardiac rehabilitation program.
- Avoid extremes of heat and cold.

H

Continued

TABLE 42   Patient & Caregiver Teaching

Heart Failure—cont'd

Ongoing Monitoring

- Know the signs and symptoms of worsening heart failure (think *FACES*: *f*atigue, limitation of *a*ctivities, chest *c*ongestion/cough, *e*dema, and *s*hortness of breath).
- Recall the symptoms experienced when illness began. Reappearance of previous symptoms may indicate a recurrence.
- Report immediately any of the following to the HCP:
  - Weight gain of 3 lb (1.4 kg) in 2 days, or 3-5 lb (1.4-2.3 kg) in a week
  - Difficulty breathing, especially with activity or when lying flat
  - Waking up breathless at night
  - Frequent dry, hacking cough, especially when lying down
  - Fatigue, weakness
  - Swelling of ankles, feet, or abdomen. Swelling of face or difficulty breathing (if taking ACE inhibitors)
  - Nausea with abdominal swelling, pain, and tenderness
  - Dizziness or fainting
- Follow up with HCP on regular basis.
- Consider joining a local support group with your family members and caregivers.

Health Promotion

- Obtain annual influenza vaccination.
- Obtain pneumococcal vaccination (see Table 27-5 in Lewis et al, *Medical-Surgical Nursing*, ed 10, p. 504, for guidelines on pneumococcal vaccination).
- Develop plan to reduce risk factors (e.g., BP control, tobacco cessation, weight reduction).

Rest

- Plan a regular daily rest and activity program.
- After exertion, such as exercise and ADLs, plan a rest period.
- Shorten working hours, or schedule rest period during working hours.
- Avoid emotional upsets. Share any concerns, fears, feelings of depression, etc., with HCP.

TABLE 42   Patient & Caregiver Teaching

Heart Failure—cont'd

Drug Therapy

- Take each drug as ordered.
- Develop a system (e.g., daily chart, weekly pillbox) to ensure that drugs have been taken.
- Count heart rate each day before taking drugs (if appropriate). Know the limits that your HCP wants for your heart rate.
- Take BP at determined intervals (if appropriate). Know your target BP limits.
- Know signs and symptoms of orthostatic hypotension and how to prevent them (see Table 32-12 in Lewis et al, *Medical-Surgical Nursing*, ed 10, p. 697).
- If taking anticoagulants, know signs and symptoms of internal bleeding (bleeding gums, increased bruises, blood in stool or urine) and actions to take.
- If taking warfarin (Coumadin), know INR results, target INR level, and how often to have INR checked .

ACE, Angiotensin-converting enzyme; *INR,* international normalized ratio.

HEMOPHILIA AND VON WILLEBRAND DISEASE

Description

Hemophilia is an X-linked recessive genetic disorder caused by a defective or deficient coagulation factor. The two major types of hemophilia that can occur in mild to severe forms are *hemophilia A* (classic hemophilia, factor VIII deficiency) and *hemophilia B* (Christmas disease, factor IX deficiency). *von Willebrand disease* is a related disorder involving a deficiency of the von Willebrand coagulation protein.

Hemophilia A is the most common form of hemophilia, accounting for about 85% of all cases. There are rare cases of acquired hemophilia A, which is due to the development of antibodies against the body's own factor VIII. von Willebrand disease is considered the most common congenital bleeding disorder in humans.

Deficiency and inheritance patterns of these three forms of inherited coagulopathy are compared in Table 43.

TABLE 43	Types of Hemophilia	
Type	**Defect/Deficiency**	**Inheritance Pattern**
Hemophilia A	Factor VIII deficiency	Recessive sex-linked (transmitted by female carriers, displayed almost exclusively in men)
Hemophilia B	Factor IX deficiency	Recessive sex-linked (transmitted by female carriers, displayed almost exclusively in men)
von Willebrand disease	vWF, variable factor VIII deficiencies; platelet dysfunction	Autosomal dominant, seen in both genders Recessive (in severe forms of the disease)

vWF, von Willebrand factor.

Clinical Manifestations and Complications

Clinical manifestations and complications related to hemophilia include (1) slow, persistent, prolonged bleeding from minor trauma and small cuts; (2) delayed bleeding after minor injuries (the delay may be several hours or days); (3) uncontrollable hemorrhage after dental extractions or irritation of the gingiva with a hard-bristle toothbrush; (4) prolonged epistaxis, especially after a blow to the face; (5) GI bleeding from ulcers and gastritis; (6) hematuria from genitourinary (GU) trauma and splenic rupture resulting from falls or abdominal trauma; (7) ecchymoses, subcutaneous hematomas, and possible compartment syndrome; (8) neurologic signs, such as pain, anesthesia, and paralysis, that may develop from nerve compression caused by hematoma formation; and (9) hemarthrosis (bleeding into the joints), which may lead to joint deformity severe enough to cause crippling (commonly in knees, elbows, shoulders, hips, and ankles).

Diagnostic Studies

Laboratory studies determine the type of hemophilia present. A factor deficiency within the intrinsic system (factor VIII, IX, XI, or XII or von Willebrand factor [vWF]) will yield the laboratory results presented in Table 30-17, Lewis et al, *Medical-Surgical Nursing,* ed 10, p. 627.

Interprofessional Care

The goal of care is to prevent and treat bleeding. People with hemophilia or von Willebrand disease require preventive care, the use of replacement therapy during acute bleeding episodes and for prophylaxis, and treatment of complications of the disease and its therapy.

- Replacement of deficient clotting factors is the primary means of supporting patients with hemophilia. In addition to treating acute crises, replacement therapy may be given before surgery and dental care as a prophylactic measure.
- For mild hemophilia A or certain subtypes of von Willebrand disease, desmopressin acetate (DDAVP), a synthetic analog of vasopressin, may be used to stimulate an increase in factor VIII.

Complications of treatment of hemophilia include development of inhibitors to factor VIII or IX, transfusion-transmitted infectious disorders, allergic reactions, and thrombotic complications with the use of factor IX because it contains activated coagulation factors.

The most common difficulty with acute management is starting factor replacement therapy too late and stopping it too soon. Generally, minor bleeding episodes should be treated for at least 72 hours. Surgery and traumatic injuries may require more prolonged support. Eventually, a patient's development of inhibitors to the factor products requires individualized expert patient management.

Nursing Management

Because of the hereditary nature of hemophilia, referral of affected people for genetic counseling before reproduction is an essential preventive measure. Counseling is especially important because people with hemophilia are living into adulthood.

Acute interventions are related primarily to controlling the bleeding and include the following:

1. Stop the topical bleeding as quickly as possible by applying direct pressure or ice, packing the area with Gelfoam or fibrin foam, and applying topical hemostatic agents, such as thrombin and fibrin sealants.
2. Administer the specific coagulation factor concentrate as ordered. Monitor the patient for signs and symptoms such as hypersensitivity.
3. When joint bleeding occurs, complete rest of the involved joint is important to prevent crippling deformities from hemarthrosis. Pack the joint in ice. Give analgesics (e.g., acetaminophen, codeine) to reduce severe pain. Aspirin and aspirin-containing compounds should never be used. As soon as bleeding ceases,

H

encourage mobilization of the affected area through range-of-motion (ROM) exercises and physical therapy. Weight bearing is avoided until all swelling has resolved and muscle strength has returned.

4. Manage life-threatening complications that may develop as a result of hemorrhage. Examples are prevention or treatment of airway obstruction from hemorrhage into the neck and pharynx and early assessment and treatment of intracranial bleeding.

▼ Patient and Caregiver Teaching

Quality of life and survival may be significantly affected by the patient's knowledge of the illness and how to live with it. Provide ongoing assessment of the patient's adaptation to the illness.

- Teach the patient with hemophilia that immediate medical attention is required for severe pain or swelling of a muscle or joint that restricts movement or inhibits sleep and for a head injury, swelling in the neck or mouth, abdominal pain, hematuria, melena, and skin wounds with continued bleeding.
- Teach the patient to perform daily oral hygiene without causing trauma.
- Advise the patient to only participate in noncontact sports (e.g., golf) and to wear gloves when doing household chores, to prevent cuts or abrasions from knives, hammers, and other tools.
- The patient should wear a medical identification (Medic Alert) tag to ensure that HCPs know about the hemophilia in case of an accident.
- Many patients or their caregivers can be taught to self-administer the factor replacement therapies at home.

HEMORRHOIDS

Description

Hemorrhoids are dilated veins that may be internal (occurring above the internal sphincter) or external (occurring outside the external sphincter).

Pathophysiology

Hemorrhoids develop because of increased anal pressure and weakening of the connective tissue that supports the hemorrhoidal veins. Weakened supporting tissue allows for downward displacement of the hemorrhoidal veins, causing them to dilate. An intravascular clot in the venule results in a *thrombosed* external hemorrhoid.

Hemorrhoids are the most common reason for bleeding with defecation. Hemorrhoids may be precipitated by many factors, including pregnancy, obesity, prolonged constipation, straining in an effort to defecate, heavy lifting, prolonged standing and sitting, and portal hypertension (as found in cirrhosis).

Clinical Manifestations

Classic manifestations of hemorrhoids include bleeding, anal pruritus, prolapse, and pain.

- *Internal hemorrhoids* cause pain if they become constricted. Internal hemorrhoids can prolapse into the anal canal or externally, causing a sense of pressure with defecation and a protruding mass.
- *External hemorrhoids* are reddish blue and seldom bleed. There may be itching, burning, and edema. They usually do not cause pain and inflammation unless a thrombosis (blood clot) is present. Thrombosed hemorrhoids are bluish purple masses palpable at the anal orifice. The clot can erode through the overlying stretched skin, causing bleeding with defecation. Constipation or diarrhea can aggravate the symptoms.

Diagnostic Studies

- *Internal hemorrhoids* are diagnosed by digital examination, anoscopy, and sigmoidoscopy.
- *External hemorrhoids* can be diagnosed by visual inspection and digital examination.

Interprofessional Care

Therapy is directed toward the causes of the condition and the patient's symptoms. A high-fiber diet and increased fluid intake prevent constipation and reduce straining. Ointments, creams, suppositories, and pads that contain antiinflammatory agents (e.g., hydrocortisone) or astringents and anesthetics (e.g., witch hazel, benzocaine) may be used to shrink mucous membranes and relieve discomfort. The use of topical corticosteroids such as hydrocortisone agents should be limited to 1 week or less to prevent side effects such as contact dermatitis and mucosal atrophy. Stool softeners may ease defecation. Sitz baths help relieve pain.

- External hemorrhoids are usually managed by conservative therapy unless they become thrombosed. For internal hemorrhoids, nonsurgical approaches (band ligation, infrared coagulation, cryotherapy, laser treatment) can be used.
- Hemorrhoidectomy (surgical excision of hemorrhoids) is reserved for patients with severe symptoms related to multiple

H

thrombosed hemorrhoids or marked protrusion. Surgical removal may be done by cautery, clamp, or excision. Hemorrhoids may recur. Occasionally, anal strictures develop and dilation is necessary.

Nursing Management

Nursing care includes teaching measures to prevent constipation, avoidance of prolonged standing or sitting, proper use of over-the-counter preparations, and instructions on when to seek medical care (e.g., excessive pain and bleeding, prolapsed hemorrhoids).

- Severe pain caused by sphincter spasm is common after a hemorrhoidectomy. Most patients initially receive an opioid and NSAID in conjunction with topical preparations that provide anesthesia or reduce internal sphincter spasms, such as calcium channel blockers (e.g., nifedipine with lidocaine, diltiazem), or nitroglycerin preparations.
- Packing inserted into the rectum to absorb drainage is usually removed the first or second postoperative day. Provide privacy. Assess for rectal bleeding.
- Sitz baths are started 1 or 2 days after surgery. Initially, do not leave the patient alone because of the possibility of weakness or fainting. A sponge ring in the bath helps relieve pressure on the area.
- A stool softener such as docusate sodium (Colace) may be ordered. If the patient does not have a bowel movement within 2 or 3 days, an oil retention enema is given.
- The patient usually dreads the first bowel movement and often resists the urge to defecate. Give pain medication before the bowel movement to reduce discomfort.

▼ **Patient and Caregiver Teaching**

After surgery:

- Teach the importance of diet, sitz baths, symptoms of complications (especially bleeding), and avoidance of constipation and straining.

HEPATITIS, VIRAL

Description

Hepatitis is an inflammation of the liver. Viral infection is the most common cause of hepatitis. The types of viral hepatitis are A, B, C, D, E, and G. They differ in their modes of transmission and disease course (Table 44). Other viruses known to damage the liver include cytomegalovirus, Epstein-Barr virus, herpesvirus, coxsackievirus, and rubella virus.

TABLE 44 Characteristics of Hepatitis Viruses

Incubation Period and Mode of Transmission	Sources of Infection	Infectivity
Hepatitis A virus (HAV) *Incubation:* 15-50 days (average, 28) *Transmission:* • Fecal-oral (primarily fecal contamination and oral ingestion)	• Crowded conditions (e.g., day care, nursing home) • Poor personal hygiene • Poor sanitation • Contaminated food, milk, water, shellfish • Persons with subclinical infections, infected food handlers, sexual contacts, IV drug users	• Most infectious during 2 wk before onset of symptoms • Infectious until 1-2 wk after the start of symptoms
Hepatitis B virus (HBV) *Incubation:* 45-180 days (average, 56-96) *Transmission:* • Percutaneous (parenteral) or permucosal exposure to blood or blood products • Sexual contact • Perinatal transmission	• Contaminated needles, syringes, and blood products • Sexual activity with infected partners • Asymptomatic carriers • Tattoos or body piercing with contaminatec needles • HBV-infected mother (perinatal transmission)	• Before and after symptoms appear • Infectious for 4-6 mo • Carriers continue to be infectious for life

Continued

H

TABLE 44 **Characteristics of Hepatitis Viruses—cont'd**

Incubation Period and Mode of Transmission	Sources of Infection	Infectivity
Hepatitis C virus (HCV)	• Blood and blood products	• 1-2 wk before symptoms appear
Incubation: 14-180 days (average 56)	• Needles and syringes	• Continues during clinical course
Transmission:	• Sexual activity with infected partners	• 75%-85% go on to develop chronic hepatitis C and remain infectious
• Percutaneous (parenteral) or mucosal exposure to blood or blood products		
• High-risk sexual contact		
• Perinatal contact		
Hepatitis D virus (HDV)	• Same as for HBV	• Blood infectious at all stages of HDV infection
Incubation: 2-26 wk	• Can cause infection only when HBV is present	
Transmission:	• Routes of transmission same as for HBV	
• HBV must precede HDV		
• Chronic carriers of HBV always at risk		
Hepatitis E virus (HEV)	• Contaminated water, poor sanitation	• Not known
Incubation: 15-64 days (average, 26-42 days)	• Found in Asia, Africa, and Mexico	• May be similar to HAV
Transmission: Fecal-oral route	• Not common in United States	
• Outbreaks associated with contaminated water supply in developing countries		

Hepatitis A

Hepatitis A viral infection can cause a mild flu-like illness with jaundice. It can also cause acute liver failure, but does not result in chronic (long-term) infection.

Hepatitis A virus (HAV) is a ribonucleic acid (RNA) virus transmitted primarily through fecal contamination of food or drinking water. Transmission occurs in food handling and among family members, institutionalized individuals, and children in day care centers.

- Detection of hepatitis A IgM indicates acute hepatitis. Anti-HAV (antibody to HAV) immunoglobulin (Ig) M appears in the serum as the stool becomes negative for the virus. Hepatitis A IgG indicates past infection.
- Hepatitis A vaccination and thorough hand washing are the best measures to prevent outbreaks.

Hepatitis B

Hepatitis B virus (HBV) is a blood-borne pathogen that can cause either acute or chronic disease. The incidence of HBV infection has decreased because of the widespread use of the HBV vaccine.

- HBV is a deoxyribonucleic acid (DNA) virus. It can be transmitted several ways, including (1) perinatally to infants by mothers infected with HBV to their infants; (2) percutaneously (e.g., IV drug use, accidental needlestick punctures); and (3) via small cuts on mucosal surfaces and exposure to infectious blood, blood products, or other body fluids (e.g., semen, vaginal secretions, saliva).

Hepatitis C

Infection with the hepatitis C virus (HCV) can result in both acute and chronic illness.

- Acute HCV, which is usually asymptomatic, can be difficult to detect unless diagnosed with laboratory testing.
- Chronic HCV results in a potentially progressive liver disease, with 20% to 30% of the patients developing cirrhosis. Hepatitis C is the most common cause of chronic liver disease and the most common indication for liver transplantation in the United States.

Hepatitis D

Hepatitis D virus (HDV), also called *delta virus,* cannot survive on its own and requires HBV to replicate. It can be acquired at the same time as HBV, or a person with HBV can be infected with HDV at a later time. HDV is transmitted percutaneously.

- HDV can cause a spectrum of illness ranging from an asymptomatic chronic carrier state to acute liver failure. There is no vaccine for HDV. However, vaccination against HBV reduces the risk of HDV co-infection.

Hepatitis E

Hepatitis E virus (HEV) is an RNA virus transmitted by the fecal-oral route. The usual mode of transmission is drinking contaminated water. Hepatitis E infection occurs primarily in developing countries, with epidemics reported in India, Asia, Mexico, and Africa.

For a more complete description of each hepatitis virus, see Lewis et al, *Medical-Surgical Nursing,* ed 10, pp. 974 to 981.

Pathophysiology

In viral hepatitis, hepatocytes become targets of the virus in one of two ways: through direct action of the virus (as in HCV infection) or through a cell-mediated immune response to the virus (as in HBV infection). The destruction of hepatocytes leads to liver-related dysfunction in bile production, coagulation, blood glucose, and protein metabolism. Detoxification and processing of drugs, hormones, and metabolites may also be disrupted.

- Liver cells can regenerate and, if no complications occur, resume their normal appearance and function.
- Antigen-antibody complexes may form circulating immune complexes in the early phases of hepatitis and activate the complement system. Manifestations of this activation are rash, angioedema, arthritis, fever, and malaise.

Clinical Manifestations

A large number of patients with acute hepatitis have no symptoms. Manifestations of viral hepatitis may be classified into acute and chronic phases.

The *acute phase* usually lasts 1 to 6 months.

- During the incubation period, symptoms may include intermittent or ongoing anorexia, lethargy, nausea, vomiting, low-grade fever, skin rashes, diarrhea or constipation, malaise, fatigue, myalgias, arthralgias, other flu-like symptoms, and right upper quadrant tenderness (caused by liver inflammation).
- Physical examination may reveal hepatomegaly, lymphadenopathy, and sometimes splenomegaly. This is the period of maximal infectivity for hepatitis A.
- The acute phase may be *icteric* (jaundice) or anicteric. Jaundice, a yellowish discoloration of body tissues, results from an alteration in normal bilirubin metabolism or flow of bile into the hepatic or biliary duct systems. The urine may darken because of excess bilirubin excreted by the kidneys. If conjugated bilirubin cannot flow out of the liver because of bile duct obstruction, stools will be light or clay-colored. Pruritus, caused by bile salts beneath the skin, may result if cholestasis is present.

- The convalescence following the acute phase begins as jaundice is disappearing and lasts weeks to months, with an average of 2 to 4 months. During this period the patient's major complaints are malaise and easy fatigability. Hepatomegaly remains for several weeks.

In the *chronic phase,* patients may be asymptomatic. Others, however, may have intermittent or ongoing malaise, fatigue, myalgias, arthralgias, and hepatomegaly.

Complications

Most patients with acute viral hepatitis recover completely with no complications. The overall mortality rate for acute hepatitis is less than 1%. Complications include acute liver failure, chronic hepatitis, cirrhosis of the liver (see Cirrhosis, p. 136), and hepatocellular carcinoma (see Liver Cancer, p. 392).

The disappearance of jaundice does not mean the patient has totally recovered. Some HBV infections and the majority of HCV infections result in chronic (lifelong) viral infection.

Diagnostic Studies

The only definitive way to distinguish among the various types of viral hepatitis is by testing the patient's blood for the specific antigen or antibody. Table 45 presents the serologic tests for the different types of viral hepatitis. In addition, liver function tests show significant abnormalities. Physical assessment may reveal hepatic tenderness, hepatomegaly, and splenomegaly.

Interprofessional Care

There is no specific treatment for acute viral hepatitis. Most patients can be managed at home. Emphasis is on providing adequate nutrition and measures to rest the body while the liver cells regenerate. The degree of rest ordered depends on symptom severity; usually, alternating periods of activity with rest is adequate.

Drug Therapy

There are no specific drug therapies for the treatment of acute hepatitis A infection. Supportive drug therapy may include antiemetics for nausea, such as prochlorperazine, promethazine, or ondansetron (Zofran).

Treatment of acute hepatitis B is indicated only in patients with severe hepatitis and liver failure. Drug therapy for chronic HBV infection is focused on decreasing the hepatitis B viral load and liver enzyme levels and on slowing the rate of disease progression. Current drug therapies for chronic HBV infection suppress viral replication and prevent complications of hepatitis B. First-line

H

TABLE 45 Diagnostic Tests for Viral Hepatitis

Virus	Test(s)	Significance
A	Anti-HAV immunoglobulin M (IgM)	Acute infection
	Anti-HAV immunoglobulin G (IgG)	Previous infection or immunization Not routinely done in clinical practice
B	HBsAg (hepatitis B surface antigen)	Marker of infectivity Present in acute or chronic infection Positive in chronic carriers
	Anti-HBs (hepatitis B surface antibody)	Indicates previous infection with HBV or immunization
	HBeAg (hepatitis B e antigen)	Indicates high infectivity Used to determine the clinical management of patients with chronic hepatitis B
	Anti-HBe (hepatitis B e antibody)	Indicates previous infection In chronic hepatitis B, indicates a low viral load and low degree of infectivity
	Anti-HBc (antibody to hepatitis B core antigen) IgM	Indicates acute infection Does not appear after vaccination
	Anti-HBc IgG	Indicates previous infection or ongoing infection with hepatitis B Does not appear after vaccination
	HBV DNA quantitation	Indicates active ongoing viral replication Best indicator of viral replication and effectiveness of therapy in patients with chronic hepatitis B
	HBV genotyping	Indicates the genotype of HBV

TABLE 45 **Diagnostic Tests for Viral Hepatitis—cont'd**		
Virus	**Test(s)**	**Significance**
C	Anti-HCV (antibody to HCV)	Marker for acute or chronic infection with HCV
	HCV RNA quantitation	Indicates active ongoing viral replication
	HCV genotyping	Indicates the genotype of HCV
D	Anti-HDV	Present in patients with past or current infection with HDV
	HDV Ag (hepatitis D antigen)	Present within a few days after infection
E*	Anti-HEV IgM and IgG	Present 1 wk to 2 mo after illness onset
	HEV RNA quantitation	Indicates active ongoing viral replication

A, Hepatitis A virus (HAV); *B*, hepatitis B virus (HBV); *C*, hepatitis C virus (HCV); *D*, hepatitis D virus (HDV); *E*, hepatitis E virus (HEV).
*Currently, no serologic tests to diagnose HEV infection are commercially available in the United States. However, diagnostic tests are available in research laboratories to detect IgM and IgG anti-HEV and HEV RNA levels.

therapies include primarily nucleoside and nucleotide analogs and occasionally interferon therapy.

- Nucleoside and nucleotide analogs suppress HBV replication by inhibiting viral DNA synthesis. Drugs such as lamivudine (Epivir), adefovir (Hepsera), entecavir (Baraclude), tenofovir (Viread), and telbivudine (Tyzeka) can reduce viral load and liver damage.

In people with acute hepatitis C, treatment with pegylated interferon within the first 12 to 24 weeks of infection has shown a marked reduction in the development of chronic hepatitis C. Treatment of chronic hepatitis C is based on the genotype of the HCV and the severity of liver disease. Drug therapy is directed at eradicating the virus through the use of direct-acting antivirals (DAAs) and preventing HCV-related complications.

Drug therapy is also used for prevention of HAV and HBV infection.

- Immune globulin (IG) provides temporary (1 to 2 months) passive immunity and is effective for preventing hepatitis A if

H

given within 2 weeks after exposure. Although IG may not prevent infection in all people, it may modify the illness to a subclinical infection.

- IG is recommended for people who do not have anti-HAV antibodies and are exposed because of close contact with people who have HAV or foodborne exposure.
- A combined HAV and HBV vaccine is available for people older than 18 years of age. The vaccine is given in a series of three IM injections in the deltoid muscle. The vaccine is more than 95% effective.
- For postexposure prophylaxis, the vaccine and hepatitis B IG (HBIG) are used. HBIG contains antibodies to HBV and confers temporary passive immunity. HBIG is recommended for post-exposure prophylaxis in cases of needlestick, mucous membrane contact, or sexual exposure and for infants born to mothers who are seropositive for HBsAg.

Nutritional Therapy

No special diet is required in the treatment of viral hepatitis. Emphasize a well-balanced diet that the patient can tolerate. Vitamin supplements, particularly B-complex vitamins and vitamin K, are frequently used. If anorexia, nausea, and vomiting are severe, IV solutions of glucose or supplemental enteral nutrition therapy may be used.

Nursing Management

Goals

The patient with viral hepatitis will have relief of discomfort, be able to resume normal activities, and return to normal liver function without complications.

Nursing Diagnoses

- Imbalanced nutrition: less than body requirements
- Activity intolerance
- Risk for impaired liver function

Nursing Interventions

During acute intervention, assess for the presence and degree of jaundice. Provide comfort measures to relieve pruritus, headache, and arthralgias.

- Ensuring that the patient receives adequate nutrition is not always easy. Small, frequent meals may be preferable to three large ones and may also help prevent nausea. Include measures to stimulate the appetite, such as mouth care, antiemetics, and attractively served meals in pleasant surroundings in your plan of care.
- Assess the patient's response to rest and activity, and modify plans accordingly.

- Emotional rest is as essential as physical rest. Bed rest may produce anxiety and extreme restlessness in some patients. Diversional activities, such as reading and hobbies, may help.

Viral hepatitis is a community health problem. Your role is important in the prevention and control of this disease (see Lewis et al, *Medical-Surgical Nursing,* ed 10, pp. 982 to 984, for a summary of preventive measures).

Hepatitis A.   Vaccination is the best protection against HAV infection. Preventive measures include personal and environmental hygiene and health education to promote good sanitation. Hand washing is essential and is probably the most important precaution. Teach about careful hand washing after bowel movements and before eating.

Hepatitis B.   The best way to reduce HBV infection is to identify those at risk, screen them for HBV, and vaccinate those who are not infected. Teach individuals at high risk of contracting HBV to reduce risks. Good hygienic practices, including hand washing and using gloves when expecting contact with blood, are important.

- Close contacts and sexual partners of the patient with hepatitis B who are HBsAg-negative and antibody-negative should be vaccinated. A condom is advised for sexual intercourse. Razors, toothbrushes, and other personal items should not be shared.

Hepatitis C.   There currently is no hepatitis C vaccine available. Primary measures to prevent HCV transmission are similar to those for HBV, including the screening of blood, organ, and tissue donors; use of infection control measures; and modification of high-risk sexual behavior.

During acute intervention, assess for the presence and degree of jaundice. Provide comfort measures to relieve pruritus, headache, and arthralgias.

- Ensuring that the patient receives adequate nutrition is not always easy. Small, frequent meals may be preferable to three large ones and may also help prevent nausea. Include measures to stimulate the appetite, such as mouth care, antiemetics, and attractively served meals in pleasant surroundings in your plan of care.
- Assess the patient's response to rest and activity, and modify plans accordingly.
- Emotional rest is as essential as physical rest. Bed rest may produce anxiety and extreme restlessness in some patients. Diversional activities, such as reading and hobbies, may help.

▼ Patient and Caregiver Teaching
- Teach the patient and caregivers how to prevent transmission
- Caution the patient about overexertion.

- Teach the patient and caregivers the symptoms to report. Assess the patient for manifestations of complications such as bleeding or encephalopathy.
- Instruct the patient to have regular follow-up for at least 1 year. Teach the patient the symptoms of recurrent hepatitis B and C and the need for follow-up evaluations. All patients with chronic HBV or HCV infection should avoid alcohol because it can accelerate disease progression.
- Teach the patient who is receiving drug therapy for the treatment of hepatitis B or C about the drug(s).

HERNIA

Description

A *hernia* is a protrusion of the viscus (internal organ such as the intestine) through an abnormal opening or a weakened area in the wall of the cavity in which it is normally contained. A hernia may occur in any part of the body, but it usually occurs within the abdominal cavity.

- Hernias that easily return to the abdominal cavity are called *reducible*. The hernia can be reduced manually or may reduce spontaneously when the person lies down.
- Irreducible, or incarcerated, hernias cannot be placed back into the abdominal cavity and have abdominal contents trapped in the opening. When the hernia is irreducible and intestinal flow and blood supply are obstructed, the hernia is *strangulated*. See Intestinal Obstruction, p. 363.

Types

Types of hernias include hiatal, inguinal, femoral, umbilical, and ventral (incisional). See Hiatal Hernia, p. 306.

- *Inguinal hernia* is the most common type of hernia and occurs at the point of weakness in the abdominal wall where the spermatic cord in men or the round ligament in women emerges. Inguinal hernia is more common in men.
- *Femoral hernia* occurs when there is a protrusion through the femoral ring into the femoral canal. It easily becomes strangulated and occurs more frequently in women.
- *Umbilical hernia* occurs when the rectus muscle is weak (as with obesity) or the umbilical opening fails to close after birth.
- *Ventral* or *incisional hernia* is caused by a weakness of the abdominal wall at the site of a previous incision or stoma. It occurs most commonly in patients who are obese, who have had multiple surgical procedures in the same area, or who have

had inadequate wound healing because of poor nutrition or infection.

Clinical Manifestations

A hernia is often readily visible, especially with abdominal muscle tension. Pain may worsen with activities that increase intraabdominal pressure, such as lifting, coughing, and straining.

- A strangulated hernia causes severe pain with symptoms of a bowel obstruction, such as vomiting, cramping abdominal pain, and distention.
- Strangulated hernias or painful, inflamed hernias that cannot be reduced require emergency surgery.

Diagnosis is based on history and physical examination findings. Ultrasound, CT, and MRI can assist in identifying a hernia and determining the contents.

Interprofessional Care

Laparoscopic surgery is the treatment of choice for hernias. The surgical repair of a hernia, known as a *herniorrhaphy,* is usually an outpatient procedure. Reinforcement of the weakened area with wire, fascia, or mesh is known as a *hernioplasty.* Strangulated hernias are treated immediately with resection of the involved area so that necrosis and gangrene do not occur, and in some cases with a temporary colostomy.

Nursing Management

After a hernia repair, the patient may have difficulty voiding. Measure intake and output and observe for a distended bladder.

- Scrotal edema is a painful complication after an inguinal hernia repair. Elevation of the scrotum with a scrotal support and application of an ice bag may help relieve pain and edema.
- Encourage deep breathing, but not coughing. Teach patients to splint the incision and keep the mouth open when coughing or sneezing.
- The patient may be restricted from heavy lifting (>10 lb) for 6 to 8 weeks.

HERPES, GENITAL

Description

Genital herpes infection is a common, lifelong, and incurable infection. Two strains of herpes cause genital infections: herpes simplex virus type 1 (HSV-1) and herpes simplex virus type 2 (HSV-2). Although both forms of HSV may cause genital infection, HSV-1 is more commonly associated with oral lesions and HSV-2 is more common in the genitals. However, an increasing proportion of genital herpes infections are caused by HSV-1.

More than 24 million people in the United States have HSV-2. Rates of new infections are high, partly because of the fact that an estimated 80% of those infected with genital HSV-2 have never received a clinical diagnosis and are unaware that they are capable of transmitting the virus.

Pathophysiology

The herpes simplex virus (HSV) enters through the mucous membranes or breaks in the skin during contact with an infected person. HSV then reproduces inside the cell and spreads to surrounding cells. The virus next enters the peripheral or autonomic nerve endings and ascends to the sensory or autonomic nerve ganglion, where it often becomes dormant. Viral reactivation (recurrence) may occur when the virus travels down to the initial site of infection.

When a person is infected with HSV, the virus usually persists within the individual for life. Transmission of HSV occurs through direct contact with skin or mucous membranes when an infected individual is symptomatic or through asymptomatic viral shedding.

Both HSV-1 and HSV-2 can cause either genital or orolabial infections. There is no absolute, single site for either virus.

- HSV-1 infections are more common "above the waist," involving the gingivae, dermis, upper respiratory tract, and, rarely the CNS. Among young women, HSV-1 is more commonly associated with genital infection than HSV-2.
- HSV-2 almost always infects sites "below the waist"—the genital tract or perineum.

Clinical Manifestations

In the *primary (initial) episode* of genital herpes, most people do not have recognizable symptoms of infection. If symptoms do occur, they follow a series of stages. During the *prodromal* stage, the period before lesions appear, the patient may have burning, itching, or tingling at the site of inoculation. In the *vesicular* stage, a few to multiple small, often painful vesicles (blisters) may appear on the buttock, inner thigh, penis, scrotum, vulva, perineum, perianal region, vagina, or cervix. The vesicles contain large quantities of infectious viral particles. Next, in the *ulcerative* stage, the lesions rupture and form shallow, moist ulcerations Finally, crusting and epithelialization of the erosions occur.

- Primary infections tend to be associated with local inflammation and pain, regional (inguinal node) lymphadenopathy, and systemic flu-like symptoms including fever, headache, malaise, and myalgia.

- Urination may be painful from urine touching active lesions. Urinary retention may occur as a result of HSV urethritis or cystitis. A purulent vaginal discharge may develop with HSV cervicitis.

Recurrent genital herpes occurs in many individuals during the year after the primary episode. The symptoms of recurrent episodes are less severe, and the lesions usually heal more quickly. HSV-1 genital infections recur less frequently than HSV-2 genital infections, and over time, both decrease in frequency.

- Common triggers of recurrence include stress, fatigue, sunburn, general illness, immunosuppression, and menses. Many patients can predict a recurrence by noticing early prodromal symptoms of tingling, burning, and itching at the site where lesions will eventually appear. Symptoms of recurrent episodes are less severe, and the lesions usually heal within 8 to 12 days. With time the recurrent lesions will generally occur less frequently.
- The greatest risk for transmitting infection exists when active lesions are present. However, it is possible to transmit the virus when no visible lesions or symptoms are present. HSV transmission occurs most commonly during these asymptomatic periods.

Complications

- Both HSV-1 and HSV-2 can cause rare but serious complications such as blindness, encephalitis (inflammation of the brain), and aseptic meningitis (inflammation of the linings of the brain).
- Autoinoculation can result in the development of lesions in the buttocks, groin, thighs, fingers, and eyes.
- Pregnant women with HSV can transmit the virus to the baby, most commonly if the virus is shed while the infant passes though the birth canal. Women with a primary episode of HSV near the time of delivery have the highest risk of transmitting genital herpes to the neonate. An active genital lesion at the time of delivery is usually an indication for cesarean delivery.

Diagnostic Studies

- Diagnosis is usually based on the patient's symptoms and history.
- Highly accurate serologic tests are available for the diagnosis of HSV-1 and HSV-2. These type-specific immunoassays test for the presence of antibodies to HSV.

H

- A viral culture of the active lesion can also be used to isolate the virus.

Interprofessional Care
Drug Therapy

Three antiviral agents are available for the treatment of HSV: acyclovir (Zovirax), valacyclovir (Valtrex), and famciclovir (Famvir). These drugs inhibit herpetic viral replication and are prescribed for primary and recurrent infections. These drugs do not cure HSV but shorten the duration of viral shedding and healing time of genital lesions and reduce outbreaks by 75%. Continued use of oral acyclovir for up to 5 years is safe and effective. IV acyclovir is reserved for severe or life-threatening infections.

Nursing Management

The primary goal is to keep lesions clean and dry. Teach patients with active outbreaks to maintain good genital hygiene and wear loose-fitting cotton undergarments.

- Techniques to reduce pain on urination include pouring water onto the perineal area while voiding to dilute the urine or voiding in the shower. Pain may require a local anesthetic such as lidocaine gel or analgesics such as ibuprofen, acetaminophen, acetaminophen with codeine, or aspirin.
- Ice packs to the affected area can provide some relief.
- See Sexually Transmitted Infections, p. 562.

HIATAL HERNIA

Description

Hiatal hernia is herniation of a portion of the stomach into the esophagus through an opening or hiatus in the diaphragm. It is also referred to as diaphragmatic hernia or esophageal hernia. Hiatal hernias are common among older adults and occur more frequently in women than in men. Hiatal hernias are classified into two types (Fig. 11).

- A *sliding hernia* is the most common type. It occurs at the junction of the stomach and esophagus located above the hiatus of the diaphragm. A part of the stomach "slides" through the hiatal opening in the diaphragm. This occurs when the patient is supine, and it usually goes back into the abdominal cavity when the patient is standing upright.

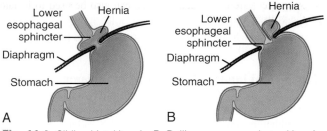

Fig. 11 **A,** Sliding hiatal hernia. **B,** Rolling or paraesophageal hernia.

- A *paraesophageal* or *rolling hernia* occurs at the esophagogastric junction where the fundus and the greater curvature of the stomach roll up through the diaphragm to form a pocket alongside the esophagus.

Pathophysiology

Many factors contribute to the development of hiatal hernia. Structural changes, such as weakening of the muscles in the diaphragm around the esophagogastric opening, occur with aging. Factors that increase intraabdominal pressure including obesity, pregnancy, ascites, tumors, intense physical exertion, and frequent heavy lifting may also predispose patients to development of a hiatal hernia.

Clinical Manifestations

Signs and symptoms of hiatal hernia are similar to those described for gastroesophageal reflux disease (GERD). Some people are asymptomatic.

- Heartburn is common, especially after a meal or after lying supine. Bending over may cause a severe burning pain, which is usually relieved by sitting or standing. Large meals, alcohol, and smoking may precipitate pain.
- Nocturnal attacks are common, especially if the person has eaten before lying down.

Complications may include GERD, esophagitis, hemorrhage from erosion, stenosis, ulcerations of the herniated portion of the stomach, strangulation of the hernia, and regurgitation with tracheal aspiration.

H

Diagnostic Studies

- Barium swallow (esophagram) may show gastric mucosa protrusion through the esophageal hiatus. See also tests done for GERD, p. 240.

Nursing and Interprofessional Management

Conservative therapy for hiatal hernia is similar to that for GERD (p. 241). Teach the patient to reduce intraabdominal pressure by eliminating constricting garments and avoiding lifting and straining.

Surgical approaches include reduction of the herniated stomach into the abdomen, *herniotomy* (excision of the hernia sac), *herniorrhaphy* (closure of the hiatal defect), an antireflux procedure, and *gastropexy* (attachment of the stomach subdiaphragmatically to prevent reherniation).

- Laparoscopically performed Nissen and Toupet fundoplication techniques are the standard antireflux surgeries for hiatal hernia.

HODGKIN'S LYMPHOMA

Description

Hodgkin's lymphoma, also called Hodgkin's disease, is a malignant condition characterized by proliferation of abnormal, giant, multinucleated cells called *Reed-Sternberg cells,* which are located in lymph nodes. The disease accounts for 11% of all lymphomas and has a bimodal age-specific incidence, occurring most frequently in people 15 to 30 years of age and in those older than 55 years. In adults it is twice as prevalent among men as among women. Each year, approximately 9190 new cases of Hodgkin's lymphoma are diagnosed and approximately 1100 deaths occur. However, long-term survival exceeds 80% for all stages.

Pathophysiology

Although the cause of Hodgkin's lymphoma remains unknown, several key factors are thought to play a role in its development. The main interacting factors include infection with the Epstein-Barr virus, genetic predisposition, and exposure to occupational toxins.

In Hodgkin's lymphoma the normal structure of the lymph nodes is destroyed by hyperplasia of monocytes and macrophages. The disease is believed to arise at a single location (it originates in the cervical lymph nodes in 80% of patients) and then spreads along adjacent lymphatics. It eventually infiltrates other organs, especially the lungs, spleen, and liver.

Clinical Manifestations

The initial manifestation is most often an enlargement of the cervical, axillary, or inguinal lymph nodes. The enlarged nodes are not painful unless pressure is exerted on adjacent nerves.

- The patient may note weight loss, fatigue, weakness, fever, chills, tachycardia, or night sweats. A group of initial findings, including fever, night sweats, and weight loss (referred to as *B symptoms*), correlate with a worse prognosis.
- Generalized pruritus without skin lesions may develop. Cough, dyspnea, stridor, and dysphagia may all reflect mediastinal node involvement.
- In more advanced disease, there may be hepatomegaly and splenomegaly. Anemia results from increased destruction and decreased production of erythrocytes. Intrathoracic involvement may lead to superior vena cava syndrome. Enlarged retroperitoneal nodes may cause palpable abdominal masses or interfere with renal function.
- Jaundice may result from liver involvement.
- Spinal cord compression leading to paraplegia may occur with extradural involvement.

Diagnostic Studies

Peripheral blood analysis, excisional lymph node biopsy, bone marrow examination, and radiologic studies are important means of evaluating Hodgkin's lymphoma.

- Microcytic hypochromic anemia, leukopenia, and thrombocytopenia may develop, usually as a consequence of treatment, advanced disease, or hypersplenism (related to the disease process).
- Other blood studies may show elevated erythrocyte sedimentation rate, elevated alkaline phosphatase from liver and bone involvement, hypercalcemia from bone involvement, and hypoalbuminemia from liver involvement.
- Positron emission tomography (PET) scans with or without CT scan are used to stage and then assess response to therapy. The scans may show increased uptake of carbohydrate by cancer cells (by PET) and masses (by CT) such as mediastinal lymphadenopathy, renal displacement caused by retroperitoneal node enlargement, abdominal lymph node enlargement, or liver, spleen, bone, and brain infiltration.

H

Interprofessional Care

Treatment decisions are made based on the clinical stage of the disease. The standard for chemotherapy is the ABVD regimen: doxorubicin (formerly marketed as Adriamycin), bleomycin, vinblastine, and dacarbazine, given for two to eight cycles of treatment, depending on disease stage and prognosis.

Combination chemotherapy works well because as in leukemia, the drugs used have an additive antitumor effect without increasing side effects. As with leukemia, therapy must be aggressive. Therefore potentially life-threatening problems are encountered in an attempt to achieve a remission.

A variety of chemotherapy regimens and newer agents, such as brentuximab vedotin (Adcetris), are used to treat patients who have relapsed or refractory disease. Ideally, once remission is obtained, a treatment option with the goal of cure may be intensive chemotherapy with the use of autologous or allogeneic hematopoietic stem cell transplantation.

The role of irradiation as a supplement to chemotherapy varies depending on site of disease and the presence of resistant disease after chemotherapy.

Nursing Management

Nursing care for patients with Hodgkin's lymphoma is primarily based on managing problems related to the disease, such as pain, and side effects of therapy, such as pancytopenia.

- Because the survival of patients with Hodgkin's lymphoma depends on their response to treatment, support the patient through the consequences of treatment.
- Psychosocial considerations are as important as they are with leukemia (see Leukemia, p. 386). However, the prognosis with Hodgkin's lymphoma is better than that with many forms of cancer or leukemia. The physical, psychologic, social, and spiritual consequences of the patient's disease must be addressed.
- Delayed consequences of the disease and treatment, such as secondary malignancies and long-term endocrine, cardiac, and pulmonary toxicities, may not be apparent for many years. The most common secondary malignancies are lung and breast cancer. Encourage close follow-up and screening for early detection.

HUMAN IMMUNODEFICIENCY VIRUS INFECTION

Description

Human immunodeficiency virus (HIV) is a retrovirus that causes immunosuppression. Persons with HIV infection are more susceptible to other infections that are normally controlled through immune responses. The term HIV disease is used interchangeably with HIV infection. With advances in treatment, HIV is managed as a chronic disease.

Pathophysiology

HIV is a ribonucleic acid (RNA) virus. Like all viruses, HIV cannot replicate unless it is in a living cell. HIV infects human cells that have $CD4^+$ receptors on their surfaces. These include lymphocytes, monocytes/macrophages, astrocytes, and oligodendrocytes. Immune dysfunction in HIV disease is caused predominantly by destruction of $CD4^+$ T cells (also known as T-helper cells or $CD4^+$ lymphocytes).

HIV destroys about 1 billion $CD4^+$ T cells every day. For many years the body can produce new $CD4^+$ T cells to replace the destroyed cells. However, over time the ability of HIV to destroy $CD4^+$ T cells exceeds the body's ability to replace the cells. The decline in the $CD4^+$ T cell count impairs immune function. Generally, the immune system remains healthy with more than 500 $CD4^+$ T cells/μL. Immune problems begin to occur when the count drops below 500 $CD4^+$ T cells/μL. Severe problems develop with fewer than 200 $CD4^+$ T cells/μL.

With HIV, a point is eventually reached where so many $CD4^+$ T cells have been destroyed that not enough are left to regulate immune responses. This allows opportunistic diseases (infections and cancers that occur in immunosuppressed patients) to develop. Opportunistic diseases are the main cause of disease, disability, and death in patients with HIV infection.

HIV can be transmitted through contact with infected blood, semen, vaginal secretions, or breast milk. HIV transmission occurs through sexual intercourse with an infected partner; exposure to HIV-infected blood or blood products; and perinatal transmission during pregnancy, at delivery, or through breastfeeding. HIV is not spread through casual contact.

H

Clinical Manifestations

The typical course of untreated HIV infection follows the pattern shown in Fig. 12. It is important to remember that disease

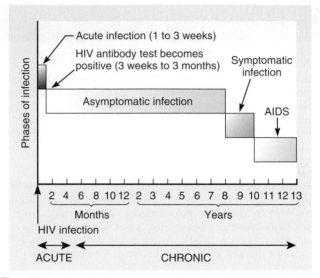

Fig. 12 Timeline for the spectrum of untreated HIV infection. The timeline represents the course of untreated illness from the time of infection to clinical manifestations of disease.

progression is highly individualized and that treatment can significantly alter the pattern. HIV infections are divided into acute and chronic stages.

Acute Infection

During acute HIV infection, HIV-specific antibodies are produced (seroconversion) and a mononucleosis-like syndrome of fever, lymphadenopathy, pharyngitis, headache, malaise, nausea, and/or a diffuse rash may occur.

- Symptoms generally occur 2 to 4 weeks after initial infection and last for 1 to 3 weeks.
- During this time a high viral load is noted and CD4+ T cell counts fall temporarily but quickly return to baseline. Many people, including HCPs, mistake acute HIV symptoms for a bad case of the flu. Individuals are most infectious during the acute infection stage because of the high amounts of circulating HIV.

Chronic Infection

There are three stages of chronic infection: asymptomatic infection, symptomatic infection, and acquired immunodeficiency syndrome (AIDS). The interval between untreated HIV infection and a diagnosis of AIDS is about 10 years.

- *Asymptomatic infection*—during this time CD4$^+$ lymphocyte counts remain above 500 cells/µL (normal or slightly decreased) and the viral load in the blood is low. At this point, individuals have no symptoms or relatively limited and vague signs of infection.
- *Symptomatic infection* occurs as the CD4$^+$ T cell count drops to 200 to 500 cells/µL and the viral load increases. Symptoms such as persistent fever, frequent night sweats, chronic diarrhea, recurrent headaches, and severe fatigue may develop.
- *AIDS* is characterized by severe immune system suppression and CD4$^+$ T cell counts below 200 cells/µL. A diagnosis of AIDS is made when an HIV-infected patient meets criteria established by the Centers for Disease Control and Prevention (CDC), which include the development of at least one of these conditions:
  1. CD4$^+$ lymphocyte count less than 200/µL
  2. Development of opportunistic infection (see Table 14-11, Lewis et al, *Medical-Surgical Nursing,* ed 10, p. 222)
  3. Development of opportunistic cancer (e.g., Kaposi sarcoma)
  4. *Wasting syndrome* (defined as a loss of 10% or more of ideal body mass)

Diagnostic Studies
Screening
The most useful screening tests are those that detect HIV-specific antibodies. A major problem is that there is a delay of several weeks after infection before antibodies can be detected.

- Standard antibody tests can be completed on blood or saliva.
  - *Rapid tests* are highly accurate and can be done in a variety of settings (mobile health units or HCP offices, or even within the privacy of an individual's home). Results are typically available within 20 minutes. Rapid tests are screening tests for antibodies, not for antigen.
  - In-home HIV test kits are available. Testing is done on saliva.
- Combination antibody and antigen tests (also known as fourth-generation tests) are able to detect HIV earlier than previous versions of HIV screening tests. The fourth-generation test decreases the window period to within 3 weeks after infection.

Progression of Human Immunodeficiency Virus Infection
- CD4$^+$ T cell count and viral load monitor progression of infection.

- WBC count, RBC count, and platelets decrease with progression of HIV.

Interprofessional Care

Treatment focuses on (1) monitoring HIV disease progression and immune function; (2) initiating and monitoring antiretroviral therapy (ART); (3) preventing, detecting, and treating opportunistic diseases; (4) managing symptoms; (5) preventing or decreasing the complications of treatment; and (6) preventing further transmission of HIV infection.

Drug Therapy

Goals of drug therapy in HIV infection are to decrease the viral load, maintain or increase CD4+ T cell counts, prevent HIV-related symptoms and opportunistic diseases, delay disease progression, and prevent HIV transmission.

Using drugs from different classes in combination therapy can inhibit viral replication in several ways, making it difficult for the virus to recover and decreasing the likelihood of drug resistance.

- Resistance develops rapidly when ART drugs are used alone or taken in inadequate doses. The most effective means to suppress HIV replication is using at least three effective ART drugs from at least two different drug classes in optimum schedules and at full dosages (Table 46).
- Many ART agents cause dangerous and potentially lethal interactions when used in combination with other commonly used drugs, including over-the-counter preparations and herbal therapies.

Opportunistic diseases associated with HIV infection can be delayed or prevented with adequate ART, vaccines (including hepatitis B, influenza, and pneumococcal), and disease-specific prevention measures.

Nursing Management

Goals

The patient with HIV infection will adhere to drug regimens; adopt a healthy lifestyle that includes avoiding exposure to other sexually transmitted infections and blood-borne diseases; protect others from HIV infection; maintain or develop healthy and supportive relationships; maintain activities and productivity; explore spiritual issues; come to terms with issues related to disease, disability, and death; and cope with symptoms caused by HIV disease and its treatments.

Text continued on p. 318

TABLE 46 Drug Therapy

Human Immunodeficiency Virus (HIV) Infection

Drug Classification	Mechanism of Action	Examples
Entry inhibitors	Prevent binding of HIV to cells, thus preventing entry of HIV into cells where replication would occur	enfuvirtide (Fuzeon) maraviroc (Selzentry)
Reverse transcriptase inhibitors		
Nucleoside reverse transcriptase inhibitors (NRTIs)	Insert a piece of DNA into the developing HIV DNA chain, blocking further development of the chain and leaving the production of the new strand of HIV DNA incomplete	zidovudine (Retrovir) didanosine (Videx, Videx-EC [timed-release]) stavudine (Zerit) lamivudine (Epivir) abacavir (Ziagen) emtricitabine (Emtriva)
Non-nucleoside reverse transcriptase inhibitors (NNRTIs)	Inhibit the action of reverse transcriptase	nevirapine (Viramune XR) delavirdine (Rescriptor) efavirenz (Sustiva) etravirine (Intelence) rilpivirine (Edurant)

Continued

H

TABLE 46 Drug Therapy

Human Immunodeficiency Virus (HIV) Infection—cont'd

Drug Classification	Mechanism of Action	Examples
Nucleotide reverse transcriptase inhibitor (NtRTI)	Combines with reverse transcriptase enzyme to block the process needed to convert HIV RNA into HIV DNA	tenofovir (Viread)
Integrase inhibitors	Bind with integrase enzyme and prevent HIV from incorporating its genetic material into the host cell	raltegravir (Isentress) elvitegravir (Vitekta*) dolutegravir (Tivicay)
Protease inhibitors (PIs)	Prevent the protease enzyme from cutting HIV proteins into the proper lengths needed to allow viable virions to assemble and bud out from the cell membrane	saquinavir (Invirase) indinavir (Crixivan) ritonavir (Norvir)† nelfinavir (Viracept) atazanavir (Reyataz) fosamprenavir (Lexiva) tipranavir (Aptivus) darunavir (Prezista) lopinavir + ritonavir (Kaletra)

| Fixed-dose combination products | More than one drug combined into a single tablet. Drugs may be from the same or different classes | Atripla (tenofovir DF + emtricitabine + efavirenz)
Combivir (lamivudine + zidovudine)
Complera (tenofovir DF + emtricitabine + rilpivirine)
Epzicom (abacavir + lamivudine)
Triumeq (abacavir + lamivudine + dolutegravir)
Trizivir (abacavir + lamivudine + zidovudine)
Truvada (tenofovir DF + emtricitabine)
Descovy (tenofovir AF + emtricitabine)
Stribild (tenofovir DF + emtricitabine + elvitegravir + cobicistat‡)
Evotaz (atazanavir + cobicistat‡)
Prezcobix (darunavir + cobicistat‡)
Genvoya (tenofovir AF + emtricitabine + elvitegravir + cobicistat‡) |

DF, Disoproxil fumarate.

*Vitekta must be administered with a boosted HIV protease inhibitor. Elvitegravir in other fixed dose combinations can be given with either a protease inhibitor or cobicistat.

†Most often used in low doses with other PIs to boost effect.

‡Cobicistat is a pharmacologic booster that enhances the potency of some HIV antiretrovirals. It has no direct effects against HIV.

H

Nursing Interventions

The complexity of HIV disease is related to its chronic nature. As with most chronic and infectious diseases, primary prevention and health promotion are the most effective health care strategies. See Table 14-15 in Lewis et al, *Medical-Surgical Nursing*, ed 10, p. 227 for a summary of interventions and strategies that highlight nursing goals, assessments, and interventions throughout the course of HIV infection.

HIV infection is preventable. Avoiding and/or modifying risky behaviors are the most effective prevention tools. Provide culturally sensitive, language-appropriate, and age-specific teaching and behavior change counseling.

- Early intervention after detection of HIV infection can promote health and limit disability. It should focus on early detection of symptoms, opportunistic diseases, and psychosocial problems.

Useful interventions for HIV-infected patients include nutritional support; moderation or elimination of alcohol, tobacco, and drug use; keeping recommended vaccines up to date; adequate rest, exercise, and stress reduction; avoiding exposure to new infectious agents; mental health counseling; and getting involved in support groups and community activities.

- Teach patients to recognize symptoms that may indicate disease progression and/or drug side effects so that prompt medical care can be initiated.
- During acute exacerbations of opportunistic diseases or adverse effects of treatment, symptomatic care may include teaching and treatment for diarrhea, pneumonia, fatigue, wasting syndrome, and ADC.
- The focus of end-of-life care is on patient comfort, facilitation of emotional and spiritual issues, and helping significant others deal with grief and loss.

▼ Patient and Caregiver Teaching

HIV education emphasizes prevention and risk reduction. Teach the proper use and placement of male and female condoms and recommend decreasing the number of sex partners. Refer patient to support services for substance use reduction and access to sterile drug equipment. For an infected patient, teaching is directed toward health promotion, managing the problems caused by HIV infection, and maximizing quality of life.

- Teach advantages and disadvantages of new treatments, including drug therapy, dangers of nonadherence to therapeutic regimens, how and when to take each medication, drug interactions to avoid, and side effects that need to be reported to the HCP. Tables 14-13, 14-16, and 14-17, Lewis et al, *Medical-Surgical*

Nursing, ed 10, pp. 224, 228, and 229, provide guidance for patient teaching in these areas.

- Teach energy conservation measures and the use of assistive devices to increase safety and decrease fatigue.
- Discuss infection control measures with the patient, caregivers, family, and visitors.
- Provide information about support groups and community resources.

HUNTINGTON'S DISEASE

Description

Huntington's disease (HD) is a genetically transmitted, autosomal dominant disorder that affects men and women equally across races. The age at onset of HD is usually between 35 and 45 years. Offspring of a person with this disease have a 50% risk of inheriting it.

Pathophysiology

As in Parkinson's disease, the pathologic process in HD involves the basal ganglia and extrapyramidal motor system. However, instead of a deficiency of dopamine (DA), HD involves a deficiency of the neurotransmitters acetylcholine (ACh) and γ-aminobutyric acid (GABA). The net effect is an excess of DA, leading to symptoms that are the opposite of those of parkinsonism.

Clinical Manifestations

Manifestations include a movement disorder and cognitive and psychiatric disorders. The movement disorder is characterized by abnormal and involuntary writhing, twisting movements of the face, limbs, and body *(chorea)*. The movements worsen as the disease progresses.

- Facial movements involving speech, chewing, and swallowing are affected and increase the risk for aspiration and malnutrition. The gait deteriorates and ambulation eventually becomes impossible.
- Psychiatric symptoms are frequently present in the early stage of the disease, often before the onset of motor symptoms. Depression is common. Other psychiatric symptoms include anxiety, agitation, impulsivity, apathy, social withdrawal, and obsessiveness.
- Cognitive deterioration is more variable and involves perception, memory, attention, and learning.

Eventually all psychomotor processes, including the ability to eat and talk, are impaired. Death usually occurs 10 to 20 years after the onset of symptoms, most commonly due to pneumonia and often by suicide.

Diagnosis

The diagnostic process begins with a review of family history and clinical symptoms. Genetic testing confirms the presence of the disease in a person with symptoms.

- People who are asymptomatic but who have a family history of HD face the dilemma of whether or not to be genetically tested. If the test result is positive, the person will develop HD, but when and to what extent the disease will develop cannot be determined.

Nursing and Interprofessional Management

Because there is no cure, interprofessional care is palliative. Tetrabenazine (Xenazine) is used to decrease the amount of DA available at brain synapses, thereby reducing the involuntary movements of chorea.

- Other useful drugs include antipsychotics such as haloperidol [Haldol]) and risperidone (Risperdal), benzodiazepines such as diazepam (Valium) and clonazepam (Klonopin), aripripazole (Abilify), and DA-depleting agents such as reserpine.
- Cognitive disorders are treated with nondrug therapies (e.g., counseling). The psychiatric disorders can be treated with selective serotonin uptake inhibitors such as sertraline (Zoloft) and paroxetine (Paxil).

The goal of nursing management is to provide the most comfortable environment possible for the patient and caregiver by maintaining physical safety, treating physical symptoms, and providing emotional and psychologic support.

- Because of the choreic movements, caloric requirements may be as high as 4000 to 5000 cal/day to maintain body weight. As the disease progresses, meeting caloric needs becomes a greater challenge when the patient has difficulty swallowing and holding the head still. Depression and mental deterioration can also compromise nutritional intake.
- Advance directives and end-of-life issues need to be discussed with the patient and caregiver.

HYPERPARATHYROIDISM

Description

Hyperparathyroidism is a condition involving increased secretion of parathyroid hormone (PTH). PTH helps regulate serum calcium and phosphate levels by stimulating bone resorption, renal tubular reabsorption of calcium, and activation of vitamin D. Oversecretion of PTH is associated with increased serum calcium levels. Hyperparathyroidism is more common in women than in men.

Hyperparathyroidism is classified as primary, secondary, or tertiary.

- *Primary hyperparathyroidism* is caused by an increased secretion of PTH leading to disorders of calcium, phosphate, and bone metabolism. The most common cause is a benign tumor (adenoma) in the parathyroid gland. Previous head and neck irradiation may be a risk factor for a parathyroid adenoma.
- *Secondary hyperparathyroidism* is a compensatory response to conditions that induce or cause hypocalcemia, the main stimulus of PTH secretion. These conditions include vitamin D deficiencies, malabsorption, chronic kidney disease, and hyperphosphatemia.
- *Tertiary hyperparathyroidism* occurs when hyperplasia of the parathyroid glands occurs in combination with loss of negative feedback from circulating calcium levels. This causes autonomous secretion of PTH even with normal calcium levels. It is observed in the patient who has had a kidney transplant after a long period of dialysis treatment for chronic kidney disease.

Pathophysiology

Excessive levels of circulating PTH usually lead to hypercalcemia and hypophosphatemia, with multiple body systems affected (see Table 49-12, Lewis et al, *Medical-Surgical Nursing,* ed 10, p. 1172).

- Decreased bone density can occur as a result of the effect of PTH on osteoclastic (bone resorption) and osteoblastic (bone formation) activity.
- In the kidneys, excess calcium cannot be reabsorbed, which leads to hypercalciuria. The excess urinary calcium, along with a large amount of urinary phosphate, can lead to formation of calculi.

Clinical Manifestations

Manifestations are associated with hypercalcemia and range from no symptoms to overt symptoms. Loss of appetite, constipation, fatigue, emotional disorders, shortened attention span, and muscle

H

weakness, particularly in the proximal muscles of the lower extremities, are often noted.

Complications include osteoporosis, renal failure, kidney stones, pancreatitis, cardiac changes, and long bone, rib, and vertebral fractures.

Diagnostic Studies
- PTH levels are elevated.
- Serum calcium levels are elevated with decreased phosphorus levels.
- Urine calcium, serum chloride, serum uric acid, and serum creatinine are elevated.
- Serum amylase (if pancreatitis is present) and alkaline phosphatase (if bone disease is present) are both elevated.
- Bone density tests can detect bone loss.
- MRI, CT scan, and ultrasound can be used to localize adenoma.

Interprofessional Care
Treatment objectives are to relieve the symptoms and prevent complications caused by excess PTH. The choice of therapy depends on the urgency of the clinical situation, degree of hypercalcemia, and underlying cause of the disorder.
- The most effective treatment of primary and secondary hyperparathyroidism is partial or complete surgical removal of the parathyroid glands. The procedure most commonly used involves outpatient endoscopy.
- Severe hypercalcemia is managed with IV sodium chloride solution and loop diuretics such as furosemide to increase the urinary excretion of calcium.

A conservative management approach is used in patients who are asymptomatic or have mild symptoms of hyperparathyroidism. This includes an annual examination with tests for serum PTH, calcium, phosphorus, and alkaline phosphatase levels and renal function; x-rays to assess for metabolic bone disease; and measurement of urinary calcium excretion. Dietary measures include high fluid and moderate calcium intake.
- X-rays and dual-energy x-ray absorptiometry (DXA) assess for metabolic bone loss.
- Bisphosphonates (e.g., alendronate [Fosamax]) inhibit osteoclastic bone resorption and improve bone mineral density. Phosphates are given if the patient has normal renal function and low serum phosphate levels.
- Calcimimetic agents (e.g., cinacalcet [Sensipar]) increase the sensitivity of the calcium receptor on the parathyroid gland, resulting in decreased PTH secretion and calcium blood levels.

Nursing Management

Nursing care after surgery is similar to that for the patient after thyroidectomy (see Hyperthyroidism, p. 332). The major postoperative complications are hemorrhage and fluid and electrolyte disturbances. Tetany is usually apparent early in the postoperative period but may develop over several days. Mild tetany, characterized by an unpleasant tingling of the hands and around the mouth, may be present but should resolve without problems. IV calcium should be readily available for use if tetany becomes more severe (e.g., muscular spasms or laryngospasms).

- Monitor intake and output to evaluate fluid status.
- Assess calcium, potassium, phosphate, and magnesium levels frequently.

▼ **Patient and Caregiver Teaching**

- Assist the patient with hyperparathyroidism to adapt the meal plan to his or her lifestyle. A referral to a dietitian may be useful.
- Because immobility can aggravate bone loss, stress the importance of an exercise program.
- Encourage the patient to keep annual appointments.
- Instruct the patient regarding the symptoms of hypocalcemia or hypercalcemia and to report them when they occur.

HYPERTENSION

Description

One in three adults in the United States has *hypertension,* or high BP. Hypertension is one of the most important modifiable risk factors that can lead to the development of cardiovascular disease (CVD). As BP increases, so does the risk of myocardial infarction (MI), heart failure, stroke, and renal disease.

Hypertension is defined as a persistent systolic BP (SBP) of 140 mm Hg or greater, diastolic BP (DBP) of 90 mm Hg or greater, or current use of an antihypertensive drug. *Prehypertension* is defined as SBP 120 to 139 mm Hg or DBP 80 to 89 mm Hg. Classification of hypertension for adults according to stages is described in Table 47.

- The classification is based on the average of two or more properly measured BP readings on two or more office visits.

Isolated systolic hypertension (ISH) is defined as an average SBP of 140 mm Hg or more, coupled with an average DBP of less than 90 mm Hg. SBP increases with aging. DBP rises until approximately age 55 and then declines. Control of ISH decreases the incidence of stroke, heart failure, and death.

H

TABLE 47	Classification of Hypertension		
Category	**SBP (mm Hg)**		**DBP (mm Hg)**
Normal	<120	and	<80
Prehypertension	120-139	or	80-89
Hypertension, stage 1	140-159	or	90-99
Hypertension, stage 2	≥160	or	≥100

From the National Heart, Lung, and Blood Institute: *Seventh report of the Joint National Committee on Detection, Evaluation, and Treatment of High Blood Pressure* (JNC-7), NIH Publication No. 04-5230, Bethesda, Md, 2004, The Institute. Retrieved from *www.nhlbi.nih.gov/guidelines/hypertension/jnc7full.pdf*. *DBP,* Diastolic blood pressure; *SBP,* systolic blood pressure.

Hypertension can be classified as primary (essential or idiopathic) or secondary. *Primary hypertension* accounts for 90% to 95% of all cases of hypertension. Although the exact cause of primary hypertension is unknown, several contributing factors have been identified. These include changes in endothelial function related to vasoconstricting or vasodilating agents, increased SNS activity, overproduction of sodium-retaining hormones, increased sodium intake, greater-than-ideal body weight, diabetes, tobacco use, and excessive alcohol intake.

Secondary hypertension is elevated BP with a specific cause that can often be identified and corrected. This type of hypertension accounts for 5% to 10% of hypertension in adults. Causes of secondary hypertension include coarctation or congenital narrowing of the aorta, renal artery stenosis, endocrine disorders such as Cushing syndrome, cirrhosis, neurologic disorders such as brain tumors and head injury, sleep apnea, and pregnancy-induced hypertension. Treatment of secondary hypertension is directed at removing or treating the underlying cause.

Pathophysiology of Primary Hypertension

The hemodynamic hallmark of hypertension is persistently increased systemic vascular resistance (SVR). Table 48 presents factors that relate to the development of primary hypertension or contribute to its consequences.

Clinical Manifestations

Hypertension is often called the "silent killer" because it is frequently asymptomatic until it becomes severe and target organ disease has occurred. A patient with severe hypertension may experience a variety of symptoms secondary to effects on blood

TABLE 48	Risk Factors for Primary Hypertension
Risk Factor	**Description**
Age	SBP rises progressively with increasing age. After age 50, SBP >140 mm Hg is a more important cardiovascular risk factor than DBP.
Alcohol	Excessive alcohol intake is strongly associated with hypertension. Patients with hypertension should limit their daily intake to 1 oz of alcohol.
Tobacco use	Smoking tobacco greatly ↑ risk of cardiovascular disease. People with hypertension who smoke tobacco are at even greater risk for cardiovascular disease.
Diabetes mellitus	Hypertension is more common in diabetics. When hypertension and diabetes coexist, complications (e.g., target organ disease) are more severe.
Elevated serum lipids	↑ Levels of cholesterol and triglycerides are primary risk factors in atherosclerosis. Hyperlipidemia is more common in people with hypertension.
Excess dietary sodium	High sodium intake can • Contribute to hypertension in some patients • Decrease the effectiveness of certain antihypertensive drugs
Gender	Hypertension is more prevalent in men in young adulthood and early middle age (<55 yr of age). After age 64, hypertension is more prevalent among women. (See Gender Differences box, Lewis et al, *Medical-Surgical Nursing*, ed 10, p. 682.)
Family history	History of a close blood relative (e.g., parents, sibling) with hypertension is associated with ↑ risk for developing hypertension.
Obesity	Weight gain is associated with increased frequency of hypertension. Risk is greatest with central abdominal obesity.
Ethnicity	Incidence of hypertension is two times higher in African Americans than in whites. (See Cultural & Ethnic Health Disparities box, Lewis et al, *Medical-Surgical Nursing*, ed 10, p. 682.)

H

Continued

TABLE 48	Risk Factors for Primary Hypertension—cont'd
Risk Factor	**Description**
Sedentary lifestyle	Regular physical activity can help control weight and reduce cardiovascular risk. Physical activity may ↓ BP.
Socioeconomic status	Hypertension is more prevalent in lower socioeconomic groups and among the less educated.
Stress	People exposed to repeated stress may develop hypertension more frequently than others. People who develop hypertension may respond differently to stress than those who do not develop hypertension.

DBP, Diastolic blood pressure; *SBP,* systolic blood pressure.

vessels in the various organs and tissues or to the increased workload of the heart. These secondary symptoms include fatigue, reduced activity tolerance, dizziness, palpitations, angina, and dyspnea.

The most common complications of hypertension are target organ diseases occurring in the heart (hypertensive heart disease), brain (cerebrovascular disease), peripheral vasculature (peripheral vascular disease), kidney (nephrosclerosis), and eyes (retinal damage).

Hypertensive Heart Disease

Hypertension is a major risk factor for coronary artery disease (CAD). The mechanisms by which hypertension contributes to the development of atherosclerosis are not fully known. The "response-to-injury" theory of atherogenesis suggests that hypertension disrupts the coronary artery endothelium. This results in a stiff arterial wall with a narrowed lumen and accounts for a high rate of CAD, angina, and MI. Sustained high BP also increases the cardiac workload and produces left ventricular hypertrophy (LVH). Progressive LVH, especially in association with CAD, is associated with the development of heart failure.

Heart failure occurs when the heart's compensatory adaptations are overwhelmed and the heart can no longer pump enough blood to meet the body's demands.

- The patient may complain of shortness of breath on exertion, paroxysmal nocturnal dyspnea, and fatigue.

Cerebrovascular Disease

Atherosclerosis is the most common cause of cerebrovascular disease. Atherosclerotic plaques are commonly distributed at the bifurcation of the common carotid artery. Portions of the atherosclerotic plaque, or the blood clot that forms on the plaque, may break off and travel to intracerebral vessels, producing a thromboembolism. The patient may experience transient ischemic attacks or a stroke.

Peripheral Vascular Disease

Hypertension speeds up the process of atherosclerosis in peripheral blood vessels, leading to the development of aortic aneurysm, aortic dissection, and peripheral vascular disease. *Intermittent claudication* (ischemic muscle pain precipitated by activity and relieved with rest) is a classic symptom of peripheral vascular disease.

Nephrosclerosis

Hypertension is one of the leading risk factors for chronic kidney disease, especially among African Americans. Some degree of renal disease is usually present in the hypertensive patient, even one with a minimally elevated BP. This disorder is the result of ischemia caused by the narrowing of renal blood vessels. This leads to the destruction of glomeruli, atrophy of tubules, and eventual death of nephrons. These changes may eventually lead to renal failure. The earliest symptom of renal disease is usually nocturia.

Retinal Damage

The appearance of the retina provides important information about the severity and duration of hypertension. The blood vessels of the retina can be directly visualized with an ophthalmoscope. Damage to the retinal vessels provides an indication of related vessel damage in the heart, brain, and kidneys. Symptoms of severe retinal damage include blurring of vision, retinal hemorrhage, and loss of vision.

Diagnostic Studies

Accurate measurement of BP is essential in assessing and monitoring hypertension. Basic laboratory studies are performed to evaluate target organ disease, determine overall cardiovascular risk, or establish baseline levels before initiating therapy.

- Routine urinalysis, blood urea nitrogen (BUN), and serum creatinine levels to screen for renal involvement
- Serum electrolytes, especially potassium levels, to detect hyperaldosteronism
- Blood glucose level to assess for diabetes mellitus
- Lipid profile to assess for risk factors for atherosclerosis
- ECG for baseline cardiac status

Interprofessional Care

Treatment goals include achieving and maintaining goal BP and reducing cardiovascular risk and target organ disease. Lifestyle modifications are indicated for all patients with prehypertension and hypertension. These modification measures include weight reduction, a Dietary Approaches to Stop Hypertension (DASH) eating plan, dietary sodium reduction, regular physical activity, moderation of alcohol consumption, management of psychosocial risk factors, and avoidance of tobacco use.

- Dietary therapy consists of restricting sodium intake to less than 2300 mg/day and following the DASH eating plan, which emphasizes fruits, vegetables, fat-free or low-fat milk and milk products, whole grains, fish, poultry, beans, seeds, and nuts. Compared with the typical American diet, the plan contains less red meat, salt, sweets, added sugars, and sugar-containing beverages and is rich in vegetables, fruit, and nonfat dairy products. Men should limit their intake of alcohol to no more than two drinks per day, and women and lighter-weight men to no more than one drink per day.
- Adults should perform moderate-intensity aerobic physical activity for at least 30 minutes most days (i.e., more than 5 days per week) or vigorous-intensity aerobic activity for at least 20 minutes 3 days a week.
- Muscle-strengthening activities should also be performed using the major muscles of the body at least twice a week. Flexibility and balance exercises are recommended at least twice a week for older adults, especially for those at risk for falls. Advise sedentary people to increase activity levels gradually.
- Psychosocial risk factors (e.g., depression, social isolation, low socioeconomic status) can contribute to the risk of developing CVD and to a poorer prognosis and clinical course in patients with CVD. Screening for these factors is important. Make appropriate referrals (e.g., counseling) when indicated.
- Nicotine contained in tobacco causes vasoconstriction and increases BP in hypertensive people. Strongly encourage everyone, especially a hypertensive patient, to avoid tobacco use.

The following are recommendations for antihypertensive drug therapy from the JNC 8:

- In patients 60 years of age or older, start drug treatment for BP of 150 mm Hg or more systolic or 90 mm Hg or more diastolic, and treat to goal BP less than those thresholds
- In patients younger than 60 years, treatment initiation and goals should be 140/90 mm Hg, the same threshold used in patients

18 years or older with either chronic kidney disease (CKD) or diabetes.

Findings from the SPRINT study indicate that treatment of systolic BP to less than 120 mm Hg (rather than 140 mm Hg) reduced the rates of major cardiovascular events by almost one-third and the risk of death by almost one-fourth. These data may result in changes to the JNC 8 guidelines.

Drug Therapy

The drugs currently available for treating hypertension have two main actions: reducing SVR and decreasing the volume of circulating blood.

- Drugs used in the treatment of hypertension include diuretics, adrenergic (SNS) inhibitors, direct vasodilators, angiotensin-converting enzyme (ACE) inhibitors, A-II receptor blockers (ARBs), and calcium channel blockers. (See Table 32-7, Lewis et al, *Medical-Surgical Nursing,* ed 10, pp. 691 to 693, for a description of antihypertensive drug therapy.)
- Most patients who have hypertension require two or more antihypertensive drugs to achieve their goal BP.
- Once antihypertensive therapy is started, most patients should return for follow-up and adjustment of drug regimens at monthly intervals until the goal BP is reached.

Nursing Management

Goals

The patient with hypertension will achieve and maintain goal BP; understand and follow the therapeutic plan; experience minimal or no unpleasant side effects of therapy; and be confident of ability to manage and cope with this condition.

Nursing Diagnoses/Collaborative Problems

- Ineffective health management
- Anxiety
- Sexual dysfunction
- Risk for decreased cardiac perfusion
- Risk for ineffective renal perfusion
- Potential complication: stroke
- Potential complication: hypertensive crisis

Nursing Interventions

You are in an ideal position to assess for the presence of hypertension, identify risk factors for hypertension and CAD, and teach the patient about these conditions.

Initially, take the BP in both arms to note any differences. Atherosclerosis in the subclavian artery can cause a falsely low reading on the side where the narrowing occurs. Use the arm with the highest BP and take at least two readings, at least 1 minute apart.

Assess for orthostatic (or postural) changes in BP and pulse in older adults, people taking antihypertensive drugs, and patients who report symptoms consistent with reduced BP on standing (e.g., light-headedness, dizziness, syncope).

Your primary nursing responsibilities for long-term management of hypertension are to assist the patient in reducing BP and adhering to the treatment plan. Your nursing actions include evaluating therapeutic effectiveness, detecting and reporting any adverse treatment effects, assessing and enhancing adherence, and patient and caregiver teaching.

▼ **Patient and Caregiver Teaching**

Help the patient and caregivers understand that hypertension is a chronic illness that cannot be cured. Emphasize that it can be controlled with drug therapy, diet changes, physical activity, periodic follow-up, and other relevant lifestyle modifications (Table 49).

TABLE 49   Patient & Caregiver Teaching

Hypertension

When teaching the patient and/or caregivers about hypertension, include the following information.

General Instructions
1. Provide the patient's BP reading and explain what it means (e.g., high, low, normal, borderline). Encourage the patient to monitor BP at home and instruct the patient to call HCP if BP exceeds high or low limits set by HCP.
2. Hypertension is usually asymptomatic, and symptoms (e.g., nosebleeds) do not reliably indicate BP levels.
3. Hypertension means high BP and does not relate to a "hyper" personality.
4. Long-term therapy and follow-up care are necessary to treat hypertension. Therapy involves lifestyle changes (e.g., weight management, sodium reduction, smoking cessation, regular physical activity), and, in most cases, drugs.
5. Therapy will not cure hypertension but should control it.
6. Controlled hypertension usually results in an excellent prognosis and a normal lifestyle.
7. Explain the potential dangers of uncontrolled hypertension (e.g., target organ disease).

TABLE 49 Patient & Caregiver Teaching

Hypertension—cont'd

Instructions Related to Drugs

1. Be specific about the names, actions, dosages, and side effects of prescribed drugs.
2. Help the patient plan regular and convenient times for taking drugs and measuring BP.
3. Do not stop drugs abruptly, because withdrawal may cause a severe hypertensive reaction.
4. Do not double up on doses when a dose is missed.
5. If BP increases, the patient should not take an increased drug dosage before consulting with the HCP.
6. Do not take a drug belonging to someone else.
7. Supplement diet with foods high in potassium (e.g., citrus fruits, green leafy vegetables) if taking potassium-wasting diuretics.
8. Avoid hot baths, excessive amounts of alcohol, and strenuous exercise within 3 hours of taking drugs that promote vasodilation.
9. Many drugs cause orthostatic hypotension. The effects of orthostatic hypotension can be reduced by rising slowly from bed, sitting on the side of the bed for a few minutes, standing slowly, and beginning to move if no symptoms develop (e.g., dizziness, light-headedness). Do not stand still for prolonged periods. Do leg exercises to increase venous return before standing or sleep with the head of the bed raised. Do lie or sit down when dizziness occurs.
10. Many drugs cause sexual problems (e.g., erectile dysfunction, decreased libido). Consult with the health care provider about changing drugs or dosages if sexual problems develop.
11. The side effects of some drugs may decrease with time.
12. Be careful about taking potentially high-risk, over-the-counter preparations, such as high-sodium antacids, appetite suppressants, and cold and sinus drugs. Read warning labels and consult with a pharmacist.

H

HYPERTHYROIDISM

Description

Hyperthyroidism is hyperactivity of the thyroid gland with a sustained increase in synthesis and release of thyroid hormones. The most common form of hyperthyroidism is Graves' disease. Other causes include toxic nodular goiter, thyroiditis, pituitary tumors, and thyroid cancer. *Thyrotoxicosis* is hypermetabolism that results from excess circulating levels of thyroxine (T_4), triiodothyronine (T_3), or both. Hyperthyroidism and thyrotoxicosis usually occur together as in Graves' disease. Graves' disease accounts for up to 80% of the cases of hyperthyroidism. Hyperthyroidism occurs in more women than in men, with the highest frequency in people 20 to 40 years old.

- Because hyperthyroidism may be precipitated by iodinated contrast media used in CT scans and other radiologic studies, patients at risk for hyperthyroidism should be monitored closely after iodinated contrast media exposure.

Pathophysiology

Graves' disease is an autoimmune disease of unknown etiology marked by diffuse thyroid enlargement and excessive thyroid hormone secretion. The patient develops antibodies to the thyroid-stimulating hormone (TSH) receptor. These antibodies attach to receptors and stimulate the thyroid gland to release T_3, T_4, or both. The excessive release of thyroid hormones leads to the clinical manifestations associated with thyrotoxicosis.

- The disease is characterized by remissions and exacerbations that may progress to thyroid tissue destruction, causing hypothyroidism.
- Precipitating factors, such as insufficient iodine supply, infection, and stressful life events, may interact with genetic factors to cause Graves' disease. Cigarette smoking increases the risk of Graves' disease and the development of eye problems associated with the disease.

Clinical Manifestations

Manifestations of hyperthyroidism are related to the effect of excess thyroid hormones.

- Inspection or palpation of the thyroid gland may reveal a goiter. Auscultation of the thyroid gland may reveal bruits, a reflection of increased blood supply.
- *Exophthalmos,* or eyeball protrusion, is caused by impaired venous drainage from the orbit, leading to increased deposits of

fat and edema fluid in the orbital tissues. This sign is a classic finding in Graves' disease. When the eyelids do not close completely, exposed corneal surfaces become dry and irritated. Serious consequences, such as corneal ulcers and eventual loss of vision, can occur. Ocular muscle changes result in muscle weakness, causing diplopia.

- A patient with advanced disease may exhibit many symptoms, whereas a patient in the early stages of hyperthyroidism may only exhibit weight loss and increased nervousness.

Other manifestations of hyperthyroidism are summarized in Table 49-5, Lewis et al, *Medical-Surgical Nursing,* ed 10, p. 1164.

Complications

Acute thyrotoxicosis (also called thyrotoxic crisis, thyroid storm) is a severe and rare condition that occurs when excessive amounts of thyroid hormones are released into the circulation. Although this is considered a life-threatening emergency, death is rare when treatment is initiated early. Thyrotoxicosis is thought to result from stressors (e.g., infection, trauma, surgery) in a patient with preexisting hyperthyroidism.

In acute thyrotoxicosis, symptoms of hyperthyroidism are prominent and severe. Manifestations include severe tachycardia, heart failure, shock, hyperthermia (with temperatures up to 106° F [41.1° C]), agitation, delirium, seizures, abdominal pain, vomiting, diarrhea, and coma.

- Treatment is aimed at reducing circulating thyroid hormone levels by appropriate drug therapy, fever reduction, fluid replacement, and elimination or management of the initiating stressor or stressors.

Diagnostic Studies

- Diagnosis is confirmed with findings of decreased serum TSH levels and elevated free thyroxine (T_4) levels.
- Radioactive iodine uptake (RAIU) differentiates Graves' disease from other forms of thyroiditis.

Interprofessional Care

The goal of management is to block the adverse effects of thyroid hormones, suppress oversecretion of thyroid hormone, and prevent complications. There are several treatment options including antithyroid medications, radioactive iodine therapy, and surgical intervention.

Drug Therapy

Drugs used in the treatment of hyperthyroidism are useful in treating thyrotoxic states, but they are not curative.

H

Antithyroid Drugs. The first-line antithyroid drugs commonly used are propylthiouracil and methimazole (Tapazole). These drugs inhibit the synthesis of thyroid hormones. Indications for use include Graves' disease in the young patient, hyperthyroidism during pregnancy, or achieving a euthyroid state before surgery or radiation therapy. Propylthiouracil, which blocks the peripheral conversion of T_4 to T_3, is first-line treatment for thyrotoxic crisis.

Iodine. In large doses, iodine (e.g., Lugol's solution, saturated solution of potassium iodide [SSKI]) inhibits the synthesis of T_3 and T_4 and blocks the release of these hormones into circulation. Iodine decreases thyroid vascularity, making surgery safer and easier.

β-Adrenergic Blockers. β-Adrenergic blockers (e.g., propranolol [Inderal]) are used to block the effects of sympathetic nervous stimulation, thereby decreasing tachycardia, nervousness, irritability, and tremors.

Radioactive Iodine. Radioactive iodine (RAI) limits thyroid hormone secretion by damaging or destroying thyroid tissue. RAI has a delayed response and the maximum effect may not be seen for up to 3 months. This treatment results in hypothyroidism for 80% of patients. Other drug therapy may be used until the effects of radiation become apparent.

Surgical Therapy

Thyroidectomy is indicated for individuals who (1) have a large goiter causing tracheal compression, (2) are unresponsive to antithyroid therapy, or (3) have thyroid cancer. A subtotal thyroidectomy involves the removal of a significant portion (90%) of the thyroid gland. A minimally invasive endoscopic or robotic thyroidectomy can be performed for patients with small nodules (less than 3 cm) without evidence of malignancy.

Nutritional Therapy

There is a high potential for nutritional deficits when an increased metabolic rate is present. A high-calorie diet (4000 to 5000 cal/day) may be needed to satisfy hunger and prevent tissue breakdown. This can be accomplished with six full meals each day and snacks high in protein, carbohydrates, minerals, and vitamins.

- Teach the patient to avoid highly seasoned and high-fiber foods because these foods can further stimulate the already hyperactive GI tract. Provide substitutes for caffeine-containing liquids such as coffee, tea, and cola because the stimulating effects of these fluids increase restlessness and sleep disturbances.
- Refer the patient to a dietitian for help in meeting individual nutritional needs.

Nursing Management

Goals

The patient with hyperthyroidism will experience relief of symptoms, have no serious complications related to the disease or treatment, maintain nutritional balance, and cooperate with the therapeutic plan.

Nursing Diagnoses

- Activity intolerance
- Imbalanced nutrition: less than body requirements

Nursing Interventions

Acute thyrotoxicosis requires aggressive treatment, often in an intensive care unit. Administer medications (previously discussed) that block thyroid hormone production and the sympathetic nervous system.

Provide supportive therapy to the patient, including monitoring for cardiac dysrhythmias and decompensation, ensuring adequate oxygenation, and giving IV fluids to replace fluid and electrolyte losses. This is especially important in the patient who experiences fluid losses because of vomiting and diarrhea.

Provision of adequate rest may be a challenge because of the patient's irritability and restlessness. Provide a calm, quiet room because increased metabolism and sensitivity of the sympathetic nervous system cause sleep disturbances.

- Interventions may include placing the patient in a cool room away from very ill patients and noisy, high-traffic areas; using light bed coverings and changing the linen frequently if the patient is diaphoretic; encouraging and assisting with exercise involving large muscle groups (tremors can interfere with small-muscle coordination) to allow the release of nervous tension and restlessness; and establishing a supportive, trusting relationship to help the patient cope with aggravating events and lessen anxiety.

If exophthalmos is present, there is a potential for corneal injury. The patient may also have orbital pain. Interventions to relieve eye discomfort and prevent corneal ulceration include applying artificial tears to soothe and moisten conjunctival membranes, elevating the patient's head to reduce periorbital edema, and providing dark glasses to reduce glare and prevent irritation from smoke, air currents, dust, and dirt. If the eyelids cannot be closed, lightly tape them shut for sleep. To maintain flexibility, teach the patient to exercise intraocular muscles several times each day by turning the eyes in the complete range of motion.

H

Nursing Management: Patient Having Thyroid Surgery

When a subtotal thyroidectomy is the treatment of choice, the patient must be adequately prepared to avoid postoperative complications.

- Preoperative teaching includes instructing the patient how to support the head manually while turning in bed to minimize stress on the surgery suture line. Range-of-motion (ROM) exercises of the neck should be practiced and the patient should be told that talking is likely to be difficult for a short time after surgery.
- Recurrent laryngeal nerve damage leads to vocal cord paralysis. If both cords are paralyzed, spastic airway obstruction will require an immediate tracheostomy.
- Respiration may become difficult because of excess swelling of the neck, hemorrhage, and hematoma formation.
- Laryngeal stridor (harsh, vibratory sound) may occur during respiration as a result of edema of the laryngeal nerve or because of tetany, which occurs if the parathyroid glands are removed or damaged during surgery. To treat tetany, IV calcium salts such as calcium gluconate should be available.

Important nursing interventions after a thyroidectomy include the following:

- Assess the patient every 2 hours for 24 hours for signs of hemorrhage or tracheal compression, such as irregular breathing, neck swelling, frequent swallowing, choking, blood on the dressings, and sensation of fullness at the incision site. Expect some hoarseness for 3 or 4 days after surgery because of edema.
- Place the patient in a semi-Fowler's position and support the head with pillows. Avoid flexion of the neck and any tension on the suture lines.
- Monitor vital signs and calcium levels. Check for signs of tetany secondary to hypoparathyroidism (e.g., tingling of toes, fingers, or around the mouth; muscular twitching; apprehension) and by evaluating any difficulty in speaking and hoarseness.
- Control postoperative pain by giving medication.
- If postoperative recovery is uneventful, the patient ambulates within hours after surgery and is permitted fluids as soon as tolerated. A soft diet starts the day after surgery.

▼ **Patient and Caregiver Teaching**

Follow-up care is important for the patient who has undergone thyroid surgery.

- Thyroid hormone balance should be monitored periodically to ensure that normal function has returned.
- Caloric intake must be reduced substantially below the amount that was required before surgery to prevent weight gain.

- Adequate iodine is necessary to promote thyroid function, but excesses inhibit the thyroid. Seafood once or twice per week or the normal use of iodized salt should provide sufficient intake.
- Encourage regular exercise to help stimulate the thyroid.
- Teach the patient to avoid high environmental temperatures because they inhibit thyroid regeneration.

If a complete thyroidectomy has been performed, instruct the patient about the need for lifelong thyroid replacement therapy. Teach the patient the signs and symptoms of thyroid failure and instruct him or her to contact the HCP if these develop.

HYPOPARATHYROIDISM

Description

Hypoparathyroidism is an uncommon condition characterized by inadequate circulating parathyroid hormone (PTH) that results in hypocalcemia. PTH resistance at the cellular level may also occur. This is caused by a genetic defect resulting in hypocalcemia in spite of normal or high PTH levels and is often associated with hypothyroidism and hypogonadism.

Pathophysiology

The most common cause of hypoparathyroidism is the accidental removal of parathyroids or damage to the vascular supply of the glands during neck surgery (e.g., thyroidectomy).

- Idiopathic hypoparathyroidism resulting from absence, fatty replacement, or atrophy of the glands is a rare disease that usually occurs early in life and may be associated with other endocrine disorders.
- Severe hypomagnesemia (e.g., malnutrition, renal failure) also leads to suppression of PTH secretion.

Clinical Manifestations

Clinical manifestations of acute hypoparathyroidism are caused by hypocalcemia (see Table 49-12, Lewis et al, *Medical-Surgical Nursing*, ed 10, p. 1172).

Sudden decreases in calcium concentration cause tetany, characterized by lip tingling and extremity stiffness. Painful tonic spasms of smooth and skeletal muscles can cause dysphagia and laryngospasms that compromise breathing.

Abnormal laboratory findings include decreased serum calcium and PTH levels and increased serum phosphate levels.

H

Nursing and Interprofessional Management

Treatment goals for the patient with hypoparathyroidism are to treat acute complications such as tetany, maintain normal serum calcium levels, and prevent long-term complications. Emergency treatment of tetany after surgery requires the administration of IV calcium.

- Give IV calcium slowly. Use ECG monitoring during calcium administration because high serum calcium levels can cause hypotension, serious cardiac dysrhythmias, or cardiac arrest.
- Rebreathing may partially relieve acute neuromuscular symptoms associated with hypocalcemia such as generalized muscle cramps or mild tetany. Instruct the patient (if able to cooperate) to breathe into and out of a paper bag or breathing mask.

▼ **Patient and Caregiver Teaching**

The patient with hypoparathyroidism needs instruction in the management of long-term nutrition and drug therapy.

- Oral calcium supplements of at least 1.5 to 3 g/day in divided doses, magnesium supplements, and vitamin D are usually prescribed.
- A high-calcium meal plan includes foods such as dark green vegetables, soybeans, and tofu. Tell the patient that foods containing oxalic acid (e.g., spinach, rhubarb), phytic acid (e.g., bran, whole grains), and phosphorus reduce calcium absorption.
- Instruct the patient about the need for lifelong treatment and follow-up care including monitoring of calcium levels three or four times a year.

HYPOTHYROIDISM

Description

Hypothyroidism is a deficiency of thyroid hormone that causes a general slowing of the metabolic rate. About 4% of the U.S. population has mild hypothyroidism, with about 0.3% having more severe disease. Hypothyroidism is more common in women than men.

Pathophysiology

Hypothyroidism can be *primary* (related to destruction of thyroid tissue or defective hormone synthesis) or *secondary* (related to pituitary disease with decreased thyroid-stimulating hormone [TSH] secretion or hypothalamic dysfunction with decreased thyrotropin-releasing hormone [TRH] secretion). Hypothyroidism can be transient, related to thyroiditis or discontinuing thyroid hormone therapy.

■ Iodine deficiency is the most common cause of hypothyroidism worldwide. In the United States, the most common cause of primary hypothyroidism is atrophy of the thyroid gland. This atrophy is the end result of Hashimoto's thyroiditis or Graves' disease. These autoimmune diseases destroy the thyroid gland.

■ Hypothyroidism may also develop as a result of treatment for hyperthyroidism, specifically thyroidectomy or radioactive iodine (RAI) therapy. Drugs such as amiodarone (Cordarone), which contains iodine or lithium that block hormone production, can cause hypothyroidism.

■ Hypothyroidism that develops in infancy (cretinism) is caused by thyroid hormone deficiencies during fetal or early neonatal life.

Clinical Manifestations

Regardless of the cause, hypothyroidism has common features. Manifestations vary depending on the severity and duration of thyroid deficiency, as well as the patient's age at onset of the deficiency.

Hypothyroidism has systemic effects characterized by a slowing of body processes. The patient is often fatigued and lethargic and experiences personality and mental changes including impaired memory, slowed speech, decreased initiative, and somnolence. Many individuals appear depressed. Weight gain is most likely a result of decreased metabolic rate.

■ Hypothyroidism is associated with decreased cardiac output, decreased cardiac contractility, and coronary atherosclerosis. Anemia is a common feature. Increased serum cholesterol and triglyceride levels and the accumulation of mucopolysaccharides in the intima of small blood vessels can result in coronary atherosclerosis.

■ GI motility is decreased in hypothyroidism and *achlorhydria* (absence or decreased secretion of hydrochloric acid) is common. Constipation is common and may progress to obstipation.

■ In the older adult, typical manifestations include fatigue, cold and dry skin, hair loss, constipation, hoarseness, and cold intolerance.

■ Those with severe long-standing hypothyroidism may display *myxedema*, which alters the physical appearance of the skin and subcutaneous tissues with manifestations of puffiness, facial and periorbital edema, and a masklike affect. Myxedema occurs with the accumulation of hydrophilic mucopolysaccharides in

the dermis and other tissues. Individuals with hypothyroidism
may describe an altered self-image.

Other manifestations of hypothyroidism are summarized in
Table 49-5, Lewis et al, *Medical-Surgical Nursing,* ed 10, p. 1164.

Complications

The mental sluggishness, drowsiness, and lethargy of hypothyroidism may progress gradually or suddenly to a notable impairment
of consciousness or coma. This situation, termed *myxedema coma,*
constitutes a medical emergency.

- Myxedema coma can be precipitated by infection, drugs (especially opioids, tranquilizers, and barbiturates), exposure to cold,
  and trauma. It is characterized by subnormal temperature, hypotension, and hypoventilation.
- For the patient to survive, vital functions must be supported and
  IV thyroid hormone replacement administered.

Diagnostic Studies

- Serum TSH and free thyroxine (FT$_4$) are the most reliable indicators of thyroid function.
- Serum TSH levels help determine the cause of hypothyroidism.
  If high, the defect is in the thyroid; if low, it is in the pituitary
  or hypothalamus.
- The presence of thyroid antibodies suggests an autoimmune
  origin of the hypothyroidism.
- Elevated cholesterol and triglycerides, anemia, and increased
  creatine kinase can occur.

Interprofessional Care

The treatment goal is the restoration of the euthyroid state as safely
and rapidly as possible with hormone therapy. A low-calorie diet
is indicated to promote weight loss or prevent weight gain.

Levothyroxine (Synthroid) is the drug of choice to treat hypothyroidism. In the young, otherwise healthy patient, the maintenance replacement dosage is adjusted according to the patient's
response and laboratory findings. The initial dosages are low to
avoid increases in resting heart rate and BP. In the patient with
compromised cardiac status, careful monitoring is needed when
starting and adjusting the dosage because the usual dose may
increase myocardial oxygen demand, causing angina and cardiac
dysrhythmias. Levothyroxine has a peak of action of 1 to 3 weeks.
In the patient without side effects the dose is increased at 4- to
6-week intervals.

Liotrix is a synthetic mix of levothyroxine (T$_4$) and liothyronine
(T$_3$) in a 4:1 combination. Liotrix, with a fast onset of action and

a peak of 2 to 3 days, can be used in acutely ill individuals with hypothyroidism.

It is important that the patient take replacement medication regularly. Lifelong thyroid therapy is usually required.

Nursing Management

Goals
The patient with hypothyroidism will experience relief of symptoms, maintain a euthyroid state, maintain a positive self-image, and comply with lifelong thyroid therapy.

Nursing Diagnoses
- Activity intolerance
- Impaired memory
- Overweight or obesity
- Constipation

Nursing Interventions
Most individuals with hypothyroidism are treated on an outpatient basis. The patient who develops myxedema coma requires acute nursing care, often in an ICU setting. Mechanical respiratory support and cardiac monitoring are frequently necessary. Give thyroid hormone therapy and all other medications IV because severe gastric hypomotility may prevent the absorption of oral preparations. Monitor core temperature because the patient with myxedema coma is often hypothermic.

- Use gentle soap and moisturize frequently to prevent skin breakdown. Frequent changes in patient positioning and a low-pressure mattress can also assist in maintaining skin integrity.
- Monitor the patient's progress, vital signs, body weight, fluid intake and output, and visible edema. Cardiac assessment is especially important because the cardiovascular response to hormone therapy determines the medication regimen.
- Note energy level and mental alertness, which should increase within 2 to 14 days and continue to rise steadily to normal levels.

▼ Patient and Caregiver Teaching
Initially the hypothyroid patient may have difficulty processing complex instructions. It is important to provide written instructions, repeat the information often, and assess the patient's comprehension level.

- Stress the need for receiving lifelong drug therapy and avoiding abrupt discontinuation of drugs. Instruct the patient in expected and unexpected side effects. In the teaching plan, include the signs and symptoms of hypothyroidism or hyperthyroidism that indicate hormone imbalance.

H

- Teach the patient to immediately contact an HCP if signs of overdose appear, such as orthopnea, dyspnea, rapid pulse, chest pain, palpitations, nervousness, or insomnia.
- The patient with diabetes mellitus should test his or her capillary blood glucose at least daily because a return to the euthyroid state frequently increases insulin requirements.
- Thyroid preparations potentiate the effects of other common drugs, such as anticoagulants, antidepressants, and digitalis compounds. Instruct the patient on the toxic signs and symptoms of these medications.
- Medication interactions are an important reason for patients to consult their HCP before switching brands of thyroid replacement medication. Switching brands may alter bioavailability of the drug and physiologic response.

INCREASED INTRACRANIAL PRESSURE

Description

Increased intracranial pressure (ICP) is a potentially life-threatening situation that results from an increase in any or all of the three components within the skull: brain tissue, blood, and cerebrospinal fluid (CSF).

Pathophysiology

Common causes of increased ICP include a mass lesion (e.g., hematoma, contusion, abscess, tumor) and cerebral edema (associated with brain tumors, hydrocephalus, head injury, or brain inflammation). These cerebral insults, which may result in hypercapnia, cerebral acidosis, impaired autoregulation, and systemic hypertension, increase the formation and spread of cerebral edema. This edema distorts brain tissue, further increasing the ICP, and leads to even more tissue hypoxia and acidosis.

Regardless of the cause, cerebral edema results in an increase in tissue volume that has the potential to increase ICP. The extent and severity of the original insult are factors that determine the degree of cerebral edema. Fig. 13 illustrates the progression of increased ICP.

There are three types of cerebral edema: vasogenic, cytotoxic, and interstitial. More than one type may occur in the same patient.

- *Vasogenic cerebral edema,* the most common type of edema, occurs mainly in the white matter and is characterized by leakage of large molecules from capillaries into extracellular space. This edema may produce a continuum of manifestations

PATHOPHYSIOLOGY MAP

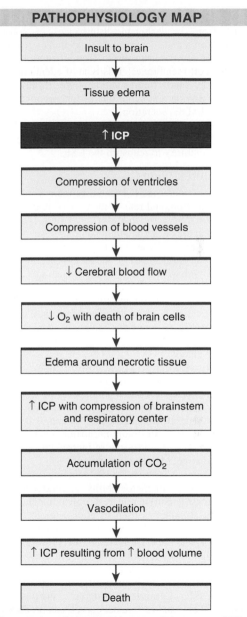

Fig. 13 Progression of increased intracranial pressure (ICP).

ranging from headache to disturbances in consciousness, including coma and focal neurologic deficits.

- *Cytotoxic cerebral edema* results from disruption of the integrity of the cell membranes. This type of edema develops from destructive lesions or trauma to brain tissue resulting in cerebral hypoxia or anoxia and syndrome of inappropriate antidiuretic hormone (SIADH) secretion.
- *Interstitial cerebral edema* is usually a result of hydrocephalus. It can be due to excess CSF production, obstruction of CSF flow, or an inability to reabsorb the CSF.

Clinical Manifestations

Manifestations of increased ICP can take many forms, depending on the cause, location, and rate of increase of ICP.

- *Change in level of consciousness* (LOC). LOC is a sensitive and reliable indicator of the patient's neurologic status. Changes in LOC may be dramatic, as in coma, or subtle, such as a change in orientation or a decrease in the level of attention.
- *Changes in vital signs.* Manifestations such as *Cushing's triad* (systolic hypertension with widening pulse pressure, bradycardia with a full and bounding pulse, and irregular respirations) may be present but often do not appear until ICP has been increased for some time or is markedly increased (e.g., with head trauma). The effect of increased ICP on the hypothalamus can cause a change in body temperature.
- *Ocular signs.* Compression of the oculomotor nerve (cranial nerve [CN] III) results in dilation of the pupil on the same side (ipsilateral) as the mass lesion, sluggish or no response to light, an inability to adduct and move the eye upward, and ptosis of the eyelid. A fixed, unilaterally dilated pupil is a neurologic emergency that indicates brain herniation. Other cranial nerves may also be affected, with signs of blurred vision, diplopia, and changes in extraocular eye movements.
- *Decrease in motor function.* As ICP continues to rise, the patient manifests changes in motor ability. A contralateral (opposite side of the mass lesion) hemiparesis or hemiplegia may develop. If a painful stimulus is used to elicit a motor response, the patient may localize to the stimulus or withdraw from it. *Decorticate* (flexor) and *decerebrate* (extensor) posturing may also be elicited by noxious stimuli (see Fig. 56-5, Lewis et al, *Medical-Surgical Nursing,* ed 10, p. 1318).
- *Headache.* Although the brain itself is insensitive to pain, compression of other intracranial structures, such as the walls of arteries and veins and the cranial nerves, can produce headache. A nocturnal headache or a headache in the morning is cause for

concern and may indicate a tumor or other space-occupying lesion that is causing increased ICP. Straining, agitation, or movement may accentuate the pain.

■ *Vomiting.* Vomiting, usually not preceded by nausea, is often a nonspecific sign of increased ICP.

The major complications of uncontrolled increased ICP are inadequate cerebral perfusion and cerebral herniation.

Diagnostic Studies

■ MRI, CT scan, and positron emission tomography (PET) can be used to diagnose the cause of increased ICP.

■ Other tests may include cerebral angiography, electroencephalography (EEG), ICP measurement, brain tissue oxygenation measurement via the LICOX catheter, transcranial Doppler studies, and evoked potential studies.

Interprofessional Care

The goals of management of increased ICP are to (1) identify and treat the underlying cause of increased ICP and (2) support brain function. The earlier the condition is recognized and treated, the better the patient outcome. A careful history helps direct the search for the underlying cause.

Ensuring adequate oxygenation to support brain function is important. Arterial blood gas (ABG) analysis guides the O_2 therapy. To meet the goal of maintaining the partial pressure of O_2 in arterial blood (PaO_2) at 100 mm Hg or greater and to keep the partial pressure of CO_2 in arterial blood ($PaCO_2$) in normal range at 35 to 45 mm Hg, an endotracheal tube or tracheostomy and mechanical ventilation may be necessary.

■ If the condition is caused by a mass lesion, such as a tumor or hematoma, surgical removal of the mass is the best management (see Brain Tumors, p. 82).

Drug Therapy

Drug therapy plays an important part in the management of increased ICP.

■ IV mannitol (Osmitrol) (25%) is an osmotic diuretic that decreases ICP in two ways: plasma expansion and osmotic effect. The immediate plasma-expanding effect reduces the hematocrit and blood viscosity, thereby increasing cerebral blood flow and cerebral oxygenation. The osmotic effect causes fluid to move from the tissue into the blood vessels, resulting in a decrease in total brain fluid content.

■ Hypertonic saline is another drug treatment used to manage increased ICP. It produces massive movement of water out of edematous swollen brain cells and into the blood vessels.

- Corticosteroids (e.g., dexamethasone) are used to treat vasogenic edema surrounding tumors and abscesses but are not
  recommended for traumatic brain injury. Corticosteroids stabilize the cell membrane and inhibit the synthesis of prostaglandins. These drugs also improve cerebral blood flow and restore
  autoregulation.
- Metabolic demands such as fever (temperatures above 38°C),
  agitation/shivering, pain, and seizures can also increase ICP.
  The interprofessional team should plan to reduce these metabolic demands in order to lower the ICP in the at-risk patient.
- High-dose barbiturates (e.g., pentobarbital [Nembutal]) are
  used in patients with increased ICP refractory to other treatments. These drugs lower cerebral metabolism, which causes a
  decrease in ICP.

Nutritional Therapy
The patient with increased ICP is in a hypermetabolic and hyper-
catabolic state that increases the need for glucose to provide the
necessary fuel for metabolism of the injured brain. If the patient
cannot maintain an adequate oral intake, other means of meeting
the nutritional requirements, such as enteral or parenteral nutrition,
should be started. Current fluid therapy is directed at keeping
patients normovolemic.

Nursing Management
Goals
The overall goals are that the patient with increased ICP will have
ICP within normal limits, maintain a patent airway, demonstrate
normal fluid and electrolyte balance, and have no complications
secondary to immobility and decreased LOC.

Nursing Diagnoses
- Risk for ineffective cerebral tissue perfusion
- Decreased intracranial adaptive capacity
- Risk for disuse syndrome

Nursing Interventions
Respiratory Function.   Maintenance of a patent airway is critical
in patients with increased ICP and is a primary nursing responsibility. As the LOC decreases, the patient is at increased risk for airway
obstruction.

- Be alert to altered breathing patterns. Snoring sounds indicate
  obstruction and require immediate intervention. An oral airway
  facilitates breathing and provides an easier suctioning route in
  the comatose patient.
- In general, any patient with a Glasgow Coma Scale score of 8
  or less (see Glasgow Coma Scale, p. 767) or an altered LOC

who is unable to maintain a patent airway or effective ventilation needs intubation and mechanical ventilation.

- Prevent hypoxia and hypercapnia. Proper positioning of the head is important.
- Elevation of the head of the bed by 30 degrees enhances respiratory exchange and aids in decreasing cerebral edema.
- Suctioning and coughing can cause transient increases in ICP and decreases in PaO_2. Suctioning should be kept to a minimum.
- Try to prevent abdominal distention, which can interfere with respiratory function. Insertion of a nasogastric tube to aspirate the stomach contents can prevent distention, vomiting, and possible aspiration. In patients with facial and skull fractures, a nasogastric tube is contraindicated, and oral insertion of a gastric tube is preferred.
- ABGs should be measured and evaluated regularly. The appropriate ventilatory support can be ordered on the basis of the PaO_2 and $PaCO_2$ values.

Fluid and Electrolyte Balance. Fluid and electrolyte disturbances can have an adverse effect on ICP. Closely monitor IV fluids. Intake and output, with insensible losses and daily weights taken into account, are important parameters in the assessment of fluid balance.

- Electrolyte determinations should be made daily. It is especially important to monitor serum glucose, sodium, potassium, magnesium, and osmolality. Monitor urinary output for problems related to syndrome of inappropriate antidiuretic hormone (SIADH) and diabetes insipidus (DI) (see Diabetes Insipidus, p. 166).

Monitoring Intracranial Pressure. ICP monitoring is used in combination with other physiologic parameters to guide the care of the patient and assess the patient's response to routine care. Valsalva maneuver, coughing, sneezing, hypoxemia, and arousal from sleep are factors that can increase ICP. (See Intracranial Pressure Monitoring, p. 770.) Methods of monitoring ICP are discussed in detail in Chapter 56, Lewis et al, *Medical-Surgical Nursing,* ed 10.

Body Position. Maintain the patient with increased ICP in the head-up position. Take care to prevent extreme neck flexion, which can cause venous obstruction and contribute to elevated ICP. Adjust the body position to decrease the ICP maximally and to improve cerebral perfusion pressure (CPP).

- Take care to turn the patient with slow, gentle movements, because rapid changes in position may increase ICP. Prevent discomfort in turning and positioning the patient because pain or agitation also increases pressure. Increased intrathoracic pressure contributes to increased ICP by impeding venous return. Thus coughing, straining, and the Valsalva maneuver should be avoided. Avoid extreme hip flexion to decrease the risk of raising the intraabdominal pressure, which increases ICP.

Protection From Injury. The patient with increased ICP and decreased LOC needs protection from self-injury. Confusion, agitation, and the possibility of seizures increase the risk of injury. Use restraints judiciously in the agitated patient. The patient can benefit from a quiet, nonstimulating environment. Touch and talk to the patient, even one who is in a coma.

Psychologic Considerations. Anxiety over the diagnosis and prognosis for the patient with neurologic problems can be distressing to the patient, caregiver, family, and nursing staff. Provide support and short, simple explanations to patients and families.

Assess the family members' desire and need to assist in providing care for the patient and allow for their participation as appropriate.

INFLAMMATORY BOWEL DISEASE

Description

Inflammatory bowel disease (IBD) is a chronic inflammation of the GI tract characterized by periods of remission interspersed with periods of exacerbation. The cause is unknown, and there is no cure. IBD is classified as either *Crohn's disease* or *ulcerative colitis* on the basis of clinical manifestations (Table 50). Ulcerative colitis is usually limited to the colon. Crohn's disease can involve any segment of the GI tract from the mouth to the anus.

Both ulcerative colitis and Crohn's disease commonly occur during the teenage years and early adulthood, and both have a second peak incidence in the sixth decade of life. IBD occurs more commonly in people of white and Ashkenazic Jewish origin than in other racial and ethnic groups. Many people with IBD have a family member with the disorder.

Pathophysiology

IBD is an autoimmune disease involving an immune reaction to a person's own intestinal tract. Some agent or a combination of agents triggers an overactive, inappropriate, sustained immune response. The resulting inflammation causes widespread tissue destruction.

Evidence suggests that IBD is caused by a combination of factors, including environmental factors, genetic predisposition,

TABLE 50 Comparison of Ulcerative Colitis and Crohn's Disease

Characteristic	Ulcerative Colitis	Crohn's Disease
Clinical		
Usual age at onset	Teens to mid-30s After 60	Teens to mid-30s After 60
Diarrhea	Common	Common
Abdominal pain	Common, severe constant	Common, cramping
Fever (intermittent)	During acute attacks	Common
Weight loss	Rare	Common, may be severe
Rectal bleeding	Common	Sometimes
Tenesmus	Common	Rare
Malabsorption and nutritional deficiencies	Minimal incidence	Common
Pathologic		
Location	Usually starts in rectum and spreads in a continuous pattern up the colon	Occurs anywhere along GI tract Most frequent site is distal ileum.
Small bowel involvement	Minimal	Common
Distribution	Continuous areas of inflammation	Healthy tissue interspersed with areas of inflammation (skip lesions)
Depth of involvement	Mucosa	Entire thickness of bowel wall (transmural)
Cobblestoning of mucosa	Rare	Common
Pseudopolyps	Common	Rare

Continued

TABLE 50 **Comparison of Ulcerative Colitis and Crohn's Disease—cont'd**

Characteristic	Ulcerative Colitis	Crohn's Disease
Complications		
Perianal abscess and fistulas	Rare	Common
Strictures	Occasional	Common
Clostridium difficile infection	Increased incidence and severity	Increased incidence and severity
Perforation	Common (because of toxic megacolon)	Common (because inflammation involves entire bowel wall)
Toxic megacolon	More common	Rare
Carcinoma	Increased incidence of colorectal cancer after 10 yr of disease	Increased incidence of small intestinal cancer
		Increased incidence of colorectal cancer but not as much as with ulcerative colitis

and alterations in immune function. The pattern of inflammation differs between Crohn's disease and ulcerative colitis.

Crohn's Disease

The inflammation in *Crohn's disease* involves all layers of the bowel wall and can occur anywhere in the GI tract from the mouth to the anus. It most commonly involves the distal ileum and proximal colon. Segments of normal bowel can occur between diseased portions, the so-called *skip lesions*.

- Typically, ulcerations are deep and longitudinal and penetrate between islands of inflamed edematous mucosa, causing the classic cobblestone appearance.
- Strictures at the areas of inflammation can cause bowel obstruction.
- Because the inflammation goes through the entire wall, microscopic leaks can allow bowel contents to enter the peritoneal cavity and form abscesses or produce peritonitis.

- Fistulas can develop between adjacent areas of bowel, between bowel and bladder, and between bowel and vagina.

Ulcerative Colitis

Ulcerative colitis usually starts in the rectum and moves in progressive fashion toward the cecum. Although mild inflammation sometimes occurs in the terminal ileum, ulcerative colitis is a disease of the colon and rectum.

- Inflammation and ulcerations occur in the mucosal layer, the innermost layer of the bowel wall. Because inflammation does not extend through all of the bowel layers, fistulas and abscesses are rare.
- Areas of inflamed mucosa form pseudopolyps, which are tongue-like projections into the bowel lumen.

Clinical Manifestations

Manifestations are often the same (diarrhea, bloody stools, weight loss, abdominal pain, fever, and fatigue) in both conditions. Bloody stools are more common with ulcerative colitis, and weight loss is more common in Crohn's disease because inflammation of the small intestine impairs nutrient absorption. Both forms of IBD are chronic disorders with mild to severe acute exacerbations that occur at unpredictable intervals over many years.

Crohn's Disease

Diarrhea and colicky abdominal pain are common symptoms of Crohn's disease.

- If the small intestine is inflamed, weight loss occurs from malabsorption.
- Rectal bleeding sometimes occurs with Crohn's disease, although not as often as with ulcerative colitis.

Ulcerative Colitis

The primary symptoms of ulcerative colitis are bloody diarrhea and abdominal pain. Pain may range from the mild, lower abdominal cramping associated with diarrhea to the severe, constant abdominal pain associated with acute perforations.

- With *mild disease,* diarrhea may consist of one or two semi-formed stools daily that contain small amounts of blood. The patient may have no other manifestations.
- In *moderate disease,* there is increased stool output (up to 10 stools/day), increased bleeding, and systemic signs and symptoms (fever, malaise, mild anemia, anorexia).
- In *severe disease,* diarrhea is bloody, with mucus in the stool, and occurs 10 to 20 times a day. In addition, fever, weight loss (more than 10% of total body weight), anemia, tachycardia, and dehydration are present.

Complications

Patients with IBD experience both local (confined to the GI tract) and systemic complications.

- GI tract complications include hemorrhage, strictures, perforation (with possible peritonitis), abscesses, fistulas, CDI, and colonic dilation (toxic megacolon).
- Toxic megacolon is more common with ulcerative colitis, whereas abscesses and perianal fistulas occur more often with Crohn's disease.
- Hemorrhage may lead to anemia and is corrected with blood transfusions and iron supplements.
- People with a history of IBD are at increased risk for colorectal cancer, whereas those with Crohn's disease are at increased risk for small intestine cancer.

Some people with IBD suffer from systemic complications including joint, eye, mouth, kidney, bone, vascular, and skin problems. Circulating factors such as cytokines trigger inflammation in these areas. Routine liver function tests are important because primary sclerosing cholangitis, a complication of IBD, can lead to liver failure.

Diagnostic Studies

Diagnosis of IBD includes ruling out other diseases with similar symptoms and then determining whether the patient has Crohn's disease or ulcerative colitis.

- Laboratory studies may indicate electrolyte disturbances, anemia, leukocytosis, hypoalbuminemia, and an elevated erythrocyte sedimentation rate.
- Stool is examined for blood, pus, and mucus and cultured to rule out infectious diarrhea.
- Double-contrast barium enema, small bowel series, transabdominal ultrasound, CT scan, and MRI are useful for IBD diagnosis.
- Colonoscopy allows examination of the entire large intestine.

Interprofessional Care

The goals of treatment are to rest the bowel, control inflammation, combat infection, correct malnutrition, alleviate stress, provide symptomatic relief, and improve quality of life.

A variety of drugs are available to treat IBD. Hospitalization is indicated if the patient does not respond to drug therapy, the disease is severe, or complications are suspected.

Drug Therapy

Drugs are used to induce and maintain a remission of IBD. Drugs are chosen on the basis of the location and severity of inflammation. Five major classes of medications used to treat IBD are aminosalicylates, antimicrobials, corticosteroids, immunosuppressants, and biologic and targeted therapy agents (Table 51).

Surgical Therapy

Many patients with Crohn's disease will eventually require surgery for complications, such as strictures, bleeding, obstructions, or fistulas.

- When segments of the intestine are removed, the remaining intestine is reanastomosed. Unfortunately, the disease often recurs at the anastomosis site.
- The main surgical treatment for Crohn's disease is strictureplasty to widen areas of narrowed bowel.

In ulcerative colitis, surgery is indicated if the patient fails to respond to conservative treatment; if exacerbations are frequent and debilitating; or if massive hemorrhage, perforation, strictures, intestinal obstruction, dysplasia, or carcinoma develops. Because ulcerative colitis affects only the colon, a total proctocolectomy is curative.

- Surgical procedures include total colectomy with rectal mucosal stripping and ileoanal reservoir, total proctocolectomy with permanent ileostomy, and total proctocolectomy with continent ileostomy.

For descriptions of these procedures, see Lewis et al, *Medical-Surgical Nursing,* ed 10, pp. 948 to 949.

Nutritional Therapy

Diet is an important component of the treatment of IBD. Consult a dietitian regarding dietary recommendations. The goals of diet management are to provide adequate nutrition without exacerbating symptoms, correct and prevent malnutrition, replace fluid and electrolyte losses, and prevent weight loss.

- Nutritional deficiencies are due to decreased oral intake, blood loss, and, depending on the location of the inflammation, malabsorption of nutrients.
- During an acute exacerbation, patients with IBD may not be able to tolerate a regular diet. Liquid enteral feedings are preferred over parenteral nutrition because atrophy of the gut and bacterial overgrowth occur when the GI tract is not used.
- There are no universal food triggers for IBD, but individuals may find that certain foods initiate diarrhea. A food diary helps to identify problem foods to avoid.

Nursing Management

Goals

The patient with IBD will experience a decrease in the number and severity of acute exacerbations, maintain normal fluid and

TABLE 51   Drug Therapy

Inflammatory Bowel Disease

Class	Action	Examples
5-Aminosalicylates (5-ASA)	Decrease inflammation by suppressing proinflammatory cytokines and other inflammatory mediators	*Systemic:* sulfasalazine (Azulfidine), mesalamine (Pentasa), olsalazine (Dipentum), balsalazide (Colazal) *Topical:* mesalamine enema (Rowasa), mesalamine suppositories (Canasa)
Antimicrobials	Prevent or treat secondary infection	metronidazole (Flagyl), ciprofloxacin (Cipro), clarithromycin (Biaxin)
Corticosteroids	Decrease inflammation	*Systemic:* corticosteroids (prednisone, budesonide [Uceris]) (oral); hydrocortisone or methylprednisolone (IV for severe disease) *Topical:* hydrocortisone suppository or foam (Cortifoam) or enema (Cortenema)
Immunosuppressants	Suppress immune response	azathioprine (Imuran), 6-mercaptopurine, methotrexate, cyclosporine
Biologic and targeted therapy agents (immunomodulators)	Inhibit the cytokine tumor necrosis factor (TNF) Prevent migration of leukocytes from bloodstream to inflamed tissue	infliximab (Remicade), adalimumab (Humira), certolizumab pegol (Cimzia), golimumab (Simponi) natalizumab (Tysabri), vedolizumab (Entyvio)

electrolyte balance, be free from pain or discomfort, adhere to medical regimens, maintain nutritional balance, and have an improved quality of life.

Nursing Diagnoses

- Diarrhea
- Imbalanced nutrition: less than body requirements
- Ineffective coping

Nursing Interventions

During the acute phase, focus your attention on hemodynamic stability, pain control, fluid and electrolyte balance, and nutritional support. Maintain accurate intake and output records and monitor the number and appearance of stools.

- It is important that you establish rapport and encourage the patient to talk about self-care strategies. An explanation of all procedures and treatment will help to build trust and allay apprehension.
- Many patients experience intermittent exacerbations and remissions of symptoms. Given the chronicity and uncertainty related to the frequency and severity of flares, the patient may experience frustration, depression, and anxiety. Psychotherapy, behavioral therapies, and support groups may help patients deal with their feelings about the disease and help to manage their symptoms.
- Severe fatigue limits the patient's energy for physical activity. Nutritional deficiencies and anemia may leave the patient feeling weak and listless. Rest is important because patients may lose sleep because of frequent episodes of diarrhea and abdominal pain. Schedule activities around rest periods.
- Until diarrhea is controlled, help the patient stay clean, dry, and free of odor. Place a deodorizer in the room. Meticulous perianal skin care using plain water (no harsh soap) together with a skin barrier prevents skin breakdown. Dibucaine (Nupercainal), witch hazel, sitz baths, and other soothing compresses or prescribed ointments may reduce irritation and anal discomfort.

▼ Patient and Caregiver Teaching

The patient and caregivers may need help in setting realistic short- and long-term goals.

- Your teaching should include (1) the importance of rest and diet management, (2) perianal care, (3) drug action and side effects, (4) symptoms of disease recurrence, (5) when to seek medical care, and (6) use of diversional activities to reduce stress.
- Excellent teaching resources are available from the Crohn's and Colitis Foundation of America (*www.ccfa.org*).

INTERSTITIAL CYSTITIS/PAINFUL BLADDER SYNDROME

Description

Interstitial cystitis (IC) is a chronic, painful inflammatory disease of the bladder characterized by symptoms of urgency/frequency and pain in the bladder and/or pelvis. *Painful bladder syndrome* (PBS) is suprapubic pain related to bladder filling.

- The term *interstitial cystitis/painful bladder syndrome* (IC/PBS) refers to cases of urinary pain that cannot be attributed to other causes such as infection or urinary calculi. It is more common in women than in men.

The etiology of IC/PBS remains unknown, with possible causes including neurogenic hypersensitivity of the lower urinary tract, alterations in mast cells in the muscle and/or mucosal layers of the bladder, infection with an unusual organism (e.g., slow-growing virus), and production of a toxic substance in the urine. The bladder wall may be irritated and inflamed and can become scarred.

Clinical Manifestations

Two primary clinical manifestations of IC are pain and bothersome lower urinary tract symptoms (e.g., frequency, urgency).

- The pain is usually located in the suprapubic area but may involve the vagina, labia, or entire perineal region. It varies in degree from moderate to severe and is exacerbated by bladder filling, postponed urination, physical exertion, pressure against the suprapubic area, certain foods, or emotional distress. The pain is transiently relieved by urination.
- People with severe cases may urinate as often as 60 times/day including nighttime urination.
- Women report that pain occurs premenstrually and is aggravated by sexual intercourse or emotional stress. Some patients experience symptoms that disappear after a period of weeks to months, whereas others have persistent symptoms for months to years.

Diagnostic Studies

IC/PBS is a diagnosis of exclusion.

- History and physical examination are necessary to rule out other disorders that produce somewhat similar symptoms, such as UTI or endometriosis.
- Cystoscopic examination may reveal a small bladder capacity and superficial ulceration with bladder filling.

Interprofessional Care

No single treatment consistently reverses or relieves symptoms. Elimination of foods and beverages that are likely to irritate the bladder may provide some relief from symptoms. Typical bladder irritants include caffeine; alcohol; citrus products; aged cheeses; nuts; foods containing vinegar or hot peppers; and foods or beverages likely to lower urinary pH (including fruits such as cranberries).

- An over-the-counter (OTC) dietary supplement, calcium glycerophosphate (Prelief), alkalinizes the urine and can provide relief from the irritating effects of certain foods.
- Because stress can exacerbate IC/PBS, relaxation techniques (e.g., sitz baths, application of heat or cold to perineum or bladder, relaxation breathing, imagery) may be helpful.
- Using lubrication or altering positions may decrease pain associated with sexual intercourse.

Two tricyclic antidepressants, amitriptyline and nortriptyline, are used to reduce the burning pain and urinary frequency. In IC, pentosan (Elmiron) is used to enhance the protective effects of the glycosaminoglycan layer of the bladder. These drugs provide relief over weeks to months, but immediate relief for an acute exacerbation of symptoms may require a short course of opioid analgesics.

Several agents may be instilled directly into the bladder through a small catheter.

- Dimethyl sulfoxide (DMSO) acts by desensitizing pain receptors in the bladder wall.
- Heparin and hyaluronic acid also may be instilled into the bladder to enhance the protective properties of the glycosaminoglycan layer of the bladder and relieve symptoms.

Several surgical procedures, such as urinary diversion or fulguration and resection of ulcers, can be used in an attempt to relieve severe, debilitating pain.

Nursing Management

Assess characteristics of the pain associated with IC/PBS. Ask the patient about specific dietary or lifestyle factors that exacerbate or alleviate pain. Instruct the patient to keep a bladder log or voiding diary over a period of at least 3 days to determine voiding frequency and patterns of nocturia.

Instruct the patient to maintain good nutrition, particularly in light of the dietary restrictions often necessary to control IC-related pain.

- Advise the patient to take a multivitamin containing no more than the recommended dietary allowance for essential vitamins and to avoid high-potency vitamins that may irritate the bladder.
- Advise the patient to avoid clothing that creates suprapubic pressure, including pants with tight belts or restrictive waistlines.
- Written educational materials concerning diet, ways to cope with the need for frequent urination, and strategies for coping with the emotional burden of IC/PBS are available from the Interstitial Cystitis Association *(www.ichelp.com)*.

INTERVERTEBRAL DISC DISEASE

Description

Intervertebral disc disease is a condition that involves the deterioration, herniation, or other dysfunction of the intervertebral discs. Disc disorders can affect the cervical, thoracic, and lumbar spine.

Pathophysiology

Intervertebral discs separate the vertebrae of the spinal column and provide shock absorption for the spine. *Degenerative disc disease* (DDD) results from increased wear and tear on the intervertebral discs with aging (Fig. 14). The discs lose their elasticity, flexibility, and shock-absorbing abilities. Unless it is accompanied by pain, this wear-and-tear condition is a normal process.

The discs become thinner as the nucleus pulposus (gelatinous center of the disc) starts to dry out and shrink. This change limits the disc's ability to distribute pressure between vertebrae. The pressure is then transferred to the annulus fibrosus (strong outside portion of the disc), causing progressive destruction.

- When the disc is damaged, the nucleus pulposus may seep through a torn or stretched annulus. This is called a *herniated disc* (slipped disc), a condition in which a spinal disc herniates and bulges outward between the vertebrae.

A herniated disc can result from natural degeneration with age or repeated stress and trauma to the spine. The nucleus pulposus may first bulge and then it can herniate, placing pressure on nearby nerves. The most common sites of rupture are the lumbosacral discs, specifically, L4-5 and L5-S1.

- Disc herniation may be the result of spinal stenosis, in which narrowing of the spinal canal creates bulging of the intervertebral disc.

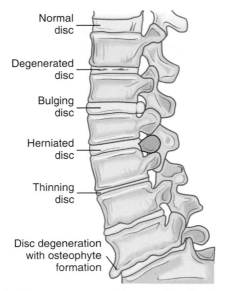

Normal disc
Degenerated disc
Bulging disc
Herniated disc
Thinning disc
Disc degeneration with osteophyte formation

Fig. 14 Common causes of degenerative disc damage.

Clinical Manifestations

Lumbar Disc Disease

The most common manifestation is low back pain. Radicular pain that radiates down the buttock and below the knee along the distribution of the sciatic nerve generally indicates disc herniation. The straight-leg raising test may be positive, indicating nerve root irritation. Back or leg pain may be reproduced by raising the leg and flexing the foot at 90 degrees.

- Reflexes may be depressed or absent, depending on the spinal nerve root involved. Paresthesia or muscle weakness in the legs, feet, or toes may occur.
- Multiple nerve root (cauda equina) compression may be marked by severe low back pain, progressive weakness, increased pain, or bowel/bladder incontinence. This condition is a medical emergency that requires surgical decompression to reduce pressure on the nerves.

Cervical Disc Disease

Pain often radiates into the arms and hands, following the pattern of the involved nerve. Reflexes may not be present, and the hand-grip is often weak.

Diagnostic Studies
- X-rays are done to detect any structural defects.
- A myelogram, MRI, or CT scan is helpful in localizing the damaged site.
- An epidural venogram or diskogram may be necessary if other diagnostic studies are inconclusive.
- Electromyography (EMG) of the extremities can be performed to determine the severity of nerve irritation or to rule out other conditions such as peripheral neuropathy.

Interprofessional Care
Conservative Therapy
The patient with suspected disc damage is usually managed first with conservative therapy. This includes limitation of extremes of spinal movement (brace/corset/belt), local heat or ice, ultrasound and massage, traction, and transcutaneous electrical nerve stimulation (TENS). Drug therapy includes nonsteroidal antiinflammatory drugs (NSAIDs), short-term opioids, corticosteroids, antidepressants, and muscle relaxants. Epidural corticosteroid injections may be effective in reducing inflammation and relieving acute pain.
- When symptoms subside, patients begin back-strengthening exercises twice per day, to continue for a lifetime. Teach the patient the principles of good body mechanics, discouraging extreme flexion and torsion.
- Most patients heal with conservative treatment after 6 months.

Surgical Therapy
Surgery for a damaged disc is generally considered when diagnostic tests indicate that the problem is not responding to conservative treatment, and the patient is in consistent pain and/or has a persistent neurologic deficit.
- An *intradiscal electrothermoplasty* (IDET) is a minimally invasive outpatient procedure for treatment of back and sciatica pain. A needle is inserted into the affected disc with x-ray guidance. The heated wire threaded through the needle destroys the small nerve fibers that have grown into the disc.
- A similar outpatient technique is *radiofrequency discal nucleoplasty,* in which a special radiofrequency probe inserted into the disc is used to break up the molecular bonds of the gel in the nucleus.
- A third procedure is the use of an *interspinous process decompression system* (X Stop). This titanium device fits onto a mount that is placed on vertebrae in the lower back. The device works by lifting the vertebrae off the pinched nerve. The X Stop is used in patients with pain due to lumbar spinal stenosis.

- *Diskectomy* can also be performed to decompress the nerve root. Microsurgical diskectomy is a version of the standard procedure in which the surgeon uses a microscope for better visualization of the disc.
- A *percutaneous diskectomy* is an outpatient surgical procedure that is done by using fluoroscopy and passing a tube through retroperitoneal soft tissues to the lateral border of the disc. A laser is used to destroy the damaged portion of the disc.
- A common traditional procedure for lumbar disc disease is a *laminectomy*. Part of the posterior arch of the vertebra (referred to as the lamina) is surgically excised to gain access to and remove all or part of the protruding disc. A short hospital stay is usually required.
- A *spinal fusion* may be needed if the spine is unstable. The spine is stabilized by creating an ankylosis (fusion) of adjacent vertebrae with a bone graft from the patient's fibula or iliac crest (autograft) or from donated cadaver bone (allograft). Metal fixation with rods, plates, or screws may be implanted. A posterior lumbar interbody fusion may be performed to provide extra support for bone grafting or a prosthetic device. Bone morphogenetic protein (BMP), a genetically engineered protein, may be used to stimulate bone growth of the graft in spinal fusions.
- Artificial disc replacement surgery for patients with DDD includes the use of the Charité disc for lower disc damage and the Prestige cervical disc system.

Nursing Management: Vertebral Disc Surgery

After vertebral disc surgery, postoperative nursing interventions mainly focus on maintaining proper alignment of the spine until healing has occurred. Depending on the type and extent of surgery and the surgeon's preference, the patient may be able to dangle the legs over the side of the bed, stand, or even ambulate the same day of surgery.

After lumbar fusion, place pillows under the thighs when the patient is supine and between the legs when the patient is in the side-lying position to provide comfort and ensure alignment.

- The patient often fears turning or any movement that increases pain. Offer reassurance to the patient that the proper technique is being used to maintain body alignment.
- Postoperatively, most patients will require opioids, such as morphine IV for 24 to 48 hours. Patient-controlled analgesia (PCA) allows for maintaining optimal analgesic levels.
- Once oral fluids are tolerated, the patient may be switched to oral drugs such as acetaminophen with codeine, hydrocodone,

or oxycodone (Percocet). Diazepam (Valium) may be prescribed for muscle relaxation.

Because the spinal canal may be entered during the surgical procedure, there is potential for cerebrospinal fluid (CSF) leakage. Immediately report CSF leakage on the dressing or severe headache.

- Frequently monitor the peripheral neurologic signs of the patient after spinal surgery. Movement of arms and legs and assessment of sensation should at least equal preoperative status. Paresthesias, such as numbness and tingling, may not be relieved immediately after surgery. Document any new muscle weakness or paresthesias and report them to the surgeon.

Paralytic ileus and interference with bowel function may occur for several days and may manifest as nausea, abdominal distention, and constipation. Assess whether the patient is passing flatus, has bowel sounds in all quadrants, and has a flat, soft abdomen. Stool softeners (e.g., docusate sodium [Colace]) may aid in relieving and preventing constipation.

- Emptying the bladder may be difficult due to activity restrictions, opioids, or anesthesia. Encourage men to dangle their legs over the side of the bed or stand to urinate if allowed by the surgeon. Urge patients to use a bedside commode or ambulate to the bathroom, when allowed, to promote bladder emptying. Intermittent catheterization or an indwelling urinary catheter may be needed by patients who have difficulty urinating.

Additional nursing responsibilities are required if the patient has also had a spinal fusion. Because a bone graft is usually involved, the postoperative healing time is prolonged compared with that for a laminectomy. Limited activity over an extended time may be necessary. A rigid orthosis (thoracic-lumbar-sacral orthosis or chair-back brace) is often used during this period.

After cervical spine surgery, be alert for symptoms of spinal cord edema such as respiratory distress and a worsening neurologic status of the upper extremities. The patient's neck may be immobilized in either a soft or a hard cervical collar.

In addition to the primary surgical site, regularly assess the donor site for the bone graft. The donor site usually causes greater postoperative pain than the fused area. A pressure dressing is applied to the donor site to prevent excessive bleeding. If the donor site is the fibula, include neurovascular extremity assessments postoperatively.

- Instruct the patient to avoid sitting or standing for prolonged periods. Encourage activities that include walking, lying down, and shifting weight from one foot to the other when standing.

- Teach the patient to think through an activity before starting a task requiring bending or stooping. Any twisting movement of the spine is contraindicated. The thighs and knees, rather than the back, should be used to absorb the shock of activity and movement.
- A firm mattress or bed board is essential.

INTESTINAL OBSTRUCTION

Description

Intestinal obstruction occurs when intestinal contents cannot pass through the GI tract. The obstruction may occur in the small intestine or colon and can be partial or complete, simple or strangulated. A partial obstruction usually resolves with conservative treatment, whereas a complete obstruction usually requires surgery. A simple obstruction has an intact blood supply, and a strangulated one does not.

Causes of intestinal obstruction can be classified as mechanical or nonmechanical (Fig. 15).

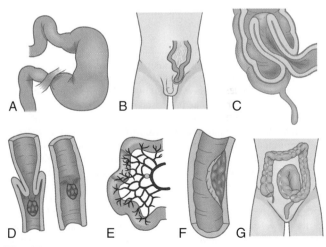

Fig. 15 Bowel obstructions. **A,** Adhesions. **B,** Strangulated inguinal hernia. **C,** Ileocecal intussusception. **D,** Intussusception from polyps. **E,** Mesenteric occlusion. **F,** Neoplasm. **G,** Volvulus of the sigmoid colon.

- *Mechanical obstruction* is a physical obstruction of the intestinal lumen that mostly occurs in the small intestine. Surgical adhesions, the most common cause of small bowel obstructions, can develop within days of surgery or several years later. Other causes of small intestinal obstruction are hernia, strictures from Crohn's disease, and intussusception after bariatric abdominal surgery. The most common cause of colon obstruction is colorectal cancer (malignant obstruction), followed by diverticular disease and sigmoid volvulus. A volvulus is a twisting of the bowel on itself that can result in intestinal obstruction.
- *Nonmechanical obstruction* occurs with reduced or absent peristalsis secondary to altered neuromuscular transmission of the parasympathetic innervation to the bowel and may result from a neuromuscular or vascular disorder. *Paralytic (adynamic) ileus* (lack of intestinal peristalsis and bowel sounds) is the most common form of nonmechanical obstruction. It occurs to some degree after any abdominal surgery. Other causes of paralytic ileus include inflammatory reactions (e.g., acute pancreatitis, acute appendicitis), electrolyte abnormalities (especially hypokalemia), and thoracic or lumbar spinal fractures. *Vascular obstructions* are rare and are caused by an interference with the blood supply to a portion of the bowel. The most common causes are emboli and atherosclerosis of the mesenteric arteries.

Pathophysiology

When fluid, gas, and intestinal contents accumulate proximal to the obstruction, distention occurs and the distal bowel collapses. As the proximal bowel becomes increasingly distended, the intraluminal bowel pressure rises. The increased pressure leads to an increase in capillary permeability and extravasation of fluids and electrolytes into the peritoneal cavity. Retention of fluid in the intestine and peritoneal cavity leads to a severe reduction in circulating blood volume and results in hypotension and hypovolemic shock.

- In the most dangerous situation, the bowel becomes so distended that the blood flow is arrested, causing edema, cyanosis, and gangrene of bowel segment. This is called intestinal strangulation or *intestinal infarction*. If it is not corrected quickly, the bowel will become necrotic and rupture, leading to infection, septic shock, and death.
- Location of the obstruction determines the extent of fluid, electrolyte, and acid-base imbalances. With a high obstruction (e.g., upper duodenum), metabolic alkalosis may result from the loss

of gastric HCl acid through vomiting or nasogastric (NG) intubation and suction. When the obstruction is in the small intestine, dehydration occurs rapidly. If the obstruction is below the proximal colon, solid fecal material accumulates until symptoms of discomfort appear.

Clinical Manifestations

- Manifestations vary depending on the location of the obstruction. The most important early manifestations of a small bowel obstruction are colicky abdominal pain, nausea, vomiting, and abdominal distention.
- Patients with obstructions in the proximal small intestine rapidly develop nausea and vomiting, which is sometimes projectile and contains bile. Vomiting usually relieves abdominal pain in higher intestinal obstructions. Vomiting from more distal obstructions of the small intestine is more gradual in onset and more fecal- and foul-smelling.
- Persistent, colicky abdominal pain, abdominal distention, constipation (new-onset), and lack of flatus are manifestations of lower intestinal obstruction.
- With mechanical obstruction, pain comes and goes in waves. By contrast, paralytic ileus produces a more constant, generalized discomfort. Strangulation causes severe, constant pain that is rapid in onset.
- Abdominal distention is usually absent or minimally noticeable in proximal small intestine obstructions and markedly increased in lower intestinal obstructions. Abdominal tenderness and rigidity are usually absent unless strangulation or peritonitis has occurred.
- Auscultation of bowel sounds reveals high-pitched sounds above the area of obstruction. Bowel sounds may also be absent. *Borborygmi* (audible abdominal sounds caused by hyperactive intestinal motility) are often noted by the patient. The patient's temperature rarely rises above 100° F (37.8° C) unless strangulation or peritonitis has occurred.

Diagnostic Studies

- CT scans and abdominal x-rays are used.
- Sigmoidoscopy or colonoscopy may provide direct visualization of an obstruction in the colon.
- An elevated WBC count may indicate strangulation or perforation.
- Elevated hematocrit (Hct) values may reflect hemoconcentration.

- Decreased hemoglobin (Hgb) and Hct values may indicate bleeding from a neoplasm or strangulation with necrosis.
- Serum electrolytes, blood urea nitrogen (BUN), and serum creatinine are monitored frequently to assess the degree of dehydration.

Interprofessional Care

Treatment of a bowel obstruction depends on the cause. If a strangulated obstruction or perforation is present, the patient will require emergency surgery to relieve the obstruction and survive. Some obstructions due to surgical adhesions may resolve without surgery. Initial treatment of bowel obstruction caused by adhesions includes placing the patient on NPO status, inserting an NG tube, IV fluid therapy, adding potassium to IV fluids after verifying renal function, and analgesics for pain control.

- The treatment goal for the patient with a malignant bowel obstruction is to regain patency and resolve the obstruction. Stents can be placed via endoscopic or fluoroscopic procedures for palliative purposes or until surgery can be performed.
- If the obstruction does not resolve within 24 hours or if the patient's condition deteriorates, surgery is performed to relieve the obstruction.
- Surgery may involve simply resecting the obstructed segment of bowel and anastomosing the remaining healthy bowel back together. Partial or total colectomy, colostomy, or ileostomy may be required when extensive obstruction or necrosis is present.
- Occasionally obstructions can be removed nonsurgically. Colonoscopy offers a means to remove polyps, dilate strictures, and remove or destroy tumors with a laser.

Nursing Management

Goals

The patient with an intestinal obstruction will have relief from the obstruction and a return to normal bowel function, minimal to no discomfort, and normal fluid and electrolyte and acid-base status.

Nursing Diagnoses

- Acute pain
- Deficient fluid volume

Nursing Interventions

Assess the patient regularly and notify the surgeon of changes in vital signs, changes in bowel sounds, decreased urine output, increased abdominal distention, and pain.

- Maintain a strict intake and output record including emesis and tube drainage.
- Monitor the patient closely for signs of dehydration and electrolyte imbalances. A patient with a high intestinal obstruction is more likely to have metabolic alkalosis. A patient with a low obstruction is at greater risk for metabolic acidosis.
- The patient is often restless, changing position to relieve the pain. Provide comfort measures and promote a restful environment.
- Nursing care of the patient after surgery for an intestinal obstruction is similar to the care of the patient after a laparotomy (see Abdominal Pain, Acute, p. 3).

IRRITABLE BOWEL SYNDROME

Description

Irritable bowel syndrome (IBS) is a disorder characterized by chronic abdominal pain or discomfort and alteration of bowel patterns. Diarrhea or constipation may predominate or they may alternate. As a functional GI disorder, IBS has no known organic cause. IBS is more frequently diagnosed in women than in men.

Patients often report a history of GI infections and food intolerances. However, the role of food allergies in IBS is unclear.

- Psychologic stressors (e.g., depression, anxiety, sexual abuse, posttraumatic stress disorder) are associated with the development and exacerbation of IBS.
- In addition to abdominal pain and diarrhea or constipation, patients commonly experience abdominal distention, excessive flatulence, bloating, urgency, and sensation of incomplete evacuation. Non-GI symptoms may include fatigue and sleep disturbances.

There are no specific physical findings with IBS. The key to accurate diagnosis is a thorough history and physical examination. Diagnostic tests are selectively used to rule out other disorders including colorectal cancer, inflammatory bowel disease, endometriosis, and malabsorption disorders (e.g., celiac disease).

Symptom-based criteria for IBS are referred to as the Rome III criteria, which include the following: the presence of abdominal pain and/or discomfort for at least 3 months that is associated with two or more of the following: improvement with defecation, change in stool frequency at onset, or change in the stool appearance at onset. Other common manifestations include abdominal distention, nausea, flatulence, bloating, urgency, mucus in the stool, and sensation of incomplete evacuation. Non-GI symptoms may include fatigue, headache, and sleep disturbances.

Nursing and Interprofessional Management

Treatment is directed at psychologic and dietary factors and drugs to regulate stool output. Patients are more likely to improve with treatment if they have a trusting relationship with their HCP. Encourage the patient to verbalize concerns.

- Because treatment is often focused on symptoms, patients may benefit from keeping a diary of symptoms, diet, and episodes of stress to help identify factors that seem to trigger the IBS symptoms.
- As tolerated, encourage the patient to increase dietary intake of fiber to at least 20 g/day or to use a bulking agent such as Metamucil. Increases in dietary fiber should be instituted gradually, to avoid bloating and abdominal discomfort from gas.
- Review foods that are high in fermentable oligo-, di-, and monosaccharides and polyols (FODMAPs) and teach patients to follow a low-FODMAP diet. Examples of food components to limit are fructans (found in wheat, rye, onions, garlic, and legumes), galactans, lactose (found in milk and yogurt), fructose (found in honey, apples, pears, and high-fructose corn syrup), sorbitol, and xylitol.
- Advise the patient whose primary symptoms are abdominal distention and flatulence to avoid common gas-producing foods such as broccoli or cabbage. Yogurt may be better tolerated than milk products. Probiotics may be used because alterations in intestinal bacteria are believed to exacerbate the condition.
- Drug therapy is individualized. Antispasmodic drugs (hyoscamine, dicyclomine [Bentyl]) decrease GI motility and smooth muscle spasms, reducing pain and diarrhea. Another option for IBS with severe pain and diarrhea is alosetron (Lotronex). Loperamide (Imodium A-D), a synthetic opioid that slows intestinal transit, may be used to treat diarrhea when it occurs. Lubiprostone (Amitiza) is approved for the treatment of women with IBS-related constipation. Linaclotide (Linzess) is approved for the treatment of IBS with constipation but is contraindicated in patients with a history of mechanical obstruction or prior bowel surgery.

Psychologic therapies include cognitive-behavioral therapy, stress management techniques, acupuncture, and hypnosis. Low doses of tricyclic antidepressants and selective serotonin reuptake inhibitors (SSRIs) may reduce symptoms. No single therapy has been found to be effective for all patients with IBS.

KIDNEY CANCER

Kidney cancer arises from the cortex or pelvis (and calyces). Adenocarcinoma (renal cell carcinoma), the most common type, is twice as frequent in men as in women. It is typically discovered when the person is 50 to 70 years old. The most significant risk factor is cigarette smoking. Other risk factors include family history (first-degree relatives), obesity, hypertension, and exposure to cadmium, asbestos, and gasoline.

Early-stage kidney cancer usually has no symptoms. The most common later manifestations are hematuria, flank pain, and a palpable mass in the flank or abdomen. Other symptoms include weight loss, fever, hypertension, and anemia. Local extension of kidney cancer into the renal vein and vena cava is common. The most common sites of metastases are lungs, liver, and long bones.

- Diagnosis is based on CT scan and ultrasound, which differentiates between a solid mass tumor and a cyst. Angiography, biopsy, and MRI are also used in diagnosis. Radionuclide scanning is used to detect metastases.

Nursing and Interprofessional Management

Preventive measures, such as quitting smoking, maintaining a healthy weight, controlling BP, and reducing or avoiding exposure to toxins, can help reduce the incidence of kidney cancer. Patients in high-risk groups should be aware of their increased risk for kidney cancer. Teach them about symptoms (e.g., hematuria, hypertension).

- Partial nephrectomy or *simple total nephrectomy* (for smaller tumors) or a radical nephrectomy (for larger tumors) is the treatment for some renal cancers. *Radical nephrectomy* involves removal of the kidney, adrenal gland, surrounding fascia, part of the ureter, and draining lymph nodes. Nephrectomy can be performed by a conventional (open) approach or laparoscopically.
- Kidney cancer is relatively resistant to most chemotherapy drug and radiation therapy. Chemotherapy drugs include 5-fluorouracil (5-FU), floxuridine, and gemcitabine (Gemzar). Radiation therapy is used palliatively in inoperable cases and when there is metastasis to bone or lungs.
- Immunotherapy, with agents including α-interferon and interleukin-2 (IL-2), is another treatment in metastatic disease.
- Targeted therapy is the preferred treatment for metastatic kidney cancer. Kinase inhibitors, which block certain proteins (kinases) that play a role in tumor growth and cancer progression, include sunitinib (Sutent), sorafenib (Nexavar), and axitinib (Inlyta).

Bevacizumab (Avastin) and pazopanib (Votrient) inhibit the formation of new blood vessels to supply the tumor. Temsirolimus (Torisel) and everolimus (Afinitor) inhibit a specific protein that regulates cell growth and metabolism.

KIDNEY DISEASE, CHRONIC

Description

Chronic kidney disease (CKD) involves progressive, irreversible loss of kidney function. CKD can be defined as either the presence of kidney damage or a decreased glomerular filtration rate (GFR) to less than 60 mL/min/1.73 m^2 for more than 3 months. The classification of CKD is presented in Table 52. The last stage of kidney failure, termed *end-stage renal disease* (ESRD), occurs when the GFR is less than 15 mL/min. At this point, renal replacement therapy (dialysis or transplantation) is required.

Although CKD has many causes, the leading causes are diabetes mellitus (in about 50% of the cases) and hypertension (in about 25%). One of every nine Americans has CKD. Over half a million Americans are receiving treatment (dialysis, transplantation).

Because the kidneys are highly adaptive, kidney disease is often not recognized until there is considerable nephron loss. CKD is often underdiagnosed and undertreated because patients are often asymptomatic. It has been estimated that about 70% of people with CKD are unaware that they have the disease.

Prognosis and course of CKD are highly variable depending on the etiology, patient's condition and age, and adequacy of health care. Some individuals live normal, active lives with compensated renal failure, whereas others may rapidly progress to ESRD.

Clinical Manifestations

As kidney function deteriorates, every body system becomes affected. Manifestations are a result of retained substances including urea, creatinine, phenols, hormones, water, and electrolytes (see Fig. 46-2 in Lewis et al, *Medical-Surgical Nursing,* ed 10, p. 1077). Uremia is a syndrome in which kidney function declines to the point that symptoms develop in multiple body systems. It often occurs when the GFR is less than 10 mL/min. Manifestations of uremia vary among patients according to the etiology of kidney disease, comorbid conditions, age, and degree of adherence to the prescribed medical regimen.

- *Urinary system.* As CKD progresses, patients have increasing difficulty with fluid retention and require diuretic therapy. After a period on dialysis, patients may develop anuria.

TABLE 52 Stages of Chronic Kidney Disease

Description	GFR (mL/min/1.73 m^2)	Clinical Action Plan
Stage 1		
Kidney damage with normal or ↑ GFR	≥90	Diagnosis and treatment CVD risk reduction Slow progression
Stage 2		
Kidney damage with mild ↓ GFR	60-89	Estimation of progression
Stage 3a		
Moderate ↓ GFR	45-59	Evaluation and treatment of complications
Stage 3b		
Moderate ↓ GFR	30-44	More aggressive treatment of complications
Stage 4		
Severe ↓ GFR	15-29	Preparation for renal replacement therapy (dialysis, kidney transplantation)
Stage 5		
Kidney failure	<15 (or dialysis)	Renal replacement therapy (if uremia is present and patient desires treatment)

Source: Kidney Disease: Improving Global Outcomes (KDIGO) CKD Work Group: KDIGO 2012 Clinical Practice Guideline for the Evaluation and Management of Chronic Kidney Disease, *Kidney Int Suppl* 3(1):1, 2013.

- *Metabolic disturbances.* As GFR decreases, blood urea nitrogen (BUN) and serum creatinine levels increase. Serum creatinine and creatinine clearance determinations (calculated GFR) are considered more accurate indicators of kidney function. As BUN increases, nausea, vomiting, lethargy, fatigue, impaired thought processes, and headaches become common.
- *Electrolyte and acid-base imbalances.* Hyperkalemia results from decreased renal excretion, breakdown of cellular protein, bleeding, and metabolic acidosis. Sodium may be elevated, normal, or low in kidney failure. Sodium retention can contribute to edema, hypertension, and heart failure. Metabolic acidosis results from the kidneys' impaired ability to excrete excess acid and from the defective reabsorption and regeneration of bicarbonate.
- *Altered carbohydrate metabolism and elevated triglycerides.* Mild to moderate hyperglycemia and hyperinsulinemia occur. Insulin and glucose metabolism may improve after the initiation of dialysis. Patients with diabetes who develop uremia may require less insulin than before the onset of CKD. This is because insulin, which depends on the kidneys for excretion, remains in circulation longer.
- *Hematologic system.* Anemia results from a lack of erythropoietin. Bleeding tendencies occur because of a defect in platelet function. Cellular and humoral immune responses are suppressed, resulting in increased susceptibility to infection.
- *Cardiovascular system.* The most common cause of death in patients with CKD is cardiovascular disease. Vascular calcification and arterial stiffness are major contributors to cardiovascular disease in CKD. Hypertension is highly prevalent among patients with CKD because hypertension is both a cause and a consequence of CKD. Hypertension is aggravated by sodium retention and increased extracellular fluid volume.
- *Musculoskeletal system.* CKD mineral and bone disorder is a common complication of CKD and results in skeletal complications such as *osteomalacia* (which results from demineralization from slow bone turnover and defective mineralization of newly formed bone) and *osteitis fibrosa* (decalcification of the bone and replacement of bone tissue with fibrous tissue).

Additional systemic signs include pulmonary edema, constipation, peripheral neuropathy, pruritus, infertility, and personality and behavior changes.

Diagnostic Studies

- Urinalysis detects RBCs, WBCs, casts, protein, and glucose.
- BUN and serum creatinine are elevated.

- GFR, obtained from 24-hour urine creatinine clearance measures, is decreased.
- Hematocrit (Hct) and hemoglobin (Hgb) levels are decreased.
- Ultrasound can be used to detect obstructions and kidney size.
- Kidney biopsy provides a definitive diagnosis.

Interprofessional Care

The focus in CKD is to preserve existing kidney function, reduce the risks of cardiovascular disease (CVD), prevent complications, and provide for the patient's comfort. It is important that patients with CKD receive appropriate follow-up care with referral to a nephrologist early in the course of the disease. A focus on stages 1 through 4 (Table 52) before the need for dialysis (stage 5) includes the control of hypertension, hyperparathyroid disease, anemia, hyperglycemia, and dyslipidemia. This section focuses primarily on the drug and nutritional aspects of care.

- Acute hyperkalemia may require treatment with IV glucose and insulin to move potassium into the cells, or IV 10% calcium gluconate. Sodium polystyrene sulfonate, a cation-exchange resin, is used to lower potassium levels in stage 4 CKD. Dialysis may be required to decrease potassium if dysrhythmias are present.
- Control and treatment of hypertension is discussed in Hypertension, p. 323. Treatment of hypertension includes weight loss (if obese), therapeutic lifestyle changes (e.g., exercise, avoidance of alcohol, smoking cessation), diet recommendations, and administration of antihypertensive agents. Drugs most commonly used include diuretics, β-adrenergic blockers, calcium channel blockers, angiotensin-converting enzyme (ACE) inhibitors, and angiotensin receptor blockers.
- Phosphate binders such as calcium carbonate (e.g., Caltrate) and calcium acetate are used to bind phosphate in the bowel, which is then excreted in the stool. Phosphate binders that do not contain calcium include sevelamer (Renagel) and lanthanum (Fosrenol).
- Exogenous erythropoietin (epoetin alfa [Epogen, Procrit]) is used to treat the anemia of CKD.

Many drugs are partially or totally excreted by the kidneys. CKD causes decreased elimination, leading to drug accumulation and the potential for drug toxicity. Drugs of particular concern include digoxin, diabetic agents (metformin, glyburide), antibiotics (e.g., vancomycin, gentamicin), and opioids.

Nutritional Therapy

The diet for CKD is designed to maintain good nutrition (see Table 46-10 for specific recommended restrictions in Lewis et al,

Medical-Surgical Nursing, ed 10, p. 1082). Refer patients with CKD to a dietitian for nutritional teaching. For CKD stages 1 to 4, many HCPs encourage a normal protein intake. However, teach patients to avoid high-protein diets and supplements, because they may overstress the diseased kidneys. Nutritional therapy also includes the restriction of water, sodium, potassium, and phosphate.

Nursing Management

Goals

The patient with chronic kidney disease will demonstrate the knowledge and ability to comply with the therapeutic regimen, participate in decision making for the plan of care and future treatment modality, demonstrate effective coping strategies, and continue with activities of daily living (ADLs) within physiologic limitations.

Nursing Diagnoses

- Excess fluid volume
- Imbalanced nutrition: less than body requirements
- Risk for electrolyte imbalance

Additional information on nursing diagnoses for the patient with CKD is presented in eNursing Care Plan 46-1 (available on the website).

Nursing Interventions

Individuals at risk for CKD include those diagnosed with diabetes or hypertension and people with a history (or a family history) of kidney disease or repeated urinary tract infections. These individuals should have regular checkups that include routine urinalysis and calculation of GFR.

- Individuals at risk need to take measures to prevent or delay the progression of CKD, including glycemic control for patients with diabetes; BP control; and lifestyle modifications, including smoking cessation.
- When potentially nephrotoxic drugs are prescribed, monitor the patient's renal function with serum creatinine, BUN, and GFR.
- Advise patients with diabetes to report any changes in urine appearance (color, odor), frequency, or volume to the HCP.
- Inform the patient that if dialysis is chosen, the option of transplantation still remains, and if a transplanted organ fails, the patient can return to dialysis.

Even though transplantation offers the best therapeutic management for patients with kidney failure, the critical shortage of donor organs limits this option.

It is important to respect the patient's choice to not receive treatment. Patients may initiate a conversation about palliative care.

TABLE 53   Patient & Caregiver Teaching

K

Chronic Kidney Disease

Include the following information in the teaching plan for the patient and caregivers.

1. Dietary (protein, sodium, potassium, phosphate) and fluid restrictions
2. Difficulties in modifying diet and fluid intake
3. Signs and symptoms of electrolyte imbalance, especially high potassium levels
4. Alternative ways of reducing thirst, such as sucking on ice cubes, lemon, or hard candy
5. Rationales for prescribed drugs and common side effects. *Examples*:
   - Phosphate binders (including calcium supplements used as phosphate barriers) should be taken with meals.
   - Calcium supplements prescribed to treat hypocalcemia should be taken on an empty stomach (but not at the same time as iron supplements).
   - Iron supplements should be taken between meals.
6. The importance of reporting any of the following:
   - Weight gain >4 lb (2 kg)
   - Increasing BP
   - Shortness of breath
   - Edema
   - Increasing fatigue or weakness
   - Confusion or lethargy
7. Need for support and encouragement. Share concerns about lifestyle changes, living with a chronic illness, and decisions about type of dialysis or transplantation.

Listen to the patient and caregivers, allowing them to do most of the talking, and pay special attention to their hopes and fears.

▼ **Patient and Caregiver Teaching**

Teach the patient and family about the diet, drugs, and follow-up medical care (Table 53).

- Teach the patient to take daily BPs and identify the signs and symptoms of fluid overload and hyperkalemia and other electrolyte imbalances.
- A dietitian should meet with the patient and caregiver on a regular basis for nutritional planning. Because patients with CKD take many drugs, a pillbox organizer or a list of the drugs and the times of administration may be helpful. Instruct the

patient to avoid over-the-counter drugs such as nonsteroidal antiinflammatory drugs (NSAIDs) and magnesium-based laxatives and antacids.

KIDNEY INJURY, ACUTE

Description

Acute kidney injury (AKI) is the term used to encompass the entire range of the syndrome ranging from a slight deterioration in kidney function to severe impairment.

AKI is characterized by a rapid loss of kidney function demonstrated by a rise in serum creatinine and/or a reduction in urine output. Evidence of severity can range from a small increase in serum creatinine or reduction in urine output to the development of azotemia (an accumulation of nitrogenous waste products [urea nitrogen, creatinine] in the blood).

Although AKI is potentially reversible, it has a high mortality rate. AKI usually affects people with other life-threatening conditions. Most commonly, AKI follows severe, prolonged hypotension or hypovolemia or exposure to a nephrotoxic agent.

Pathophysiology

AKI is categorized as prerenal, intrarenal (or intrinsic), or postrenal (Fig. 16).

- *Prerenal* causes of AKI involve factors external to the kidneys that reduce renal blood flow and lead to decreased glomerular perfusion and filtration. In prerenal oliguria, there is no damage to the kidney tissue (parenchyma). The oliguria is caused by a decrease in circulating blood volume (e.g., severe dehydration, decreased cardiac output) and is reversible with treatment. Prerenal conditions can lead to intrarenal disease if renal ischemia is prolonged.
- *Intrarenal* causes include conditions that cause direct damage to the kidney tissue, resulting in impaired nephron function. Intrarenal AKI is usually caused by prolonged ischemia, nephrotoxins (e.g., antibiotics), myoglobin released from necrotic muscle cells, or hemoglobin released from hemolyzed RBCs. Primary renal diseases such as systemic lupus erythematosus and glomerulonephritis may also cause AKI. *Acute tubular necrosis* (ATN) is the most common cause of intrarenal AKI and is primarily the result of ischemia, nephrotoxins, or sepsis.
- *Postrenal* causes involve mechanical obstruction of urinary outflow. As the flow of urine is obstructed, urine refluxes into the renal pelvis, impairing kidney function. The most common

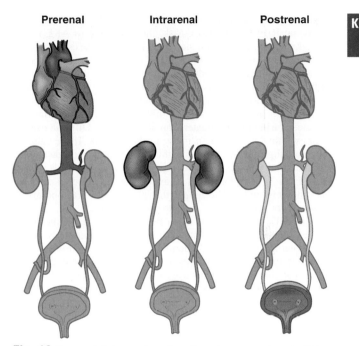

Prerenal **Intrarenal** **Postrenal**

Fig. 16 Prerenal, intrarenal, and postrenal causes of acute kidney injury (AKI).

causes are prostate cancer, benign prostatic hyperplasia (BPH), urinary tract calculi, trauma, and extrarenal tumors. Bilateral ureteral obstruction leads to *hydronephrosis* (kidney dilation), increase in hydrostatic pressure, and tubular blockage, resulting in a progressive decline in kidney function. If bilateral obstruction is relieved within 48 hours of onset, complete recovery is likely. After 12 weeks, recovery is unlikely. Prolonged obstruction can lead to tubular atrophy and irreversible kidney fibrosis.

Clinical Manifestations

Clinically, AKI may progress through three phases: oliguric, diuretic, and recovery. In some situations the patient does not recover from AKI, and chronic kidney disease (CKD) results (see Kidney Disease, Chronic, p. 370).

The diagnosis and staging of AKI are standardized using the mnemonic RIFLE (Table 54): *R*isk, the first stage of AKI, is followed by *i*njury, the second stage; AKI then increases in severity to the final or third stage, *f*ailure. The two outcome variables are *l*oss and *e*nd-stage kidney disease.

Oliguric Phase

The most common initial manifestation of AKI is oliguria, a reduction in urine output to less than 400 mL/day. Nonoliguria AKI indicates a urine output greater than 400 mL/day. Oliguria usually occurs within 1 to 7 days of injury to the kidneys. If the cause is ischemia, oliguria often occurs within 24 hours. By contrast, when nephrotoxic drugs are involved, onset may be delayed for up to a week. The oliguric phase lasts on average about 10 to 14 days but can last for months. The longer this phase lasts, the poorer the prognosis for recovery of complete renal function.

About 50% of patients will not be oliguric, making the initial diagnosis more difficult. Changes in urine output generally do not correspond to changes in glomerular filtration rate (GFR).

- A urinalysis may show casts, RBCs, WBCs, a specific gravity fixed at around 1.010, and urine osmolality around 300 mOsm/kg (300 mmol/kg). This is the same specific gravity and osmolality as for plasma.
- Fluid retention occurs as urinary output decreases. Neck veins may become distended with a bounding pulse, and edema and hypertension may develop. Fluid overload can lead to heart failure, pulmonary edema, and pericardial and pleural effusions.
- Metabolic acidosis results when the kidneys cannot synthesize ammonia (needed for hydrogen ion excretion) or excrete acid products of metabolism. The serum bicarbonate level decreases because bicarbonate is depleted in buffering hydrogen ions. The patient may develop Kussmaul (rapid, deep) respirations to increase the excretion of carbon dioxide.
- Serum sodium and potassium levels are altered. Damaged tubules cannot conserve sodium. Urinary excretion of sodium may increase, resulting in normal or below-normal levels of serum sodium. In AKI the serum potassium level increases because the kidney's normal ability to excrete potassium is impaired. Because cardiac muscle is intolerant of acute increases in potassium, treatment is essential when hyperkalemia develops.
- Leukocytosis is often present. The most common cause of death in AKI is infection.
- Blood urea nitrogen (BUN) and serum creatinine levels are elevated in kidney failure.

TABLE 54   RIFLE Classification for Staging Acute Kidney Injury

	GFR Criteria	Urine Output Criteria	Clinical Example
Risk	Serum creatinine increased × 1.5 OR GFR decreased by 25%	Urine output <0.5 mL/kg/hr for 6 hr	• The patient is a 68-year-old African-American woman with type 2 diabetes, hypertension, CAD, and CKD. • She is scheduled to undergo emergency coronary artery bypass grafting. • Serum creatinine is 1.8 mg/dL (increased), and she weighs 60 kg. • Calculated GFR is 35 mL/min /1.73². • She has stage 3b CKD.
Injury	Serum creatinine increased × 2 OR GFR decreased by 50%	Urine output <0.5 mL/kg/hr for 12 hr	• *During surgery:* She experiences hypotension for a sustained period. • Acute tubular necrosis is diagnosed. • *After surgery:* Serum creatinine is 3.6 mg/dL and urine output is reduced to 28 mL/hr.

Continued

TABLE 54 RIFLE Classification for Staging Acute Kidney Injury—cont'd

	GFR Criteria	Urine Output Criteria	Clinical Example
Failure	Serum creatinine increased × 3 OR GFR decreased by 75% OR Serum creatinine >4 mg/dL with acute rise of ≥0.5 mg/dL	Urine output <0.3 mL/kg/hr for 24 hr (oliguria) OR Anuria for 12 hr	• *At 72 hours after surgery:* In ICU, she develops ventilator-associated pneumonia and sepsis. • Serum creatinine rises to 5.2 mg/dL and urine output drops to 10 mL/hr. • BP remains low despite dopamine therapy.
Loss	Persistent acute kidney failure Complete loss of kidney function for >4 wk	—	• Continuous venovenous hemodialysis is started. • After 3 wk of therapy, she has a cardiopulmonary arrest and does not survive.
End-stage renal disease	Complete loss of kidney function for >3 mo	—	—

GFR, glomerular filtration rate.

- Neurologic changes can occur as nitrogenous waste products accumulate in the brain and other nervous tissue. Manifestations can be as mild as fatigue and difficulty concentrating and can escalate to seizures, stupor, and coma.

Diuretic Phase

During the diuretic phase, daily urine output of 1 to 3 L/day occurs but may reach 5 L/day or more. The kidneys have recovered the ability to excrete wastes but not to concentrate urine.

- The diuretic phase may last 1 to 3 weeks, with the patient's acid-base, electrolyte, and waste product values beginning to normalize. Because of large losses of fluid and electrolytes, monitor the patient for hyponatremia, hypokalemia, and dehydration.

Recovery Phase

The recovery phase begins when the GFR increases, allowing the BUN and serum creatinine levels to decrease. Kidney function may take up to 12 months to stabilize.

- The outcome of AKI is influenced by the patient's overall health, severity of renal failure, and number and type of complications. Some patients progress to ESRD. Patients who recover may achieve clinically normal kidney function but remain in an early stage of CKD.

Diagnostic Studies

- History is essential to determine the etiology.
- Urine output and serum creatinine help to make the diagnosis.
- Urinalysis is done to assess sediment, casts, hematuria, pyuria, and crystals.
- Urine osmolality, sodium content, and specific gravity help in differentiating the cause.
- Ultrasound and renal scan are used to assess renal blood flow, tubular function, and the collecting system.
- CT scan can identify lesions, masses, obstructions, and vascular abnormalities.

Interprofessional Care

Because AKI is potentially reversible, the primary goals of treatment are to eliminate the cause, manage the signs and symptoms, and prevent complications while the kidneys recover. The first step is to determine if there is adequate intravascular volume and cardiac output (CO) to ensure adequate perfusion of the kidneys.

- Diuretic therapy may be administered and usually includes loop diuretics (e.g., furosemide [Lasix], bumetanide [Bumex]) or an osmotic diuretic (e.g., mannitol). If AKI is already established, forcing fluids and diuretics will not be effective.

- Closely monitor fluid intake during the oliguric phase.
- Hyperkalemia is one of the most serious complications because it can cause cardiac dysrhythmias. Both insulin and sodium bicarbonate temporarily shift potassium into the cells, but it eventually shifts back out. Calcium gluconate raises the threshold at which dysrhythmias occur. Only sodium polystyrene sulfonate (Kayexalate) and dialysis actually remove potassium from the body.

If conservative therapy is not effective in treating AKI, renal replacement therapy (RRT) is used. The most common indications for RRT in AKI are (1) volume overload, resulting in compromised cardiac and/or pulmonary status; (2) elevated serum potassium level; (3) metabolic acidosis (serum bicarbonate level less than 15 mEq/L [15 mmol/L]); (4) BUN level greater than 120 mg/dL (43 mmol/L); (5) significant change in mental status; and (6) pericarditis, pericardial effusion, or cardiac tamponade.

- Peritoneal dialysis is considered a viable option for renal replacement, although it is infrequently used.
- Intermittent hemodialysis (HD) (4 hours daily, every other day, or three or four times per week) and continuous renal replacement therapy (CRRT) have both been used effectively. CRRT is provided continuously over approximately 24 hours through cannulation of an artery and a vein, or of two veins.

Nutritional Therapy

The challenge of nutritional management is to provide adequate calories to prevent catabolism despite the restrictions that prevent electrolyte and fluid disorders and azotemia. Adequate energy should primarily be from carbohydrate and fat sources to prevent ketosis from endogenous fat breakdown and gluconeogenesis from muscle protein breakdown.

- To maintain adequate caloric intake, 30 to 35 kcal/kg and 0.8 to 1.0 g protein/kg is recommended to prevent the further breakdown of body protein for energy purposes. Essential amino acid supplements can be given for amino acid and caloric supplementation.
- Potassium and sodium are regulated in accordance with plasma levels. Sodium is restricted as needed to prevent edema, hypertension, and heart failure.
- Fat emulsion IV infusions given as a nutritional supplement provide a good source of nonprotein calories.

If a patient cannot maintain adequate oral intake, enteral nutrition is the preferred route for nutritional support (see Enteral Nutrition, p. 706). When the gastrointestinal tract is not functional, parenteral nutrition is necessary for the provision of adequate nutrition (see Parenteral Nutrition, p. 731).

K

Nursing Management

Goals

The patient with AKI will recover without any loss of kidney function, maintain normal fluid and electrolyte balance, have decreased anxiety, and adhere to and understand the need for follow-up care.

Nursing Diagnoses/Collaborative Problem

- Risk for infection
- Excess fluid volume
- Fatigue
- Anxiety
- Potential complication: dysrhythmias

Nursing Interventions

Prevention and early recognition of AKI are essential because of the high mortality rate. These efforts are primarily directed toward (1) identifying and monitoring high-risk populations, (2) controlling exposure to industrial chemicals and nephrotoxic drugs, and (3) preventing prolonged episodes of hypotension and hypovolemia. In the hospital the factors that increase the risk for developing AKI are advanced age, massive trauma, extensive burns, cardiac failure, obstetric complications, and preexisting chronic kidney disease.

- Carefully monitor intake and output and electrolyte balance. Record extrarenal losses of fluid from vomiting, diarrhea, and hemorrhage.
- Prompt replacement of significant fluid losses helps prevent ischemic tubular damage associated with trauma, burns, and extensive surgery. Intake and output records and the patient's weight provide valuable indicators of fluid volume status.
- Monitor renal function in individuals taking potentially nephrotoxic drugs. Caution the patient about the use of over-the-counter analgesics (especially nonsteroidal antiinflammatory drugs [NSAIDs]), because these may worsen kidney function in the patient with mild CKD.
- Angiotensin-converting enzyme (ACE) inhibitors can also decrease perfusion pressure and cause hyperkalemia. If other measures such as diet modification, diuretics, and sodium bicarbonate cannot control hyperkalemia, the ACE inhibitor may need to be reduced or eliminated.

You have an important role in managing fluid and electrolyte balance during the oliguric and diuretic phases. Observing and recording accurate intake and output are essential.

- Assess for the common signs and symptoms of hypervolemia (in the oliguric phase) or hypovolemia (in the diuretic phase), potassium and sodium disturbances, and other electrolyte imbalances that may occur in AKI.

- Because infection is the leading cause of death in AKI, meticulous aseptic technique is critical. A patient with renal failure who has an infection may not have an elevated temperature.
- If antibiotics are used to treat infection, the type, frequency, and dosage must be carefully considered, because the kidneys are the primary route of excretion for many antibiotics.
- Perform skin care and take measures to prevent pressure ulcers, because mobility may be impaired. Mouth care is important to prevent stomatitis.

▼ Patient and Caregiver Teaching

- Once kidney function has returned, follow-up care and regular evaluation of renal function are necessary.
- Teach the patient the signs and symptoms of recurrent renal disease. Emphasize measures to prevent recurrence of AKI.
- The long-term convalescence of 3 to 12 months may cause psychosocial and financial hardships for both the patient and family. Make appropriate referrals for counseling.
- If the kidneys do not recover, a transition to chronic dialysis or possible future transplantation may be indicated.

LACTASE DEFICIENCY

Description

Lactase deficiency is a condition in which the lactase enzyme that breaks down lactose into two simple sugars (glucose and galactose) is deficient or absent.

Primary lactase insufficiency is most commonly a result of genetic factors. People in certain ethnic or racial groups, especially those with Asian or African ancestry, develop low lactase levels in childhood. Less common causes include low lactase levels resulting from premature birth and congenital lactase deficiency, a rare genetic disorder. Lactose malabsorption can also occur when conditions leading to bacterial overgrowth promote lactose fermentation in the small bowel, and when intestinal mucosal damage interferes with absorption (e.g., inflammatory bowel disease, celiac disease).

Clinical Manifestations

Manifestations of lactose intolerance include bloating, flatulence, crampy abdominal pain, and diarrhea. Diarrhea results from the excess undigested lactose in the small intestine. The lactose attracts water molecules, which prevents water being properly absorbed. Symptoms generally occur within 30 minutes to several hours after drinking a glass of milk or ingesting a milk product.

Diagnostic Studies

Many lactose-intolerant people are aware of their milk intolerance and avoid milk and milk products. Lactose intolerance is diagnosed by a lactose tolerance test, lactose hydrogen breath test, or genetic testing.

Nursing and Interprofessional Management

Treatment consists of eliminating lactose from the diet by avoiding milk and milk products and/or replacing lactase with commercially available preparations. Teach the patient the importance of adherence to the diet.

- A lactose-free diet may be gradually advanced to a low-lactose diet.
- Many lactose-intolerant people can tolerate small amounts of lactose.
- Because avoiding milk and milk products can lead to calcium deficiency, supplements may be necessary to prevent osteoporosis.
- Lactase enzyme (Lactaid), available as an over-the-counter product, is mixed with milk and breaks down lactose before the milk is ingested. A number of milk products pretreated with lactase enzyme are available.

LEIOMYOMAS

Leiomyomas (uterine fibroids) are common benign smooth muscle tumors in the uterus. The cause of leiomyomas is unknown. They appear to depend on estrogen and progesterone, because they grow slowly during the reproductive years and undergo atrophy after menopause.

A majority of women with leiomyomas do not have symptoms. Those who develop symptoms commonly present with abnormal uterine bleeding, pain, or symptoms associated with pelvic pressure. Pain is associated with infection or twisting of the pedicle from which the tumor is growing. Pressure on surrounding organs may result in rectal, bladder, and lower abdominal discomfort.

Diagnosis is based on the characteristic pelvic examination findings of an enlarged uterus distorted by nodular masses. Treatment depends on the patient's symptoms, age, and desire to bear children, and the location and size of the tumor or tumors. If the symptoms are minimal, the HCP may elect to monitor the patient.

- The most common treatment for uterine fibroids is hormonal therapy using oral contraceptives to slow tumor growth as well as to manage abnormal uterine bleeding.

- Persistent heavy menstrual bleeding causing anemia and large or rapidly growing tumors are indications for surgery. Leiomyomas are removed by hysterectomy or myomectomy. A myomectomy (removal of only the fibroid tumor) is performed for women who wish to have children.
- Uterine artery embolization is an alternative treatment for uterine fibroids. Embolic material (small plastic or gelatin beads) injected into the uterine artery blocks uterine blood flow to shrink the fibroid.

LEUKEMIA

Description

Leukemia is a general term used to describe a group of malignant disorders affecting the blood and blood-forming tissues of the bone marrow, lymph system, and spleen. It results in an accumulation of dysfunctional cells secondary to loss of regulation in cell division. Although leukemia is often thought of as a disease of children, the number of adults affected is 9 times that of children.

Regardless of the specific type, leukemia has no single cause. Most types of leukemia result from a combination of factors including genetic and environmental influences.

Classification

Leukemia can be classified as acute versus chronic disease and by the type of WBC involved. By combining the acute and chronic categories with the cell type involved, four major types of leukemia can be identified. Table 55 summarizes the relative incidence and features of the four types of leukemia.

Acute myelogenous leukemia (AML) represents only one fourth of all leukemias, but it makes up approximately 80% of the acute leukemias in adults. Its onset is often abrupt and dramatic. A patient may have serious infections and abnormal bleeding from onset of the disease. AML is characterized by uncontrolled proliferation of myeloblasts, the precursors of granulocytes. There is hyperplasia of the bone marrow. Clinical manifestations are usually related to replacement of normal hematopoietic cells in the marrow by leukemic myeloblasts and, to a lesser extent, to infiltration of other organs and tissue.

Acute lymphocytic leukemia (ALL) is the most common type of leukemia in children and accounts for about 20% of acute leukemia cases in adults. In ALL, immature lymphocytes proliferate in the bone marrow; most are of B cell origin. Fever is present in most patients at time of diagnosis. Signs and symptoms may appear

L

TABLE 55 Types of Leukemia

Type	Age at Onset	Clinical Manifestations	Diagnostic Findings
Acute myelogenous leukemia (AML)	Accounts for 15%-20% of acute leukemia in children and 80% in adults Increase in incidence with advancing age after 60 yr	Fatigue and weakness, headache, mouth sores, anemia, bleeding, fever, infection, sternal tenderness, gingival hyperplasia, mild hepatosplenomegaly (in one third of patients)	Low RBC count, Hgb, Hct, platelet count Low to high WBC count with myeloblasts High LDH Hypercellular bone marrow with myeloblasts
Acute lymphocytic leukemia (ALL)	Dual peak prevalence between ages 2 and 5 and after age 50	Fever, pallor, bleeding, anorexia, fatigue and weakness Bone, joint, and abdominal pain Generalized lymphadenopathy, infections, weight loss, hepatosplenomegaly, headache, mouth sores Neurologic manifestations: CNS involvement; increased intracranial pressure (nausea, vomiting, lethargy, cranial nerve dysfunction) secondary to meningeal infiltration	Low RBC count, Hgb, Hct, platelet count Low, normal, or high WBC count High LDH Transverse lines of rarefaction at ends of metaphysis of long bones on x-ray Hypercellular bone marrow with lymphoblasts Lymphoblasts also possible in cerebrospinal fluid Presence of Philadelphia chromosome (20%-25% of patients)

Continued

TABLE 55 Types of Leukemia—cont'd

Type	Age at Onset	Clinical Manifestations	Diagnostic Findings
Chronic myelogenous leukemia (CML)	Increase in incidence with advancing age with median age at diagnosis of 65 Rare in children	No symptoms early in disease Fatigue and weakness, fever, sternal tenderness, weight loss, joint pain, bone pain, massive splenomegaly, increase in sweating	Low RBC count, Hgb, Hct High platelet count early, lower count later ↑ banded neutrophils and myeloblasts and often basophils, normal number of lymphocytes, and normal or low number of monocytes Nucleated red cells are common Low leukocyte alkaline phosphatase Presence of Philadelphia chromosome in 90% of patients
Chronic lymphocytic leukemia (CLL)	Increase in incidence with advancing age after 65 yr, with predominance in men	Frequently no symptoms Detection of disease often during examination for unrelated condition, chronic fatigue, anorexia, splenomegaly and lymphadenopathy, hepatomegaly May progress to fever, night sweats, weight loss, fatigue, and frequent infections	Mild anemia and thrombocytopenia with disease progression Total WBC count >100,000/μL Increase in peripheral lymphocytes and lymphocytes in bone marrow May have autoimmune hemolytic anemia, idiopathic thrombocytopenic purpura, and hypogammaglobulinemia

CNS, Central nervous system; *LDH,* lactate dehydrogenase

abruptly with bleeding or fever, or their onset may be insidious, with progressive weakness, fatigue, and bleeding tendencies.

Chronic myelogenous leukemia (CML) is caused by excessive development of mature neoplastic granulocytes in the bone marrow. CML usually has a chronic stable phase that lasts for several years, followed by development of an acute aggressive phase (blastic phase).

- The Philadelphia chromosome, which is present in 90% to 95% of patients with CML, is a diagnostic hallmark of CML. In addition, its presence is an important indicator of residual disease or relapse after treatment.

Chronic lymphocytic leukemia (CLL) is the most common leukemia in adults, and is characterized by the production and accumulation of functionally inactive but long-lived, small, mature-appearing lymphocytes. The B lymphocyte is usually involved. Lymph node enlargement (lymphadenopathy) is present throughout the body. Because CLL is usually a disease of older adults, treatment decisions must be made by considering disease progression and treatment of side effects. Many individuals in the early stages of CLL require no treatment. Others may be followed closely and receive treatment only when the disease progresses; approximately 30% will require immediate intervention at time of diagnosis.

Clinical Manifestations

Although the manifestations of leukemia are varied, they relate to problems caused by bone marrow failure and the formation of leukemic infiltrates (Table 55). The patient is predisposed to development of anemia, thrombocytopenia, and decreased number and function of WBCs.

- WBC infiltration into the patient's organs leads to problems such as splenomegaly, hepatomegaly, lymphadenopathy, bone pain, meningeal irritation, and oral lesions.

Diagnostic Studies

- Peripheral blood evaluation and bone marrow examination are the primary methods of diagnosing and classifying the types of leukemia.
- Morphologic, histochemical, immunologic, and cytogenetic methods are all used to identify leukemic cell types and stage of development.
- Studies such as lumbar puncture and CT scan can detect leukemic cells outside the blood and bone marrow.
- The malignant cells in most patients with leukemia have specific cytogenetic abnormalities that are associated with distinct

subsets of the disease. These cytogenetic abnormalities have diagnostic, prognostic, and therapeutic importance.

Interprofessional Care

Care first focuses on the goal of attaining remission.

- In some cases, such as nonsymptomatic patients with CLL, watchful waiting with active supportive care may be appropriate.
- Because cytotoxic chemotherapy is the mainstay of treatment for some patients, you must understand the principles of cancer chemotherapy, including cellular kinetics, the use of multiple drugs rather than single agents, and the cell cycle (see Chemotherapy, p. 694).
- Corticosteroids and radiation therapy may have a role in therapy for the patient with leukemia. Total body radiation may be used to prepare a patient for bone marrow transplantation, or radiation may be restricted to certain areas (fields), such as the liver, spleen, or other organs affected by infiltrates.
- In ALL, prophylactic intrathecal methotrexate or cytarabine is given to decrease central nervous system (CNS) involvement, which is common in this type of leukemia. When CNS leukemia does occur, cranial radiation may be given. Immunotherapy and targeted therapy may be indicated for specific types of leukemia (see Lewis et al, *Medical-Surgical Nursing,* ed 10, p. 638).

Chemotherapeutic agents used to treat leukemia vary. Combination chemotherapy is the mainstay of treatment for leukemia. The three purposes for using multiple drugs are to (1) decrease drug resistance, (2) minimize drug toxicity to the patient by using multiple drugs with varying toxicities, and (3) interrupt cell growth at multiple points in the cell cycle.

Hematopoietic stem cell transplantation (HSCT) is another type of therapy used for patients with different forms of leukemia. The goal of HSCT is to totally eliminate leukemia cells from the body using combinations of chemotherapy with or without total body radiation. This treatment also eradicates the patient's hematopoietic stem cells, which are then replaced with those of a human leukocyte antigen (HLA)-matched sibling, with those of a volunteer donor (allogeneic) or an identical twin (syngeneic), or with the patient's own (autologous) stem cells that were removed (harvested) before the intensive therapy. (See content on HSCT in Lewis et al, *Medical-Surgical Nursing,* ed 10, pp. 638 to 639.)

The primary complications of patients with allogeneic HSCT are graft-versus-host disease (GVHD), relapse of leukemia (especially ALL), and infection (especially interstitial pneumonia). Because

HSCT has serious associated risks, the patient must weigh the significant risks of treatment-related death or treatment failure (relapse) against the hope of cure.

Nursing Management

Goals

The patient with leukemia will understand and cooperate with the treatment plan, experience minimal side effects and complications associated with both the disease and its treatment, and feel hopeful and supported during periods of treatment, relapse, or remission.

See nursing care plans available on the website for anemia (eNursing Care Plan 30-1), thrombocytopenia (eNursing Care Plan 30-2), and neutropenia (eNursing Care Plan 30-3).

Nursing Diagnoses

Nursing diagnoses related to leukemia include those appropriate for anemia (see Anemia, p. 29), thrombocytopenia (see Thrombocytopenic Purpura, p. 629), and neutropenia (see content on neutropenia in Lewis et al, *Medical-Surgical Nursing,* ed 10, pp. 632 to 634).

Nursing Interventions

The nursing role during acute phases of leukemia is extremely challenging because the patient has many physical and psychosocial needs. As with other forms of cancer, the diagnosis of leukemia can evoke great fear and be equated with death.

- Help the patient realize that although the future may be uncertain, one can have a meaningful quality of life while in remission or with disease control.
- Families also need help in adjusting to the stress of the abrupt onset of serious illness and losses imposed by the sick role. The diagnosis of leukemia often brings with it the need to make difficult decisions at a time of profound stress for the patient and family.
- You are an important advocate in helping the patient and family understand the complexities of treatment decisions and manage the side effects and toxicities. A patient may require protective isolation or may need to temporarily geographically relocate to an appropriate treatment center. This situation can lead a patient to feel deserted and isolated at a time when support is most needed.

From a physical care perspective, you are challenged to make assessments and plan care to help the patient deal with the severe side effects of chemotherapy. The life-threatening results of bone marrow suppression (anemia, thrombocytopenia, neutropenia) require aggressive nursing interventions.

Review all drugs being administered. Assess laboratory data reflecting the effects of the drugs. Patient survival and comfort during aggressive chemotherapy are significantly affected by the quality of nursing care.

▼ **Patient and Caregiver Teaching**

Teach the patient and caregivers to understand the importance of continued diligence in disease management and the need for follow-up care.

Involving the patient in survivor networks, support groups, or services may help the patient to adapt to living with a life-threatening illness. Exploring community resources (e.g., American Cancer Society, Leukemia Society) may reduce the financial burden and feelings of dependence. Also provide the resources for spiritual support.

LIVER CANCER

Description

Primary *liver cancer* (hepatocellular carcinoma [HCC]) is the fifth most common cancer in the world and the second most common cause of cancer death worldwide. It is the most common cause of death in patients with cirrhosis.

The incidence of HCC is rising in the United States because of the large number of patients infected with chronic hepatitis C. Cirrhosis caused by hepatitis C is the most common cause of HCC in the United States, followed by alcoholic cirrhosis. Other primary liver tumors are cholangiomas or bile duct cancers.

Metastatic carcinoma of the liver is more common than primary carcinoma. The liver is a common site of metastatic cancer growth because of its high rate of blood flow and extensive capillary network. Primary liver tumors commonly metastasize to the lung.

- The prognosis for patients with liver cancer is poor. The cancer grows rapidly, and death may occur within 6 to 12 months as a result of hepatic encephalopathy or massive blood loss from GI bleeding.

Clinical Manifestations

Liver cancer can be difficult to diagnose and differentiate from cirrhosis because of similar clinical manifestations (e.g., hepatomegaly, splenomegaly, fatigue, jaundice, weight loss, peripheral edema, ascites, portal hypertension).

- Other common manifestations include dull abdominal pain in the epigastric or right upper quadrant region, anorexia, nausea and vomiting, and increased abdominal girth.

Diagnostic Studies

- Ultrasound, CT, and MRI are used to screen and diagnose liver cancer.
- A percutaneous biopsy is performed if the results of diagnostic imaging studies are inconclusive.
- Serum α-fetoprotein (AFP) is often elevated.

Nursing and Interprofessional Management

Treatment depends on the size and number of tumors, metastasis beyond the liver, and the patient's age and overall health. In general, management is similar to that for cirrhosis (see Cirrhosis, p. 136). Surgical liver resection (partial hepatectomy) offers the best chance for a cure. However, only about 15% of patients have sufficient healthy liver tissue for this to be an option.

- For those patients who have early-stage liver cancer, liver transplantation offers an option with good prognosis.
- Other treatment options are radiofrequency ablation, chemoembolization, and alcohol injection.
- In patients with advanced HCC, sorafenib (Nexavar) is typically the first-line treatment. This kinase inhibitor, a type of targeted therapy agent, blocks proteins (kinases) that play a role in tumor growth and cancer progression.

Nursing interventions focus on keeping the patient as comfortable as possible. Because the patient with liver cancer manifests the same problems as the patient with advanced liver disease, the nursing interventions discussed for cirrhosis of the liver apply (see Cirrhosis, pp. 141-143).

LOW BACK PAIN, ACUTE

Description

Low back pain is common and has affected 80% of adults in the United States at least once during their lifetime. Risk factors associated with low back pain include cigarette smoking, stress, poor posture, lack of muscle tone, and excess weight. Jobs that require repetitive heavy lifting, vibration (e.g., jackhammer operator), and extended periods of sitting are also associated with low back pain. Low back pain is most often caused by a musculoskeletal problem.

- Health care personnel who engage in direct patient care activities are at high risk for low back pain. Lifting and moving patients, excessive bending or leaning forward, and frequent twisting can result in low back pain.

Pathophysiology

Low back pain is a common problem because the lumbar region
(1) bears most of the weight of the body, (2) is the most flexible
region of the spinal column, (3) contains nerve roots that are at risk
for injury or disease, and (4) has a naturally unstable biomechanical
structure. The causes of low back pain of musculoskeletal origin
include acute lumbosacral strain, instability of lumbosacral bony
mechanism, osteoarthritis of the lumbosacral vertebrae, degenerative disc disease, and herniation of the intervertebral disc.

Acute low back pain lasts 4 weeks or less. It is caused by trauma
or activity that causes undue stress on the lower back. Often symptoms do not appear at the time of injury but develop later because
of swelling or a gradual increase in pressure on the nerve by an
intervertebral disc.

- Symptoms may range from muscle ache to shooting or stabbing
  pain, limited flexibility and/or range of motion, or inability to
  stand upright.
- Few definitive diagnostic abnormalities are present with nerve
  irritation and muscle strain. One test is the straight-leg-raising
  test. MRI and CT scans are generally not done unless trauma or
  systemic disease (e.g., cancer, spinal infection) is suspected.

Interprofessional Care

If the acute muscle spasms and accompanying pain are not severe
and unbearable, the patient may be treated on an outpatient basis
with nonsteroidal antiinflammatory drugs (NSAIDs), muscle relaxants, massage and back manipulation, acupuncture, and use of
alternating heat and cold compresses. Severe pain may require a
brief course of corticosteroids or opioid analgesics.

Some people may need a brief period (1 to 2 days) of rest at
home, but prolonged bed rest should be avoided. Most patients do
better if they continue their regular activities. Patients should
refrain from activities that increase the pain, including lifting,
bending, twisting, and prolonged sitting. Most symptoms subside
within 2 weeks.

Nursing Management

As a role model, use proper body mechanics at all times. This
includes increasing the patient's bed height, bending at the knees,
asking for help in lifting and moving patients, and using lifting
devices.

Primary nursing responsibilities in acute low back pain are to
assist the patient to maintain activity limitations, promote comfort,

and teach the patient about the health problem and appropriate exercises.

- Referral to a physical therapist or personal trainer to address posture as well as core and abdomen strength may be appropriate. Ensure that the patient understands the type and frequency of exercise prescribed, as well as the rationale for the program.

▼ **Patient and Caregiver Teaching**

Assess the patient's use of body mechanics and offer advice when the person does activities that could produce back strain (Table 56).

TABLE 56 Patient & Caregiver Teaching

Low Back Problems

Include the following instructions when teaching the patient and caregivers how to manage low back problems.

Do

- Maintain healthy body weight.
- Maintain a neutral pelvic position if standing. Place one foot on a low stool if standing for long periods.
- Choose a seat with good lower back support, armrests, and a swivel base. Place a pillow at the lumbar spine to maintain normal curvature. Keep knees and hips level.
- Sleep in a side-lying position with knees and hips bent, and a pillow between the knees for support.
- Sleep on back with a lift under knees and legs or on back with 10-inch-high pillow under knees to flex hips and knees.
- Use proper body mechanics when lifting heavy objects. Bend at the knees, not at the waist, and stand up slowly while holding object close to your body.
- Participate in regular strength and flexibility training and low-impact aerobic exercise.
- Use local heat and cold application to relieve muscle tension.

Do Not

- Lean forward without bending knees.
- Lift anything above level of elbows.
- Stand unmoving for prolonged time.
- Sleep on abdomen or on back or side with legs out straight.
- Exercise without consulting HCP if having severe pain.
- Exceed prescribed amount and type of exercises without consulting HCP.
- Smoke or use tobacco products.

- Advise patients to maintain a healthy weight. Excess body weight stresses the lower back and weakens abdominal muscles that support the lower back.
- The position assumed while sleeping is also important in preventing low back pain. Advise patients to avoid sleeping in a prone position because it produces excessive lumbar lordosis, placing excessive stress on the lower back. Encourage the patient to sleep in a supine or side-lying position, with knees and hips flexed, to prevent unnecessary pressure on support muscles, ligaments, and lumbosacral joints. Recommend using a firm mattress.

LOW BACK PAIN, CHRONIC

Description

Chronic low back pain lasts more than 3 months or involves repeated incapacitating episodes. It is often progressive.

Causes, which can be difficult to determine, include (1) degenerative conditions such as arthritis or disc disease; (2) osteoporosis or other metabolic bone diseases; (3) weakness from the scar tissue of prior injury; (4) chronic strain on lower back muscles from obesity, pregnancy, or stressful postures on the job; and (5) congenital spine problems.

Spinal stenosis is a narrowing of the spinal canal. When it occurs in the lumbar area of the spine, it is a common cause of chronic low back pain. Spinal stenosis can be an acquired or an inherited condition.

- A common acquired cause is osteoarthritis in the spine. Arthritic changes (bone spurs, calcification of spinal ligaments, degeneration of discs) narrow the space around the spinal canal and nerve roots, eventually leading to compression. Inflammation caused by the compression results in pain, weakness, and numbness.
- Inherited conditions that lead to spinal stenosis include congenital spinal stenosis and scoliosis.

The pain associated with lumbar spinal stenosis often starts in the low back and then radiates to the buttock and leg. It is worse with walking and prolonged standing. Numbness, tingling, weakness, and sensation of heaviness in the legs and buttocks may also be present. Decrease in pain when the patient bends forward or sits down is often a sign of spinal stenosis.

- In most cases, spinal stenosis progresses slowly and does not cause paralysis.

Interprofessional Care

Treatment regimens are similar to those recommended for acute low back pain. Pain and stiffness are managed with mild analgesics, such as nonsteroidal antiinflammatory drugs (NSAIDs). Antidepressants such as duloxetine (Cymbalta) may help with pain management and sleep problems. The antiseizure drug gabapentin (Neurontin) may improve walking and relieve leg symptoms.

- Weight management, sufficient rest periods, local heat/cold application, and exercise and activity throughout the day help keep the muscles and joints mobilized.
- Complementary and alternative therapies such as biofeedback, acupuncture, and yoga may help to reduce the pain.
- Minimally invasive treatments, such as epidural corticosteroid injections and implanted devices that deliver pain medication, may be used for patients with chronic low back pain that does not respond to the usual therapeutic options.
- Surgery may be indicated in patients with severe chronic low back pain who do not respond to conservative care and/or have continued neurologic deficits. (See the Surgical Therapy section in Intervertebral Disc Disease, pp. 360-361.)

LUNG CANCER

Description

Lung cancer is the leading cause of cancer-related death in the United States and accounts for 28% of all cancer deaths. Female smokers have a higher risk of developing lung cancers than male smokers.

- Smoking is responsible for approximately 80% to 90% of all lung cancers. Tobacco smoke contains 60 carcinogens and causes changes in the bronchial epithelium, which usually returns to normal when smoking is discontinued.

Assessment of lung cancer risk is based on smoking exposure, with patients assigned to one of three categories: (1) smokers, people who are currently smoking; (2) nonsmokers, people who formerly smoked; and (3) never-smokers. The risk of developing lung cancer is directly related to total exposure to tobacco smoke, measured by total number of cigarettes smoked in a lifetime, age at smoking onset, depth of inhalation, tar and nicotine content, and the use of unfiltered cigarettes. Sidestream smoke (smoke from burning cigarettes, cigars) contains the same carcinogens found in mainstream smoke (smoke inhaled and exhaled by the smoker).

- Other causes of lung cancer include high levels of pollution, radiation (especially radon exposure), and asbestos. Heavy or prolonged exposure to industrial agents such as ionizing radiation, coal dust, uranium, formaldehyde, and arsenic can also increase the risk of lung cancer.

- Genetic, hormonal, and molecular influences may contribute to differences in lung cancer incidence, risk factors, and survival between men and women.

Pathophysiology

Most primary lung tumors are believed to arise from mutated epithelial cells. The development of mutations that are caused by carcinogens is influenced by various genetic factors. Once started, tumor development is promoted by epidermal growth factor. These cells grow slowly, taking 8 to 10 years for a tumor to reach 1 cm in size, the smallest lesion detectable on an x-ray. Lung cancers occur primarily in the segmental bronchi or beyond and have a preference for the upper lobes of the lungs.

Primary lung cancers are categorized into two broad types: *non–small cell lung cancer* (NSCLC) (80%) and *small cell lung cancer* (SCLC) (20%). Lung cancers metastasize primarily by direct extension and by way of the blood and lymph system. Common sites for metastasis are the liver, brain, bones, and adrenal glands.

Clinical Manifestations

Manifestations are usually nonspecific, appear late in the disease process, and depend on the type of primary lung cancer, its location, and metastatic spread.

- One of the most common first manifestations reported is a persistent cough. Blood-tinged sputum may be produced because of bleeding caused by the malignancy.
- The patient may complain of dyspnea or wheezing. Chest pain, if present, may be localized or unilateral, ranging from mild to severe.

Later manifestations include nonspecific symptoms and signs such as anorexia, fatigue, weight loss, and nausea and vomiting. Hoarseness may be present as a result of laryngeal nerve involvement. Unilateral paralysis of the diaphragm, dysphagia, and superior vena cava obstruction may occur because of intrathoracic spread of malignancy. There may be palpable lymph nodes in the neck or axillae. Mediastinal involvement may lead to pericardial effusion, cardiac tamponade, and dysrhythmias.

Paraneoplastic syndrome is caused by *humoral* factors *(hormones, cytokines)* excreted by tumor cells or by an *immune response* against the tumor. SCLCs are most often associated with the paraneoplastic syndrome. Symptoms of paraneoplastic syndrome may manifest before the diagnosis of the cancer.

- Examples of paraneoplastic syndrome are hypercalcemia, syndrome of inappropriate antidiuretic hormone (SIADH) secretion, hematologic disorders, and neurologic syndromes. These conditions may stabilize with treatment of the underlying neoplasm.

Diagnostic Studies

- Chest x-ray is used for diagnosis and assessing for metastasis.
- Biopsy is necessary for a definitive diagnosis. If thoracentesis is performed to relieve a pleural effusion, the fluid is also analyzed for malignant cells.
- Additional diagnostic tests include bone scans, CT scans, MRI, positron emission tomography (PET), blood tests, renal function tests, and pulmonary function tests.

Staging of NSCLC is performed according to the tumor-node-metastasis (TNM) staging system (see TNM Classification System, p. 781).

Interprofessional Care

Surgical resection is the treatment of choice in NSCLC stages I and IIIA without mediastinal involvement, because resection provides the best chance for a cure. For other NSCLC stages, patients may require surgery in conjunction with radiation therapy and/or chemotherapy and targeted therapy. Many NSCLCs are not resectable at the time of diagnosis. Surgical procedures that may be performed include pneumonectomy (removal of one entire lung), lobectomy (removal of one or more lung lobes), and segmental or wedge resection procedures.

Radiation therapy may be used for both NSCLC and SCLC (see Radiation Therapy, p. 733).

- Radiation relieves symptoms of dyspnea and hemoptysis from bronchial obstruction tumors and treats superior vena cava syndrome.
- Radiation can be used to treat the pain of metastatic bone lesions or cerebral metastasis, to reduce tumor mass preoperatively, or as an adjuvant measure postoperatively.

Stereotactic radiotherapy (SRT) uses high doses of radiation delivered accurately to the tumor. SRT provides an option for patients with early-stage lung cancers who are not surgical candidates for other medical reasons.

Chemotherapy is the primary treatment for SCLC. It may be used for nonresectable tumors or as an adjuvant therapy to surgery in NSCLC. A variety of chemotherapy drugs and multidrug regimens (i.e., protocols) have been used (see Chemotherapy, p. 694).

One type of targeted therapy for patients with NSCLC is erlotinib (Tarceva), which blocks signals for growth in cancer cells. Other drugs, such as bevacizumab (Avastin), inhibit new blood vessel growth (angiogenesis).

Immunotherapy with nivolumab (Opdivo) and pembrolizumab (Keytruda) may be used to boost the immune response and can shrink some tumors or slow their growth.

Nursing Management

Goals
The patient with lung cancer will have adequate airway clearance, effective breathing patterns, adequate oxygenation of tissues, minimal to no pain, and a realistic attitude about treatment and prognosis.

Nursing Diagnoses
- Ineffective airway clearance
- Ineffective breathing pattern
- Impaired gas exchange
- Anxiety

Nursing Interventions
Care of the patient with lung cancer initially involves support and reassurance during the diagnostic evaluation. Individualized care will depend on the plan for treatment.

- Assessment and symptom management are pivotal.
- For many individuals who have lung cancer, little can be done to significantly prolong their lives. Radiation therapy and chemotherapy can provide palliative relief from distressing symptoms. Constant pain may become a major problem.
- Provide patient comfort, monitor for side effects of prescribed medications, foster appropriate coping strategies for patient and caregiver, assess smoking cessation readiness, and help patients access resources to deal with the illness.

▼ Patient and Caregiver Teaching
- A wealth of material is available to the smoker who is interested in smoking cessation. See pp. 146 to 148 in Lewis et al, *Medical-Surgical Nursing,* ed 10.
- Encourage the patient and family to provide a smoke-free environment. This may include smoking cessation for multiple family members. If the treatment plan includes the use of home oxygen, instruct the patient and family on the safe use of oxygen.
- Teach the patient to recognize signs and symptoms that may indicate progression or recurrence of disease.

LYME DISEASE

Description

Lyme disease is an infection caused by the spirochete *Borrelia burgdorferi* and transmitted through the bite of an infected deer tick. The tick typically feeds on mice, dogs, cats, cows, horses, deer, and humans. Wild animals do not exhibit the illness, but clinical Lyme disease does occur in domestic animals. Person-to-person transmission does not occur.

The summer months are the peak season for human infection. Most U.S. cases occur in three areas: along the Northeastern states from Virginia to Maine, in the Midwestern states of Wisconsin and Minnesota, and along the northwestern coast of California and Oregon. More than 30,000 cases are reported annually in the United States. Reinfection is not uncommon.

Clinical Manifestations

The most characteristic sign is erythema migrans (EM), a skin lesion that occurs at the site of the tick bite within 3 to 30 days after exposure.

- The EM lesion begins as a central red macule or papule that slowly expands to include a red outer ring of up to 12 inches, resembling a bull's-eye. It may be warm to the touch but is not itchy or painful. The rash is often accompanied by flu-like symptoms, such as fever, headache, fatigue, stiff neck, swollen lymph nodes, and migratory joint and muscle pain. Loss of tone in facial muscles can manifest as Bell's palsy.
- Symptoms generally resolve over a period of weeks or months, even without treatment.
- The untreated spirochete can disseminate within several weeks or months to the heart, joints, and CNS. Cardiac manifestations such as heart block and myocarditis may require hospitalization. About 60% of persons with untreated infection develop chronic arthritic pain and swelling in the large joints, primarily the knee. Chronic neurologic complaints include short-term memory loss, cognitive impairment, shooting pains, and numbness and tingling in the feet.

Diagnostic Studies

Diagnosis is often based on clinical manifestations, in particular the EM lesion, and a history of exposure in an endemic area.

- CBC and erythrocyte sedimentation rate (ESR) are usually normal.

- A two-step laboratory testing process is recommended to confirm the diagnosis. The first step is the enzyme immunoassay (EIA), a test that will have positive results for most people with Lyme disease. If the EIA is positive or inconclusive, a Western blot test can confirm the infection.
- In individuals with neurologic involvement, cerebrospinal fluid should also be examined.

Nursing and Interprofessional Management

Active lesions can be treated with oral antibiotics. Doxycycline (Vibramycin), cefuroxime (Ceftin), and amoxicillin are often effective in early-stage infection and in preventing disease progression. Doxycycline is preferred because it treats both Lyme disease and human granulocytic anaplasmosis, which can be transmitted as a co-infection with a single tick bite. Doxycycline is effective in preventing Lyme disease when given within 3 days after the bite of a deer tick.

- Approximately 10% to 20% of people treated with antibiotics for Lyme disease may experience lingering fatigue or joint and muscle pain. The International Lyme and Associated Diseases Society supports a diagnosis of chronic Lyme disease in these cases and recommends extended antibiotic treatment until the patient experiences subjective improvement.
- Patient and caregiver teaching for the prevention of Lyme disease in endemic areas focuses on strategies for avoiding tick bites, as outlined in Table 64-13, Lewis et al, *Medical-Surgical Nursing,* ed 10, p. 1535.

MACULAR DEGENERATION

Description

Age-related *macular degeneration* (AMD) is a degeneration of the retina involving the macula that results in varying degrees of central vision loss. It is the most common cause of irreversible central vision loss in people over 60 years old in the United States. AMD is divided into two classic forms: *dry* (atrophic), which is more common, and *wet* (exudative), which is more severe. Wet AMD accounts for 90% of the cases of AMD-related blindness.

Pathophysiology

AMD is related to retinal aging. Increased risk factors for AMD include white ethnicity, family history of AMD, chronic inflammation conditions, smoking, and hypertension. Nutritional deficiencies of vitamins C, E, and beta-carotene, and zinc may play a role in the progression of AMD.

- In *dry AMD,* people notice that reading and other close-vision tasks become more difficult. This form starts with the abnormal accumulation of yellowish extracellular deposits called *drusen* in the retinal pigment epithelium. Atrophy and degeneration of macular cells then result, leading to slowly progressive and painless vision loss.
- *Wet AMD* is characterized by the growth of new blood vessels in an abnormal location in the retinal epithelium. As the new blood vessels leak, scar tissue gradually forms.

Clinical Manifestations

The patient may experience blurred and darkened vision, *scotomas* (blind spots in the visual fields), or *metamorphopsia* (distortion of vision). Acute vision loss may occur from either the dry or wet forms of AMD.

Diagnostic Studies

- Visual acuity measurement
- Ophthalmoscopic examination to look for drusen and other changes in the fundus
- Amsler grid test to define the involved area and provide a baseline for future comparison
- Fundus photography and IV fluorescein angiography to further define the extent and type of AMD
- Retinal anatomy can also be determined using optical coherence tomography (OCT) or scanning laser ophthalmoscopy.

Nursing and Interprofessional Management

Visual prognosis varies greatly for people with AMD. Limited treatment options for patients with wet AMD include several medications (i.e., ranibizumab [Lucentis], bevacizumab [Avastin], and pegaptanib [Macugen]) injected directly into the vitreous cavity. These drugs are selective inhibitors of endothelial growth factor and help to slow vision loss.

- Photodynamic therapy is used in wet AMD to destroy abnormal blood vessels without permanent damage to the retinal pigment epithelium and photoreceptor cells.
- Patients at risk for AMD (in consultation with their HCP) should consider supplements of vitamins and minerals.
- Many patients with low-vision assistive devices can continue reading and retain a license to drive during the daytime and at lower speeds.

The permanent loss of central vision associated with AMD has significant psychosocial implications for nursing care. Nursing management of the patient with uncorrectable visual impairment is discussed in Lewis et al, *Medical-Surgical Nursing,* ed 10, pp. 369 to 370, and is appropriate for the patient with AMD. It is especially important to avoid giving patients the impression that "nothing can be done" about their problem. Although therapy will not recover lost vision, much can be done to augment the remaining vision.

MALIGNANT MELANOMA

Description

Malignant melanoma is a tumor arising in cells producing melanin, usually the melanocytes of the skin. Melanoma, the deadliest form of skin cancer, can metastasize to any organ, including the brain and heart.

The exact cause of melanoma is unknown. Ultraviolet (UV) radiation from the sun is the main cause of melanoma, but artificial sources of UV radiation such as sunlamps and tanning booths can play a role. UV radiation damages the deoxyribonucleic acid (DNA) in skin cells, causing mutations in the genetic code. People with fair skin and eyes, a prior diagnosis of melanoma, or a first-degree relative diagnosed with melanoma have an increased risk. Immunosuppression and dysplastic nevi also increase the risk of melanoma.

Clinical Manifestations

About 25% of melanomas occur in existing nevi or moles; about 20% occur in dysplastic nevi. Melanoma frequently occurs on the lower legs in women and on the trunk, head, and neck in men. Because most melanoma cells continue to produce melanin, melanoma tumors are often brown or black.

- Individuals should consult an HCP immediately if a mole or lesion shows any of the clinical signs of melanoma (see Fig. 23-2, Lewis et al, *Medical-Surgical Nursing,* ed 10, p. 410). These ABCDE signs include **a**symmetry, **b**order irregularity, **c**olor varied from one area of the lesion to another, **d**iameter greater than 6 mm, and **e**volving, changing appearance.
- Any sudden or progressive increase in the size, color, or shape of a mole should be checked. When melanoma begins in the skin, it is called *cutaneous melanoma.* Melanoma can also occur in the eyes, ears, gastrointestinal tract, and oral and genital mucous membranes.

Interprofessional Care

Suspicious pigmented lesions should be biopsied using an excisional biopsy technique. The most important prognostic factor is tumor thickness at the time of diagnosis.

- Two methods are used to determine tumor thickness: the *Breslow measurement,* which indicates tumor depth in millimeters, and the *Clark level,* which indicates the depth of invasion of the tumor. The higher the number, the deeper the melanoma.

Treatment depends on the site of the original tumor, stage of the cancer, and patient's age and general health. Initial treatment of malignant melanoma is surgical excision. Melanoma that has spread to the lymph nodes or nearby sites usually requires additional therapy, such as chemotherapy, immunotherapy, targeted therapy, and/or radiation therapy.

Chemotherapy includes dacarbazine (DTIC) and temozolomide (Temodar). Adding combinations of cisplatin, carmustine, carboplatin, or vincristine improves response rate.

Immunotherapy can include cytokines (α-interferon, interleukin-2), programmed cell death protein 1 (PD-1) inhibitors, and cytotoxic T-lymphocyte–associated protein 4 (CTLA-4) inhibitors. PD-1 inhibitors include nivolumab (Opdivo) and pembrolizumab (Keytruda). Ipilimumab (Yervoy) is a CTLA-4 inhibitor.

Targeted therapy for melanoma includes BRAF and MEK inhibitors. These drugs include vemurafenib (Zelboraf), dabrafenib (Tafinlar), trametinib (Mekinist), and cobimetinib (Cotellic).

Cutaneous melanoma is nearly 100% curable by excision if diagnosed at stage 0. The presence of metastasis in the sentinel lymph node is the most important prognostic factor for recurrence. If metastasis to other organs is found (stage IV), treatment then becomes palliative.

▼ **Patient and Caregiver Teaching**

Emphasize the importance of protection from the damaging effects of the sun, such as wearing a large-brimmed hat, sunglasses, and a long-sleeved shirt of a lightly woven fabric.

- Inform patients that the rays of the sun are most dangerous at midday. Recommend that patients use a broad-spectrum sunscreen with a minimum sun protection factor (SPF) of 15 on a daily basis. Sunscreens with an SPF of 15 or higher filter 92% of UV type B (UVB) rays and make sunburn unlikely when applied appropriately. Sunscreen should be reapplied every 2 hours.
- Teach patients to self-examine their skin at least monthly to detect new or persistent skin lesions.

MALNUTRITION

Description

Malnutrition is an excess, deficit, or imbalance of essential nutrients. Malnutrition is also described as undernutrition or overnutrition. *Undernutrition* describes a state of poor nourishment as a result of inadequate diet or diseases that interfere with appetite and assimilation of ingested food. *Overnutrition* refers to the ingestion of more food than is required for body needs, as in obesity.

- The incidence of hospitalized patients who are malnourished or at nutritional risk is 30% to 50%. The prevalence of malnutrition in older adults ranges from 6% (community-dwelling older adults) to 50% (rehabilitation settings).

The following etiology-based terminology indicates the interaction and importance of inflammation on nutritional status:

- Starvation-related malnutrition, or primary protein-calorie malnutrition (PCM), occurs when nutritional needs are not met. It is a clinical state in which there is chronic starvation without inflammation (e.g., anorexia nervosa).
- Chronic disease–related malnutrition, or secondary PCM, is associated with conditions that impose sustained inflammation of a mild to moderate degree. This occurs when tissue needs are not met, although the dietary intake would be satisfactory under normal conditions. Conditions associated with this type of malnutrition include organ failure, cancer, rheumatoid arthritis, obesity, and metabolic syndrome.
- Acute disease- or injury-related malnutrition is associated with a marked inflammatory response after major infection, burn, trauma, or surgery.

Many factors contribute to the development of malnutrition, including socioeconomic factors, physical illnesses, incomplete diets, and drug-nutrient interactions.

Pathophysiology of Starvation

Initially, the body selectively uses carbohydrates (glycogen), rather than fat and protein, to meet metabolic needs. This may deplete glycogen stores in the liver and muscles within 18 hours.

- When carbohydrate stores are depleted, skeletal protein begins to be converted to glucose for energy, resulting in a negative nitrogen balance. Within 5 to 9 days, the body mobilizes fat to supply energy.
- In prolonged starvation, fat provides up to 97% of calories, conserving protein. Depletion of fat stores depends on the

amount available. Fat stores are generally used up in 4 to 6 weeks. Once fat stores are used, body proteins, including those in internal organs and plasma, are the only remaining source of energy.

The liver is the body organ that loses the most mass during protein deprivation. It gradually becomes infiltrated with fat secondary to decreased synthesis of lipoproteins. If dietary protein and other necessary constituents are not given, death will rapidly ensue.

Clinical Manifestations

Manifestations of malnutrition range from mild to emaciation and death. The most obvious clinical manifestations on physical examination are apparent in the skin (dry and scaly skin, brittle nails, rashes, hair loss), mouth (crusting and ulceration, changes in tongue), muscles (decreased mass and weakness), and CNS (mental changes such as confusion, irritability).

- The person is more susceptible to infection. Both humoral and cell-mediated immunity are deficient. Leukocytes decrease in the peripheral blood. Phagocytosis is impaired as a result of the lack of energy necessary to drive the process. Many malnourished persons are also anemic.

Diagnostic Studies

- Serum albumin and prealbumin levels are decreased.
- C-reactive protein (CRP) and serum potassium are often elevated.
- RBC count and hemoglobin (Hgb) levels indicate the presence and degree of anemia.
- WBC count and total lymphocyte count are decreased.
- Liver enzyme studies may be elevated.
- Waist circumference and waist-to-hip ratio help evaluate the response to therapy.

Nursing and Interprofessional Management

Nutritional screening identifies individuals who are malnourished or at risk for malnutrition and determines if a more detailed nutritional assessment is necessary. Hospital-specific screening tools are based on common admission assessment criteria that typically include history of weight loss, intake before admission, use of nutritional support, chewing or swallowing issues, and skin breakdown.

Obtaining an accurate measure of body weight and height and recording this information are critical components of nutritional assessment. *Body mass index* (BMI) is a measure of weight in proportion to height. BMIs outside the normal weight range are associated with increased morbidity and mortality.

Goals

The patient with malnutrition will gain weight, consume a specified number of calories per day, and have no adverse consequences related to malnutrition or nutritional therapies.

Nursing Diagnoses

- Imbalanced nutrition: less than body requirements
- Feeding self-care deficit
- Deficient fluid volume
- Risk for impaired skin integrity

Nursing Interventions

Identify patients who are at risk and determine why they are at risk. Identify nutritional risk factors and why they exist. In states of increased stress, such as surgery, severe trauma, and sepsis, more calories and protein are needed.

- Daily weights provide an ongoing record of body weight change. To obtain an accurate weight, weigh the patient at the same time each day, using the same scale, with the patient wearing the same type or amount of clothing.
- You and the dietitian can assist the patient and caregiver in the selection of high-calorie and high-protein foods.
- If the patient is unable to consume enough nutrition with a high-calorie, high-protein diet, oral liquid nutritional supplements can be added.
- Encourage the family to bring the patient's favorite food while the patient is hospitalized.

Some patients may benefit from appetite stimulants, such as megestrol acetate (Megace) or dronabinol (Marinol), to improve nutritional intake. If the patient is still unable to take in enough calories, enteral feedings may be considered (see Enteral Nutrition, p. 706). Parenteral nutrition (PN) might be initiated if enteral feedings are not feasible (see Parenteral Nutrition, p. 731).

▼ Patient and Caregiver Teaching

- Teach the patient and caregivers the importance of good nutrition and the rationale for recording the daily weight, intake, and output.
- Assess the ability of the patient and caregiver to comply with the dietary instructions related to past eating habits, religious and ethnic preferences, age, income, other resources, and state of health.
- Ensure proper follow-up care such as visits by the home health nurse and outpatient dietitian referrals.

MÉNIÈRE'S DISEASE

Description

Ménière's disease is an inner ear disease characterized by episodic vertigo, tinnitus, sensation of aural fullness, and fluctuating sensorineural hearing loss. Sudden, severe attacks of vertigo with nausea and vomiting are incapacitating. Symptoms usually begin between the ages of 30 and 60 years.

Pathophysiology

An excessive volume of endolymph ruptures the membranous labyrinth, mixing high-potassium endolymph with low-potassium perilymph.

Clinical Manifestations

- Attacks may occur without warning or be preceded by an aura consisting of a sense of fullness in the ear, increasing tinnitus, and muffled hearing.
- The patient may report a whirling sensation and the feeling of being pulled to the ground ("drop attack").
- Autonomic signs and symptoms include pallor, sweating, nausea, and vomiting.
- Duration of an attack may be hours or days, and attacks may occur several times per year. The clinical course is highly variable.
- Low-pitched tinnitus may be present continuously in the affected ear, or it may be intensified during an attack.
- Hearing loss fluctuates, worsening with each vertigo attack, with the risk of progression to permanent hearing loss.

Diagnostic Studies

- Audiogram results demonstrate mild, low-frequency hearing loss.
- Vestibular tests may isolate the cause of vertigo.
- Glycerol test supports the diagnosis if hearing improvement occurs.

Nursing and Interprofessional Management

During an acute attack, antihistamines, anticholinergics, and benzodiazepines can decrease the abnormal sensation and lessen symptoms such as nausea and vomiting. Acute vertigo is treated symptomatically with bed rest, sedation, and antiemetics or antivertigo drugs for motion sickness. Diazepam (Valium), meclizine (Antivert), and fentanyl with droperidol may be used to reduce the vertigo. Most patients respond to the prescribed drugs but must learn to live with the unpredictability of the attacks and the loss of hearing.

- During an acute attack, a patient needs reassurance that the condition is not life-threatening.
- Focus on providing only essential care, because movement aggravates vertigo.
- Side rails should be up and the bed in low position if the patient is in bed. Avoid the use of lights and television, which exacerbate symptoms. Have an emesis basin available because vomiting is common. Assist with ambulation because unsteadiness remains after an attack.

Management between attacks may include calcium channel blockers, diuretics, antihistamines, and a low-sodium diet.

With frequent incapacitating attacks and reduced quality of life, surgical therapy is indicated. Surgical options include endolymphatic shunt, vestibular nerve resection, and labyrinth ablation. Careful management can decrease the possibility of progressive sensorineural loss in many patients.

MENINGITIS, BACTERIAL

Description

Meningitis is an acute inflammation of the meningeal tissues surrounding the brain and spinal cord. Older adults and people who are debilitated are more often affected than the general population. College students living in dormitories and individuals living in institutions (e.g., prisoners) are also at a high risk for contracting meningitis.

Bacterial meningitis is considered a medical emergency. If it is left untreated, the mortality rate approaches 100%. Bacterial meningitis must be reported to the Centers for Disease Control and Prevention (CDC). See Table 34, p. 210, for a comparison of meningitis and encephalitis.

Pathophysiology

Meningitis usually occurs in the fall, winter, or early spring and is often secondary to viral respiratory disease. *Streptococcus pneumoniae* and *Neisseria meningitidis* are the leading causes of bacterial meningitis. *N. meningitidis* has at least 13 different subtypes (serogroups), with five of them (A, B, C, Y, W) causing most cases. Organisms usually gain entry to the central nervous system (CNS) through the upper respiratory tract or bloodstream, but they may enter by direct extension from penetrating wounds of the skull or through fractured sinuses in basal skull fractures.

The inflammatory response to the infection tends to increase cerebrospinal fluid (CSF) production with a moderate increase in intracranial pressure (ICP). The purulent secretion produced by bacteria quickly spreads to other areas of the brain through the CSF.

- All patients with meningitis must be observed closely for manifestations of increased ICP, which is thought to be a result of swelling around the dura and increased CSF volume. (See Increased Intracranial Pressure, p. 342.)

Clinical Manifestations

Fever, severe headache, nausea, vomiting, and *nuchal rigidity* (resistance to flexion of the neck) are key signs.

- Photophobia, a decreased level of consciousness (LOC), and signs of increased ICP may also be present.
- If the infecting organism is the meningococcus, a skin rash is common and petechiae may be seen on the trunk, lower extremities, and mucous membranes.
- Seizures occur in one third of all cases of meningitis.
- Coma is associated with a poor prognosis and occurs in 5% to 10% of patients with bacterial meningitis.

Complications

The most common acute complication of bacterial meningitis is increased ICP. Another complication is residual neurologic dysfunction of one or more cranial nerves.

- The optic nerve (CN II) is compressed by increased ICP. Papilledema is often present, and blindness may occur.
- When the oculomotor (CN III), trochlear (CN IV), and abducens (CN VI) nerves are irritated, ocular movements are affected. Ptosis, unequal pupils, and diplopia are common.
- Irritation of the trigeminal nerve (CN V) results in sensory losses and loss of the corneal reflex. Irritation of the facial nerve (CN VII) may produce facial paresis. Irritation of the vestibulocochlear nerve (CN VIII) causes tinnitus, vertigo, and deafness.
- Hemiparesis, dysphasia, and hemianopsia may also occur, with these signs usually resolving over time.
- Acute cerebral edema may cause seizures, optic nerve palsy, bradycardia, hypertensive coma, and death.
- Headaches may occur for months after the diagnosis of meningitis until the irritation and inflammation have completely resolved.
- A noncommunicating hydrocephalus may occur if the exudate causes adhesions that prevent the normal flow of the CSF from the ventricles. CSF reabsorption by the arachnoid villi may also

be obstructed by the exudate. Surgical implantation of a shunt is the only treatment.

■ A complication of meningococcal meningitis is *Waterhouse-Friderichsen syndrome*. The syndrome is manifested by petechiae, disseminated intravascular coagulation (DIC), and adrenal hemorrhage.

Diagnostic Studies

When a patient has manifestations suggestive of bacterial meningitis, a blood culture and CT scan should be done. Diagnosis is usually verified by doing a lumbar puncture with analysis of the CSF.

■ CSF, sputum, and nasopharyngeal secretions are used to identify the causative organism.
■ Skull x-rays may detect infected sinuses.
■ CT scans may reveal increased ICP or hydrocephalus.

Interprofessional Care

Prevention of respiratory tract infections through vaccination programs for pneumococcal pneumonia and influenza is important. Three kinds of meningococcal vaccines are available. They protect against all serogroups of meningococcal disease that are most commonly seen in the United States, but they will not prevent all cases.

Rapid diagnosis based on a history and physical examination is crucial because the patient is usually in a critical state when health care is sought. When meningitis is suspected, antibiotic therapy is instituted after collection of culture specimens, even before the diagnosis is confirmed. Penicillin, ampicillin, vancomycin, ceftriaxone (Rocephin), or cefotaxime (Claforan) are some commonly prescribed drugs for treating bacterial meningitis. Dexamethasone may also be prescribed before or with the first dose of antibiotics.

Nursing Management
Goals
The patient with meningitis will have a return to maximal neurologic functioning, resolution of infection, and control of pain and discomfort.
Nursing Diagnoses
■ Decreased intracranial adaptive capacity
■ Risk for ineffective cerebral tissue perfusion
■ Acute pain
■ Hyperthermia
Nursing Interventions
Prevention of respiratory infections through vaccination programs for pneumococcal pneumonia and influenza is very important.

Early and vigorous treatment of respiratory and ear infections is important. People who have had close contact with anyone who has meningitis should be given prophylactic antibiotics.

The patient with meningitis is acutely ill. The fever is high, and head pain is severe. Irritation of the cerebral cortex may result in seizures with changes in mental status and level of consciousness (LOC). The severity of manifestations is dependent on the level of ICP.

- Assess and record vital signs, neurologic status, fluid intake and output, skin, and lung fields at regular intervals based on the patient's condition.
- Head and neck pain secondary to movement require attention. Codeine provides some pain relief without undue sedation for most patients. A darkened room and cool cloth over the eyes relieve the discomfort of photophobia. For the delirious patient, additional low lighting may be necessary to decrease hallucinations.
- All patients suffer some degree of mental distortion and hypersensitivity and may be frightened and misinterpret the environment. Make every attempt to minimize environmental stimuli and prevent injury.

If seizures occur, take protective measures. Administer antiseizure medications as ordered. Problems associated with increased ICP need to be managed (see Increased Intracranial Pressure, p. 342).

Fever must be vigorously treated because it increases cerebral edema and the frequency of seizures. Aspirin or acetaminophen may be used to reduce fever. If the fever is resistant to aspirin or acetaminophen, more vigorous means are necessary, such as use of a cooling blanket. If a cooling blanket is not available, tepid sponge baths with water may be effective. Because high fever greatly increases the metabolic rate, the patient should be assessed for dehydration and adequacy of intake. Supplemental feeding (e.g., enteral nutrition) to maintain adequate nutritional intake may be necessary.

- Meningitis generally requires respiratory isolation until the cultures are negative. Meningococcal meningitis is highly contagious, whereas other causes of meningitis may pose minimal to no infection risk with patient contact.
- After the acute period has passed, stress the importance of good nutrition with an emphasis on a high-protein, high-caloric diet in small, frequent feedings.
- Muscle rigidity may persist in the neck and backs of the legs. Progressive range-of-motion (ROM) exercises and warm baths are useful. Have the patient gradually increase activity as tolerated, but encourage adequate rest and sleep.

- Residual effects can result in sequelae such as dementia, seizures, deafness, hemiplegia, and hydrocephalus. Assess vision,
  hearing, cognitive skills, and motor and sensory abilities after
  recovery with appropriate referrals as indicated.
- Throughout the acute and convalescent periods, be aware of the
  anxiety and stress experienced by the caregiver and other family
  members.
- A general nursing care plan for the person with bacterial meningitis is available in eNursing Care Plan 56-2, available on the
  website.

METABOLIC SYNDROME

Description
Metabolic syndrome is a group of metabolic risk factors that
increase an individual's chance of developing cardiovascular
disease, stroke, and diabetes mellitus. About one in three adults
have metabolic syndrome. The syndrome is more prevalent among
people 60 years of age and older.

Metabolic syndrome is characterized by a cluster of health problems, including obesity, hypertension, abnormal lipid levels, and
high blood glucose.

Pathophysiology
The main underlying risk factor for metabolic syndrome is insulin
resistance related to excessive visceral fat (Fig. 17). Insulin resistance is diminished ability of the body's cells to respond to the
action of insulin. The pancreas compensates by secreting more
insulin, resulting in hyperinsulinemia.

Other characteristics of metabolic syndrome include hypertension, increased risk for clotting, and abnormalities in cholesterol
levels. The net effect of these conditions is an increased prevalence
of coronary artery disease.

- African Americans, Hispanics, Native Americans, and Asians
  are at an increased risk for metabolic syndrome.
- Environmental factors that influence the chances of having the
  syndrome are the same as those involved in the development of
  obesity.
- Metabolic syndrome is also associated with aging.

Clinical Manifestations
Manifestations include impaired fasting blood glucose, hypertension, abnormal cholesterol levels, and obesity. Patients with this

PATHOPHYSIOLOGY MAP

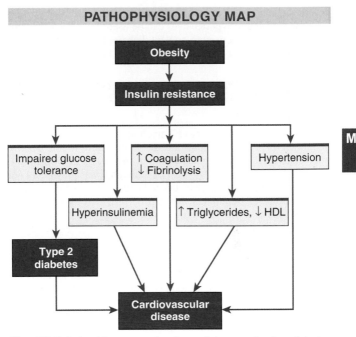

Fig. 17 Relationship among insulin resistance, obesity, diabetes mellitus, and cardiovascular disease. *HDL,* High-density lipoprotein.

syndrome are at a higher risk for heart disease, stroke, diabetes, renal disease, and polycystic ovary syndrome.

Nursing and Interprofessional Management

Lifestyle modifications are the first-line interventions to reduce the risk factors for metabolic syndrome. Management or reversal of metabolic syndrome can be achieved by reducing the major risk factors for cardiovascular disease: reducing low-density lipoprotein (LDL) cholesterol, stopping smoking, lowering BP, and reducing glucose levels. For long-term risk reduction, weight should be decreased, physical activity increased, and healthy dietary habits established.

You can assist patients by providing information on healthy diets, exercise, and positive lifestyle changes. Although there is no specific medication for metabolic syndrome, cholesterol-lowering medication and antihypertensives can be used. Metformin (Glucophage) has also been used to prevent diabetes by lowering glucose levels and enhancing the sensitivity of cells to insulin.

MULTIPLE MYELOMA

Description

Multiple myeloma, or plasma cell myeloma, is a condition in which neoplastic plasma cells infiltrate the bone marrow and destroy bone. The disease is twice as common in men as in women and usually develops after age 40 years. Although it was previously not considered curable, the 5-year survival rate is close to 45% because of the variety of treatments that can be provided throughout the course of the disease.

Pathophysiology

The cause of multiple myeloma is unknown. Exposure to radiation, organic chemicals (e.g., benzene), herbicides, and insecticides may play a role. Obesity, genetic factors, and viral infection may also influence the risk of developing multiple myeloma.

Instead of plasma cells producing antibodies to fight different infections, myeloma tumors produce monoclonal antibodies (immunoglobulins). *Monoclonal* means they are all of one kind, making them ineffective and even harmful. Not only do they not fight infections, but they also infiltrate the bone marrow. These monoclonal proteins (called M proteins) are made up of two light chains and two heavy chains. *Bence Jones proteins* are the light chain part of these monoclonal antibodies. They show up in the urine in many patients with multiple myeloma.

Production of excessive and abnormal amounts of interleukins (IL-4, IL-5, IL-6) also contributes to the pathologic process of bone destruction. The body's normal immune response is compromised by the reduction in number of normal plasma cells.

- Ultimately the end-organ effects of myeloma are seen in the bones and kidneys and possibly the spleen, lymph nodes, and liver.

Clinical Manifestations

Multiple myeloma develops slowly and insidiously.

- The patient often does not manifest symptoms until the disease is advanced, at which time skeletal pain is the major symptom. Pain in the pelvis, spine, and ribs is common.

- Diffuse osteoporosis develops as the myeloma protein destroys bone. Osteolytic lesions are seen on x-rays in the skull, vertebrae, and ribs. Vertebral destruction can lead to vertebral collapse with compression of the spinal cord.
- Loss of bone integrity can lead to the development of pathologic fractures. Bone degeneration causes calcium loss from bones, resulting in hypercalcemia. Hypercalcemia may cause renal, GI, or neurologic changes, such as polyuria, anorexia, confusion, and ultimately seizures, coma, and cardiac problems.
- The high levels of M protein can result in renal failure from renal tubular obstruction and interstitial nephritis.
- The patient may display manifestations of anemia, thrombocytopenia, and granulocytopenia, all of which are related to the replacement of normal bone marrow with plasma cells.

Diagnostic Studies

- Pancytopenia, hyperuricemia, hypercalcemia, and elevated creatinine may be found.
- Excessive production and secretion of monoclonal (M) protein is found in blood and urine.
- The light-chain part of the M protein (called Bence Jones protein) can be detected in the urine.
- Bone marrow examination shows significantly increased numbers of plasma cells.
- Skeletal bone surveys, MRI, and/or positron emission tomography (PET) and CT scans show distinct lytic areas of bone erosions; generalized thinning of the bones or fractures, especially in the vertebrae, ribs, pelvis, and bones of the thigh and upper arms.
- The simplest measure of prognosis in multiple myeloma is based on blood levels of two markers: β_2-microglobulin and albumin. In general, higher levels of these two markers are associated with a poorer prognosis.

Interprofessional Care

The therapeutic approach involves managing both the disease and its symptoms. Multiple myeloma is seldom cured, but treatment can relieve symptoms, produce remission, and prolong life. Current treatment options include "watchful waiting" (for early multiple myeloma), chemotherapy, immunotherapy and targeted therapy, and hematopoietic stem cell transplantation (HSCT).

Ambulation and adequate hydration are used to treat hypercalcemia, dehydration, and potential renal damage. Weight bearing helps the bones reabsorb some calcium, and fluids dilute calcium and prevent protein precipitates from causing renal tubular obstruction.

Control of pain and prevention of pathologic fractures are other goals of interprofessional care. Analgesics, orthopedic supports, and localized radiation help reduce skeletal pain. Surgical procedures, such as vertebroplasty, may be done to support degenerative vertebrae.

Chemotherapy with corticosteroids is usually the first treatment recommended and is used to reduce the number of plasma cells (see Chemotherapy, p. 694). The chemotherapy regimen usually includes a corticosteroid (dexamethasone or prednisone) plus one or two agents such as melphalan (Alkeran), vincristine, cyclophosphamide, doxorubicin, and bendamustine (Treanda). High-dose chemotherapy followed by HSCT has evolved as the standard of care in eligible patients.

Immunotherapy and targeted therapy are also used to treat multiple myeloma. Immunomodulator drugs include thalidomide (Thalidomide), lenalidomide (Revlimid), and pomalidomide (Pomalyst). Proteosome inhibitors include bortezomib (Velcade) and carfilzomib (Kyprolis). Panobinostat (Farydak) is a drug that can affect which genes are active inside of cells.

Drugs may be used to treat the complications of multiple myeloma. For example, allopurinol (Zyloprim) may be given to reduce hyperuricemia, and IV furosemide (Lasix) promotes renal excretion of calcium. Radiation therapy is another component of treatment, primarily because of its effect on localized lesions.

Nursing Management

Maintaining adequate hydration is a primary nursing consideration to minimize problems from hypercalcemia. Fluids are administered to achieve a urine output of 1.5 to 2 L/day if the patient does not already have renal compromise. Because of the myeloma proteins, the patient is at additional risk for renal dysfunction. Monitor electrolytes and fluid balance closely.

Because of the potential for pathologic fractures, use caution when moving and ambulating the patient. A slight twist or strain on a weakened bone may be sufficient to cause a fracture.

Pain management requires innovative and knowledgeable nursing interventions. Analgesics, such as nonsteroidal antiinflammatory drugs (NSAIDs), acetaminophen, or acetaminophen with codeine, may be more effective than opioids alone in diminishing bone pain. Braces, especially for the spine, may also help prevent pain.

- Assessment and prompt treatment of infection are important.
- The patient's psychosocial needs require sensitive, skilled management. Help the patient and significant others adapt to

changes fostered by chronic sickness and adjust to the losses related to the disease process, while helping to maximize functioning and quality of life.

MULTIPLE SCLEROSIS

Description

Multiple sclerosis (MS) is a chronic, progressive, degenerative disorder of the central nervous system (CNS) characterized by demyelination of the nerve fibers of the brain and spinal cord. The age at onset of MS is usually between 20 and 50 years, although it can occur in young teens and much older adults. Women are affected more often than men.

- Incidence of MS is five times higher in temperate climates, such as those found in Europe, Canada, and the northern United States, than in tropical regions.

Pathophysiology

It is unlikely that MS is related to a single cause; the disease develops in a genetically susceptible person as a result of environmental exposure, such as an infection. Multiple genes are believed to be involved in the inherited susceptibility to MS, and first-, second-, and third-degree relatives of patients with MS are at an increased risk.

MS is characterized by chronic inflammation, demyelination, and gliosis (scarring) in the CNS. The primary neuropathologic condition is an autoimmune disease caused by autoreactive T cells. An environmental factor or virus in genetically susceptible individuals may initially trigger this process. Possible precipitating factors include infection, smoking, physical injury, emotional stress, excessive fatigue, and pregnancy.

The activated T cells migrate to the CNS, causing blood-brain barrier disruption. Subsequent antigen-antibody reaction within the CNS results in an inflammatory response leading to axon demyelination.

- Initially, attacks on the neuron myelin sheaths in the brain and spinal cord result in damage to the myelin sheath. However, the nerve fiber is not affected. Transmission of nerve impulses still occurs, although transmission is slowed. The patient may complain of a noticeable impairment of function (e.g., weakness). However, the myelin can regenerate. When it does, symptoms disappear and the patient experiences a remission.
- As ongoing inflammation occurs, nearby oligodendrocytes are affected, and myelin loses the ability to regenerate. Eventually

M

damage to the underlying axon disrupts impulse transmission, resulting in permanent loss of nerve function.
- As inflammation subsides, glial scar tissue replaces the damaged tissue, leading to formation of hard, sclerotic plaques throughout the CNS white matter.

Clinical Manifestations

The onset is often insidious and gradual, with vague, intermittent symptoms. The disease may not be diagnosed until years after the onset of the first symptom.

- The disease is characterized by chronic progressive deterioration in some patients and remissions and exacerbations in others. With repeated exacerbations, the overall trend is progressive deterioration in neurologic function. Clinical manifestations vary according to areas of the CNS involved. A classification scheme with four primary patterns of MS has been developed (Table 57).
- Blurred or double vision, red-green color distortion, or even blindness in one eye may be the first symptom experienced by a person with MS.
- Many patients describe muscle weakness in the extremities as well as problems with coordination and balance. Those symptoms may even affect walking or standing. MS can cause partial or complete paralysis in the worst cases.
- Sensory symptoms include numbness and tingling, vertigo, tinnitus, decreased hearing, and chronic neuropathic pain.
- Cerebellar signs include nystagmus, ataxia, dysarthria, and dysphagia.
- Severe fatigue is aggravated by heat, humidity, deconditioning, and drug side effects.
- Bowel and bladder function can be affected if the sclerotic plaque is located in the areas of the CNS that control elimination. Problems usually include constipation and a spastic (uninhibited) bladder.
- Sexual dysfunction occurs in many people. Physiologic erectile dysfunction may result from spinal cord involvement in men. Women may experience decreased libido, difficulty with orgasmic response, painful intercourse, and decreased vaginal lubrication.
- About half of people with MS will experience some problems with cognitive function, including difficulties with short-term memory, attention, information processing, and word finding. General intellect remains unchanged and intact, including long-term memory, conversational skills, and reading comprehension.

TABLE 57	Patterns of Multiple Sclerosis
MS Category	**Characteristics**
Relapsing-remitting	Clearly defined attacks of worsening neurologic function *(relapses)* with partial or complete recovery *(remission)* Approximately 85% of people are initially diagnosed with this type of MS
Primary-progressive	Steadily worsening neurologic function from the beginning with minor improvements but no distinct relapses or remissions About 10% of people are diagnosed with this type of MS
Secondary-progressive	A relapsing-remitting initial course, followed by progression with or without occasional relapses, minor remissions, and plateaus New treatments may slow progression Most people initially diagnosed with relapsing-remitting MS eventually transition to this type
Progressive-relapsing	Progressive disease from onset, with clear acute relapses, with or without full recovery Periods between relapses are characterized by continuing progression Only 5% of people experience this type of MS

M

The average life expectancy after the onset of symptoms is more than 25 years. Death usually occurs because of the infectious complications (e.g., pneumonia) of immobility or because of unrelated disease.

Diagnostic Studies

Because there is no definitive diagnostic test for MS, factors considered are history, clinical manifestations, and results of diagnostic testing.

- MRI of the brain and spinal cord may show the presence of plaques, inflammation, atrophy, and tissue breakdown and destruction.

- Cerebrospinal fluid (CSF) analysis may show an increase in immunoglobulin G (IgG) or the presence of oligoclonal banding.
- Evoked potentials are often delayed as a result of decreased nerve conduction from the eye and ear to the brain.

A diagnosis of MS requires evidence of at least two inflammatory demyelinating lesions in at least two different locations within the CNS, along with evidence of damage or an attack occurring at different times (usually 1 month or more apart). In addition, all other possible diagnoses must have been ruled out.

Interprofessional Care

Because there is currently no cure for MS, interprofessional care is aimed at treating the disease process and providing symptomatic relief.

Drug Therapy

Disease-modifying therapy is more effective when initiated early in the course of MS. The initial treatment of MS is the use of immunomodulator drugs to modify the disease progression and prevent relapses. These drugs include interferon β-1b (Betaseron, Extavia), interferon β-1a (Avonex, Rebif), and glatiramer acetate (Copaxone).

- Fingolimod (Gilenya) reduces MS disease activity by preventing lymphocytes from reaching the CNS and causing damage.
- Teriflunomide (Aubagio) is an immunomodulatory agent with antiinflammatory properties.
- For more active and aggressive forms of MS, natalizumab (Tysabri), alemtuzumab (Lemtrada), mitoxantrone, and dimethyl fumarate (Tecfidera) may be used. Natalizumab is given when patients have had an inadequate response to other drugs. Alemtuzumab is generally reserved for patients who have an inadequate response to two or more drugs indicated for the treatment of MS. Mitoxantrone, an antineoplastic medication, has serious adverse effects, including cardiotoxicity, leukemia, and infertility. Dimethyl fumarate activates the Nrf2 pathway. This pathway provides a way for cells in the body to defend themselves against inflammation and oxidative stress caused by MS.
- Corticosteroids (e.g., methylprednisolone, prednisone) are the most helpful agents for treating acute exacerbations of the disease by reducing edema and acute inflammation at the site of demyelination. However, these drugs do not affect the ultimate outcome or degree of residual neurologic impairment from the exacerbation.

Many other drugs are used to treat the symptoms of MS. Antispasmodics are used for spasticity. Amantadine and CNS stimulants (methylphenidate [Ritalin] and modafinil [Provigil]) are used to alleviate fatigue. Anticholinergics are used to treat bladder symptoms. Donepezil (Aricept), an acetylcholinesterase inhibitor, is used to treat cognitive impairment. Tricyclic antidepressants and antiseizure drugs are used for chronic pain.

Other Therapy
Surgical intervention (e.g., neurectomy, rhizotomy, cordotomy), dorsal-column electrical stimulation, or intrathecal baclofen (Lioresal) delivered by pump may be required if spasticity is not controlled with antispasmodics. Tremors that become unmanageable with pharmacologic therapy are sometimes treated by thalamotomy or deep brain stimulation.

M

Neurologic function sometimes improves with physical therapy and speech therapy. Exercise decreases spasticity, increases coordination, and retrains unaffected muscles to substitute for impaired ones. An especially beneficial type of physical therapy is water exercise.

Nursing Management
Goals
The patient with MS will maximize neuromuscular function, maintain independence in activities of daily living for as long as possible, manage disabling fatigue, optimize psychosocial well-being, adjust to the illness, and reduce factors that precipitate exacerbations.

Nursing Diagnoses
- Impaired physical mobility
- Impaired urinary elimination
- Ineffective health management

Nursing Interventions
The patient with MS should be aware of triggers that may cause exacerbations or worsening of the disease. Exacerbations of MS are triggered by infection (especially upper respiratory and urinary tract infections), trauma, childbirth, stress, fatigue, and climatic changes. Assist the patient to identify particular triggers and develop ways to avoid them or minimize their effects.

- During the diagnostic phase, the patient needs reassurance that even though there is a tentative diagnosis of MS, certain diagnostic studies must be made to rule out other neurologic disorders. The patient with recently diagnosed MS may need assistance with the grieving process.
- During an acute exacerbation, the patient may need to be immobile and confined to bed. The focus of nursing intervention at this phase is to prevent complications of immobility.

▼ Patient and Caregiver Teaching

- Teach about building a general resistance to illness. This includes avoiding fatigue, extremes of heat and cold, and exposure to infection.
- Teach the patient to achieve a good balance of exercise and rest, eat nutritious and well-balanced meals, and minimize caffeine intake.
- Patients should know their treatment regimens, the side effects of drugs, and drug interactions with over-the-counter preparations.
- Bladder control is a major problem for many patients. Although anticholinergics may be beneficial for some patients to decrease spasticity, you may need to teach others self-catheterization.
- Increasing dietary fiber may help some patients avoid constipation.

The National Multiple Sclerosis Society and its local chapters can offer a variety of services to meet the needs of MS patients and their families.

MYASTHENIA GRAVIS

Description

Myasthenia gravis (MG) is an autoimmune disease of the neuromuscular junction characterized by fluctuating weakness of certain skeletal muscle groups. The mean age at onset in women is 28 years, with a mean age at onset in men of 42 years.

Pathophysiology

MG is caused by an autoimmune process in which antibodies are produced that attack acetylcholine (ACh) receptors. A reduction in the number of ACh receptor sites at the neuromuscular junction prevents ACh molecules from attaching to receptors and stimulating muscle contraction. Anti-ACh receptor antibodies are detectable in the serum of most patients with MG. Thymic hyperplasia and tumors are common in patients with MG, suggesting that autoantibody production occurs in the thymus.

Clinical Manifestations

The primary feature is fluctuating weakness of skeletal muscle. This weakness increases with muscle use throughout the day. Strength is usually restored after a period of rest. The muscles most often involved are those used for moving the eyes and eyelids, chewing, swallowing, speaking, and breathing.

- At onset, only the ocular muscles are involved for many patients, with bilateral ptosis and constant or transient diplopia as a result.
- Facial mobility and expression can be impaired. There may be difficulty in chewing and swallowing food. Speech is affected, and the voice often fades during conversations.
- No other signs of neural disorder accompany MG. There is no sensory loss, reflexes are normal, and muscle atrophy is rare.
- The course of the disease is highly variable. Some patients may have short-term remissions, others may stabilize, and still others may have severe progressive involvement.
- Exacerbations of MG can be precipitated by respiratory infection, surgery, emotional distress, pregnancy, exposure to drugs that may increase myasthenic weakness, or beginning treatment with corticosteroids. The major complications of MG result from muscle weakness affecting swallowing and breathing. An acute exacerbation of MG that results in aspiration, respiratory infection, and respiratory insufficiency is known as a *myasthenic crisis*.

Diagnostic Studies

The diagnosis of MG can be made on the basis of history and physical examination.

- Electromyography (EMG) may show a decremental response to repeated stimulation of the hand muscles, indicating muscle fatigue.
- The Tensilon test reveals improved muscle contractility after an IV injection of the anticholinesterase agent edrophonium chloride.
- If a confirmed diagnosis of MG has been made, a chest CT scan may be done to evaluate the thymus.

Interprofessional Care

Drug Therapy

Drug therapy for MG includes anticholinesterase drugs, alternate-day corticosteroids, and immunosuppressants.

- Acetylcholinesterase is the enzyme that breaks down ACh in the synaptic cleft. Acetylcholinesterase inhibitors prolong the action of ACh and facilitate transmission of impulses at the neuromuscular junction. Pyridostigmine (Mestinon) is the most successful drug in this group.
- Corticosteroids (prednisone) are used to suppress the immune response. Drugs such as azathioprine (Imuran), mycopheno-late (CellCept), and cyclosporine may also be used for immunosuppression.

M

Other Therapies
Because the presence of the thymus gland in the patient with MG
appears to enhance the production of ACh receptor antibodies,
removal of the thymus gland results in improvement in a majority
of patients.
- Plasmapheresis and IV immunoglobulin G can provide a short-
  term improvement in symptoms and is indicated for patients in
  crisis or in preparation for surgery when corticosteroids must
  be avoided.

Nursing Management
Goals
The patient with MG will have a return of normal muscle endur-
ance, manage fatigue, avoid complications, and maintain a quality
of life appropriate to disease course.
Nursing Diagnoses
- Ineffective airway clearance
- Impaired verbal communication
- Activity intolerance
- Disturbed body image
Nursing Interventions
The patient with MG who is admitted to the hospital usually has a
respiratory tract infection or is in acute myasthenic crisis. Nursing
care is aimed at maintaining adequate ventilation, continuing drug
therapy, and watching for side effects of therapy. Be able to distinguish cholinergic from myasthenic crisis, because the causes and
treatment of the two differ greatly (Table 58).
- Care focuses on reducing the impact of neurologic deficits on
  activities of daily living.
- Scheduling doses of medication so that peak action is reached
  at mealtime may make eating less difficult. Teach the patient
  about a balanced diet of foods that can be chewed and swallowed. Semisolid foods may be easier to eat than solids or
  liquids.
- Arrange diversional activities that require little physical effort
  and match the interests of the patient.
▼ Patient and Caregiver Teaching
Teaching should focus on following the medical regimen, avoiding
potential adverse reactions to drugs, planning activities of daily
living to avoid fatigue, locating available community resources,
and managing complications of the disease and therapy (crisis
conditions).
- Explore community resources such as the Myasthenia Gravis
  Society and MG support groups.

TABLE 58 Comparison of Myasthenic and Cholinergic Crises

	Myasthenic Crisis	Cholinergic Crisis
Cause(s)	Exacerbation of myasthenia by precipitating factors or occurring after failure to take drug as prescribed or with drug dose too low	Overdose of anticholinesterase drugs resulting in increased ACh at the receptor sites, remission (spontaneous or after thymectomy)
Differential Diagnosis	Improved strength after IV administration of anticholinesterase drugs	Weakness within 1 hr after ingestion of anticholinesterase
	Increased weakness of skeletal muscles manifesting as ptosis, bulbar signs (e.g., difficulty swallowing, difficulty articulating words), or dyspnea	Increased weakness of skeletal muscles manifesting as ptosis, bulbar signs, dyspnea; smooth muscle effects: pupillary miosis, salivation, diarrhea, nausea or vomiting, abdominal cramps, increased bronchial secretions, sweating, lacrimation

ACh, Acetylcholine.

MYOCARDIAL INFARCTION

Myocardial infarction is part of the spectrum referred to as acute coronary syndrome. See Acute Coronary Syndrome, p. 5, for the discussion of this disorder.

MYOCARDITIS

Description

Myocarditis is a focal or diffuse inflammation of the myocardium that has been associated with viral, bacterial, and fungal infections and with radiation therapy, pharmacologic and chemical factors, and autoimmune disorders. Coxsackieviruses A and B are the most common etiologic agents.

Pathophysiology

When the myocardium becomes infected, the causative agent invades the myocytes and causes cellular damage and necrosis. The immune response is activated, cytokines and oxygen free radicals are released, and an autoimmune response occurs, resulting in further destruction of myocytes. Myocarditis results in cardiac dysfunction and possibly dilated cardiomyopathy (see Cardiomyopathy, p. 106).

Clinical Manifestations

Clinical manifestations of myocarditis are variable, ranging from a benign course without overt symptoms to severe heart involvement or sudden cardiac death. Fever, fatigue, malaise, myalgias, pharyngitis, dyspnea, lymphadenopathy, and nausea and vomiting are early systemic manifestations of the viral illness.

- *Early:* Cardiac signs appear 7 to 10 days after viral infection and include pericardial chest pain with a pericardial friction rub and effusion.
- *Late:* Cardiac signs relate to the development of heart failure and may include S_3, crackles, jugular venous distention, syncope, peripheral edema, and angina.

Diagnostic Studies

- ECG changes are often nonspecific and reflect associated pericardial involvement, including diffuse ST-segment abnormalities. Dysrhythmias and conduction disturbances may be present.
- Laboratory findings are often inconclusive, with mild to moderate leukocytosis and atypical lymphocytes, increased erythrocyte sedimentation rate (ESR) and C-reactive protein (CRP) levels, elevated levels of cardiac biomarkers such as troponin, and elevated viral titers. (Virus is generally present in tissue and fluid samples only during the initial 8 to 10 days of illness.)
- Histologic confirmation is through an endomyocardial biopsy. A biopsy done during the initial 6 weeks of acute illness is most diagnostic because this is the period during which lymphocytic infiltration and myocyte damage indicative of myocarditis are present.
- Echocardiography, radionuclide scans, and MRI are used to evaluate cardiac function.

Interprofessional Care

The treatment for myocarditis consists of managing associated symptoms.

- Digoxin improves heart contractility and reduces ventricular rate but is used cautiously in patients with myocarditis because of the heart's increased sensitivity to the adverse effects of this drug (e.g., dysrhythmias, potential toxicity).
- Angiotensin-converting enzyme (ACE) inhibitors and β-adrenergic blockers are used if the heart is enlarged or to treat heart failure.
- Diuretics reduce fluid volume and decrease preload. If hypotension is not present, nitroprusside and milrinone may be used to reduce afterload and improve cardiac output by decreasing systemic vascular resistance.

Immunosuppressive agents may reduce myocardial inflammation and prevent irreversible heart damage. However, the use of these agents for the treatment of myocarditis remains controversial because the drugs may also lead to a recurrence.

General supportive measures for the management of myocarditis include oxygen therapy, bed rest, and restricted activity. In cases of severe heart failure, intraaortic balloon pump therapy and ventricular assist devices may be required.

Nursing Management

Focus your interventions on instituting measures to decrease cardiac workload (e.g., use of semi-Fowler's position, spaced activity and rest periods, provisions for a quiet environment). Carefully monitor medications that increase the heart's contractility and decrease the preload or afterload.

The patient may be anxious about the diagnosis of myocarditis and recovery. Assess the level of anxiety, institute measures to decrease anxiety, and keep the patient and caregivers informed about the therapeutic plan.

The patient who receives immunosuppressive therapy is at an increased risk for infection. Monitor for complications and provide the patient with proper infection control procedures.

NAUSEA AND VOMITING

Description

Nausea and vomiting are the most common manifestations of GI diseases. Although each manifestation can occur independently, they are closely related and usually treated as one problem. Nausea and vomiting occur in a wide variety of GI disorders and in conditions unrelated to GI disease, including pregnancy, infection, central nervous system (CNS) disorders (e.g., meningitis), cardiovascular problems (e.g., myocardial infarction [MI], heart failure

[HF]), metabolic disorders (e.g., diabetes mellitus), side effects of drugs (e.g., chemotherapy, digitalis), and psychologic factors (e.g., stress, fear).

Nausea is a feeling of discomfort in the epigastrium with a conscious desire to vomit. Anorexia usually accompanies nausea.

Regurgitation is an effortless process in which partially digested food slowly comes up from the stomach.

Vomiting (emesis) is a complex act that results in the forceful ejection of partially digested food and secretions from the upper GI tract. *Projectile vomiting* is a forceful expulsion of stomach contents without nausea.

Pathophysiology

A vomiting center in the brainstem coordinates the multiple components involved in vomiting. Neural impulses reach the vomiting center by way of afferent pathways through branches of the autonomic nervous system. Receptors for these afferent fibers are located in the GI tract, kidneys, heart, and uterus. When stimulated, these receptors relay information to the vomiting center, which initiates the vomiting reflex. In addition, the chemoreceptor trigger zone (CTZ) located in the brain responds to chemical stimuli of drugs and toxins. Once stimulated (e.g., in motion sickness), the CTZ transmits impulses directly to the vomiting center.

The simultaneous closure of the glottis, deep inspiration with contraction of the diaphragm in the inspiratory position, closure of the pylorus, relaxation of the stomach and lower esophageal sphincter, and contraction of the abdominal muscles with increasing intraabdominal pressure force stomach contents up and out of the mouth.

- ■ Early morning vomiting is common in pregnancy. Emotional stressors may elicit vomiting during or immediately after eating. Cyclic vomiting syndrome consists of recurring episodes of nausea, vomiting, and fatigue that last from a few hours up to 10 days.

Clinical Manifestations

When nausea and vomiting occur over a long period, dehydration can develop rapidly. Water and essential electrolytes (e.g., potassium, sodium, chloride, hydrogen) are lost. As vomiting persists, the patient may have severe electrolyte imbalances, extracellular fluid volume loss, decreased plasma volume, and eventually circulatory failure.

- Metabolic alkalosis may result from loss of gastric HCl acid. Less frequently, metabolic acidosis can occur when the contents of the small intestine are vomited.
- Weight loss may occur in a short time with severe vomiting.

The threat of pulmonary aspiration is a concern when vomiting occurs in older or unconscious patients or those with other conditions that impair the gag reflex. To prevent aspiration, put the patient who cannot adequately manage self-care in a semi-Fowler's or side-lying position.

Interprofessional Care

The goals of management are to determine and treat the underlying cause of nausea and vomiting and to provide symptomatic relief. Assess the patient for precipitating factors and describe the contents of the emesis.

The use of drugs in the treatment of nausea and vomiting depends on the cause of the problem. Using antiemetics before determining the cause can mask the underlying disease process and delay diagnosis and treatment. Many antiemetic drugs act in the CNS via the CTZ to block the neurochemicals that trigger nausea and vomiting.

- Drugs may include anticholinergics (e.g., scopolamine), antihistamines (e.g., promethazine), phenothiazines (e.g., prochlorperazine), and butyrophenones (e.g., droperidol). Other drugs with antiemetic effects include benzamides (metoclopramide [Reglan]), 5-hydroxytryptamine [5-HT] (serotonin) receptor antagonists (e.g., ondansetron [Zofran]), and neurokinin-1 receptor antagonists (e.g., aprepitant [Emend]). A comprehensive list of drugs used for nausea and vomiting is included in Table 41-1, Lewis et al, *Medical-Surgical Nursing,* ed 10, p. 895.

The patient with severe vomiting requires IV fluid therapy with electrolyte and glucose replacement until able to tolerate oral intake. Some patients may need a nasogastric (NG) tube and suction to decompress the stomach. Once symptoms have subsided, oral nutrition beginning with clear liquids is started. Water is the initial fluid of choice for oral rehydration. Have the patient sip small amounts of fluid (5 to 15 mL) every 15 to 20 minutes. Other options include carbonated beverages with the carbonation removed at room temperature and warm tea. As the patient's condition improves, provide a diet high in carbohydrates and low in fat.

Alternative therapies such as acupressure or acupuncture have been effective in reducing postoperative nausea and vomiting.

N

Patients may use herbs such as ginger and peppermint oil. Relaxation breathing exercises, changes in body position, or exercise may help some patients.

Nursing Management
Goals
The patient with nausea and vomiting will experience minimal or no nausea and vomiting, have normal electrolyte levels and hydration status, and return to a normal pattern of fluid balance and nutrient intake.

Nursing Diagnoses
- Nausea
- Deficient fluid volume
- Imbalanced nutrition: less than body requirements

Nursing Interventions
For persistent vomiting, the patient is kept NPO and given IV fluids until a diagnosis is confirmed. An NG tube connected to suction may be necessary. Secure the NG tube to prevent tube movement in the nose and throat that can stimulate nausea and vomiting.

- Record intake and output, position the patient to prevent aspiration, and monitor vital signs.
- Assess for signs of dehydration, and observe for changes in the patient's physical comfort and mentation. Provide physical and emotional support and maintain a quiet, odor-free environment.

▼ Patient and Caregiver Teaching
- Provide explanations for diagnostic tests and procedures.
- Instruct the patient and caregiver how to manage the unpleasant sensations of nausea, methods to prevent nausea and vomiting, and strategies to maintain fluid and nutritional intake.
- Use of relaxation techniques, frequent rest periods, effective pain management strategies, and diversional tactics can prevent or reduce nausea and vomiting.
- Cleansing the face and hands with a cool washcloth and providing mouth care between episodes provide comfort.
- When food is identified as the precipitating cause of nausea and vomiting, help the patient identify the specific food and when it was eaten, prior history with that food, and whether anyone else who ate the food is sick.

A patient may be reluctant to resume fluid intake because of fear of nausea recurring. Suggest clear liquids, cola beverages, sports drinks, tea or broth, dry crackers or toast, and then plain gelatin. Bland foods such as pasta, rice, cereal, baked potato, or cooked chicken are generally well tolerated in small amounts.

NEPHROTIC SYNDROME

Description

Nephrotic syndrome results when the glomerulus of the kidney is excessively permeable to plasma protein, causing proteinuria and leading to low plasma albumin and tissue edema. Common causes include primary glomerular disease (e.g., focal glomerulonephritis), infections (e.g., hepatitis, streptococcal), neoplasms (e.g., Hodgkin's lymphoma), allergens (e.g., bee sting), drugs (e.g., nonsteroidal antiinflammatory drugs [NSAIDs]), and multisystem diseases (e.g., diabetes mellitus, systemic lupus erythematosus [SLE]).

Pathophysiology and Clinical Manifestations

The increased glomerular membrane permeability found in nephrotic syndrome is responsible for massive excretion of protein in the urine. This results in decreased serum protein and subsequent edema formation, including ascites and anasarca.

- Diminished plasma oncotic pressure from the decrease in serum proteins stimulates hepatic lipoprotein synthesis, which results in hyperlipidemia. Fat bodies (fatty casts) in the urine cause urine to appear foamy.
- Immune responses are altered in nephrotic syndrome. As a result, infection is a major cause of morbidity and mortality.
- Calcium and skeletal abnormalities may occur, including hypocalcemia, blunted calcemic response to parathyroid hormone, hyperparathyroidism, and osteomalacia.
- Hypercoagulability results from the urinary loss of anticoagulant proteins. Hypercoagulability with thromboembolism is potentially the most serious complication of nephrotic syndrome. The renal vein is the most common site for thrombus formation. Pulmonary emboli occur in about 40% of nephrotic patients with thrombosis.

Characteristic manifestations include peripheral edema, massive proteinuria, hypertension, hyperlipidemia, and hypoalbuminemia. Laboratory findings include decreased serum albumin, decreased total serum protein, and elevated serum cholesterol.

Interprofessional Care

The goals are to relieve the symptoms and cure or control the primary disease. Corticosteroids and cyclophosphamide may be used. Prednisone is effective to varying degrees for some causes of nephrotic syndrome (e.g., membranous glomerulonephritis, lupus nephritis). Management of diabetes and treatment of edema are also important.

Management of edema includes the cautious use of angiotensin-converting enzyme (ACE) inhibitors, NSAIDs, low sodium intake (2 to 3 g/day), and a low- to moderate-protein diet (1 to 2 g/kg/day). Some patients may need thiazide or loop diuretics. The treatment of hyperlipidemia includes lipid-lowering agents, such as colestipol (Colestid) and lovastatin.

Nursing Management

The major focus of care is related to edema. Assess the edema by weighing the patient daily, accurately recording intake and output, and measuring abdominal girth or extremity size. Monitor effectiveness of diuretic therapy. Clean edematous skin carefully. Avoid trauma to the skin.

Patients have the potential to become malnourished from anorexia and the loss of protein in the urine. Serve small, frequent meals in a pleasant setting to encourage better dietary intake.

- Teach the patient to avoid exposure to people with known infections.
- Support for the patient in coping with an altered body image is essential because of the embarrassment often associated with the edematous appearance.

NON-HODGKIN'S LYMPHOMAS

Description

Non-Hodgkin's lymphomas (NHLs) are a heterogeneous group of malignant neoplasms of B, T, or natural killer (NK) cell origin. NHLs affect all ages. B cell lymphomas constitute about 88% of all NHLs.

NHLs are categorized by the level of differentiation, cell of origin, and rate of cellular proliferation. A variety of clinical presentations and courses are recognized, from indolent (slowly developing) to rapidly progressive disease. NHL is the most commonly occurring hematologic cancer and the fifth leading cause of cancer death.

Pathophysiology

The cause of NHL is usually unknown. NHLs may result from chromosomal translocations, infections, environmental factors, and immunodeficiency states. Chromosomal translocations have an important role in the pathogenesis of many NHLs. Some viruses and bacteria are implicated in the pathogenesis of NHL, including Epstein-Barr virus, hepatitis B and C viruses, *Helicobacter pylori, Campylobacter jejuni,* and *Borrelia burgdorferi.*

Environmental factors linked to the development of NHL include exposure to chemicals (e.g., pesticides, herbicides, solvents, organic chemicals, wood preservatives). NHL is also more common in individuals with inherited immunodeficiency syndromes and those who have used immunosuppressive medications (e.g., to prevent rejection after organ transplantation or to treat autoimmune disorders) or have received chemotherapy or radiation therapy.

Although there is no hallmark feature in NHL, all NHLs involve lymphocytes arrested in various stages of development. *Diffuse large B cell lymphoma,* the most common aggressive lymphoma, is a neoplasm that originates in the lymph nodes, usually in the neck or abdomen. *Burkitt's lymphoma* is the most highly aggressive type of NHL and is thought to originate from B cell blasts in the lymph nodes.

Clinical Manifestations

NHLs can originate outside the lymph nodes and the method of spread can be unpredictable. The majority of patients have widely disseminated disease at the time of diagnosis.

- The primary manifestation is painless lymph node enlargement. Because the disease is usually disseminated when diagnosed, other symptoms are present depending on where the disease has spread (e.g., hepatomegaly with liver involvement, neurologic symptoms with CNS disease). NHL can also manifest nonspecifically with airway obstruction, renal failure, pericardial tamponade, and GI complaints.
- Patients with high-grade (very aggressive) lymphomas may have lymphadenopathy and constitutional ("B") symptoms, such as fever, night sweats, and weight loss.
- An overlap exists between leukemia and NHL because both involve proliferation of lymphocytes or their precursors. A leukemia-like picture with peripheral lymphocytosis and bone marrow involvement may be present in about 20% of adults with some types of NHL.

Diagnostic Studies

Diagnostic studies for NHL resemble those used for Hodgkin's lymphoma. However, because NHL is more often found in extranodal sites, more diagnostic studies may be done, such as MRI or lumbar puncture to rule out CNS disease, a bone marrow biopsy to determine bone marrow infiltration, or a barium enema, upper endoscopy, or CT to visualize suspected GI involvement.

Lymph node biopsy establishes cell type and pattern. Prognosis is based on the histopathology.

Nursing and Interprofessional Management

Treatment for NHL involves chemotherapy and sometimes radiation therapy (see Chemotherapy, p. 694; Radiation Therapy, p. 733). Ironically, aggressive lymphomas are more responsive to treatment and more likely to be cured. Indolent lymphomas have a naturally long course but are more difficult to treat effectively.

- Rituximab (Rituxan), a monoclonal antibody against the CD20 antigen on the surface of normal and malignant B lymphocytes, is used to treat NHL.
- Numerous chemotherapy combinations have been used to try to overcome the resistant nature of this disease (see Table 30-29, Lewis et al, *Medical-Surgical Nursing,* ed 10, p. 644).
- Hematopoietic stem cell transplantation in NHL may be of benefit in certain subtypes with aggressive or refractory lymphoma.
- Other therapies for some types of NHL include the monoclonal antibody ibritumomab tiuxetan (Zevalin).
- For more diffuse disease, treatment may include phototherapy, α-interferon, oral bexarotene (Targretin), vorinostat (Zolinza), or denileukin diftitox (Ontak).
- Complete remissions are uncommon, but a majority of patients respond with improvement in symptoms.

Nursing care for patients with NHL is similar to that for patients with Hodgkin's lymphoma. It is largely based on managing problems related to the disease (pain, spinal cord compression, tumor lysis syndrome), pancytopenia, and other effects of therapy.

- The patient undergoing external beam radiation therapy has special nursing needs. The skin in the radiation field requires attention. Concepts related to safety issues regarding radiation therapy are important in the plan of care (see Chapter 15, Lewis et al, *Medical-Surgical Nursing,* ed 10).
- Psychosocial considerations are important. Help the patient and family understand the disease, treatment, and expected and potential side effects.
- As in Hodgkin's lymphoma, evaluation of patients with NHL for long-term effects of therapy is important because the delayed consequences of disease and treatment may not become apparent for many years.

OBESITY

Description

Obesity is an excessively high amount of body fat or adipose tissue. Obesity is a major health problem because it increases the risk of numerous other diseases such as diabetes and cancer.

The magnitude of the obesity problem is a public health crisis with significant geographic, racial and ethnic, and income disparities. Currently, about 34% of adults in the United States are obese. Obesity rates are highest in the South and among African Americans, Hispanics, and lower-income, less-educated Americans.

- Attitudes about obesity can create biases and discrimination against people who are obese. Obesity needs to be viewed and treated as a chronic disease.
- Reversing the childhood obesity crisis is key to addressing the overall obesity epidemic. One in ten children become obese as early as ages 2 to 5. Nearly one third of children and teens are currently obese or overweight. It is estimated that almost half of overweight adults were overweight in childhood and two thirds of obese children remained obese into adulthood.

The most common measure of obesity is the *body mass index* (BMI). BMI is calculated by dividing a person's weight (in kilograms) by the square of the height in meters.

- Individuals with a BMI less than 18.5 kg/m^2 are considered underweight, whereas a BMI between 18.5 and 24.9 kg/m^2 reflects a normal body weight. A BMI of 25 to 29.9 kg/m^2 is classified as being *overweight* and people with values at 30 kg/m^2 or above are considered *obese*. The term *extreme obesity* is used for those with a BMI greater than 40 kg/m^2.
- The waist-to-hip ratio (WHR) is another method used to assess obesity. This ratio is a method of describing the distribution of both subcutaneous and visceral adipose tissue and is calculated by using the waist measurement divided by the hip measurement. A WHR less than 0.8 is optimal. A WHR greater than 0.8 indicates more truncal fat, which puts the individual at greater risk for health complications.
- Individuals with fat located primarily in the abdominal area (*apple-shaped body*) are at greater risk for obesity-related complications than those whose fat is primarily located in the upper legs (*pear-shaped body*).

O

Pathophysiology

The cause of obesity involves significant genetic/biologic suscep-tibility factors that are highly influenced by environmental and psychosocial factors.

Most obese people have *primary obesity,* which is excess calorie intake over energy expenditure for the body's metabolic demands. Others have *secondary obesity,* which can result from various con-genital anomalies, chromosomal anomalies, metabolic problems, central nervous system lesions and disorders, or drugs (e.g., corti-costeroids, antipsychotics).

- Neuropeptide Y, produced in the hypothalamus, is a powerful appetite stimulant. When it is imbalanced, it leads to overeating and obesity. Hormones and peptides produced in the gut and adipocyte cells affect the hypothalamus and have a critical role in appetite and energy balance.

The two major consequences of obesity are due to the sheer increase in fat mass and the production of adipokines produced by fat cells. Adipocytes produce at least 100 different proteins. These proteins (secreted as enzymes), adipokines, growth factors, and hormones, contribute to the development of insulin resistance and atherosclerosis.

Environmental factors include greater access to prepackaged and fast foods, larger portion sizes, lack of physical activity and sed-entary recreation, and high-calorie foods that may be more acces-sible to those of low socioeconomic status.

- The association of food with comfort, reward, pleasure, and fun is a powerful incentive for overeating.

Diagnostic Studies

- History and physical examination are done to assess the extent and duration of obesity.
- Laboratory tests of liver function, fasting glucose level, triglyc-eride level, and low- and high-density lipoprotein cholesterol levels assist in evaluating the cause and effects of obesity.
- Classifications of body weight and obesity are defined by BMI, standardized height-weight charts, or waist-hip ratio.

Interprofessional Care

- A multifaceted approach needs to be taken with attention to nutritional therapy, exercise, behavior modification, and for some, medication or surgical intervention. Stress healthy eating habits and adequate physical activity as lifestyle patterns to develop and maintain. Restricting dietary intake so that it is below energy requirements is a cornerstone for any weight loss or maintenance program. A good weight loss plan should contain foods from the basic food groups (see Fig. 39-3, Lewis et al, *Medical-Surgical Nursing,* ed 10, p. 861).

- Setting a realistic and healthy goal, such as losing 1 to 2 lb/wk, should be mutually agreed on at the beginning of a weight loss program.
- During plateau periods, when no weight is lost for several days to several weeks, patients need encouragement and support to prevent giving up on the weight loss plan.
- Exercise is an essential part of a weight control program. Patients should exercise daily, preferably 30 minutes to an hour. Exercise is especially important in maintaining weight loss.
- People who participate in a behavioral therapy program are more successful in maintaining their losses over an extended time than those who do not participate in such training.
- The person who is on a weight control program may be encouraged to join a support or self-help group if the support of others having the same experiences is helpful.

Drug Therapy

Medications, if used, should be part of a comprehensive weight-reduction program that includes reduced-calorie diet, exercise, and behavior modification. Drugs should be reserved for adults with a BMI of 30 kg/m^2 or greater (obese) or adults with a BMI of 27 kg/m^2 or greater (overweight) who have at least one weight-related condition such as hypertension, type 2 diabetes, or dyslipidemia. The drugs currently approved by the U.S. Food and Drug Administration (FDA) for treatment of obesity are presented in Table 59.

Surgical Therapy

Bariatric surgery, surgery on the stomach and/or intestines to help a person with extreme obesity lose weight, has become a viable option for treating obesity. Surgery is currently the only treatment that has been found to have a successful and lasting impact for sustained weight loss for individuals with extreme obesity.

- Bariatric surgeries are categorized as restrictive, malabsorptive, or a combination of restrictive and malabsorptive. In restrictive procedures, the stomach is reduced in size (less food eaten). In malabsorptive procedures, the small intestine is shortened or bypassed (less food absorbed). A majority of procedures are performed laparoscopically.
- Common restrictive surgeries include adjustable gastric banding and vertical sleeve gastrectomy. These surgeries are discussed further on pp. 885 to 887 in Lewis et al, *Medical-Surgical Nursing,* ed 10.

The Roux-en-Y gastric bypass (RYGB) procedure is a combination of restrictive and malabsorptive surgery. This surgical

TABLE 59 Drug Therapy

Obesity

Drug	Mechanism of Action	Nursing Considerations
orlistat (Xenical, Alli [low-dose form available over the counter])	• Blocks fat breakdown and absorption in intestine • Inhibits the action of intestinal lipases, resulting in undigested fat excreted in feces	• Associated with leakage of stool, flatulence, diarrhea, and abdominal bloating, especially if a high-fat diet is consumed • Severe liver injury may occur. • Fat-soluble vitamins may need to be supplemented.
lorcaserin (Belviq)	• Selective serotonin (5-HT) agonist • Suppresses appetite and creates a sense of satiety	• Common side effects are headache, dizziness, fatigue, nausea, dry mouth, and constipation.
bupropion/ naltrexone (Contrave)	• *bupropion*: antidepressant • *naltrexone*: opioid antagonist	• Common side effects are nausea, constipation, headache, vomiting, dizziness, insomnia, dry mouth, and diarrhea. • Suicidal thoughts and behaviors and neuropsychiatric reactions can occur. • Can increase BP and heart rate and should not be used in patients with uncontrolled hypertension. • Can cause seizures and must not be used in patients who have seizure disorders.
phentermine/ topiramate (Qsymia)	• *phentermine*: sympathomimetic anorectic • *topiramate*: antiseizure drug that induces satiety	• Common side effects are paresthesias, dizziness, insomnia, constipation, and dry mouth. • Must not be used in patients with glaucoma or hyperthyroidism. • Can increase heart rate and should not be used in patients with uncontrolled hypertension or heart disease.
liraglutide (Saxenda)	• Glucagon-like peptide 1 (GLP-1) agonist • Induces satiety	• Used to treat type 2 diabetes. • Needs to be injected. • Side effects include thyroid tumors and pancreatitis.

procedure is the most common bariatric procedure performed in the United States and is considered the gold standard among bariatric procedures.

- This procedure involves creating a small gastric pouch and attaching it directly to the small intestine using a Y-shaped limb of the small bowel. After the procedure, food bypasses 90% of the stomach, the duodenum, and a small segment of jejunum.
- A complication of the RYGB is *dumping syndrome,* in which gastric contents empty too rapidly into the small intestine, overwhelming its ability to digest nutrients. Signs and symptoms can include vomiting, nausea, weakness, sweating, faintness, and diarrhea.

An alternative to gastrointestinal restriction or bypass surgery is the Maestro Rechargeable System. It consists of a pacemaker-like electrical pulse generator, wire leads, and electrodes that are implanted in the abdomen. Intermittent electrical pulses to the vagus nerve signal to the brain that the stomach feels empty or full.

Cosmetic surgeries may be used to reduce fatty tissue and skinfolds. These procedures include a *lipectomy* (adipectomy) to remove unsightly adipose folds and *liposuction* for cosmetic purposes.

Nursing Management
Goals
The overall goals are that the patient with obesity will modify eating patterns, participate in a regular physical activity program, achieve weight loss to a specified level, maintain weight loss at a specified level, and minimize or prevent health problems related to obesity.

Nursing Interventions
Together with other members of the interprofessional team, you have a major role in planning for and managing the care of an obese patient. It is essential that you have a nonjudgmental approach in helping patients manage their problems related to obesity.

- Exploring an individual's motivation for weight loss is essential for overall success.
- Focusing on the reasons for wanting to lose weight may help patients develop strategies for a weight loss program. The supervised plan of care must be directed at two different processes: (1) successful weight loss, which requires a short-term energy deficit, and (2) successful weight control, which requires long-term behavior changes.

Preoperative care for gastric surgery includes planning for the special needs of an obese patient, such as the availability of a larger-sized BP cuff, hospital gown, bed, and chair. Consider how the patient will be weighed, transported through the hospital, and turned. Instruct the patient in the proper coughing technique, deep breathing, use of an incentive spirometer, and methods of turning and positioning to prevent pulmonary complications after surgery.

Postoperative care focuses on careful assessment and immediate intervention for cardiopulmonary complications, deep vein thrombosis, anastomosis leaks, and electrolyte imbalances. Facilitate patient respiratory efforts (elevating the head of the bed, turning, coughing, deep breathing); monitor for wound infection, dehiscence, and delayed healing; and promote early ambulation. Patients experience considerable abdominal pain after surgery. Give pain medications as necessary during the immediate postoperative period.

- Some patients express guilt feelings concerning the fact that the only way they could lose weight was by surgical means rather than by the "sheer willpower" of reduced dietary intake. Be ready to provide support so that the patient does not dwell on negative feelings.
- Emphasize the importance of long-term follow-up care, in part because of potential complications late in the recovery period. Encourage patients to adhere strictly to the prescribed diet and inform the HCP of any changes in their physical or emotional condition.

OBSTRUCTIVE SLEEP APNEA

Description

Obstructive sleep apnea (OSA), also called *obstructive sleep apnea–hypopnea syndrome,* is characterized by partial or complete upper airway obstruction during sleep. *Apnea* is the cessation of spontaneous respirations lasting longer than 10 seconds. *Hypopnea* is a condition characterized by shallow respirations (30% to 50% reduction in airflow).

- Sleep apnea occurs in 2% to 10% of Americans. Risk increases with age greater than 65 years, craniofacial abnormalities that affect the upper airway, acromegaly, obesity, and tobacco smoking. OSA patients with excessive daytime sleepiness have increased mortality.

Pathophysiology

Airflow obstruction occurs when (1) narrowing of the air passages with relaxation of muscle tone during sleep leads to apnea and hypopnea and (2) the tongue and soft palate fall backward and partially or completely obstruct the pharynx.

- Each obstruction may last 10 to 90 seconds. During the apneic period, hypoxemia and hypercapnia may cause the person to arouse briefly and snort or gasp without fully awakening.
- Apnea and arousal cycles occur as many as 200 to 400 times during 6 to 8 hours of sleep.

Clinical Manifestations

Manifestations of sleep apnea include frequent arousals during sleep, insomnia, excessive daytime sleepiness, and witnessed apneic episodes. A bed partner may complain about the person's loud snoring. Other symptoms include morning headaches, personality changes, and irritability.

- Untreated sleep apnea may cause hypertension, right-sided heart failure from pulmonary hypertension, and cardiac dysrhythmias. Chronic sleep loss can lead to decreased ability to concentrate, impaired memory, failure to accomplish daily tasks, and interpersonal difficulties.

Diagnostic Studies

- Sleep and medical history
- Polysomnography. OSA is defined as more than five apnea/hypopnea events per hour accompanied by a 3% to 4% decrease in O_2 saturation.

Nursing and Interprofessional Management
Conservative Treatment

Conservative home treatment for mild sleep apnea (5 to 10 apnea/hypopnea events per hour) includes sleeping on one's side rather than the back, elevating the head of the bed, and avoiding sedatives or alcoholic beverages 3 to 4 hours before sleep. Because excessive weight worsens sleep apnea, refer patient to a weight loss program if indicated.

- Continuous positive airway pressure (CPAP) is often used for patients with severe symptoms (more than 15 apnea/hypopnea events per hour). A nasal mask, nasal pillows, or full-face mask is worn attached to a high-flow blower (see Fig. 7-5, Lewis et al, *Medical-Surgical Nursing,* ed 10, p. 97). CPAP reduces apnea episodes, daytime sleepiness, and fatigue.
- Using a special mouth guard during sleep to prevent airflow obstruction may reduce symptoms.
- Opioid analgesics and sedating medications may worsen OSA symptoms by depressing respiration.
- When hospitalized, patients with OSA should continue CPAP use.

Surgery

If conservative measures fail, surgery may be done. Two common procedures are uvulopalatopharyngoplasty and genioglossal advancement and hyoid myotomy. Radiofrequency ablation may also be used.

- Postoperative complications include airway obstruction or hemorrhage.
- Patients are usually discharged within 1 day after surgery. Tell patients to expect a sore throat and to reduce foul breath odor by rinsing with diluted mouthwash and then salt water after several days. Snoring may persist until inflammation has subsided.

ORAL CANCER

Description

There are two types of *oral cancer:* oral cavity cancer, which starts in the mouth, and oropharyngeal cancer, which develops in the part of the throat just behind the mouth (the oropharynx). *Head and neck squamous cell carcinoma* (HNSCC) is a broad term for cancers of the oral cavity, pharynx, and larynx that account for 90% of malignant oral tumors.

- Cancer of the lip has a more favorable prognosis because the lesions are visible and are usually diagnosed earlier.
- The 5-year survival rate is 83% for localized cancer and 61% for all stages of cancer of the oral cavity and pharynx combined.

Pathophysiology

Oral cancer has a number of predisposing factors including prolonged sun exposure, tobacco use (cigar, cigarette, pipe, snuff), and frequent alcohol consumption. Human papillomavirus (HPV)-associated oropharyngeal cancer is associated with multiple sexual partners, especially multiple oral sex partners.

Clinical Manifestations

Common manifestations include the following:

- *Leukoplakia,* called "smoker's patch," is a whitish precancerous lesion on the mucosa of the mouth or tongue that results from chronic irritation, especially from smoking. The patch may become keratinized (hard and leathery) and is then sometimes described as hyperkeratosis.

- *Erythroplakia* is a red velvety patch on the mouth or tongue. More than 50% of cases of erythroplakia progress to squamous cell carcinoma.

Patients may report nonspecific symptoms such as chronic sore throat, sore mouth, and voice changes. Some patients with oral cancer have an asymptomatic neck mass. Later symptoms of oral cancer are pain, dysphagia (difficulty swallowing), and difficulty in moving the jaw (e.g., chewing, speaking).

Cancer of the lip usually appears as an indurated, painless lip ulcer. The first sign of tongue cancer is an ulcer or area of thickening. Soreness or pain of the tongue may occur, especially on eating hot or highly seasoned foods.

- Later symptoms and signs of tongue cancer include increased salivation, slurred speech, dysphagia, toothache, and earache.

Diagnostic Studies

- Biopsy of suspected lesion
- Oral exfoliative cytology and toluidine blue test are used to screen for oral cancer.
- Once cancer is diagnosed, CT scan, MRI, and positron emission tomography (PET) are used in staging.

Interprofessional Care

Management usually consists of surgery, radiation therapy, and/or chemotherapy. Surgery remains the most effective treatment. Some patients with small tumors in the mouth and throat are candidates for minimally invasive robotic-assisted surgery. Many surgeries are radical procedures involving extensive resections. Some examples are hemiglossectomy (removal of one half of the tongue), glossectomy (removal of the entire tongue), and radical neck dissection (wide excision of the lymph nodes and their lymphatic channels). A tracheostomy (see Tracheostomy, p. 735) is commonly done with radical neck dissection.

Chemotherapy and radiation therapy are used together when there are positive margins, bone erosion, or positive lymph nodes (see Chemotherapy, p. 694, and Radiation Therapy, p. 733). Chemotherapy agents used include 5-fluorouracil (5-FU), methotrexate, cisplatin, carboplatin, paclitaxel (Taxol), docetaxel (Taxotere), cetuximab (Erbitux), and bleomycin.

Palliative treatment is used when the prognosis is poor, the cancer is inoperable, or the patient decides against surgery. If it becomes difficult for the patient to swallow, placing a gastrostomy will allow for adequate nutritional intake. Frequent oral suctioning may be needed.

Nursing Management
Goals
The patient with carcinoma of the oral cavity will have a patent airway, be able to communicate, have adequate nutritional intake to promote wound healing, and have relief of pain and discomfort.
Nursing Diagnoses
- Imbalanced nutrition: less than body requirements
- Chronic pain
- Anxiety
- Ineffective health maintenance
Nursing Interventions
You have a significant role in early detection and treatment of oral cancer. Identify patients at risk (users of tobacco products, alcoholics, those with poor dental hygiene, pipe smokers) and provide information regarding predisposing factors. Inform the patient who smokes about smoking cessation programs available in the community. Warn adolescents and teenagers about the dangers of using snuff or chewing tobacco.
- Refer any individual with an ulcerative lesion that does not heal within 2 to 3 weeks to an HCP.
- Teach the patient to report unexplained pain or soreness of the mouth, unusual bleeding, dysphagia, sore throat, voice changes, or swelling or lump in the neck.

See Head and Neck Cancer, p. 258, for care of the preoperative or postoperative patient with a radical neck dissection.

OSTEOARTHRITIS

Description
Osteoarthritis (OA), the most common form of joint disease, is a slowly progressive noninflammatory disorder of the diarthrodial (synovial) joints. Currently 27 million Americans are affected by OA, with the numbers expected to greatly increase as the population ages.

OA is not considered to be a normal part of the aging process, but aging is one risk factor for disease development. Cartilage destruction can actually begin between the ages of 20 and 30 years, and a majority of adults are affected by age 40. Few patients experience symptoms until after age 50 or 60 years, but more than half of those over age 65 have x-ray evidence of the disease in at least one joint. After age 50, women are more often affected than men.

- Obesity is a modifiable risk factor that contributes to hip and knee OA by increasing the mechanical stress on the joints. Regular moderate exercise, which also helps with weight control, decreases the risk for disease development and progression. Anterior cruciate ligament injury from quick stops and pivoting, as in football and soccer, has been linked to an increased risk for knee OA. Occupations that require frequent kneeling and stooping also increase the risk for knee OA.

Pathophysiology

The development of OA is complex. Genetic, metabolic, and local factors interact to cause cartilage deterioration from damage at the level of the chondrocytes. The normally smooth, white, translucent articular cartilage becomes dull, yellow, and granular as the disease progresses. Affected cartilage steadily becomes softer and less elastic. It is less able to resist wear with heavy use.

The body's attempts at cartilage repair cannot keep up with the destruction of OA. As the collagen structure of the cartilage changes, articular surfaces become cracked and worn. While central cartilage becomes thinner, cartilage at the joint edges becomes thicker, and osteophytes form. Joint surfaces become uneven, affecting the distribution of stress across the joint and causing reduced motion.

Although inflammation is not typical of OA, secondary synovitis may occur when phagocytes try to rid the joint of small pieces of cartilage torn from the joint surface. These changes cause the early pain and stiffness of OA. Pain in later disease occurs when articular cartilage is lost and bony joint surfaces rub on each other.

Clinical Manifestations

Fatigue, fever, and organ involvement are not present in OA. This is an important distinction between OA and inflammatory joint disorders such as rheumatoid arthritis (Table 60). Manifestations of OA range from mild discomfort to significant disability.

Joints

Joint pain is the primary symptom and the typical reason the patient seeks medical attention. Pain generally gets worse with joint use. In early stages of OA, joint pain is relieved by rest. However, the patient with advanced disease may complain of pain at rest or have trouble sleeping because of increased joint pain. Pain may also worsen as the barometric pressure falls before the onset of severe weather. The pain of OA may be referred to the groin, buttock, or side of the thigh or knee. Sitting down becomes difficult, as does

Parameter	Rheumatoid Arthritis	Osteoarthritis
TABLE 60	**Comparison of Rheumatoid Arthritis and Osteoarthritis**	
Age at onset	Young to middle age	Usually >40 yr
Gender	Female:male ratio is 2:1 or 3:1	Female:male ratio 2:1 after age 60; except for traumatic arthritis, men less affected until age 70 or 80
	Fewer marked sex differences after age 60	
Weight	Lost or maintained weight	Often overweight or obese
Disease	Systemic disease with exacerbations and remissions	Localized disease with variable, progressive course
Affected joints	Small joints typically affected first (PIPs, MCPs, MTPs), wrists, elbows, shoulders, knees	Weight-bearing joints of knees and hips, small joints (MCPs, DIPs, PIPs), cervical and lumbar spine
	Usually bilateral, symmetric joint involvement	Often asymmetric
Pain characteristics	Stiffness lasts 1 hr to all day and may decrease with use.	Stiffness occurs on arising but usually subsides after 30 min.
	Pain is variable, may disrupt sleep.	Pain gradually worsens with joint use and disease progression, relieved with joint rest but may disrupt sleep.

Effusions	Common	Uncommon
Nodules	Present, especially on extensor surfaces	Heberden's (DIPs) and Bouchard's (PIPs) nodes
Synovial fluid	WBC count 3000-25,000/µL with mostly neutrophils; decreased viscosity	WBC count <2000/µL (mild leukocytosis); normal viscosity
X-rays	Joint space narrowing and erosion with bony overgrowths, subluxation with advanced disease; Osteoporosis related to decreased activity, corticosteroid use	Joint space narrowing, osteophytes, subchondral cysts, sclerosis
Laboratory findings	RF-positive in 70%-90% of patients; negative titers in early disease for about 25% of patients; ANA-positive in 20%-30% of patients; Positive anti-CCP in more than 80% of patients; Elevated ESR, CRP indicative of active inflammation	RF-negative; ANA-negative; Anti-CCP-negative; Transient elevation in ESR related to synovitis

ANA, Antinuclear antibodies; *anti-CCP*, anti-citrullinated peptide; *CRP*, C-reactive protein; *DIPs*, distal interphalangeals; *ESR*, erythrocyte sedimentation rate; *MCPs*, metacarpophalangeals; *MTPs*, metatarsophalangeals; *PIPs*, proximal interphalangeals; *RF*, rheumatoid factor.

rising from a chair when the hips are lower than the knees. As OA develops in intervertebral joints of the spine, localized pain and stiffness are common.

Unlike pain, which typically worsens with activity, joint stiffness occurs after periods of rest or static position. Early-morning stiffness is common but generally resolves within 30 minutes, a feature that distinguishes OA from inflammatory arthritic disorders such as rheumatoid arthritis.

- Overactivity can temporarily increase stiffness. *Crepitation,* a grating sensation caused by loose cartilage particles in the joint cavity, can also contribute to stiffness.
- OA usually affects joints asymmetrically. The most commonly involved joints are shown in Fig. 64-2, Lewis et al, *Medical-Surgical Nursing,* ed 10, p. 1520.

Deformity

Deformity or instability associated with OA is specific to the involved joint. For example, *Heberden's nodes* occur on the distal interphalangeal joints due to osteophyte formation and loss of joint space. *Bouchard's nodes* on the proximal interphalangeal joints indicate similar disease involvement. Heberden's and Bouchard's nodes are often red, swollen, and tender. These bony enlargements do not usually cause significant loss of function.

Knee OA often leads to joint deformity as a result of cartilage loss in the medial compartment. For example, the patient becomes bow-legged (varus deformity) in response to medial joint arthritis. Lateral joint arthritis causes a "knock-knee" appearance (valgus deformity). In advanced hip OA, one of the patient's legs may become shorter as the joint space narrows.

Diagnostic Studies

- A bone scan, CT scan, or MRI may be useful to diagnose OA. X-rays also confirm disease and monitor the progression of joint damage. However, these changes do not always reflect the degree of pain the patient experiences.
- No laboratory abnormalities or biomarkers are specific diagnostic indicators. The erythrocyte sedimentation rate (ESR) is normal except in instances of acute inflammation, when minimal elevations may be noted.
- Synovial fluid analysis helps distinguish between OA and types of inflammatory arthritis. In OA, fluid remains clear yellow with little or no sign of inflammation.

Interprofessional Care

Interprofessional care focuses on managing pain and inflammation, preventing disability, and maintaining and improving joint function. Nondrug interventions are the basis of management, and drug therapy supplements nondrug treatments.

The affected joint should be rested during any periods of acute inflammation and maintained in a functional position with splints or braces if necessary. Immobilization should not exceed 1 week because joint stiffness increases with inactivity. The patient may need to modify activities or use an assistive device to decrease stress on affected joints. Teach the patient with knee OA to avoid prolonged standing, kneeling, or squatting.

- Applications of heat and cold may help reduce complaints of pain and stiffness. Heat therapy is helpful for stiffness, including hot packs, whirlpool, ultrasound, and paraffin wax baths.
- If the patient is overweight, weight reduction is critical to the treatment plan. Help the patient evaluate the current diet to make needed changes. Exercise is an important part of OA management. Aerobic conditioning, range-of-motion exercises, and specific programs for quadriceps strengthening have been beneficial for many patients with knee OA.

Complementary and alternative therapies for OA symptom management are popular with patients who have not found relief through traditional medical care. Teach the patient to carefully research any alternative therapies and avoid replacing conventional OA treatments with unproven approaches. Acupuncture may reduce arthritis pain and improve joint mobility. Massage and Tai Chi may also reduce pain and improve function. Some nutritional supplements may have antiinflammatory effects (e.g., fish oil, ginger, S-adenosyl methionine [SAM-e]). Results of studies on glucosamine and chondroitin are mixed regarding their effectiveness with OA symptoms.

Drug Therapy

Drug therapy is based on the severity of the patient's symptoms (see Table 64-3, Lewis et al, *Medical-Surgical Nursing*, ed 10, pp. 1521 to 1522). The patient with mild to moderate joint pain may receive relief from acetaminophen (Tylenol). Topical agents such as capsaicin cream (Zostrix), salicylates, camphor, eucalyptus oil, and menthol may provide temporary pain relief.

If the patient does not obtain adequate OA pain management with acetaminophen or has moderate to severe pain, a nonsteroidal antiinflammatory drug (NSAID) may provide greater relief.

- NSAID therapy is typically initiated in low-dose, over-the-counter strengths (e.g., ibuprofen, 200 mg up to four times per day), with the dose increased as the patient's symptoms indicate. If the patient is at risk for or experiences GI side effects with NSAID use, a protective agent such as misoprostol (Cytotec) may be indicated. Patients taking an anticoagulant (e.g., warfarin [Coumadin]) and an NSAID or a combination of aspirin with another NSAID are at high risk for bleeding.

- As an alternative to traditional NSAIDs, treatment with the cyclooxygenase (COX)-2 inhibitor celecoxib (Celebrex) may be considered.

Intraarticular injections of corticosteroids may decrease local inflammation and effusion. Systemic use of corticosteroids is not indicated and may actually accelerate the disease process.

- Injection of hyaluronic acid (viscosupplementation) has been a common treatment for knee OA. However, its effectiveness in treating arthritis is not clear.

Symptoms of OA are often managed conservatively for many years. However, the patient's loss of joint function, unmanaged pain, and decreased independence in self-care may prompt a recommendation for surgery. Arthroscopy has been commonly performed for patients with knee OA. For most patients, however, this procedure provides no additional benefit over physical therapy and medical treatment.

Nursing Management

Goals

The patient with OA will maintain or improve joint function through a balance of rest and activity, use joint protection measures to improve activity tolerance, achieve independence in self-care and maintain optimal role function, and use drug and nondrug strategies to manage pain satisfactorily.

Nursing Diagnoses

- Acute and chronic pain
- Impaired physical mobility
- Overweight or obesity
- Depression

Nursing Interventions

Focus community education on altering modifiable risk factors. For example, encourage the patient to lose weight and reduce occupational or recreational hazards. For athletic instruction and physical fitness programs, include safety measures that protect and reduce trauma to the joints. Traumatic joint injuries should be treated promptly to decrease the risk of developing OA.

The patient with OA is usually treated on an outpatient basis, often by an interprofessional team that includes a rheumatologist, a nurse, an occupational therapist, and a physical therapist.

- Drugs are administered for the treatment of pain and inflammation. Nondrug strategies to decrease pain and disability may include massage, use of heat (thermal packs) or cold (ice packs), meditation, and yoga.

- Home and work environment modification is essential for patient safety, accessibility, and self-care. Teach about removing scatter rugs, providing rails at the stairs and bathtub, using night-lights, and wearing well-fitting supportive shoes. Assistive devices such as canes, walkers, elevated toilet seats, and grab bars reduce joint load and promote safety.
- Sexual counseling may help the patient and his or her partner to enjoy physical closeness by introducing the idea of alternate positions and timing for intercourse.

▼ Patient and Caregiver Teaching

Patient and caregiver teaching related to OA is an important nursing responsibility.

- Provide information about the nature and treatment of the disease, pain management, posture and body mechanics, correct use of assistive devices such as a cane or walker, principles of joint protection and energy conservation, and an exercise program.
- Individualize home management goals to meet the patient's needs. Include the patient caregiver, family, and significant others in goal setting and teaching.
- Assure the patient that OA is a localized disease and that severe deforming arthritis is not the usual course. The patient may appreciate community resources such as the Arthritis Foundation's Self-Help Course *(www.arthritis.org)*.

OSTEOMALACIA

Osteomalacia is caused by vitamin D deficiency, which results in bone losing calcium and becoming soft. The disease is uncommon in the United States. It is the same disorder as rickets in children, except that the epiphyseal growth plates are closed in adults.

- Vitamin D is required for absorption of calcium from the intestine. Insufficient vitamin D intake can interfere with the normal bone mineralization; with little or no calcification, bones become soft.
- Causes include limited sun exposure (which is needed for vitamin D synthesis), GI malabsorption, extensive burns, chronic diarrhea, pregnancy, kidney disease, and drugs such as phenytoin (Dilantin).
- Severely obese people are at higher risk for developing osteomalacia due to inadequate physical activity and poor diet.

Common clinical features are bone pain and difficulty walking or rising from a chair. Other manifestations include low back and bone pain, progressive muscle weakness (especially in the pelvic girdle), weight loss, and progressive deformities of the weight-bearing bones. Fractures are common and slow to heal.

Laboratory findings often include decreased serum calcium or phosphorus levels, decreased serum 25-hydroxyvitamin D, and elevated serum alkaline phosphatase. X-rays may demonstrate the effects of generalized bone demineralization, especially a loss of calcium in the bones of the pelvis, and the presence of associated bone deformity.

- *Looser's transformation zones* (ribbons of decalcification in bone found on x-ray) are diagnostic of osteomalacia. Significant osteomalacia may exist without demonstrable x-ray changes.

Interprofessional care is directed toward the correction of the vitamin D deficiency. When vitamin D_3 (cholecalciferol) and vitamin D_2 (ergocalciferol) are used as supplements, the patient often shows a dramatic response. Calcium or phosphorus supplements may also be prescribed. Encourage consumption of eggs, meat, oily fish, and milk and breakfast cereals fortified with calcium and vitamin D. Exposure to sunlight and weight-bearing exercise are also valuable.

OSTEOMYELITIS

Description

Osteomyelitis is a severe infection of the bone, bone marrow, and surrounding soft tissue. Although *Staphylococcus aureus* is a common cause of infection, a variety of microorganisms may cause osteomyelitis (Table 61).

Pathophysiology

Infecting microorganisms can invade by indirect or direct entry. The *indirect* (hematogenous) *entry* of microorganisms most frequently affects growing bone in boys younger than 12 years old and is associated with their higher incidence of blunt trauma. Adults with genitourinary and respiratory tract infections or disorders marked by vascular insufficiency (e.g., diabetes mellitus) are at high risk for the spread of a primary infection via the blood to the bone. Highly vascular bones such as the pelvis, tibia, and vertebrae are the most common sites of infection.

Direct-entry osteomyelitis can occur at any age when an open wound (e.g., penetrating wounds, fractures) allows microorganisms to enter the body. Osteomyelitis may also be related to the presence of a foreign body, such as an implant or an orthopedic prosthetic device (e.g., plate, total joint prosthesis).

TABLE 61	Organisms Causing Osteomyelitis
Organism	**Predisposing Problem(s)**
Staphylococcus aureus	Pressure ulcer, penetrating wound, open fracture, orthopedic surgery, disorders with vascular insufficiency (e.g., diabetes, atherosclerosis)
Staphylococcus epidermidis	Indwelling prosthetic devices (e.g., joint replacements, fracture fixation devices)
Streptococcus viridans	Abscessed tooth, gingival disease
Escherichia coli	Urinary tract infection
Mycobacterium tuberculosis	Tuberculosis
Neisseria gonorrhoeae	Gonorrhea
Pseudomonas	Puncture wounds, IV drug use
Salmonella	Sickle cell disease
Fungi, mycobacteria	Immunocompromised host

After gaining entry into the blood, the microorganisms multiply, and pressure increases because of the nonexpanding nature of most bone. This leads to ischemia and vascular compromise of the periosteum.

- The infection spreads through the bone cortex and marrow cavity, ultimately resulting in cortical devascularization and necrosis. Bone death occurs as a result of ischemia.
- The areas of devitalized bone eventually separate from surrounding living bone, forming *sequestra*. The part of the periosteum that continues to have a blood supply forms new bone called *involucrum*. It is difficult for blood-borne antibiotics or defending WBCs to reach the sequestra. A sequestrum may become a reservoir for microorganisms that spread to other sites, including the lungs and brain. If the sequestrum does not resolve on its own or is not debrided surgically, a sinus tract may develop with chronic, purulent drainage.

Acute osteomyelitis refers to the initial infection or an infection of less than 1 month in duration.

Chronic osteomyelitis refers to a bone infection that persists for longer than 1 month or an infection that failed to respond to an initial course of antibiotic therapy. Chronic osteomyelitis may be a continuous, persistent problem (a result of inadequate acute treatment) or a process of exacerbations and remissions. Over time, granulation tissue turns to avascular scar tissue, providing an ideal site for microorganism growth that cannot be penetrated by antibiotics.

Clinical Manifestations
Acute Osteomyelitis
Systemic manifestations include fever, night sweats, restlessness, nausea, and malaise.
- Local manifestations include constant bone pain that is unrelieved by rest and worsens with activity; swelling, tenderness, and warmth at the infection site; and restricted movement of the affected part.
- Later signs include drainage from the sinus tracts to the skin and/or fracture site.

Chronic Osteomyelitis
Systemic signs may be less severe than those seen with the acute form.

Diagnostic Studies
- Bone or soft tissue biopsy is definitive for determining the causative microorganism.
- Blood and/or wound cultures are frequently positive for microorganisms.
- Elevated WBC and erythrocyte sedimentation rate (ESR) may be found.
- X-ray signs suggestive of osteomyelitis usually do not appear until 10 days to weeks after the appearance of clinical symptoms, by which time the disease will have progressed.
- Radionuclide bone scans (gallium and indium) are helpful in diagnosis and usually positive in the area of infection.
- MRI and CT scan may be used to help identify the extent of the infection.

Interprofessional Care
Aggressive and prolonged IV antibiotic therapy is the treatment of choice for acute osteomyelitis if bone ischemia has not occurred. If antibiotic therapy is delayed, surgical debridement and decompression are often necessary.

Patients are often discharged to home care with IV antibiotics delivered through a central venous access device (CVAD). These include centrally inserted catheters, peripherally inserted central catheters (PICCs), and implanted ports. IV antibiotic therapy may be started in the hospital and continued at home for 4 to 6 weeks or as long as 3 to 6 months. A variety of antibiotics may be prescribed, depending on the microorganism. These drugs include penicillin, nafcillin (Nafcil), neomycin, vancomycin, cephalexin (Keflex), cefazolin (Ancef), cefoxitin (Mefoxin), gentamicin, and tobramycin.

- In adults with chronic osteomyelitis, oral therapy with a fluoroquinolone (ciprofloxacin [Cipro]) for 6 to 8 weeks may be prescribed instead of IV antibiotics.
- Oral antibiotic therapy may also be given after IV therapy is complete to ensure resolution of the infection.
- Patient response to drug therapy is monitored through bone scans and ESR tests.

Surgical treatment for chronic osteomyelitis includes surgical removal of the poorly vascularized tissue and dead bone and extended use of antibiotics. Antibiotic-impregnated acrylic bead chains may be implanted during surgery.

- Intermittent or constant irrigation of the affected bone with antibiotics may also be initiated.
- Hyperbaric oxygen therapy using 100% oxygen may be administered as an adjunct therapy in refractory cases of chronic osteomyelitis.

If orthopedic prosthetic devices are a source of chronic infection, they must be removed. Muscle flaps or skin grafting provide wound coverage over the dead space (cavity) in the bone. Bone grafts may help to restore blood flow. However, flaps or grafts should never be placed in the presence of active or suspected infection. Amputation of the extremity may be indicated to preserve life or improve quality of life (see Amputation, p. 681).

- Rare complications of osteomyelitis include septicemia, septic arthritis, pathologic fractures, and amyloidosis.

Nursing Management
Goals
The patient with osteomyelitis will have satisfactory pain and fever control, not experience any complications associated with osteomyelitis, cooperate with the treatment plan, and maintain a positive outlook on the disease outcome.
Nursing Diagnoses
- Acute pain
- Ineffective health maintenance
- Impaired physical mobility
Nursing Interventions
Control of other infections (e.g., urinary and respiratory tract, deep pressure ulcers) is important in preventing osteomyelitis.

Individuals especially at risk for osteomyelitis are those who are immunocompromised, or who have diabetes, orthopedic prosthetic devices, or vascular insufficiency.

- Instruct these patients and their families regarding manifestations of osteomyelitis and to immediately tell the HCP about bone pain, fever, swelling, and restricted limb movement so that treatment can be started.

Some immobilization of the affected limb (e.g., splint, traction) is usually indicated to decrease pain. Carefully handle the involved limb to avoid excessive manipulation, which increases pain and may cause a pathologic fracture.

- Assess the patient's pain. Muscle spasms may cause minor to severe pain. Nonsteroidal antiinflammatory drugs (NSAIDs), opioid analgesics, and muscle relaxants may be prescribed to provide patient comfort. Encourage nondrug (e.g., guided imagery, relaxation breathing) approaches to pain.
- Dressings are used to absorb drainage from wounds and to debride devitalized tissue from the wound site when removed. Sterile technique is essential when changing the dressing.

The patient is frequently placed on bed rest in the early stages of acute infection. Good body alignment and frequent position changes prevent complications associated with immobility and promote comfort.

- Peak and trough blood levels of most antibiotics should be monitored to avoid adverse drug effects.

▼ **Patient and Caregiver Teaching**

- Teach patient the possible adverse and toxic reactions associated with prolonged high-dose antibiotic therapy (e.g., tobramycin, neomycin). These reactions include hearing deficit, impaired renal function, and neurotoxicity (e.g., limb weakness or numbness, cognitive changes or loss of memory, vision changes, headache, behavioral problems). Reactions associated with cephalosporins (e.g., cefazolin) include hives, severe or watery diarrhea, blood in stools, and throat or mouth sores.
- Long-term antibiotic therapy can result in an overgrowth of *Candida albicans* and *Clostridium difficile* in the genitourinary and oral cavities. Instruct the patient to report any whitish yellow, curdlike lesions to the HCP.
- If at home, instruct patient and family on management of the venous access device. Also teach how to administer the antibiotic when scheduled and the need for follow-up laboratory testing. Stress importance of continuing to take antibiotics after the symptoms have improved.
- Instruct the patient and caregiver in the technique for wound dressing changes and assist them to obtain supplies.

- The patient and caregivers are often frightened and discouraged because of the serious nature of the disease, uncertainty of the outcome, and the long, costly treatment. Continued psychologic and emotional support is an integral part of nursing management.

OSTEOPOROSIS

Description

Osteoporosis, or porous bone (fragile bone disease), is a chronic, progressive metabolic bone disease marked by low bone mass and structural deterioration of bone tissue, leading to increased bone fragility. Over 5 million people in the United States have decreased bone density or osteoporosis. One in two women and one in four men over the age of 50 will sustain an osteoporosis-related fracture during their lifetime.

Risk factors for osteoporosis are female gender, advancing age (older than 65 years), white or Asian ethnicity, family history, low body weight, postmenopausal (estrogen deficiency), sedentary lifestyle, and a diet low in calcium or vitamin D deficiency. Low testosterone levels are a major risk factor in men.

- Current guidelines recommend an initial bone density test in all women over age 65. Women who are younger than 65 and at high risk (e.g., low body weight, smoker, prior fractures) should also have a bone density test. If results are normal and the person is at low risk for osteoporosis, another test is not needed for 15 years. Testing should start earlier and be done more frequently if a person is at high risk for fractures.
- Currently there is not sufficient evidence to demonstrate significant benefit for osteoporosis screening in men.

Pathophysiology

Peak bone mass (maximum bone tissue) is typically achieved before age 20 years. It is largely determined by four factors: heredity, nutrition, exercise, and hormone function. Heredity may be responsible for up to 70% of peak bone mass.

- Bone loss from midlife (age 35 to 40 years) onward is inevitable, but the rate of loss varies. Women experience rapid bone loss when estrogen production declines at menopause. This rate of loss then slows and eventually matches the rate of bone lost by men aged 65 to 70.

Bone is continually being deposited by osteoblasts and resorbed by osteoclasts, a process called *remodeling*. Normally, the rates of bone deposition and resorption are equal, so that the total bone mass remains constant. In osteoporosis, bone resorption exceeds bone deposition.

- Specific diseases associated with osteoporosis include inflammatory bowel disease, intestinal malabsorption, kidney disease, rheumatoid arthritis, hyperthyroidism, chronic alcoholism, cirrhosis of the liver, and diabetes mellitus.
- Many drugs can interfere with bone metabolism, including corticosteroids, antiseizure drugs (phenytoin [Dilantin]), heparin, aluminum-containing antacids, certain cancer chemotherapy agents, and excessive thyroid hormones. Long-term corticosteroid use is a major contributor to osteoporosis.

Clinical Manifestations

Osteoporosis is often called the "silent disease" because bone loss occurs without symptoms. People may not know they have osteoporosis until a sudden strain, bump, or fall causes a hip, wrist, or vertebral fracture.

- The first clinical indication of osteoporosis is usually back pain or spontaneous fractures. The loss of bone mass causes the bone to become mechanically weak and prone to spontaneous fractures or fractures from minimal trauma. A person who has one spinal vertebral fracture due to osteoporosis has an increased risk for a second vertebral fracture within 1 year.
- Over time, wedging and fractures of the vertebrae produce gradual loss of height and a humped back known as "dowager's hump," or *kyphosis.*

Diagnostic Studies

Osteoporosis often goes unnoticed because it cannot be detected by conventional x-ray until 25% to 40% of the calcium in the bone is lost.

- Serum calcium, phosphorus, and alkaline phosphatase levels remain normal, although alkaline phosphatase may be elevated after a fracture.
- Bone mineral density (BMD) measurements are used to measure bone density.
  - Quantitative ultrasound (QUS) measures bone density with sound waves in the heel, kneecap, or shin.
  - One of the most common BMD studies is dual-energy x-ray absorptiometry (DXA), which measures bone density in the spine, hips, and forearm (the most common sites of fractures resulting from osteoporosis). DXA studies are also useful to evaluate changes in bone density over time and to assess the effectiveness of treatment.

- DXA results are reported as T-scores: The *T-score* is the number of standard deviations below the average for normal bone density. A T-score of greater than −1 indicates normal bone density. Osteoporosis is defined as a BMD of less than −2.5 (at least 2.5 standard deviations) below the mean BMD of young adults. A T-score between +1 and −1 is considered normal. A T-score between −1 and −2.5 indicates *osteopenia* (bone loss that is greater than normal, but not yet at the level for a diagnosis of osteoporosis). A T-score of −2.5 or lower indicates osteoporosis. The greater the negative number, the more severe the osteoporosis.
- Sometimes the HCP asks for a *Z-score* instead of a T-score. For this score, a person is compared with someone his or her own age, gender, and/or ethnic group instead of a healthy 30-year-old. Among older adults, Z-scores can be misleading because decreased bone density is common. If the Z-score is −2 or lower, it may suggest that something other than aging is causing abnormal bone loss.

Nursing and Interprofessional Management

Care of the patient with osteoporosis focuses on proper nutrition, dietary calcium and calcium supplementation, exercise, prevention of falls and fractures, and drugs. Treatment is recommended for postmenopausal women who have (1) a T-score of less than −2.5, (2) a T-score between −1 and −2.5 with additional risk factors, or (3) a prior history of a hip or vertebral fracture.
- A patient's risk of fracture due to osteoporosis can also be calculated using the Fracture Risk Assessment (FRAX) tool *(www.shef.ac.uk/FRAX)*.

Prevention and treatment of osteoporosis focus on adequate calcium intake (1000 mg/day for women ages 19 to 50 years and men ages 19 to 70 years; 1200 mg/day in women 51 years or older and men 71 years or older).
- If dietary intake of calcium is inadequate, supplemental calcium may be recommended. The amount of elemental calcium varies in different calcium preparations.
- Vitamin D is important in calcium absorption and function. Most people get enough vitamin D from their diet or naturally through synthesis in the skin from exposure to sunlight. Being in the sun for 20 minutes a day is generally enough. However, supplemental vitamin D (800 to 1000 IU) is recommended for postmenopausal women, older adults, people who are homebound or in long-term care settings, and those in northern climates, because of decreased sun exposure.

- Regular physical activity is important to build up and maintain bone mass. The best exercises are those that are weight bearing and force an individual to work against gravity, such as walking, weight training, stair climbing, and dancing. Encourage walking (for 30 minutes three times per week) over high-impact aerobics or running, both of which may put too much stress on the bones resulting in fractures.

Vertebroplasty and kyphoplasty are minimally invasive procedures that are used to treat osteoporotic vertebral fractures. In *vertebroplasty,* bone cement is injected into the collapsed vertebra to stabilize it, but it does not correct the deformity. In *kyphoplasty,* an air bladder is inserted into the collapsed vertebra and inflated to restore vertebral body height, and then bone cement is injected.

Drug Therapy

Estrogen replacement therapy and estrogen with progesterone are no longer routinely given after menopause to prevent osteoporosis, because supplemental estrogen is associated with increased risk of heart disease as well as breast and uterine cancer. If a woman is taking short-term estrogen therapy to treat menopausal symptoms such as hot flashes, she may also receive some protection against bone loss and fractures of the hip and vertebrae.

- Bisphosphonates inhibit osteoclast-mediated bone resorption and slow the cycle of bone remodeling. Although a modest increase in BMD is typical, bone remodeling may be suppressed to the extent that normal bone formation is impaired and fracture risk increases. These drugs are widely used in the prevention and treatment of osteoporosis. Common side effects are anorexia, weight loss, and gastritis. Teach the patient to take the medication correctly to improve its absorption and decrease GI side effects (especially esophageal irritation). Alendronate (Fosamax) is available as a daily or weekly oral tablet. Ibandronate (Boniva) is available as a once-per-month oral tablet or can be given every 3 months by IV infusion. The immediate-release form of risedronate (Actonel) is given daily, weekly, or monthly based on the dose. Zoledronic acid (Reclast) is approved as a once-yearly IV infusion to treat osteoporosis, or is given every 2 years to prevent the disease. Renal function tests and serum calcium must be assessed before administration of the drug.
- Calcitonin is secreted by the thyroid gland and inhibits osteoclastic bone resorption by directly interacting with active osteoclasts. Salmon calcitonin is available in intranasal form. When

calcitonin is used, calcium supplementation is necessary to prevent secondary hyperparathyroidism.

- Another group of drugs used to treat osteoporosis is the selective estrogen receptor modulators, such as raloxifene (Evista). These drugs mimic the effect of estrogen on bone by reducing bone resorption without stimulating the tissues of the breast or uterus. Raloxifene may decrease breast cancer risk. Similar to tamoxifen, it blocks the estrogen receptor sites of cancer cells.
- Teriparatide (Forteo) is a portion of human parathyroid hormone that is used for the treatment of osteoporosis by increasing the action of osteoblasts. It is the first drug for osteoporosis that stimulates new bone formation rather than just preventing further bone loss.
- Denosumab (Prolia) may be used for postmenopausal women with osteoporosis who are at high risk for fractures. It is a monoclonal antibody that binds to a protein (RANKL) involved in the formation and function of osteoclasts. Denosumab is given as a subcutaneous injection every 6 months.

Medical management of patients receiving corticosteroids includes prescribing the lowest possible dose of the drug for the shortest possible time. Ensure an adequate intake of calcium and vitamin D, including supplementation when osteoporosis drugs are prescribed. If osteopenia is evident on bone densitometry, treatment with bisphosphonates may be considered.

OVARIAN CANCER

Description

Ovarian cancer is a malignant tumor of the ovaries. It is the fifth leading cause of cancer deaths in women in the United States. Most women with ovarian cancer have advanced disease at diagnosis. It occurs most frequently in women between 55 and 65 years of age. Currently only 20% of ovarian cancers are diagnosed at an early stage.

Women who have mutations of the *BRCA* genes have an increased susceptibility to ovarian (and breast) cancer. Additional risk factors are presented in Table 62. Protective factors decrease the risk of ovarian cancer by reducing the number of ovulatory cycles and thus reduce exposure to estrogen.

Pathophysiology

The cause of ovarian cancer is unknown. About 90% of ovarian cancers are epithelial carcinomas that arise from malignant

TABLE 62   Risk Factors for Ovarian Cancer

Increased Risk	Decreased Risk (Protective)
• Family or personal history of ovarian, breast, or colon cancer • Personal history of hereditary nonpolyposis colorectal cancer • Hormone replacement therapy • Mutant *BRCA* gene • Early menarche and late menopause • Increasing age • Nulliparity • High-fat diet	• Oral contraceptive use (for >5 yr) • Breastfeeding • Multiple pregnancies • Early age at birth of first baby

transformation of the surface epithelial cells. Germ cell tumors account for another 10%.

Intraperitoneal dissemination is a common characteristic of ovarian cancer. It metastasizes to the uterus, bladder, bowel, and omentum. In advanced disease, ovarian cancer may spread to the stomach, colon, and liver.

Clinical Manifestations

Early ovarian cancer usually has no obvious symptoms. Most clinical manifestations are vague and nonspecific. These include pelvic or abdominal pain, bloating, urinary urgency or frequency, and difficulty eating or feeling full quickly.

- Late-stage disease typically manifests with abdominal enlargement with ascites (fluid in the abdominal cavity), unexplained weight loss or gain, and menstrual changes.

Diagnostic Studies

- Yearly bimanual pelvic examinations should be performed to identify an ovarian mass.
- Abdominal or vaginal ultrasound can be used to detect ovarian masses.
- An exploratory laparotomy may be used to establish the diagnosis and disease stage.
- For women at high risk for ovarian cancer, screening using a combination of the tumor marker CA-125 and ultrasound is often recommended in addition to a yearly pelvic examination.

Interprofessional Care

Women identified as being at high risk based on family and health history may require counseling regarding options such as prophylactic oophorectomy and oral contraceptives.

Most patients with ovarian cancer have widespread disease at presentation. The initial treatment for all stages of ovarian cancer is surgery, which is usually a total abdominal hysterectomy and bilateral salpingo-oophorectomy with omentectomy and removal of as much of the tumor as possible (i.e., tumor debulking).

Depending on cell differentiation and cancer stage, treatment options include intraperitoneal and systemic chemotherapy, intraperitoneal instillation of radioisotopes, and external abdominal and pelvic radiation therapy.

- The chemotherapy agents most commonly used are taxanes (paclitaxel or docetaxel) and platinum-based agents (carboplatin or cisplatin).
- Targeted therapy agents that are used to treat advanced ovarian cancer include bevacizumab (Avastin) and olaparib (Lynparza). Bevacizumab is an angiogenesis inhibitor. Olaparib is a poly ADP-ribose polymerase (PARP) inhibitor that blocks enzymes involved in repairing damaged DNA.

Nursing Management: Cancers of the Female Reproductive Tract

See Cervical Cancer, p. 117.

PAGET'S DISEASE

Description

Paget's disease (osteitis deformans) is a chronic skeletal bone disorder in which there is excessive bone resorption followed by replacement of normal marrow by vascular, fibrous connective tissue and new bone that is larger, more disorganized, and weaker. Commonly affected regions of the skeleton are the pelvis, long bones, spine, ribs, sternum, and cranium. The etiology of Paget's disease is unknown, although a viral etiology has been proposed.

Up to 40% of all patients with Paget's disease have a relative with the disorder. Men are affected twice as often as women.

Clinical Manifestations

In milder forms of Paget's disease, patients may remain free of symptoms. The disease may be discovered incidentally on x-ray or serum chemistry findings indicating a high alkaline phosphatase (ALP) level.

- Bone pain may develop gradually and progress to severe intractable pain. Other early manifestations include fatigue and progressive development of a waddling gait.
- Headaches, dementia, visual deficits, and loss of hearing can result with an enlarged, thickened skull. Increased bone volume in the spine can cause spinal cord or nerve root compression.

Pathologic fracture is the most common complication and may be the first indication of the disease. Other complications include osteosarcoma, osteoclastoma (giant cell tumor), and fibrosarcoma.

Diagnostic Studies

- Serum ALP levels are markedly elevated (indicating rapid bone turnover) in advanced disease.
- X-rays may show curvature of an affected bone and thickened bone cortex, especially in weight-bearing bones and the cranium.
- Bone scans using a radiolabeled bisphosphate demonstrate increased uptake in the affected skeletal areas.

Nursing and Interprofessional Management

Care is usually limited to symptomatic and supportive care, with correction of secondary deformities by either surgical intervention or braces.

- Bisphosphonate drugs, such as etidronate (Didronel), alendronate (Fosamax), risedronate (Actonel), and ibandronate (Boniva), are also used to retard bone resorption. Zoledronic acid (Reclast) may also be given as a bone-building drug. Calcium and vitamin D are often given to decrease hypocalcemia, a common side effect with these drugs. Monitor drug effectiveness by regular assessment of serum ALP.
- Calcitonin therapy is recommended for patients who cannot tolerate bisphosphonate drugs. Response to calcitonin therapy is not permanent and often stops when therapy is discontinued.
- Pain is usually managed with nonsteroidal antiinflammatory drugs (NSAIDs).
- Orthopedic surgery for fractures, hip and knee replacements, and knee realignment may be necessary.

A firm mattress should be used to provide back support and relieve pain. The patient may need to wear a corset or light brace to relieve back pain and to provide support when in the upright position. Teach the patient correct application of such devices, and how to regularly examine areas of the skin for friction damage.

- Good body mechanics are essential. Discourage activities such as lifting and twisting. Physical therapy may increase muscle strength.
- A healthy diet, especially as it pertains to vitamin D, calcium, and protein, is important for bone formation.
- Teach the patient to use an assistive device and make environmental changes (e.g., eliminate throw rugs) to decrease risk for falls and related fractures.

PANCREATIC CANCER

Description

Pancreatic cancer is the fourth leading cause of death from cancer in the United States, with the peak incidence between the ages of 65 and 80 years. Most pancreatic tumors are adenocarcinomas. As the tumor grows, the common bile duct becomes obstructed and obstructive jaundice develops. Tumors starting in the body or the tail of the pancreas often remain silent until their growth is advanced.

The majority of cancers have metastasized at the time of diagnosis, with a poor prognosis. Most patients die within 5 to 12 months of the initial diagnosis, and the 5-year survival rate is less than 5%.

Pathophysiology

The cause of pancreatic cancer is unknown. Risk factors are cigarette smoking, high-fat diet, diabetes mellitus, chronic pancreatitis, family history of pancreatic cancer, and exposure to chemicals such as benzidine. Smokers are two to three times more likely to develop pancreatic cancer than nonsmokers. The risk is related to both duration of smoking and number of cigarettes smoked per day.

Clinical Manifestations

Signs and symptoms of pancreatic cancer are often similar to those of chronic pancreatitis. Manifestations include abdominal pain (dull or aching), anorexia, rapid and progressive weight loss, nausea, and jaundice.

- The most common manifestations when the cancer occurs in the head of the pancreas are pain, jaundice, and weight loss.
- Pruritus may accompany obstructive jaundice. In general, pain is common and is related to the location of the malignancy. Extreme, unrelenting pain is related to extension of the cancer into the retroperitoneal tissues and nerve plexuses. The pain is frequently located in the upper abdomen or left hypochondrium

and often radiates to the back. It is commonly related to eating, and it also occurs at night.
- Weight loss is due to poor digestion and absorption caused by lack of digestive enzymes from the pancreas.

Diagnostic Studies
- Abdominal ultrasound or endoscopic ultrasound (EUS), spiral CT scan, MRI, and MR cholangiopancreatography (MRCP) are the most commonly used imaging techniques for diagnosing and staging pancreatic cancer.
- Endoscopic retrograde cholangiography (ERCP) allows for visualization and collection of secretions and tissues from the pancreatic duct and biliary system.
- CA19-9, which is elevated in pancreatic cancer, is the most commonly used tumor marker.

Interprofessional Care
Surgery provides the most effective treatment, but only 15% to 20% of patients have resectable tumors at the time of diagnosis. The classic surgery is a *radical pancreaticoduodenectomy* or *Whipple procedure*. This procedure is a resection of the proximal pancreas (proximal pancreatectomy), the adjoining duodenum (duodenectomy), the distal portion of the stomach (partial gastrectomy), and the distal segment of the common bile duct. An anastomosis of the pancreatic duct, common bile duct, and stomach to the jejunum is done.
- If the pancreatic tumor cannot be removed surgically, palliative measures may include a cholecystojejunostomy to relieve biliary obstruction and/or endoscopic placement of biliary stents.
- Radiation therapy alters survival rates little but is effective for pain relief. External irradiation is usually used, but implantation of internal radiation seeds into the tumor has also been used.
- The role of chemotherapy in pancreatic cancer is limited. Chemotherapy usually consists of fluorouracil (5-FU) and gemcitabine (Gemzar), either alone or in combination with agents such as capecitabine (Xeloda), paclitaxel (Abraxane), or erlotinib (Tarceva). Erlotinib is a targeted therapy agent.

Nursing Management
Because the patient with pancreatic cancer has many of the same problems as the patient with pancreatitis, nursing care includes the same measures (see Pancreatitis, Acute, p. 469).
- Provide symptomatic and supportive nursing care, including medications and comfort measures to relieve pain.

- Psychologic support is essential, especially during times of anxiety or depression.
- Support adequate nutrition with measures to manage anorexia, nausea, and vomiting. Offer frequent and supplemental feedings.
- Because bleeding can result from impaired vitamin K production, assess for bleeding from body orifices and mucous membranes.
- Helping the patient and caregivers through the grieving process is an important aspect of nursing care.

PANCREATITIS, ACUTE

Description

Acute pancreatitis is acute inflammation of the pancreas, varying from mild edema to severe hemorrhagic necrosis. Pancreatic enzymes spilling into the surrounding pancreatic tissue cause autodigestion and severe pain. Acute pancreatitis is most common in middle-aged men and women, with the rate three times higher in African Americans than in whites.

The severity of the disease varies according to the extent of pancreatic destruction. Some patients recover completely, others have recurring attacks, and still others develop chronic pancreatitis. Acute pancreatitis can be life-threatening.

Pathophysiology

Many factors can cause injury to the pancreas. In the United States the most common cause is gallbladder disease (gallstones), which is more common in women. The second most common cause is chronic alcohol intake, which is more common in men. Smoking is an independent risk factor for acute pancreatitis. Biliary sludge, which is a mixture of cholesterol crystals and calcium salts, is found in 20% to 40% of patients with acute pancreatitis. Acute pancreatitis attacks are also associated with hypertriglyceridemia (serum levels over 1000 mg/dL).

Less common causes of acute pancreatitis include trauma (postoperative or post-procedure after endoscopic retrograde cholangiopancreatography [ERCP]), viral infections (mumps, HIV infection), penetrating duodenal ulcers, cysts, abscesses, cystic fibrosis, certain drugs (corticosteroids, sulfonamides, NSAIDs), and metabolic disorders (hyperparathyroidism, renal failure). Autodigestion of the pancreas is precipitated by injury to pancreatic cells or activation of pancreatic enzymes in the pancreas rather than in the intestine. The pathophysiologic involvement in acute pancreatitis is classified as either *mild pancreatitis* (also known as edematous or interstitial) or *severe pancreatitis* (also called *necrotizing pancreatitis*). Patients with severe pancreatitis are at high risk for developing pancreatic necrosis, organ failure, and septic complications.

Clinical Manifestations

Abdominal pain is the predominant symptom of acute pancreatitis. The pain is usually located in the left upper quadrant but may be in the midepigastric area. The pain commonly radiates to the back because of the retroperitoneal location of the pancreas.

- The pain has a sudden onset and is described as severe, deep, piercing, and continuous or steady. It is aggravated by eating and frequently begins when the patient is recumbent; pain is not relieved by vomiting. The pain may be accompanied by flushing, cyanosis, and dyspnea.

Other manifestations of acute pancreatitis include nausea and vomiting, low-grade fever, leukocytosis, hypotension, tachycardia, and jaundice. Abdominal tenderness with muscle guarding is common. Bowel sounds may be decreased or absent. Paralytic ileus may occur and causes marked abdominal distention. The lungs are frequently involved, with crackles present.

- Intravascular damage from circulating trypsin may cause areas of cyanosis or greenish to yellow-brown discoloration of the abdominal wall. Other areas of ecchymoses are the flanks (*Grey Turner's spots* or *sign,* a bluish flank discoloration) and the periumbilical area (*Cullen's sign,* a bluish periumbilical discoloration).
- Shock may occur because of hemorrhage into the pancreas, toxemia from the activated pancreatic enzymes, or hypovolemia resulting from massive fluid shifts into the retroperitoneal space.

Complications

Local complications of acute pancreatitis are pseudocyst and abscess.

- A *pancreatic pseudocyst* is an accumulation of fluid, pancreatic enzymes, tissue debris, and inflammatory exudates surrounded by a wall. Manifestations of pseudocyst are abdominal pain, palpable epigastric mass, nausea, vomiting, and anorexia. The serum amylase level frequently remains elevated. CT, MRI, and endoscopic ultrasound (EUS) may be used in the diagnosis. The cysts usually resolve spontaneously within a few weeks but may perforate, causing peritonitis, or rupture into the stomach or the duodenum. Treatment options include surgical drainage, percutaneous catheter placement and drainage, and endoscopic drainage.

- A *pancreatic abscess* is a collection of pus resulting from extensive necrosis in the pancreas. It may become infected or perforate into adjacent organs. Manifestations include upper abdominal pain, abdominal mass, high fever, and leukocytosis. Pancreatic abscesses require prompt surgical drainage to prevent sepsis.

Systemic complications of acute pancreatitis include pleural effusion, atelectasis, pneumonia, hyperglycemia, hypotension, and hypocalcemia leading to tetany.

Diagnostic Studies

- Elevations of serum amylase and lipase are primary diagnostic findings.
- Liver enzymes, triglycerides, glucose, and bilirubin are elevated with a decrease in calcium.
- Abdominal ultrasound, x-ray, or contrast-enhanced CT scan can identify pancreatic problems.
- ERCP is used along with EUS, magnetic resonance cholangio-pancreatography (MRCP), and angiography to diagnose pancreatic problems.

Interprofessional Care

P

Goals of management for acute pancreatitis include relief of pain, prevention or alleviation of shock, reduction of pancreatic secretions, correction of fluid and electrolyte imbalances, prevention or treatment of infections, and removal of the precipitating cause, if possible.

Treatment of acute pancreatitis is focused on supportive care, including aggressive hydration, pain management, management of metabolic complications, and minimization of pancreatic stimulation. Treatment and control of pain are very important. Morphine may be used and may be combined with an antispasmodic.

- If shock is present, blood volume replacements, volume expanders, and fluids may be given.

It is important to reduce or suppress pancreatic enzymes to decrease stimulation of the pancreas and allow it to rest. Usually the patient is NPO, and nasogastric (NG) suction is used to reduce vomiting and prevent gastric digestive juices from entering the duodenum. Drugs that neutralize or suppress formation of HCl in the stomach, such as antacids, histamine H_2-receptor antagonists, and proton pump inhibitors, may also help to suppress gastric acid secretion.

- Inflamed and necrotic pancreatic tissue is a good medium for bacterial growth. Antibiotic therapy should be instituted early if an infection occurs.
- With resolution of the pancreatitis, the patient resumes oral intake. Enteral nutrition support may be needed.

When the acute pancreatitis is related to gallstones, an urgent ERCP with endoscopic sphincterotomy may be performed. This may be followed by laparoscopic cholecystectomy to reduce the potential for recurrence. Surgical intervention may be indicated when the diagnosis is uncertain and in patients who do not respond to conservative therapy. Patients with severe acute pancreatitis may require drainage of necrotic fluid collections performed surgically, under CT guidance, or endoscopically. Percutaneous pseudocyst drainage can be performed, and a drainage tube is left in place.

Several different drugs are used to prevent and treat problems associated with pancreatitis (see Table 43-19, Lewis et al, *Medical-Surgical Nursing,* ed 10, p. 1001). Currently there are no drugs that cure pancreatitis.

Nursing Management
Goals
The patient with acute pancreatitis will have relief of pain, normal fluid and electrolyte balance, minimal to no complications, and no recurrent attacks.
Nursing Diagnoses
- Acute pain
- Deficient fluid volume
- Imbalanced nutrition: less than body requirements
- Ineffective health management
Nursing Interventions
Encourage early diagnosis and treatment of biliary tract disease, such as cholelithiasis. Encourage the patient to eliminate alcohol intake, especially if there have been previous episodes of pancreatitis.

During the acute phase, a major focus of your care is pain relief. Pain and restlessness can increase the metabolic rate and stimulate pancreatic enzymes. Assess and document the duration of pain relief. Measures such as comfortable positioning, frequent changes in position, and relief of nausea and vomiting assist in reducing the restlessness that usually accompanies the pain.

- A side-lying position with the head elevated 45 degrees decreases tension on the abdomen and may help ease the pain.
- For the patient who is on NPO status or has an NG tube, provide frequent oral and nasal care to relieve dryness of the mouth and nose.

- Observe for fever and other manifestations of infection. Respiratory tract infections are common because the retroperitoneal fluid raises the diaphragm, which causes the patient to take shallow, guarded abdominal breaths. Measures to prevent respiratory tract infections include turning, coughing, deep breathing, and assuming a semi-Fowler's position.

Patients may require follow-up home care to detect complications. Physical therapy may be needed due to loss of muscle strength.

▼ **Patient and Caregiver Teaching**

- Counseling regarding abstinence from alcohol is important to prevent the patient from experiencing future attacks of acute pancreatitis and development of chronic pancreatitis.
- Because cigarettes can stimulate the pancreas, smoking should be avoided.
- Dietary teaching should include the restriction of fats because they stimulate the secretion of cholecystokinin, which then stimulates the pancreas. Encourage carbohydrates, which are less stimulating to the pancreas. Instruct the patient to avoid crash dieting and binge eating, because these can precipitate attacks.
- Instruct patient and caregiver to recognize symptoms of infection, diabetes mellitus, or *steatorrhea* (foul-smelling, frothy stools). These changes indicate possible ongoing destruction of pancreatic tissue.

PANCREATITIS, CHRONIC

Description

Chronic pancreatitis is a continuous, prolonged, inflammatory, and fibrosing process involving the pancreas. The pancreas is progressively destroyed as it is replaced by fibrotic tissue with strictures and calcifications. Chronic pancreatitis may follow acute pancreatitis or occur in the absence of any history of an acute condition.

Chronic pancreatitis can be due to alcohol abuse; obstruction caused by cholelithiasis (gallstones), tumor, pseudocysts, or trauma; or systemic diseases (e.g., systemic lupus erythematosus), autoimmune pancreatitis, or cystic fibrosis.

Pathophysiology

The most common cause of *obstructive* pancreatitis is inflammation of the sphincter of Oddi associated with cholelithiasis (gallstones). Cancer of the ampulla of Vater, duodenum, or pancreas can also cause this type of chronic pancreatitis.

The most common cause of *nonobstructive* pancreatitis (the most common type of chronic pancreatitis) is alcohol abuse. In nonobstructive pancreatitis there is inflammation and sclerosis, mainly in the head of the pancreas and around the pancreatic duct.

Clinical Manifestations

As with acute pancreatitis, a major manifestation of chronic pancreatitis is abdominal pain. The patient may have episodes of acute pain, but it usually is chronic (recurrent attacks at intervals of months or years). The attacks may become more and more frequent until the pain is almost constant, or they may diminish as the pancreatic fibrosis develops. The pain is located in the same areas as in acute pancreatitis but is usually described as a heavy, gnawing feeling or sometimes as burning and cramplike. The pain is not relieved with food or antacids.

- Other manifestations include signs and symptoms of pancreatic insufficiency, including malabsorption with weight loss, constipation, mild jaundice with dark frothy urine, steatorrhea, and diabetes mellitus. The steatorrhea may become severe, with voluminous, foul, fatty stools. Abdominal tenderness may be present.
- Complications of chronic pancreatitis may include pseudocyst formation, bile duct or duodenal obstruction, pancreatic ascites or pleural effusion, or pancreatic cancer.

Diagnostic Studies

Confirming the diagnosis of chronic pancreatitis can be challenging and is based on the patient's signs and symptoms, laboratory studies, and imaging.

- Serum amylase and lipase levels may be slightly elevated or not at all.
- Serum bilirubin and alkaline phosphatase levels may be elevated.
- Mild leukocytosis and elevated sedimentation rate may be found.
- Endoscopic retrograde cholangiopancreatography (ERCP) is used to visualize the pancreatic and biliary ductal system.
- CT, MRI, MR cholangiopancreatography (MRCP), abdominal ultrasound, and endoscopic ultrasound may be used in the diagnostic workup.

Nursing and Interprofessional Management

When the patient with chronic pancreatitis experiences an acute attack, the therapy is similar to that for acute pancreatitis. At other times the focus is on the prevention of further attacks, relief of pain, and control of pancreatic exocrine and endocrine insufficiency. Sometimes large, frequent doses of analgesics are needed to relieve the pain.

- A bland diet low in fat and high in carbohydrates, pancreatic enzyme replacement such as pancrelipase (Creon, Zenpep), and management of diabetes are measures used to control the pancreatic insufficiency.
- Treatment of chronic pancreatitis sometimes requires endoscopic therapy or surgery. When biliary disease is present or obstruction or pseudocyst develops, surgery may be indicated to divert bile flow or relieve ductal obstruction.

▼ **Patient and Caregiver Teaching**
- Instruct the patient to take measures to prevent further attacks. Dietary control, along with consistency in other treatment measures such as taking pancreatic enzymes, is essential.
- Observe the patient's stools for steatorrhea to help determine the effectiveness of the enzyme replacement. Instruct the patient and caregiver to observe the stools.
- The patient must avoid alcohol and may need assistance with this problem. If the patient is dependent on alcohol, a referral to other agencies or resources may be necessary.
- If diabetes has developed, instruct the patient regarding blood glucose testing and drug therapy (see Diabetes Mellitus, p. 166).

PARKINSON'S DISEASE

Description

Parkinson's disease (PD) is a chronic, progressive neurodegenerative disorder characterized by slowness in the initiation and execution of movement *(bradykinesia),* increased muscle tone *(rigidity),* tremor at rest, and gait disturbance. It is the most common form of *parkinsonism* (a syndrome characterized by similar symptoms).

Up to 1 million Americans are believed to be living with PD, with approximately 60,000 diagnosed each year. Incidence of PD increases with age, but an estimated 4% of people with PD are diagnosed before the age of 50 years. PD is more common in men by a ratio of 3:2.

Approximately 20% of patients with PD have a family history of PD. Many genes have been linked to the development of familial PD.

Pathophysiology

Although the exact cause of PD is unknown, a complex interplay of environmental and genetic factors is involved. About 15% of

PD patients have a family history of the disease, indicating a strong genetic basis for PD. In other people, exposure to toxins or certain viruses may trigger PD.

There are many forms of secondary (atypical) parkinsonism other than PD. Parkinson-like symptoms can occur after intoxication with a variety of chemicals, including carbon monoxide and manganese (among copper miners) and the product of meperidine analog synthesis, MPTP (1-methyl-4-phenyl-1,2,3,6-tetrahydropyridine).

Drug-induced parkinsonism can follow reserpine, methyldopa, lithium, haloperidol (Haldol), and phenothiazine therapy. It is also seen after use of amphetamine and methamphetamine.

- The pathology of PD involves the degeneration of the dopamine-producing neurons in the substantia nigra of the midbrain, which in turn disrupts the normal balance between dopamine (DA) and acetylcholine (ACh) in the basal ganglia.
- DA is a neurotransmitter essential for normal functioning of the extrapyramidal motor system, including control of posture, support, and voluntary motion. Symptoms do not occur until 80% of neurons in the substantia nigra are lost.
- *Lewy bodies,* unusual clumps of protein, are found in the brains of patients with PD. It is not known what causes these bodies to form, but their presence indicates abnormal functioning of the brain.

Clinical Manifestations

Onset of PD is gradual and insidious, and the clinical course is progressive. Classic manifestations of PD are easily remembered using the mnemonic *TRAP* (Tremor, Rigidity, Akinesia, and Postural instability). In the beginning stages, only a mild tremor, slight limp, or decreased arm swing may be evident. Later the patient may have a shuffling, propulsive gait with arms flexed and loss of postural reflexes. Some patients exhibit a slight change in speech patterns.

- *Tremor,* often the first sign, may initially be minimal, so that the patient is the only one who notices it. This tremor is more prominent at rest and is aggravated by emotional stress or increased concentration. The hand tremor is described as "pill rolling" because the thumb and forefinger appear to move in a rotary fashion as if rolling a pill, coin, or other small object. Tremor can involve the diaphragm, tongue, lips, and jaw.
- *Rigidity* is increased resistance to passive motion when the limbs are moved through their range of motion. Parkinsonian rigidity is typified by jerky (cogwheel) rigidity, as if there were intermittent catches when the joint is passively moved.

- *Akinesia* is the absence or loss of control of voluntary muscle movements. *Bradykinesia* (slow movement) is particularly evident in the loss of automatic movements, secondary to the physical and chemical alteration of the basal ganglia. In the unaffected person, automatic movements are involuntary and occur subconsciously. These include blinking of the eyelids, swinging of the arms while walking, swallowing of saliva, self-expression with facial and hand movements, and minor movement of postural adjustment. A lack of such spontaneous activity in PD accounts for the "old man" image with stooped posture, masklike face ("deadpan" expression), drooling of saliva, and shuffling gait.
- *Postural instability* is common, and patients may complain of being unable to stop themselves from going forward (propulsion) or backward (retropulsion).

Nonmotor signs and symptoms include depression, anxiety, apathy, fatigue, pain, urinary retention, erectile dysfunction, and memory changes. Sleep problems are common and include difficulty staying asleep at night, restless sleep, nightmares, and drowsiness or sudden sleep onset during the day.

Complications

As the disease progresses, complications may occur, including motor symptoms. These include dyskinesias (spontaneous, involuntary movements), weakness, dementia, depression, hallucinations, and psychosis.

- Swallowing becomes more difficult *(dysphagia)*; malnutrition or aspiration may result.
- General debilitation may lead to pneumonia, urinary tract infections, and skin breakdown.
- Orthostatic hypotension along with the loss of postural reflexes may result in fall injuries.

Diagnostic Studies

Because there is no specific diagnostic test for PD, the diagnosis is based on the history and clinical features.

- A definitive diagnosis can be made when TRAP manifestations are present.
- The ultimate confirmation is a positive response to antiparkinsonian drugs.

Interprofessional Care

Because there is no cure, management is aimed at relieving symptoms.

Drug Therapy

Drug therapy for PD is aimed at correcting the imbalance of central nervous system (CNS) neurotransmitters. Antiparkinsonian drugs either enhance the release or supply of DA (dopaminergic) or antagonize or block the effects of ACh in the striatum. Levodopa with carbidopa (Sinemet) is the primary treatment for symptomatic patients. Levodopa is a precursor of DA and can cross the blood-brain barrier. It is converted to DA in the basal ganglia. Prolonged use of levodopa can result in dyskinesias and "off/on" periods when the medication will unpredictably start or stop working. See Table 63 for the actions of drugs commonly used to manage PD.

Surgical Therapy

Surgical procedures are aimed at relieving symptoms of PD and are usually used in patients who are unresponsive to drug therapy or who have developed severe motor complications. Procedures fall into three categories: ablation (destruction), deep brain stimulation (DBS), and transplantation.

Nutritional Therapy

Malnutrition and constipation can be serious consequences of inadequate nutrition. Patients who have dysphagia and bradykinesia need appetizing foods that are easily chewed and swallowed, with adequate fiber to avoid constipation. Provide ample time for eating to avoid frustration.

Nursing Management

Goals

The patient with PD will maximize neurologic function, maintain independence in activities of daily living for as long as possible, and optimize psychosocial well-being.

TABLE 63 Drug Therapy	
Parkinson's Disease	
Drug	**Mechanism of Action**
Dopaminergics	
Dopamine Precursors	
levodopa (L-dopa) levodopa/carbidopa (Sinemet)	Converted to dopamine in basal ganglia

TABLE 63 Drug Therapy

Parkinson's Disease—cont'd

Drug	Mechanism of Action
Dopamine Receptor Agonists	
bromocriptine (Parlodel) cabergoline pramipexole (Mirapex) ropinirole (Requip, Requip XL) rotigotine (Neupro [transdermal patch])	Stimulate dopamine receptors
Dopamine Agonists	
amantadine	Blocks NMDA-type glutamate receptors, increases dopamine release, and blocks dopamine reuptake
apomorphine (Apokyn)	Stimulates postsynaptic dopamine receptors
Anticholinergics	
trihexyphenidyl benztropine (Cogentin)	Block cholinergic receptors, thus helping to balance cholinergic and dopaminergic activity
Antihistamine	
diphenhydramine	Has anticholinergic effect
Monoamine Oxidase Inhibitors	
selegiline (Eldepryl) rasagiline (Azilect)	Block breakdown of dopamine
Catechol O-Methyltransferase (COMT) Inhibitors	
entacapone (Comtan) tolcapone (Tasmar)	Block COMT and slow the breakdown of levodopa, thus prolonging the action of levodopa

NMDA, N-Methyl-D-aspartic acid.

P

Nursing Diagnoses
- Impaired physical mobility
- Impaired swallowing
- Imbalanced nutrition: less than body requirements

Nursing Interventions

Promotion of physical exercise and a well-balanced diet are major areas for nursing care. Exercise can limit the consequences of decreased mobility such as muscle atrophy, contractures, and constipation. Include exercises for overall muscle tone and to strengthen the muscles involved with speaking and swallowing.

Because PD is a chronic degenerative disorder, focus on teaching and nursing care directed toward the maintenance of good health, encouragement of independence, and avoidance of complications such as contractures.

▼ **Patient and Caregiver Teaching**
- For patients who are at risk for falling and tend to "freeze" while walking, have them think consciously about stepping over imaginary lines, practice stepping over rice kernels, rock from side to side, lift the toes when stepping, or take one step backward and two steps forward.
- Teach the patient to facilitate getting out of a chair by using an upright chair with arms and placing the back legs on small (2-inch) blocks.
- Encourage environmental alterations, such as removing rugs and excess furniture to avoid stumbling.
- Clothing can be simplified by the use of slip-on shoes and hook-and-loop (Velcro) fasteners or zippers on clothing instead of buttons and hooks.
- An elevated toilet seat can facilitate getting on and off the toilet.
- As the disease progresses, the impact on the psychologic well-being of the patient increases. Assist the patient through listening, providing education, encouraging social interactions, and referral to the American Parkinson Disease Association (*www.apdaparkinson.org*).

Family members (e.g., spouse, children) provide care for the majority of patients with PD. As the disease progresses, the caregiver burden increases and has been associated with decreases in caregiver physical and mental health. Strategies to reduce caregiver burden are described in Lewis et al, *Medical-Surgical Nursing,* ed 10, pp. 49 to 50.

PELVIC INFLAMMATORY DISEASE

Description

Pelvic inflammatory disease (PID) is an infectious condition of the pelvic cavity that may involve the fallopian tubes (salpingitis), ovaries (oophoritis), and pelvic peritoneum (peritonitis).

Pathophysiology

PID is often the result of untreated cervical infection. The organism infecting the cervix can spread into the uterus, fallopian tubes, ovaries, and peritoneal cavity. The most frequent causative organisms are *Chlamydia trachomatis* and *Neisseria gonorrhoeae*. These organisms, as well as anaerobes, mycoplasmas, streptococci, and enteric gram-negative rods, gain entrance during sexual intercourse or after pregnancy termination, pelvic surgery, or childbirth.

Clinical Manifestations

Lower abdominal pain is a common manifestation of PID.

- The pain gradually becomes constant, ranging from mild to severe. Movement such as walking and intercourse increases the pain.
- Spotting after intercourse and purulent cervical or vaginal discharge are common.
- Fever and chills may also be present.
- Women with less acute symptoms often notice increased cramping pain with menses, irregular bleeding, and some pain with intercourse. Women who have mild symptoms may go untreated because they did not seek care or the HCP misdiagnosed their complaints.

Complications

Complications of PID may include septic shock, perihepatitis, tubo-ovarian abscess, peritonitis, and embolism. PID can cause adhesions and strictures in the fallopian tubes, which may lead to ectopic pregnancy. Further damage can obstruct the fallopian tubes, causing infertility.

Diagnostic Studies

A pelvic examination is used to assist in the diagnosis of PID. Women with PID have lower abdominal tenderness, adnexal tenderness, and cervical motion tenderness.

- Diagnostic testing includes examination for *N. gonorrhoeae* and *C. trachomatis*.

P

- A pregnancy test is done to rule out ectopic pregnancy.
- When pain or obesity compromises the pelvic examination, a vaginal ultrasound may be ordered.

Interprofessional Care

PID is usually treated on an outpatient basis. With effective combination antibiotic therapy, the pain should subside. The patient should abstain from intercourse for 3 weeks. Her partner(s) must be examined and treated. An important part of care is physical rest and oral fluids. Reevaluation in 48 to 72 hours, even if symptoms are improving, is an essential part of outpatient care.

If a tubo-ovarian abscess is present, or if the patient is acutely ill or in severe pain, hospital admission is indicated. Maximum doses of IV antibiotics are given in the hospital. Corticosteroids may be added to the regimen to reduce inflammation, allowing for faster recovery and optimizing the chances for subsequent fertility. Applying heat to the lower abdomen or sitz baths may improve circulation and decrease pain. Bed rest in a semi-Fowler's position promotes drainage of the pelvic cavity by gravity; this may prevent the development of abscesses high in the abdomen. Analgesics to relieve pain and IV fluids to prevent dehydration are also used.

Surgery is indicated for abscesses that fail to resolve with IV antibiotics. An abscess may be drained using a laparoscopic approach or via laparotomy.

Nursing Management

Prevention, early recognition, and prompt treatment of vaginal and cervical infections can help prevent PID and its serious complications. Provide information regarding factors that place a woman at increased risk for PID. Urge women to seek medical attention for any unusual vaginal discharge or possible infection of their reproductive organs.

During the patient's hospitalization for PID, you have an important role in implementing drug therapy, monitoring the patient's health status, and providing symptom relief and patient teaching. Explain the need for limited activity, being in a semi-Fowler's position, and increased fluid intake. Assess the degree of abdominal pain to provide information about the effectiveness of drug therapy.

- The patient may feel guilty about having PID, especially if it was associated with a sexually transmitted infection. She may also be concerned about the complications associated with PID, such as infertility and the increased incidence of ectopic pregnancy. Discuss her feelings and concerns to assist her to cope.

PELVIC PAIN, CHRONIC

Description

Chronic pelvic pain refers to pain in the pelvic region (below the umbilicus and between the hips) that lasts 6 months or longer. The cause of chronic pelvic pain is often hard to find.

- Gynecologic causes include pelvic inflammatory disease (PID), endometriosis, ovarian cysts, uterine fibroids, pelvic adhesions, and ectopic pregnancies.
- Abdominal causes include irritable bowel syndrome, interstitial cystitis, appendicitis, and colitis.
- Psychologic factors (e.g., depression, chronic stress, history of sexual or physical abuse) may increase the risk of developing chronic pelvic pain. Emotional distress makes pain worse, and living with chronic pain contributes to emotional distress.

Clinical Manifestations and Diagnostic Studies

- Manifestations of chronic pelvic pain include severe and steady pain, intermittent pain, dull and achy pain, sensation of pelvic pressure or heaviness, and sharp pains or cramping. Pain may occur during intercourse or while having a bowel movement. In addition to a detailed history and physical examination (including a pelvic examination), the patient may be asked to keep a journal of the onset of symptoms and precipitating factors.
- Diagnostic tests may include cultures from cervix or vagina (used to detect sexually transmitted infections [STIs]), ultrasound, CT scan, or MRI to detect abnormal structures or growths.
- Laparoscopy may be used to visualize the pelvic organs. This procedure is especially useful in detecting endometriosis and chronic PID.

Interprofessional Care

If the cause of chronic pelvic pain is found, treatment focuses on that cause. If no cause can be found, treatment involves managing the pain. Over-the-counter analgesics (e.g., aspirin, ibuprofen, acetaminophen) may provide some relief. Sometimes stronger pain drugs may be needed. Birth control pills or other hormonal agents may help relieve cyclic pelvic pain related to menstrual cycles. If an infection is the source of the problem, antibiotics are used.

Laparoscopic surgery may be used to remove pelvic adhesions or endometrial tissue. As a last resort, a hysterectomy may be done.

Tricyclic antidepressants (e.g., amitriptyline, nortriptyline [Pamelor]) have pain-relieving and antidepressant effects. These

P

drugs may help relieve chronic pelvic pain even in women who do not have depression.

PEPTIC ULCER DISEASE

Description

Peptic ulcer disease is an erosion of the mucosa resulting from the digestive action of hydrochloric acid (HCl) and pepsin. Any portion of the GI tract that comes into contact with gastric secretions is susceptible to ulcer development, including the lower esophagus, stomach, and duodenum, and at the margin of a gastrojejunal anastomosis site after surgical procedures. Approximately 350,000 new cases of ulcers are diagnosed each year.

Peptic ulcers can be classified as acute or chronic, depending on the degree and duration of mucosal involvement, and gastric or duodenal, according to the location.

- An *acute ulcer* is associated with superficial erosion and minimal inflammation. It is of short duration and resolves quickly when the cause is identified and removed.
- A *chronic ulcer* is of long duration, eroding through the muscular wall with the formation of fibrous tissue. It is continuously present for many months or recurs intermittently. Chronic ulcers are more common than acute erosions.
- *Gastric* and *duodenal* ulcers, although defined as peptic ulcers, are distinctly different in etiology and incidence (Table 64). Generally, the treatment of all ulcer types is similar.

Pathophysiology

Peptic ulcers develop only in the presence of an acid environment. The back-diffusion of HCl acid into the gastric mucosa results in cellular destruction and inflammation. Histamine is released from the damaged mucosa, resulting in vasodilation and increased capillary permeability and further secretion of acid and pepsin. A variety of agents are known to destroy the mucosal barrier (see Gastritis, p. 236).

In addition to chronic gastritis, *Helicobacter pylori* is associated with peptic ulcer development. Approximately two thirds of the world's population is infected with *H. pylori*. In the stomach, the bacteria can live a long time by colonizing the gastric epithelial cells within the mucosal layer. The bacteria also produce urease, which metabolizes urea-producing ammonium chloride and other damaging chemicals. Urease also activates the immune response, with both antibody production and the release of inflammatory cytokines.

TABLE 64 Comparison of Gastric and Duodenal Ulcers

Gastric Ulcers	Duodenal Ulcers
Lesion	
Superficial, smooth margins Round, oval, or cone-shaped	Penetrating (associated with deformity of duodenal bulb from healing of recurrent ulcers)
Location of Lesion	
Predominantly antrum, also in body and fundus of stomach	First 1-2 cm of duodenum
Gastric Secretion	
Normal to decreased	Increased
Incidence	
Greater in women	Greater in men, but increasing in women (especially postmenopausal)
Peak age 50-60 yr	Peak age 35-45 yr
Increased cancer risk	No increase in cancer risk
H. pylori infection in 80%	*H. pylori* infection in 90%
↑ With incompetent pyloric sphincter and bile reflux	Associated with other diseases (e.g., chronic obstructive pulmonary disease, pancreatic disease, hyperparathyroidism, Zollinger-Ellison syndrome, chronic renal failure)
Clinical Manifestations	
Burning or gaseous pressure in epigastrium	Burning, cramping, pressure-like pain across midepigastrium and upper abdomen
	Back pain with posterior ulcers
Pain 1-2 hr after meals	Pain 2-5 hr after meals and midmorning, midafternoon, middle of night
If penetrating ulcer, aggravation of discomfort with food	Periodic and episodic
	Pain relief with antacids and food
Recurrence Rate	
High	High

P

- In one patient, *H. pylori* may lead to intestinal metaplasia in the stomach and result in chronic atrophic gastritis, whereas in other patients *H. pylori* may alter gastric secretion and produce tissue damage leading to peptic ulcer disease. Response to *H. pylori* is likely to be influenced by many factors, including genetics, environment, and diet.

Clinical Manifestations

Discomfort generally associated with gastric ulcer is located high in the epigastrium and occurs about 1 to 2 hours after meals. The pain is described as burning or gaseous. If the ulcer has eroded through the gastric mucosa, food tends to aggravate rather than alleviate the pain.

Duodenal ulcer symptoms occur when gastric acid comes in contact with the ulcer, generally 2 to 5 hours after a meal. The pain is described as "burning" or "cramplike." It is most often located in the midepigastric region beneath the xiphoid process. Duodenal ulcers can also produce back pain. A characteristic of duodenal ulcer is its tendency to occur continuously for a few weeks or months and then disappear for a time, only to recur some months later.

- Not all patients with gastric or duodenal ulcers experience pain or discomfort. Silent peptic ulcers are more likely to occur in older adults and those taking nonsteroidal antiinflammatory drugs (NSAIDs). The presence or absence of symptoms is not directly related to the size of the ulcer or the degree of healing.

Complications

Major complications of peptic ulcers are hemorrhage, perforation, and gastric outlet obstruction. All are considered emergencies and may require surgical intervention.

Hemorrhage is the most common complication. Duodenal ulcers account for a greater percentage of upper GI bleeding episodes than gastric ulcers.

Perforation, the most lethal complication, occurs when the ulcer penetrates the serosal surface, with spillage of either gastric or duodenal contents into the peritoneal cavity. The contents entering the peritoneal cavity from the stomach or the duodenum may contain saliva, food particles, HCl acid, pepsin, bacteria, bile, and pancreatic enzymes. Bacterial peritonitis may occur within 6 to 12 hours.

- Manifestations of perforation are sudden and dramatic in onset and include severe upper abdominal pain that quickly spreads throughout the abdomen. Respirations become shallow and rapid, and bowel sounds are usually absent.

Gastric outlet obstruction may occur with acute or chronic peptic ulcer disease. Obstruction in the distal stomach and duodenum is the result of edema, inflammation, or pylorospasm and fibrous scar tissue formation. Symptoms and signs include upper abdomen discomfort and swelling that worsens toward the end of the day, vomiting (often projectile), and constipation.

Diagnostic Studies

- Endoscopy is used to obtain tissue for biopsy, confirm the absence of a malignancy, obtain specimens to test for *H. pylori,* and determine the degree of ulcer healing after treatment.
- Biopsy of the antral mucosa and testing for urease (rapid urease testing) confirm a diagnosis of *H. pylori* infection. Noninvasive tests include a urea breath test, which can identify active infection.
- CBC, urinalysis, liver enzyme studies, serum amylase determination, and stool examination may be performed for further diagnostic information.

Interprofessional Care

Conservative Therapy

The aim of treatment is to decrease gastric acidity and enhance mucosal defense mechanisms. The regimen consists of rest, drug therapy, smoking cessation, and long-term follow-up care. Strict adherence to the prescribed regimen of drugs is important because ulcers frequently recur.

Drug therapy includes the use of histamine H_2-receptor antagonists (e.g., cimetidine, famotidine [Pepcid]), proton-pump inhibitors (PPIs) (e.g., omeprazole [Prilosec]), antisecretory agents (e.g., misoprostol [Cytotec]), cytoprotective agents (e.g., sucralfate [Carafate]), antacids, and anticholinergics. Aspirin and NSAIDs are discontinued for 4 to 6 weeks. When aspirin must be continued, co-administration with a PPI, H_2-receptor blocker, or misoprostol (Cytotec) may be prescribed. See Table 41-10, Lewis et al, *Medical-Surgical Nursing,* ed 10, p. 903.

The patient is given antibiotics and a PPI for 10 to 14 days to eradicate *H. pylori* infection. Because of the development of antibiotic-resistant organisms, a growing percentage of patients do not have *H. pylori* eradicated with a single round of therapy.

Healing of a peptic ulcer requires many weeks of therapy. Pain disappears after 3 to 6 days, but complete healing may take 3 to 9 weeks.

An acute exacerbation is frequently accompanied by bleeding, increased pain and discomfort, and nausea and vomiting.

- With hemorrhage, management is similar to that described for upper GI bleeding (pp. 245-246). Emergency assessment and management of the patient with a massive hemorrhage are described in Lewis et al, *Medical-Surgical Nursing,* ed 10, pp. 922 to 923.
- With perforation, the focus of therapy is to stop the spillage of gastric contents by nasogastric (NG) tube or surgery. Blood volume is replaced with IV solutions, and packed RBCs may be necessary. Broad-spectrum antibiotic therapy is started immediately to treat bacterial peritonitis. Pain medication is also given.
- With gastric outlet obstruction, the aim of therapy is to decompress the stomach using an NG tube. IV fluids and electrolytes may be given for dehydration, vomiting, and electrolyte imbalances. Pain relief results from the decompression.

Nutritional Therapy

There are no recommended dietary modifications for peptic ulcer disease. Patients are taught to eat and drink foods and fluids that do not cause distressing symptoms. Foods that commonly cause gastric irritation include caffeine; hot, spicy foods; pepper; carbonated beverages; and broth (meat extract). Teach the patient to eliminate alcohol consumption because it can delay healing.

Surgical Therapy

With the use of drug therapy and endoscopic therapy, surgery for peptic ulcer disease is uncommon. Surgery is done when the patient has complications unresponsive to medical management or when gastric cancer may be present.

Surgical procedures include partial gastrectomy, vagotomy, or pyloroplasty. Partial gastrectomy with removal of the distal two thirds of the stomach and anastomosis of the gastric stump to the duodenum is called a *gastroduodenostomy* or *Billroth I* operation; removal of the distal two thirds of the stomach with anastomosis of the gastric stump to the jejunum is called a *gastrojejunostomy* or *Billroth II* operation. *Vagotomy* (severing of the vagal nerve) is done to decrease gastric acid secretion. *Pyloroplasty* is the surgical enlargement of the pyloric sphincter to facilitate the passage of contents from the stomach.

Postoperative complications from surgery are dumping syndrome, postprandial hypoglycemia, and bile reflux gastritis.

- *Dumping syndrome* occurs when surgery drastically reduces the reservoir capacity of the stomach and causes loss of control over the amount of gastric chyme entering the small intestine. The large bolus of hypertonic fluid entering the intestine causes a fluid shift into the bowel, creating a decrease in plasma volume along with distention of the bowel lumen and rapid intestinal transit. The patient usually describes feelings of generalized weakness, sweating, palpitations, and dizziness caused by the decrease in plasma volume. The patient also complains of abdominal cramps, borborygmi, and the urge to defecate. The onset of symptoms occurs within 15 to 30 minutes of eating, and symptoms usually last about 1 hour after eating.

- *Postprandial hypoglycemia* is considered a variant of dumping syndrome, because it is the result of uncontrolled gastric emptying of a bolus of fluid high in carbohydrates, resulting in hyperglycemia and the release of excessive amounts of insulin into the circulation. Symptoms and signs are similar to those of a hypoglycemic reaction, including sweating, weakness, mental confusion, palpitations, and tachycardia. Symptoms generally occur 2 hours after eating.

- Gastric surgery that involves the pylorus can result in reflux of bile into the stomach. The major symptom of *bile reflux gastritis* is continual epigastric distress that increases after meals. Vomiting relieves distress temporarily. The administration of cholestyramine to bind with the bile salts, either before or with meals, successfully treats this problem.

Because of surgical changes, the stomach's reservoir is diminished, and meal size must be reduced accordingly. Advise the patient to limit fluids with meals. Dry foods with a low carbohydrate content and moderate protein and fat content are better tolerated initially. Dietary changes and a short rest period after each meal reduce the likelihood of dumping syndrome.

Nursing Management
Goals
The patient with peptic ulcer disease will adhere to the prescribed therapeutic regimen, experience a reduction in or absence of discomfort, exhibit no signs of GI complications, have complete healing of the peptic ulcer, and make appropriate lifestyle changes to prevent recurrence.

Nursing Diagnoses
- Acute pain
- Nausea

Nursing Interventions
During an acute phase the patient may be NPO, have an NG tube inserted and connected to intermittent suction, and have IV fluid replacement. Explain the rationale for this therapy to the patient and caregiver. The volume of fluid lost, the patient's signs and symptoms, and laboratory test results determine the type and amount of IV fluids administered. When the stomach is kept empty

of gastric secretions, the ulcer pain diminishes and ulcer healing begins. The patient's immediate environment should be quiet and restful.

If the patient has surgery, postoperative care is similar to that after abdominal laparotomy (see Abdominal Pain, Acute, p. 3). Additional considerations for a patient with a partial gastrectomy include:

- It is essential that the NG suction be working and that the tube remain patent so that accumulated gastric secretions do not put a strain on the anastomosis. Observe the gastric aspirate for color, amount, and odor.
- Observe the patient for signs of decreased peristalsis and lower abdominal discomfort that may indicate impending intestinal obstruction.
- Observe the dressing for signs of bleeding or odor and drainage indicative of an infection.
- Keep the patient comfortable and free of pain by administering prescribed drugs and by frequent changes in position.
- Encourage early ambulation.
- While the NG tube is connected to suction, maintain IV therapy. Add potassium and vitamin supplements (as ordered) to the infusion until oral feedings are resumed.
- The patient may require cobalamin therapy.

▼ **Patient and Caregiver Teaching**

General instructions should cover aspects of the disease process, drugs, possible changes in lifestyle, and regular follow-up evaluation (Table 65). Emphasize the need for long-term follow-up care, and encourage the patient to seek immediate intervention if symptoms return.

PERICARDITIS, ACUTE

Description

Pericarditis is a condition caused by inflammation of the pericardium. The pericardium provides lubrication to decrease friction between heart contractions, and helps prevent excessive dilation of the heart during diastole.

Pathophysiology

Acute pericarditis is most often idiopathic (unknown) with a variety of suspected viral causes. The coxsackievirus B group is the most commonly identified virus. Other causes include uremia, bacterial infection, acute myocardial infarction (MI), neoplasm, and trauma.

TABLE 65   Patient & Caregiver Teaching

Peptic Ulcer Disease (PUD)

Include the following instructions when teaching the patient and caregivers about management of PUD.

1. Follow dietary modifications, including avoiding foods that may cause epigastric distress such as acidic foods.
2. Avoid cigarettes. In addition to promoting ulcer development, smoking delays ulcer healing.
3. Reduce or eliminate alcohol intake.
4. Avoid OTC drugs unless approved by the HCP. Many preparations contain ingredients, such as aspirin, that should not be taken unless approved by the HCP. Check with the HCP about the use of nonsteroidal antiinflammatory drugs.
5. Do not interchange brands of antacids, H_2-receptor blockers, and proton pump inhibitors that can be purchased OTC without checking with the HCP. This can lead to harmful side effects.
6. Take all drugs as prescribed. This includes both antisecretory and antibiotic drugs. Failing to take drugs as prescribed can result in relapse.
7. It is important to report any of the following:
   • Increased nausea or vomiting
   • Increased epigastric pain
   • Bloody emesis or tarry stools
8. Stress can be related to signs and symptoms of PUD. Learn and use stress management strategies (see Chapter 6, Lewis et al, *Medical-Surgical Nursing*, ed 10, pp. 82 to 87).
9. Share concerns about lifestyle changes and living with a chronic illness.

P

Pericarditis in the patient with an acute MI may be described as two distinct syndromes. *Acute pericarditis* may occur within the initial 48- to 72-hour period after an MI. *Dressler's syndrome* (late pericarditis) appears 4 to 6 weeks after an MI.

An inflammatory response is the characteristic pathologic finding in acute pericarditis. There is an influx of neutrophils, increased pericardial vascularity, and eventual fibrin deposition on the pericardium.

Clinical Manifestations

Clinical symptoms include progressive, frequently severe sharp chest pain. The pain generally worsens with deep inspiration and in the supine position. It is relieved by sitting up and leaning forward.

■ The pain may radiate to the neck, arms, or left shoulder, making it difficult to distinguish from angina. One distinction is that pericarditis pain can be referred to the trapezius muscle (shoulder, upper back).

■ Dyspnea that accompanies acute pericarditis is related to the patient's need to breathe in rapid, shallow breaths to avoid chest pain and may be aggravated by fever and anxiety.

■ The hallmark finding is a *pericardial friction rub,* which is a scratching, grating, high-pitched sound believed to arise from friction between the roughened pericardial and epicardial surfaces. It is best heard with the stethoscope diaphragm firmly placed at the lower left sternal border of the chest with the patient leaning forward. Because it is difficult to tell a pericardial friction rub from a pleural friction rub, ask the patient to hold his or her breath. If you still hear the rub, then it is cardiac. Pericardial friction rubs may be intermittent.

Complications

Pericardial effusion is buildup of fluid in the pericardium. Large effusions may compress nearby structures. Pulmonary tissue compression can cause cough, dyspnea, and tachypnea. Phrenic nerve compression can induce hiccups, and compression of the recurrent laryngeal nerve may result in hoarseness. Heart sounds are generally distant and muffled. BP is usually maintained.

Cardiac tamponade develops as the pericardial effusion increases in volume, compressing the heart. The patient may report chest pain and is often confused, anxious, and restless. Heart sounds become muffled, pulse pressure is narrowed, and the patient develops tachypnea, tachycardia, and decreased cardiac output. Neck veins may be markedly distended because of jugular venous pressure elevation. *Pulsus paradoxus,* which may be present, is a decrease in systolic BP with inspiration that is exaggerated in cardiac tamponade. (See Table 36-5, Lewis et al, *Medical-Surgical Nursing,* ed 10, p. 785, for measurement technique.)

Diagnostic Studies

■ An ECG is useful in diagnosis, with changes (e.g., diffuse ST-segment elevation) noted in approximately 90% of the cases.

■ Echocardiography is used to determine the presence of pericardial effusion or cardiac tamponade.

■ Doppler and color M-mode imaging assess diastolic function and help to diagnose constrictive pericarditis.

■ Laboratory findings include leukocytosis and elevation of erythrocyte sedimentation rate (ESR) and C-reactive protein

(CRP). Troponin levels may be elevated in patients with ST-segment elevation and acute pericarditis, which may indicate concurrent myocardial damage.
- CT scan and MRI permit visualization of the pericardium and pericardial space.

Interprofessional Care

Management is directed toward identification and treatment of the underlying problem. Antibiotics treat bacterial pericarditis, and nonsteroidal antiinflammatory drugs (NSAIDs) (e.g., salicylates [aspirin], ibuprofen) control the pain and inflammation of acute pericarditis. Corticosteroids are generally reserved for patients with pericarditis secondary to systemic lupus erythematosus, those already taking corticosteroids for a rheumatologic or other immune system condition, or those who do not respond to NSAIDs. Colchicine, an antiinflammatory drug used to treat gout, can be used for patients who have recurrent pericarditis.
- Pericardiocentesis is usually done for pericardial effusion with acute cardiac tamponade, purulent pericarditis, and suspected neoplasm. Hemodynamic support for the patient undergoing pericardiocentesis may include administering volume expanders and inotropic agents (e.g., dopamine) and discontinuing anticoagulants.
- A *pericardial window* can be used for diagnosis or for drainage of excess fluid. This procedure involves cutting a "window" or portion of the pericardium. The opening allows the fluid to drain continuously into the peritoneum or the chest cavity.

Nursing Management

Management of the patient's pain and anxiety is the primary nursing consideration. Assess the pain to distinguish the pain of myocardial ischemia (angina) from the pain of pericarditis. Pericarditis pain is usually located in the precordium or over the left trapezius ridge and has a sharp, pleuritic quality that increases with inspiration. Relief from this pain is often obtained by sitting or leaning forward and is worse when the patient is lying flat.
- Pain relief measures include maintaining the patient on bed rest with the head of the bed elevated to 45 degrees and providing an overhead table for arm support.
- Antiinflammatory agents help alleviate the patient's pain. Because of the associated risk of GI bleeding, administer these drugs with food and instruct the patient to avoid alcohol.
- Monitor for the signs and symptoms of tamponade and prepare for possible pericardiocentesis.

- Anxiety-reducing measures for the patient include providing simple, complete explanations of all procedures performed. Such explanations are particularly important for the patient whose diagnosis is being established and for the patient who has previously experienced angina or an MI.

PERIPHERAL ARTERY DISEASE

Description

Peripheral artery disease (PAD) involves thickening of artery walls. This results in a progressive narrowing of the arteries of the upper and lower extremities. PAD is strongly related to other types of cardiovascular disease (CVD) and their risk factors. PAD prevalence increases with age.

Pathophysiology

The leading cause of PAD is atherosclerosis, which is a gradual thickening of the *intima* (the innermost layer of the arterial wall) and *media* (middle layer of the arterial wall). This results from the deposit of cholesterol and lipids within the vessel walls and leads to progressive narrowing of the artery. Although the exact cause(s) of atherosclerosis are unknown, inflammation and endothelial injury play a major role.

- Risk factors for PAD are tobacco use (most significant factor), chronic kidney disease, diabetes, hypertension, and hypercholesterolemia.
- Atherosclerosis more commonly affects certain segments of the arterial tree. These include the coronary, carotid, and lower extremity arteries. Clinical symptoms occur when vessels are 60% to 75% blocked.

Peripheral Artery Disease: Lower Extremities

Lower extremity PAD may affect the iliac, femoral, popliteal, tibial, or peroneal arteries. The femoral-popliteal area is the most common site in nondiabetic patients. Patients with diabetes tend to develop PAD in the arteries below the knee.

Clinical Manifestations

Severity of the manifestations generally depends on the site and extent of the obstruction and the amount of collateral circulation.

- The classic symptom of PAD is *intermittent claudication,* which is ischemic muscle pain that is caused by exercise, resolves within 10 minutes or less with resting, and is reproducible.

- Some individuals with PAD either have no symptoms or atypical leg symptoms (e.g., burning, hardness, heaviness, knotting, pressure, soreness, tightness, weakness) in atypical locations (e.g., ankle, foot, hamstring, hip, knee, shin).
- Paresthesia, manifested as numbness or tingling in the toes or feet, may result from nerve tissue ischemia. Reduced blood flow to neurons produces loss of pressure and deep pain sensation.
- Pallor of the foot is noted in response to leg elevation. *Reactive hyperemia* (redness) develops when the limb is allowed to hang in a dependent position *(dependent rubor)*. The skin becomes shiny and taut, and there is hair loss on the lower legs. Pedal, popliteal, or femoral pulses are diminished or absent.
- As PAD progresses and involves multiple arterial segments, continuous pain develops at rest. Rest pain most often occurs in the forefoot or toes and is aggravated by limb elevation.

The most serious complications are nonhealing arterial ulcers and gangrene, which may require lower extremity amputation.

Diagnostic Studies
- Doppler ultrasound and duplex imaging assess blood flow.
- Segmental BPs are obtained (using Doppler ultrasound and a sphygmomanometer) at the thigh, below the knee, and at ankle level while the patient is supine. A drop in segmental BP of greater than 30 mm Hg suggests PAD.
- Angiography or magnetic resonance angiography (MRA) delineates location and extent of PAD.

Interprofessional Care
The first treatment goal is to reduce cardiovascular risk factors. Tobacco cessation is essential. Aggressive lipid management is essential for all patients with PAD. Both dietary interventions and drug therapy are needed.
- Statins (e.g., simvastatin [Zocor]) and a fibric acid derivative (gemfibrozil [Lopid]) lower low-density lipoprotein (LDL) and triglyceride levels. Hypertension and diabetes mellitus also need to be properly controlled.
- Antiplatelet agents are critical for reducing the risk of CVD events and death in patients with PAD. Oral antiplatelet therapy should include 75 to 325 mg/day of aspirin. Aspirin-intolerant patients may take 75 mg of clopidogrel (Plavix) daily.
- Two drugs are available to treat intermittent claudication: cilostazol (Pletal) and pentoxifylline. Cilostazol, a phosphodiesterase inhibitor, inhibits platelet aggregation and increases vasodilation. Pentoxifylline, a xanthine derivative, improves

the deformability of RBCs and WBCs and decreases fibrinogen concentration, platelet adhesiveness, and blood viscosity.

A supervised exercise program is recommended as an initial treatment modality for all patients with intermittent claudication. Exercise should be performed for 30 to 45 minutes/day, at least 3 times/week, for a minimum of 3 months. Although walking is the most commonly prescribed exercise for patients with PAD, alternative modes of exercise (e.g., cycling) may also be recommended.

- Teach patients to adjust their overall caloric intake so that an ideal body weight can be achieved and maintained. Recommend a diet high in fruits, vegetables, and whole grains and low in cholesterol, saturated fat, and salt.
- Patients taking antiplatelet agents, nonsteroidal antiinflammatory drugs (NSAIDs) (e.g., ibuprofen), or anticoagulants (e.g., warfarin) should consult their HCP before taking any dietary or herbal supplements, because of potential interactions and bleeding risks.

Critical limb ischemia is a condition characterized by chronic ischemic rest pain lasting more than 2 weeks, arterial leg ulcers, or gangrene of the leg as a result of PAD. Conservative management goals for critical limb ischemia include protecting the patient's extremity from trauma, decreasing ischemic pain, preventing and controlling infection, and maximizing perfusion. Carefully inspect, cleanse, and lubricate both feet to prevent cracking of the skin and infection.

Interventional radiology catheter-based procedures are alternatives to open surgical approaches for treatment of lower extremity PAD.

- *Percutaneous transluminal angioplasty* uses a catheter with a cylindric balloon at the tip. The end of the catheter is advanced to the stenotic area of the artery. The balloon is inflated, compressing the atherosclerotic intimal lining.
- *Stents,* expandable metallic devices, are positioned to keep the artery open immediately after balloon angioplasty is performed. The stents may be covered with Dacron or a drug-eluting agent (e.g., paclitaxel) to reduce restenosis by limiting the amount of new tissue growth into the stent.
- *Atherectomy* removes the obstructing plaque. A directional atherectomy device uses a high-speed cutting disk that cuts long strips of the atheroma. Laser atherectomy uses ultraviolet energy to break apart the atheroma.
- Various surgical approaches can be used to improve arterial blood flow beyond a blocked artery. The most common is a peripheral arterial bypass operation with autogenous (native)

vein or synthetic graft material to bypass or carry blood around the lesion.

- Other surgical options include *endarterectomy* (opening the artery and removing the obstructing plaque) and *patch graft angioplasty* (opening the artery, removing the plaque, and sewing a patch to the opening to widen the lumen).
- Amputation may be required if tissue necrosis is extensive, gangrene or osteomyelitis develops, or all major arteries in the limb are occluded, precluding the possibility of successful surgery.

Nursing Management
Goals
The patient with lower extremity PAD will have adequate tissue perfusion, relief of pain, increased exercise tolerance, and intact, healthy skin on extremities. Additional information on care for the patient with PAD of the lower extremities is presented in eNursing Care Plan 37-1 on the website.
Nursing Diagnoses
- Ineffective peripheral tissue perfusion
- Chronic pain
- Activity intolerance
- Ineffective health management
Nursing Interventions
After surgical or radiologic intervention, check the operative extremity every 15 minutes initially and then hourly for color, temperature, capillary refill, presence of peripheral pulses, and movement and sensation. Loss of palpable pulses or a change in the Doppler sound over a pulse requires immediate notification of the physician or radiologist and prompt intervention.

After the patient leaves the recovery area, continue to monitor perfusion of the extremities and assess for potential complications such as bleeding, hematoma, thrombosis, embolization, and compartment syndrome. A dramatic increase in pain, loss of previously palpable pulses, extremity pallor or cyanosis, decreasing ankle-brachial index (ABI) on serial measurements, numbness or tingling, or a cold extremity suggests blockage of the graft or stent. Report these findings to the HCP immediately.

- Knee-flexed positions should be avoided except for exercise. Turn the patient frequently and position with pillows to support the incision. Starting on postoperative day 1, assist patient out of bed several times daily. Walking even short distances is desirable.
- Discourage prolonged sitting with leg dependency because it may cause pain and edema, increase the risk of venous

thrombosis, and place stress on the suture lines. If edema develops, position the patient supine and elevate the leg above the heart level.

▼ **Patient and Caregiver Teaching**

- Encourage supervised exercise training after a successful revascularization. Explain that exercise decreases CVD risk factors including hypertension, hyperlipidemia, obesity, and glucose levels.
- Teach foot care to all patients with PAD. Meticulous foot care is especially important in the diabetic patient with PAD.
- Tell patients to inspect their legs and feet daily for mottling, changes in skin color or texture, and reduction in hair growth. Show patients how to check skin temperature and capillary refill and to palpate pulses.
- Encourage patients to wear clean, all-cotton or all-wool socks and comfortable shoes with rounded (not pointed) toes and soft insoles. Tell patients to lace shoes loosely and to break in new shoes gradually.

PERITONITIS

Description

Peritonitis results from a localized or generalized inflammatory process involving the peritoneum. Causes are listed in Table 66. Primary peritonitis occurs when blood-borne organisms enter the peritoneal cavity. For example, the ascites that occurs with cirrhosis of the liver provides an excellent liquid environment for bacteria to flourish. Organisms can also enter the peritoneum during peritoneal dialysis. Secondary peritonitis is more common and occurs when abdominal organs perforate or rupture and release their contents (bile, enzymes, bacteria) into the peritoneal cavity.

Pathophysiology

Intestinal contents irritate the normally sterile peritoneum, producing an initial chemical peritonitis that is followed a few hours later by bacterial peritonitis. The resulting inflammatory response leads to massive fluid shifts (peritoneal edema) and formation of adhesions as the body attempts to wall off the infection.

Clinical Manifestations and Complications

- Abdominal pain is the most common symptom.
- A universal sign of peritonitis is tenderness over the involved area. Rebound tenderness, muscular rigidity, and spasm are other major signs of peritoneum irritation.

TABLE 66   Causes of Peritonitis

Primary
- Blood-borne organisms
- Genital tract organisms
- Cirrhosis with ascites

Secondary
- Appendicitis with rupture
- Blunt or penetrating trauma to abdominal organs
- Diverticulitis with rupture
- Ischemic bowel disorders
- Pancreatitis
- Perforated intestine
- Perforated peptic ulcer
- Peritoneal dialysis
- Postoperative (breakage of anastomosis)

- Abdominal distention or ascites, fever, tachycardia, tachypnea, nausea, vomiting, and altered bowel habits may also be present.
  Complications include hypovolemic shock, sepsis, intraabdominal abscess, paralytic ileus, and acute respiratory distress syndrome. If treatment is delayed, peritonitis may be fatal.

Diagnostic Studies
- CBC will determine elevations in WBC count and hemoconcentration from fluid shifts.
- Peritoneal aspiration and analysis for blood, bile, pus, bacteria, fungi, and amylase content.
- Abdominal x-ray may show dilated loops of bowel consistent with paralytic ileus, free air if perforation has occurred, or air-fluid levels if an obstruction is present.
- CT scan and ultrasound may be useful in identifying ascites or abscesses.
- Peritoneoscopy may be helpful in patients without ascites.

Interprofessional Care
Patients with milder cases of peritonitis or those who are poor surgical candidates may be managed conservatively with antibiotics, nasogastric (NG) suction, analgesics, and IV fluid administration. Surgery is indicated to locate the cause, drain purulent fluid, and repair damage (e.g., perforated organs).

Nursing Management

Goals
The patient with peritonitis will have resolution of inflammation, relief of abdominal pain, freedom from complications (especially hypovolemic shock and sepsis), and normal nutritional status.

Nursing Interventions
The patient with peritonitis is extremely ill and needs skilled supportive care. Establish IV access to replace lost fluids and deliver antibiotic therapy. Monitor the patient for pain and response to analgesics. The patient may be positioned with knees flexed to increase comfort. Sedatives may be given to allay anxiety.

- Accurate monitoring of fluid intake and output and electrolyte status is necessary to determine replacement therapy. Monitor vital signs frequently.
- Antiemetics may be administered to decrease nausea and vomiting and prevent further fluid and electrolyte losses. The patient is NPO and may have an NG tube in place to decrease gastric distention and further leakage of bowel contents into the peritoneum.
- If the patient has an open surgical procedure, drains are inserted to remove purulent drainage and excess fluid. Postoperative care is similar to that for the patient with an exploratory laparotomy (see Abdominal Pain, Acute, p. 3).

PNEUMONIA

Description
Pneumonia is an infection of the lung parenchyma. Despite new antimicrobial agents to treat pneumonia, it is still associated with significant morbidity and mortality. Pneumonia can be caused by bacteria, viruses, *Mycoplasma* organisms, fungi, parasites, and chemicals.

A clinically effective way to classify pneumonia is to classify it as *community-acquired pneumonia* (CAP) or *hospital-acquired pneumonia* (HAP). Classifying pneumonia is important because of the differences in the likely causative organisms (Table 67) and the selection of appropriate treatment.

- *CAP* is an acute infection of the lung occurring in patients who have not been hospitalized or resided in a long-term care facility within 14 days of the onset of symptoms.
- *HAP* is pneumonia in a nonintubated patient that begins 48 hours or longer after admission to a hospital and was not present at the time of admission.

TABLE 67 Organisms Causing Pneumonia	
Community-Acquired Pneumonia	**Hospital-Acquired Pneumonia**
• *Streptococcus pneumoniae** • *Mycoplasma pneumoniae* • *Haemophilus influenzae* • Respiratory viruses • *Chlamydophila pneumoniae* • *Chlamydophila psittaci* • *Coxiella burnetii* • *Legionella pneumophila* • Oral anaerobes • *Moraxella catarrhalis* • *Staphylococcus aureus* • *Pseudomonas aeruginosa* • Enteric aerobic gram-negative bacteria (e.g., *Klebsiella* species) • Fungi • *Mycobacterium tuberculosis*	• *Pseudomonas aeruginosa*† • *Escherichia coli*† • *Klebsiella pneumoniae*† • *Acinetobacter* species† • *Haemophilus influenzae* • *Staphylococcus aureus* • *Streptococcus pneumoniae* • *Proteus* species • *Enterobacter* species • Oral anaerobes

*Most common cause of community-acquired pneumonia (CAP).
†Most common causes of hospital-acquired pneumonia (HAP).

P

- *Ventilator-associated pneumonia (VAP)*, also a type of HAP, refers to pneumonia that develops more than 48 hours after endotracheal intubation.

Pathophysiology

Normally the airway distal to the larynx is sterile because of protective defense mechanisms. Pneumonia is more likely to result when defense mechanisms are incompetent or overwhelmed by infectious agents because of:

- Decreased consciousness that depresses the cough and epiglottal reflexes
- Tracheal intubation interfering with the normal cough reflex and the mucociliary escalator mechanism
- Impaired mucociliary mechanism caused by air pollution, cigarette smoking, viral upper respiratory tract infections, and normal aging changes
- Chronic diseases such as cancer, diabetes mellitus, and heart disease, which can suppress the immune system's ability to inhibit bacterial growth

Organisms that cause pneumonia reach the lungs by aspiration from the nasopharynx or oropharynx, inhalation of microbes present in the air, or hematogenous spread from a primary infection elsewhere in the body.

Specific pathophysiologic changes vary according to the offending organism. Most organisms trigger an inflammatory response in the lung. A vascular reaction occurs with increased blood flow and vascular permeability. Neutrophils, the offending organism, and fluid from surrounding blood vessels fill the alveoli, interrupting oxygen transportation, which leads to hypoxia. Mucus production is increased, which can obstruct airflow and further decrease gas exchange.

Consolidation, a feature of bacterial pneumonia, occurs when normally air-filled alveoli are filled with fluid and debris.

Complete resolution and healing occur if there are no complications. Macrophages lyse and process the debris, normal lung tissue is restored, and gas exchange returns to normal.

Clinical Manifestations and Complications

The most common presenting manifestations of pneumonia are cough, fever, shaking chills, dyspnea, tachypnea, and pleuritic chest pain.

- Cough may be or may not be productive. Sputum may appear green, yellow, or rust-colored (bloody).
- Viral pneumonia may initially seem to be influenza, with respiratory symptoms appearing and/or worsening 12 to 36 hours after onset.
- In older or debilitated patients, confusion or stupor (possibly related to hypoxia) may be the only finding.

On physical examination, fine or coarse crackles may be auscultated over the affected area. If consolidation is present, bronchial breath sounds, egophony, and increased fremitus may be noted.

Complications include *atelectasis* (collapsed, airless alveoli), *pleurisy* (inflammation of the pleura), pleural effusion, bacteremia, lung abscess, pericarditis, meningitis, sepsis, and acute respiratory failure.

Diagnostic Studies

- History, physical examination, and chest x-ray often provide enough information for making management decisions without further testing.
- Chest x-ray often shows a pattern characteristic of the infecting organism.
- Sputum culture, gram stain of sputum, and blood cultures are used to identify the causative organism.

- Arterial blood gases (ABGs) are used to assess for hypoxemia, hypercapnia, and acidosis.
- WBC count often reveals leukocytosis.

Interprofessional Care

Pneumococcal vaccine is used to prevent *Streptococcus pneumoniae* (pneumococcus) pneumonia. Vaccination is recommended for individuals 65 years of age or older and younger patients who are at high risk. A one-time repeat vaccination in 5 years is recommended for those who received their initial vaccination before the age of 65.

Currently, no definitive treatment exits for a majority of viral pneumonias. Care is generally supportive. Prompt treatment with appropriate antibiotics almost always cures bacterial pneumonia, including *Mycoplasma* pneumonia. In uncomplicated cases, the patient responds to drug therapy within 48 to 72 hours. Table 27-6 in Lewis et al, *Medical-Surgical Nursing,* ed 10, p. 504, outlines drugs for treatment of bacterial CAP.

- Supportive measures may be used, including oxygen therapy, analgesics to relieve chest pain, and antipyretics such as aspirin or acetaminophen. Individualize rest and activity to the patient's tolerance.
- Hydration is important. If the patient has heart failure, fluid intake is carefully monitored. If the patient cannot maintain adequate oral intake, IV administration of fluids and electrolytes may be necessary.
- Small, frequent meals are easier for some patients to tolerate. Offer foods high in calories and nutrients.

Nursing Management
Goals
The patient with pneumonia will have clear breath sounds, normal breathing patterns, no signs of hypoxia, normal appearance on chest x-ray, normal WBC count, and no complications related to pneumonia.
Nursing Diagnoses
- Impaired gas exchange
- Ineffective breathing pattern
- Acute pain
Nursing Interventions
Interventions focus on preventing pneumonia. If possible, exposure to upper respiratory infections (URIs) should be avoided. If a URI occurs, it should be treated promptly with supportive measures (e.g., rest, fluids). If symptoms persist for more than 7 days, the person should seek medical care. The individual at increased risk

for pneumonia should be encouraged to obtain both influenza and pneumococcal vaccines.

The eNursing Care Plan 27-1 (on the website) for a patient with pneumonia applies to individuals both at home and in the hospital.

- Place the patient with altered consciousness in positions (e.g., side-lying, upright) that will prevent or minimize aspiration. Turn and reposition the patient at least every 2 hours to facilitate adequate lung expansion and mobilization of secretions.
- The patient who has a feeding tube requires attention to prevent aspiration.
- In the ICU, strict adherence to "ventilator bundle" interventions has been shown to significantly reduce the incidence of VAP. These interventions are elevation of the head of the bed 30 to 45 degrees, daily "sedation holidays," assessment of readiness to extubate, prophylaxis for peptic ulcer disease and venous thromboembolism, and daily oral care with chlorhexidine.
- The patient who has difficulty swallowing (e.g., after a stroke) needs assistance in eating, drinking, and taking medication to prevent aspiration. After a patient has had local anesthesia to the throat, assess for a gag reflex before giving food or fluids.
- Patients with impaired mobility from any cause need assistance with turning and moving, as well as encouragement to breathe deeply at frequent intervals.
- Practice strict medical asepsis and adherence to infection control guidelines to reduce the incidence of HAP.

▼ Patient and Caregiver Teaching
- Teach the patient about the importance of taking every dose of the prescribed antibiotic, any drug–drug and food–drug interactions for the prescribed antibiotic, and the need for adequate rest to continue recovery.
- Instruct the patient to drink plenty of liquids (at least 6 to 10 glasses/day, unless contraindicated) and to avoid alcohol and smoking.
- A cool mist humidifier or warm bath may help the patient breathe easier.
- Teaching should also include information about available influenza and pneumococcal vaccines.

PNEUMOTHORAX

Description

A *pneumothorax* is a complete or partial collapse of a lung as a result of an accumulation of air in the pleural space. Pneumothorax can be classified as *open* (air entering through an opening in the chest wall) or *closed* (no external wound).

Pathophysiology

Normally, negative (subatmospheric) pressure exists between the visceral pleura (surrounding the lung) and the parietal pleura (lining the thoracic cavity), allowing the lungs to be filled by chest wall expansion. The pleural space contains only a few milliliters of lubricating fluid to reduce friction when the tissues move. When air enters the pleural space, the change in pressure (from negative to positive) causes a partial or complete lung collapse. As the volume of air in the pleural space increases, the lung volume decreases. This condition should be suspected after any blunt trauma to the chest wall.

Types of Pneumothorax

Spontaneous pneumothorax typically occurs as a result of the rupture of small blebs (air-filled sacs) located on the apex of the lung. These blebs can occur in healthy, young individuals (primary spontaneous pneumothorax) or as a result of lung disease such as chronic obstructive pulmonary disease (COPD), asthma, cystic fibrosis, and pneumonia (secondary spontaneous pneumothorax). Smoking increases the risk of bleb formation. Other risk factors include being tall and thin, male gender, family history, and previous spontaneous pneumothorax.

Traumatic pneumothorax can occur from either penetrating (open) or nonpenetrating (closed) chest trauma. Penetrating trauma (e.g., stab or gunshot wound, subclavian catheter insertion, surgical thoracotomy) allows air to enter the pleural space through an opening in the chest wall. A penetrating chest wound may be referred to as a *sucking chest wound,* because air enters the pleural space through the chest wall during each inspiration.

Tension pneumothorax occurs when air enters the pleural space but cannot escape. The continued accumulation of air in the pleural space causes increasingly elevated intrapleural pressures. This results in compression of the lung on the affected side and pressure on the heart and great vessels, pushing them away from the affected side (Fig. 18). The mediastinum shifts toward the unaffected side, compressing the "good" lung, which further compromises oxygenation. As pressure increases, venous return is decreased and cardiac output falls. Tension pneumothorax may result from either an open or a closed pneumothorax.

Hemothorax is an accumulation of blood in the pleural space resulting from injury to the chest wall, diaphragm, lung, blood vessels, or mediastinum. The patient with a traumatic hemothorax

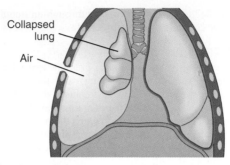

Collapsed
lung

Air

Fig. 18 Tension pneumothorax. As pleural pressure on the affected side increases, mediastinal displacement ensues, with resultant respiratory and cardiovascular compromise. Tracheal deviation is an external manifestation of the mediastinal shift.

requires immediate insertion of a chest tube for evacuation of the blood, which can be recovered and reinfused for a short time after the injury.

Clinical Manifestations

If the pneumothorax is small, only mild tachycardia and dyspnea may be present. If it is a large pneumothorax, shallow, rapid respirations, dyspnea, air hunger, and oxygen desaturation may occur.

- Chest pain and a cough with or without hemoptysis may be present.
- On auscultation, no breath sounds are detected over the affected area.
- Chest x-ray shows air or fluid in the pleural space and reduction in lung volume.

Interprofessional Care

Tension pneumothorax is a medical emergency, requiring urgent needle compression followed by chest tube insertion with water-seal drainage.

If the patient with a small pneumothorax is stable, the condition may resolve spontaneously, or the pleural space can be aspirated with a large-bore needle (thoracentesis).

The most common treatment for a pneumothorax and hemothorax is to insert a chest tube and connect it to water-seal drainage (see Chest Tubes and Pleural Drainage, p. 699). Repeated spontaneous pneumothoraces may need to be treated surgically by a partial pleurectomy, stapling, or pleurodesis to promote the adherence of pleurae to one another.

POLYCYSTIC KIDNEY DISEASE

Polycystic kidney disease (PKD) is the most common life-threatening genetic disease in the world, affecting 600,000 people in the United States. There are two forms of PKD. The *childhood form* is a rare autosomal recessive disorder that is often rapidly progressive. The *adult form* of PKD is an autosomal dominant disorder. Adult PKD is latent for many years and is usually manifested between 30 and 40 years of age. It involves both kidneys. The cortex and medulla are filled with large, thin-walled cysts that are several millimeters to several centimeters in diameter. The cysts enlarge and destroy surrounding tissue by compression.

Early in adult PKD, patients are usually asymptomatic. Symptoms appear when the cysts begin to enlarge. Often the first manifestations are headaches, urinary tract infection (UTI) or urinary calculi, hypertension, hematuria (from rupture of cysts), or pain or a sensation of heaviness in the back, side, or abdomen. Bilateral, enlarged kidneys are often palpable on physical examination.

- Chronic pain can be constant and severe.
- Usually the disease progresses to end-stage renal disease (ESRD) by age 60.
- PKD can also affect the liver (liver cysts), heart (abnormal heart valves), blood vessels (aneurysms), and intestines (diverticulosis). The most serious complication is a ruptured cerebral aneurysm.

Diagnosis is based on clinical manifestations, family history, ultrasound (best screening measure), or CT scan (more precise).

There is no specific treatment for PKD. A major aim is to prevent or treat UTIs with appropriate antibiotics. Nephrectomy may be necessary if pain, bleeding, or infection becomes a chronic, serious problem. When the patient begins to experience progressive renal failure, interventions are determined by the remaining renal function. Dialysis and kidney transplantation may be needed to treat ESRD.

Nursing measures are those used for management of ESRD (see Kidney Disease, Chronic, pp. 374-376). They include diet modification, fluid restriction, drugs (e.g., antihypertensives), and assisting the patient and family in coping with the chronic disease process and financial concerns.

- The patient with the adult form of PKD often has children by the time the disease is diagnosed. The patient needs appropriate counseling regarding plans for having more children.

P

POLYCYTHEMIA

Description

Polycythemia is the production and presence of increased number of RBCs. The increase in RBCs can be so great that blood circulation is impaired as a result of the increased blood viscosity (hyperviscosity) and volume (hypervolemia).

Pathophysiology

The two types of polycythemia are *primary polycythemia (polycythemia vera)* and *secondary polycythemia* (Fig. 19). Their etiologies and pathogeneses differ, although their complications and clinical manifestations are similar.

Polycythemia vera is a chronic myeloproliferative disorder involving increased production of not only RBCs but also WBCs and platelets. The disease develops insidiously and follows a chronic, vacillating course. The median age at diagnosis is 60 years. Patients have enhanced blood viscosity and blood volume and congestion of organs and tissues with blood. Splenomegaly and hepatomegaly are common.

- Polycythemia vera is associated with mutations in a gene that provides instructions for making a protein that promotes proliferation of cells, especially blood cells from hematopoietic stem cells.

Secondary polycythemia can be either hypoxia-driven or hypoxia-independent. In *hypoxia-driven polycythemia*, hypoxia stimulates erythropoietin (EPO) production in the kidney, which in turn stimulates RBC production. The need for O_2 may result from high altitude, pulmonary and cardiovascular disease, defective O_2 transport, or tissue hypoxia. In *hypoxia-independent polycythemia*, erythropoietin (EPO) is produced by a malignant or benign tumor tissue.

Clinical Manifestations

- Initial manifestations from hypertension caused by hypervolemia and hyperviscosity include complaints of headache, vertigo, dizziness, tinnitus, and visual disturbances.
- Manifestations caused by blood vessel distention, circulatory stasis, thrombosis, and tissue hypoxia include angina, heart failure (HF), intermittent claudication, and thrombophlebitis.
- The most common serious acute complication is stroke secondary to thrombosis.
- Hemorrhage caused by either vessel rupture from overdistention or inadequate platelet function may result in petechiae, ecchymoses, epistaxis, or GI bleeding.

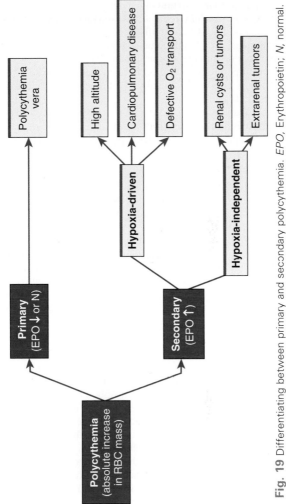

Fig. 19 Differentiating between primary and secondary polycythemia. *EPO*, Erythropoietin; *N*, normal.

Other clinical manifestations include:
- Generalized pruritus related to histamine release from an increased number of basophils
- Hepatomegaly and splenomegaly may contribute to patient complaints of satiety and sensation of fullness
- Pain from peptic ulcer caused by increased gastric secretions
- Paresthesia and erythromelalgia (painful burning and redness of the hands and feet)
- Plethora (ruddy complexion)
- Hyperuricemia resulting from an increase in RBC destruction that accompanies excessive RBC production; may cause gout

Diagnostic Studies

Diagnostic study abnormalities include:
- Elevated hemoglobin (Hgb) and RBC count with microcytosis
- Low to normal EPO level in polycythemia vera, high EPO level in secondary polycythemia
- Elevated WBC count with basophilia
- Elevated platelets (thrombocytosis) and platelet dysfunction
- Elevated leukocyte alkaline phosphatase, uric acid, and cobalamin levels
- Elevated histamine levels

Bone marrow examination in polycythemia vera shows hypercellularity of RBCs, WBCs, and platelets.

Interprofessional Care

Treatment is directed toward reducing blood volume and viscosity and bone marrow activity. Phlebotomy is the mainstay of treatment. At the time of diagnosis, 300 to 500 mL of blood may be removed every other day until the hematocrit (Hct) level is reduced to normal. An individual managed with repeated phlebotomies eventually becomes iron-deficient, although this effect is rarely symptomatic. Avoid iron supplementation.
- Hydration therapy is used to reduce the blood's viscosity.
- Myelosuppressive agents such as hydroxyurea (Hydrea), busulfan (Myleran), and chlorambucil (Leukeran) are used. Ruxolitinib (Jakafi), which inhibits expression of the *JAK2* mutation, is used when there is no response to hydroxyurea.
- Low-dose aspirin is used to prevent clotting.
- Interferon-alpha (IFN-α) is used in women of childbearing age or those with intractable pruritus.
- Anagrelide (Agrylin) may be used to reduce the platelet count and inhibit platelet aggregation.

- Allopurinol (Zyloprim) may reduce the number of acute gouty attacks caused by increased uric acid levels from cell destruction.

Nursing Management

Primary polycythemia vera is not preventable. However, because secondary polycythemia is caused by hypoxia, maintaining adequate oxygenation may prevent problems. Therefore controlling chronic pulmonary disease, stopping smoking, and avoiding high altitudes may be important.

When acute exacerbations of polycythemia vera develop, assist with or perform phlebotomies, depending on the institution's policies.

- Evaluate fluid intake and output during hydration therapy to avoid fluid overload (which further complicates circulatory congestion) and underhydration (which can make the blood even more viscous).
- If myelosuppressive agents are used, teach the patient about medication side effects.
- Assess the patient's nutritional status because inadequate food intake can result from GI symptoms of sensation of fullness, pain, and dyspepsia.
- Begin activities and/or medications to decrease thrombus formation. Initiate active or passive leg exercises and ambulation when possible.
- Because of its chronic nature, polycythemia vera requires ongoing evaluation. Phlebotomy may need to be done every 2 to 3 months. Evaluate the patient for complications.

PRESSURE ULCER

Description

A *pressure ulcer* is localized injury to the skin and/or underlying tissue (usually over a bony prominence) as a result of pressure or pressure in combination with shear. The most common sites for pressure ulcers are the sacrum and heels.

Factors influencing pressure ulcer development include amount of pressure (intensity), length of time pressure is exerted on skin (duration), and ability of patient's tissue to tolerate externally applied pressure. *Shearing force* (pressure exerted on skin when the surface layer adheres to bedding while deeper skin layers slide in the direction of body movement) and excessive moisture also contribute to pressure ulcer formation.

- Risk factors for the development of pressure ulcers include patients who are older, incontinent, unable to reposition or unaware of the need to reposition (e.g., spinal cord injury), and bed- or wheelchair-bound.

Clinical Manifestations

Pressure ulcers are staged on the basis of the visible or palpable tissue in the ulcer bed. Table 68 illustrates the pressure ulcer stages. If the pressure ulcer becomes infected, the patient may display systemic signs of infection (e.g., leukocytosis, fever).

Nursing and Interprofessional Management

Pressure ulcer management requires local wound care as well as support measures such as adequate nutrition, pain management, and pressure relief. Both conservative and surgical strategies are used in the treatment of pressure ulcers, depending on the ulcer's stage and condition.

- Stage 3 or 4 (full-skin-thickness injury) pressure ulcer acquired after admission to a health care setting is considered a serious reportable event.

Nursing Management

Goals

The patient with a pressure ulcer will have no deterioration of the ulcer, reduce or eliminate the factors that lead to pressure ulcers, not develop an infection in the pressure ulcer, have healing of pressure ulcers, and have no recurrence.

Nursing Diagnosis

- Impaired skin integrity

Nursing Interventions

Assess patients for pressure ulcer risk on admission and at periodic intervals, using a validated assessment tool such as the Braden Scale (available at www.bradenscale.com). Reposition patients frequently to prevent pressure ulcers. Although the past "standard" was every 2 hours, the frequency of turning and repositioning patients should be individualized on the basis of risk factors and the type of support surface. For example, some high-risk patients may need to be turned and repositioned every hour.

- Once a person has been identified as being at risk for a pressure ulcer, prevention strategies should be implemented. Table 69 and eNursing Care Plan 11-2 (available on the website for Lewis et al, *Medical-Surgical Nursing,* ed 10) list guidelines for preventing pressure ulcers.

TABLE 68 Staging of Pressure Ulcers

Definition and Description	Clinical Presentation
	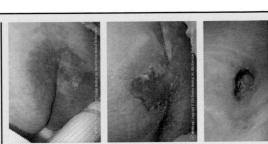

Stage/Category I: Non-Blanchable Erythema

Intact skin with non-blanchable redness of a localized area, usually over a bony prominence. Darkly pigmented skin may not have visible blanching. Its color may differ from the surrounding area. The area may be painful, firm, soft, warmer, or cooler as compared with adjacent tissue.

Stage/Category II: Partial-Thickness Injury

Partial-thickness loss of dermis presents as a shallow open ulcer with a red-pink wound bed, without slough. May also present as an intact or open/ruptured blister filled with serum or serosanguineous fluid. Presents as a shiny or dry shallow ulcer without slough or bruising. (Bruising indicates deep tissue injury.)

Stage/Category III: Full-Thickness Skin Loss

Full-thickness tissue loss. Subcutaneous fat may be visible but bone, tendon, or muscle are not exposed. Slough may be present but does not obscure depth of tissue loss. May include undermining and tunneling. The depth of a category/stage III pressure ulcer varies by anatomic location.

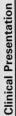

Continued

P

TABLE 68 Staging of Pressure Ulcers—cont'd

Definition and Description	Clinical Presentation
Stage/Category IV: Full-Thickness Tissue Loss Full-thickness tissue loss with exposed bone, tendon, or muscle. Slough or eschar may be present. Often includes undermining and tunneling. Depth of pressure ulcer varies by anatomic location. Ulcers can extend into muscle and/or supporting structures (e.g., fascia, tendon, or joint capsule), making osteomyelitis or osteitis likely to develop. Exposed bone/muscle is visible or directly palpable.	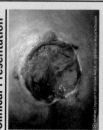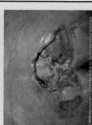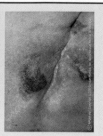
Unstageable/Unclassified: Full-Thickness Skin or Tissue Loss (Depth Unknown) Full-thickness tissue loss in which actual depth of ulcer is completely obscured by slough (yellow, tan, gray, green or brown) and/or eschar (tan, brown or black) in wound bed. Until enough slough and/or eschar are removed to expose the base of wound, the true depth cannot be determined; but it will be either a stage III or IV wound. Stable (dry, adherent, intact without erythema, or fluctuance) eschar on the heels serves as the body's "natural" (biologic) cover and should not be removed.	
Suspected Deep Tissue Injury (Depth Unknown) Purple or maroon localized area of discolored intact skin or blood-filled blister due to damage of underlying soft tissue from pressure and/or shear. The area may be preceded by tissue that is painful, firm, mushy, boggy, warmer, or cooler as compared with adjacent tissue. Deep tissue injury may be difficult to detect in individuals with dark skin tones. Evolution may include a thin blister over a dark wound bed. The wound may further evolve and become covered by thin eschar. Evolution may be rapid, exposing additional layers of tissue even with optimal treatment.	

Photos used with permission of the National Pressure Ulcer Advisory Panel.

Devices such as alternating pressure mattresses, foam mattresses with adequate stiffness and thickness, wheelchair cushions, padded commode seats, foam boots, and lift sheets are useful in reducing pressure and shearing force.

If a pressure ulcer has developed, document its size, depth, and appearance. Initiate interventions based on the ulcer's characteristics (e.g., size, stage, location, presence of infection or pain) and the patient's general clinical status.

Local ulcer care may involve debridement, wound cleaning, relief of pressure, and the application of a dressing.

- Necrotic tissue or eschar (except for dry, stable necrotic heels) must be removed by surgical, mechanical, enzymatic, or autolytic debridement methods. Once the pressure ulcer has been successfully debrided and has a clean granulating base, the goal is to provide an appropriate wound environment that supports moist wound healing and prevents disruption of newly formed granulation tissue.
- Reconstruction of the pressure ulcer site by operative repair, using skin grafts, skin flaps, musculocutaneous flaps, or free flaps, may be necessary.
- Pressure ulcers should be cleaned with noncytotoxic solutions, such as normal saline, that do not kill or damage cells.
- After cleansing the pressure ulcer, cover it with an appropriate dressing. (Dressings are discussed in Table 11-9, Lewis et al, *Medical-Surgical Nursing,* ed 10, p. 169.)
- Maintenance of adequate nutrition is an important nursing responsibility when caring for a patient with a pressure ulcer. Oral feedings must be adequate in calories, protein, fluids, vitamins, and minerals to meet the patient's nutritional requirements. Enteral feedings can be used to supplement oral feedings. If necessary, parenteral nutrition may be used.

▼ **Patient and Caregiver Teaching**

Because recurrence of pressure ulcers is common, it is extremely important to teach both the patient and caregiver about prevention techniques (Table 69).

- Teach caregiver about the etiology of pressure ulcers, prevention techniques, early signs, nutritional support, and care techniques for pressure ulcers.
- Because the patient with a pressure ulcer often requires extensive care for other health problems, the caregiver may need your psychosocial support.

TABLE 69 Patient & Caregiver Teaching

Pressure Ulcer

When teaching the patient or caregiver to prevent and care for pressure ulcers, do the following:

1. Identify and explain risk factors and etiology of pressure ulcers to patient and caregiver.
2. Assess all at-risk patients at the time of first hospital and/or home visit or whenever the patient's condition changes. Thereafter, assess at regular intervals based on care setting (every 24 hours for acute care or every visit in home care).
3. Teach the caregiver techniques for managing incontinence. If incontinence occurs, cleanse skin at time of soiling and use absorbent pads or briefs.
4. Demonstrate correct positioning to decrease risk of skin breakdown. Instruct caregiver to reposition a bed-bound patient at least every 2 hours, a chair-bound patient every hour. NEVER position the patient with weight directly on the pressure ulcer.
5. Assess resources (i.e., caregiver's availability and skill, finances, equipment) of patients requiring pressure ulcer care at home. When selecting ulcer care dressing, consider cost and amount of caregiver time required.
6. Teach patient and/or caregiver to place clean dressings over sterile dressings using "no touch" technique when changing dressings. Instruct caregiver on disposal of contaminated dressings.
7. Teach patient and caregiver to inspect skin daily. Tell them to report any significant changes to the HCP.
8. Teach patient and caregiver the importance of good nutrition to enhance ulcer healing.
9. Evaluate program effectiveness.

PROSTATE CANCER

Description

Prostate cancer is a malignant tumor of the prostate gland. It is the most common cancer among men, excluding skin cancer, and is the second leading cause of cancer death in men (exceeded only by lung cancer). Men have a 1 in 7 risk of developing prostate cancer.

- African American men have a higher incidence of prostate cancer than any other population worldwide (except Jamaican men of African descent).

Pathophysiology

Prostate cancer is a slow growing androgen-dependent cancer. Tumor spread is by three routes: direct extension, through the lymph system, or through the bloodstream. Spread by direct extension involves the seminal vesicles, urethral mucosa, bladder wall, and external sphincter. Later spread occurs through the lymphatic system to the regional lymph nodes. The bloodstream appears to be the route for spread to the pelvic bones, head of the femur, lower lumbar spine, liver, and lungs.

- The incidence of prostate cancer increases markedly after age 50, with a median age at diagnosis of 67 years.
- Dietary factors and obesity may be associated with prostate cancer. A diet high in red and processed meats and high-fat dairy products along with a low intake of vegetables and fruits may increase the risk of prostate cancer.
- There is an increased prevalence of prostate cancer among farmers and commercial pesticide applicators, possibly secondary to exposure to chemicals found in pesticides.
- Persons with a family history of prostate cancer are at increased risk.

Clinical Manifestations

Prostate cancer is usually asymptomatic in the early stages. Eventually the patient may have signs and symptoms similar to those of benign prostatic hyperplasia (BPH), including dysuria, hesitancy, dribbling, frequency, urgency, hematuria, nocturia, retention, interruption of urinary stream, and inability to urinate.

- Pain in the lumbosacral area that radiates down to the hips or legs, when coupled with urinary symptoms, may indicate metastasis. As the cancer spreads to the bones, pain can become severe, especially in the back and legs, because of spinal cord compression and bone destruction.

Diagnostic Studies

- Most men in the United States with prostate cancer are diagnosed by prostate-specific antigen (PSA) screening. Men should be informed about the potential risks (e.g., subsequent evaluation and treatment that may be unnecessary) and benefits (early detection of prostate cancer) of PSA screening before being tested. The discussion about screening should take place at (1) age 50 for men who are at average risk of prostate cancer and are expected to live at least 10 more years; (2) age 45 for men at high risk for development of prostate cancer, including African Americans and men who have a first-degree relative (father, brother, or son) diagnosed with prostate cancer at an early age (younger than age 65); and (3) age 40 for men at even higher risk (those with more than one first-degree relative who had prostate cancer at an early age). Mild elevations in PSA may occur with aging, BPH, recent ejaculation, constipation, or prostatitis, or after long bike rides. Decreases in the PSA level can occur with drugs such as finasteride (Proscar) and dutasteride (Avodart).

- When prostate cancer treatment is successful, PSA levels should fall to undetectable levels.
- On digital rectal examination (DRE), the prostate gland may feel hard, nodular, and asymmetric.
- Elevated prostatic acid phosphatase (PAP) levels are specific for prostate cancer.
- Biopsy using transrectal ultrasound can confirm the diagnosis.
- CT scan, bone scan, or MRI can assess cancer spread.
- Elevated serum alkaline phosphatase may indicate bone metastasis.

Interprofessional Care
Staging
The management of prostate cancer depends on the stage and overall health of the patient. The most common classification system for determining the extent of the prostate cancer is the tumor-node-metastasis (TNM) system (see p. 781).

The tumor is graded on the basis of tumor histology using the Gleason scale: Grade 1 represents the most well-differentiated or lowest grade (most like original cells), and grade 5 represents the most poorly differentiated (unlike original cells) or highest grade. The two most commonly occurring patterns of cells are graded with the two scores, which are then added together to create a Gleason score.

- The patient's Gleason score and PSA level at diagnosis are used with the TNM system to determine the stage of the tumor (Table 70).
- Most patients (90%) with prostate cancer are initially diagnosed when the cancer is in either a local or a regional stage. The 5-year survival rate with an initial diagnosis at these stages is 100%.

At all stages, there is more than one possible treatment option. The decision of which treatment course to pursue should be made jointly by patients, their partners, and the interprofessional team.

- A conservative approach to slow-growing tumors is active surveillance or "watchful waiting." This strategy is appropriate for

TABLE 70 **Staging of Prostate Cancer**

Stage	Tumor Size	Lymph Node Involvement	Metastasis	PSA Level	Gleason Score
I	Not felt on DRE Not seen by visual imaging	No	No	<10	≤6
II	Felt on DRE Seen by imaging Tumor confined to prostate	No	No	10-20	6-7
III	Cancer outside prostate Possible spread to seminal vesicles	No	No	Any level	Any score
IV	Any size	Any nodal involvement	Yes	Any level	Any score

DRE, Digital rectal examination; *PSA*, prostate-specific antigen.
Adapted from American Cancer Society: *How is prostate cancer staged?* Retrieved from *www.cancer.org/Cancer/ProstateCancer/DetailedGuide/prostate-cancer-staging.*

P

(1) a life expectancy of less than 10 years (low risk of dying of the disease), (2) the presence of a low-grade, low-stage tumor, and (3) serious coexisting medical conditions. Patients are monitored with frequent PSA testing and DREs. Significant changes in PSA level, DRE findings, or symptoms warrant a reevaluation of treatment options.

Surgical Therapy

With radical prostatectomy, the entire prostate gland, seminal vesicles, and part of the bladder neck (ampulla) are removed. Retroperitoneal lymph node dissection is performed only on men with a high risk for metastatic disease. Surgery is usually not considered an option for advanced-stage disease (except to relieve symptoms associated with obstruction) because metastasis has already occurred.

- Traditional approaches for radical prostatectomy are retropubic (low abdominal incision) and perineal (incision between the scrotum and anus).
- Robotic-assisted (e.g., da Vinci system) laparoscopic prostatectomy is associated with less bleeding, less pain, and a faster recovery than with other approaches.
- After surgery, the patient has a large indwelling catheter with a 30-mL balloon placed in the bladder via the urethra. A drain is left in the surgical site to aid in the removal of drainage from the area.

Two major adverse outcomes after a radical prostatectomy are erectile dysfunction and urinary incontinence. The incidence of erectile dysfunction is dependent on the patient's age, preoperative sexual functioning, whether nerve-sparing surgery was performed, and the expertise of the surgeon. A nerve-sparing technique is sometimes used to reduce the risk of erectile dysfunction. Problems with urinary control may occur for the first few months because the bladder must be reattached to the urethra after the prostate is removed. Kegel exercises strengthen the urinary sphincter and may help improve continence. Cryotherapy is a surgical technique that destroys cancer cells by freezing. The treatment takes about 2 hours, with the patient under general or spinal anesthesia.

A bilateral orchiectomy is the surgical removal of the testes that may be done alone or in combination with prostatectomy. For advanced stages of prostate cancer, an orchiectomy is one treatment option for cancer control.

Radiation Therapy

Radiation therapy is a common option for prostate cancer. Radiation therapy may be offered as the only treatment, or it may be offered in combination with surgery or hormonal therapy. Salvage radiation therapy given for cancer recurrence after a radical prostatectomy may improve survival for some men.

- External beam radiation is the most widely used method. Brachytherapy using radioactive seed implants placed in the prostate gland is best suited for patients with early-stage disease.

Drug Therapy

The types of drug therapy available for the treatment of advanced or metastatic prostate cancer are androgen deprivation (hormone) therapy, chemotherapy, or a combination of both.

Prostate cancer growth is largely dependent on the presence of androgens. Androgen deprivation therapy (ADT) is focused on reducing the levels of circulating androgens in order to reduce the tumor growth. One of the biggest challenges with ADT is that almost all tumors treated will become resistant to this therapy *(hormone-refractory)* within a few years. Androgen deprivation can be produced by inhibiting androgen production or blocking androgen receptors. See Table 54-7, Lewis et al, *Medical-Surgical Nursing,* ed 10, p. 1280, for mechanisms of action and side effects from ADT.

- Luteinizing hormone–releasing hormone (LHRH) agonists (e.g., leuprolide [Lupron, Eligard], goserelin [Zoladex], triptorelin [Trelstar]) produce a chemical castration similar to the effects of an orchiectomy.
- Androgen receptor blockers (e.g., flutamide, nilutamide [Nilandron], enzalutamide (Xtandi), bicalutamide [Casodex]) compete with circulating androgens at the receptor sites.
- Combining an androgen receptor blocker with an LHRH agonist results in combined androgen blockade.

Chemotherapy is generally reserved for patients with hormone-refractory prostate cancer (HRPC) in late-stage disease. In HRPC, the cancer is progressing despite treatment. This occurs in patients who have taken an antiandrogen for a certain period of time. The goal of chemotherapy is mainly palliative.

- Men with advanced prostate cancer who have HRPC may receive a vaccine (sipuleucel-T [Provenge]). The vaccine stimulates the patient's system against the cancer and may prolong survival.

Nursing Management

Goals

The patient with prostate cancer will be an active participant in the treatment plan, have satisfactory pain control, follow the therapeutic plan, understand the effect of the therapeutic plan on sexual function, and find a satisfactory way to manage the impact on bladder or bowel function.

Nursing Diagnoses
- Decisional conflict
- Acute pain
- Urinary retention and impaired urinary elimination
- Sexual dysfunction
- Anxiety

Nursing Interventions

One of your most important roles is to encourage patients (in consultation with their HCP) to have an annual prostate screening (PSA and DRE). See discussion of screening recommendations, pp. 517-518.

- Provide sensitive, caring support for the patient and the family to help them cope with the cancer diagnosis.
- Care during the preoperative and postoperative phases of radical prostatectomy is similar to that with surgical procedures for BPH (see pp. 75-77).
- Refer to nursing interventions for the patient undergoing radiation therapy (p. 733) and chemotherapy (p. 694).
- Pain control is the primary nursing intervention for the terminally ill patient. It is managed through ongoing pain assessment, administration of prescribed medications (both opioid and non-opioid agents), and the use of nonpharmacologic methods of pain relief (e.g., relaxation breathing).
- In advanced prostate cancer, hospice care is often appropriate and beneficial. (Hospice care is discussed in Chapter 9, Lewis et al, *Medical-Surgical Nursing,* ed 10.)

▼ **Patient and Caregiver Teaching**

Teach appropriate catheter care for the patient discharged with an indwelling catheter in place and the patient's caregiver.

- Instruct to clean the urethral meatus with soap and water once each day; maintain a high fluid intake; keep the collecting bag lower than the bladder at all times; keep the catheter securely anchored to the inner thigh or abdomen; and report any signs of bladder infection, such as bladder spasms, fever, or hematuria.
- If urinary incontinence is a problem, encourage the patient to practice pelvic floor muscle exercises (Kegel) with urination and throughout the day. Continuous practice during the 4- to 6-week healing process improves the success rate.

PSORIATIC ARTHRITIS

Psoriatic arthritis (PsA) is a progressive, inflammatory disease affecting about 30% of the people with psoriasis. *Psoriasis* is a common, benign, inflammatory skin disorder characterized by the presence of red, irritated, and scaly patches.

- Both PsA and psoriasis appear to have a genetic link with human leukocyte antigens (HLAs) in many patients. Although the exact cause of PsA is unknown, a combination of immune, genetic, and environmental factors is suspected.

PsA can occur in different forms. *Distal arthritis* primarily involves the ends of the fingers and toes, with pitting and color changes in the fingernails and toenails. *Asymmetric arthritis* involves different joints between the extremities. *Symmetric* PsA resembles rheumatoid arthritis (RA) and affects joints on both sides of the body at the same time. It accounts for about 50% of cases. *Psoriatic spondylitis* is marked by pain and stiffness in the spine and neck. *Arthritis mutilans* is the most severe form of the disease, affecting only 5% of people with psoriatic arthritis but causing complete destruction of small joints.

- On x-ray, cartilage loss and erosion are similar to those seen in RA. Advanced cases of PsA often reveal widened joint spaces.
- A "pencil in cup" deformity is common in the distal interphalangeal (DIP) joints as a result of thin, weakened bone. In this deformity, the narrowed end of the affected metacarpals or phalanges inserts into the expanded end of the other (adjacent) bone sharing the joint.
- Elevated erythrocyte sedimentation rate (ESR), elevated serum uric acid, and mild anemia are seen in some patients. Therefore, the diagnosis of gout must be excluded.

Treatment includes splinting, joint protection, and physical therapy. Nonsteroidal antiinflammatory drugs (NSAIDs) given early in the course of the disease may help with inflammation. Drug therapy also includes disease-modifying antirheumatic drugs (DMARDs) such as methotrexate, which is effective for both articular and cutaneous manifestations. Sulfasalazine, cyclosporine, and biologic response modifiers (e.g., etanercept, golimumab, adalimumab, infliximab) may also be used. Apremilast (Otezla), an inhibitor of the enzyme phosphodiesterase-4, may be given to decrease inflammation.

P

PULMONARY EMBOLISM

Description

Pulmonary embolism (PE) is the blockage of pulmonary arteries by a thrombus, fat, or air embolus or tumor tissue. Risk factors for

PE include immobility or reduced mobility, surgery within the last 3 months (especially pelvic and lower extremity surgery), history of *deep vein thrombosis* (DVT), malignancy, obesity, oral contraceptives, hormone therapy, cigarette smoking, prolonged air travel, heart failure, pregnancy, and clotting disorders.

Approximately 10% of patients with massive PE die within the first hour. Treatment with anticoagulants significantly reduces mortality.

Pathophysiology

Most PEs arise from DVT formed in the deep leg veins. An *embolus* is a mobile clot that travels with blood flow through ever-smaller blood vessels until it lodges and obstructs perfusion of the pulmonary circulation.

Clinical Manifestations

Manifestations of PE are varied and nonspecific, making diagnosis difficult.

- Dyspnea is the most common presenting symptom.
- Other signs and symptoms are hypoxemia, tachypnea, cough, chest pain, hemoptysis, crackles, wheezing, fever, accentuation of the pulmonic heart sound, tachycardia, syncope, and sudden change in mental status as a result of hypoxemia.
- Massive emboli may produce abrupt hypotension and shock.
- Small emboli may go undetected or produce vague, transient symptoms. However, in the patient with underlying cardiopulmonary disease, even small emboli may result in severe cardiopulmonary compromise.

Complications

Pulmonary infarction (death of lung tissue) is most likely when (1) the occlusion is of a large or medium-sized pulmonary vessel (more than 2 mm in diameter), (2) there is insufficient collateral blood flow from the bronchial circulation, or (3) preexisting lung disease is present. Infarction results in alveolar necrosis and hemorrhage. Concomitant pleural effusion is frequent.

Pulmonary hypertension results from hypoxemia or involvement of more than 50% of the area of the normal pulmonary bed. As a single event, an embolus rarely causes pulmonary hypertension unless it is massive. Recurrent emboli may result in chronic pulmonary hypertension, leading eventually to dilation and hypertrophy of the right ventricle. Depending on the degree of pulmonary hypertension and its rate of development, outcomes can vary, with some patients dying within months of the diagnosis and others living for decades (see Pulmonary Hypertension, p. 526).

Diagnostic Studies

- Spiral (or helical) CT scan is the most frequently used test for diagnosis of PE. If the patient cannot have the contrast media used in a spiral CT, then a ventilation-perfusion (V/Q) scan is done.
- D-dimer testing assists in screening for an embolism.
- Pulmonary angiography is the most sensitive and specific test for detection of emboli.
- Arterial blood gases (ABGs) are abnormal with pulmonary occlusion but are not diagnostic of PE.

Interprofessional Care

Objectives of treatment are to (1) prevent further growth or multiplication of thrombi in the lower extremities, (2) prevent embolization to the pulmonary vascular system from the upper or lower extremities, and (3) provide cardiopulmonary support if indicated. Supportive therapy for the patient's cardiopulmonary status varies according to the severity of the PE.

- Administration of O_2 is by mask or cannula with the concentration determined by ABG analysis. Endotracheal intubation and mechanical ventilation may be needed to maintain adequate oxygenation.
- Respiratory measures such as turning, coughing, and deep breathing are important to help prevent or treat atelectasis.
- If shock is present, vasopressor agents may be necessary to support perfusion. If heart failure is present, diuretics are used.

Immediate coagulation is required for patients with PE. Subcutaneous administration of low-molecular-weight heparin (LMWH) (e.g., enoxaparin [Lovenox], fondaparinux) has been found to be safer and more effective than using unfractionated heparin. Warfarin (Coumadin) should also be initiated at the time of diagnosis and is typically administered for 3 to 6 months. Alternatives to warfarin include apixaban (Eliquis), dabigitran (Pradaxa), and edoxaban (Savaysa).

- Fibrinolytic agents, such as the tissue plasminogen activator alteplase (Activase), dissolve the PE lesion as well as the thrombus source.

Hemodynamically unstable patients with massive PE and contraindications to fibrinolytic therapy may be candidates for immediate pulmonary embolectomy. This can be done via a vascular (catheter) or surgical approach.

- To prevent further migration of clots from the lower extremities into the pulmonary system, an inferior vena cava (IVC) filter may be surgically placed.

Nursing Management

Nursing measures aimed at prevention of PE are similar to those for prevention of DVT (see Venous Thrombosis, p. 671).

The prognosis for a patient with PE is good if therapy is promptly instituted. Keep the patient in bed in a semi-Fowler's position to facilitate breathing. Maintain an IV line for drugs and fluid therapy. Administer O_2 therapy as ordered. Carefully monitor vital signs, ABGs, cardiac rhythm, pulse oximetry, and lung sounds to assess the patient's clinical status.

- The patient is usually anxious because of pain, inability to breathe, and fear of death. Provide explanations, emotional support, and reassurance to help relieve the patient's anxiety.

▼ **Patient and Caregiver Teaching**

- Long-term management is similar to that for the patient with Venous Thrombosis (see p. 676).
- Patient teaching regarding long-term anticoagulant therapy is critical. Patients with recurrent emboli are treated indefinitely. INR (international normalized ratio) levels are obtained at intervals, and warfarin dosage is adjusted accordingly.
- Discharge planning is aimed at limiting the progression of the condition and preventing complications and recurrence. Reinforce the need for the patient to return to the HCP for regular follow-up examinations.

PULMONARY HYPERTENSION

Description

Pulmonary hypertension is elevated pulmonary pressures resulting from increased resistance to blood flow through the pulmonary circulation. Pulmonary hypertension can occur as a primary disease (idiopathic pulmonary arterial hypertension) or as a secondary complication of a respiratory, cardiac, autoimmune, hepatic, or connective tissue disorder (secondary pulmonary arterial hypertension).

Idiopathic pulmonary arterial hypertension (IPAH) is pulmonary hypertension that occurs without an apparent cause. (It was previously known as *primary pulmonary hypertension* [PPH].) It has been associated with connective tissue diseases, cirrhosis, and HIV infection, but the exact relationship between these disorders and IPAH remains unclear. If untreated, this disorder can be rapidly progressive, causing right-sided heart failure and death within a few years. Although new drug therapy has greatly improved survival, the disease remains incurable.

Pathophysiology

The pathophysiology of IPAH is poorly understood. Some type of insult (e.g., hormonal, mechanical) to the pulmonary endothelium may occur, causing a cascade of events leading to vascular scarring, endothelial dysfunction, and smooth muscle proliferation. IPAH affects females more often than males.

Clinical Manifestations

Classic manifestations are dyspnea on exertion and fatigue. Exertional chest pain, dizziness, and syncope are other symptoms. As the disease progresses, dyspnea occurs at rest. Pulmonary hypertension increases the workload of the right ventricle and causes right ventricular hypertrophy (a condition called *cor pulmonale*) (see Cor Pulmonale, p. 152) and eventually heart failure (see Heart Failure, p. 274).

- Right-sided cardiac catheterization is the definitive test to diagnose any type of pulmonary hypertension.
- Confirmation of IPAH requires a thorough workup to exclude conditions that may cause secondary pulmonary arterial hypertension. Diagnostic evaluation includes ECG, chest x-ray, pulmonary function testing, echocardiogram, and CT scan.

Nursing and Interprofessional Management

Although IPAH has no cure, treatment can relieve symptoms, improve quality of life, and prolong life. Drug therapy consists of several drug classifications that promote vasodilation of the pulmonary blood vessels, reduce right ventricular overload, and reverse remodeling. See Table 27-27, Lewis et al, *Medical-Surgical Nursing*, ed 10, p. 532.

- Diuretics are used to manage peripheral edema.
- Anticoagulants are beneficial in pulmonary complications related to thrombus formation.
- Use of low-flow O_2 provides symptomatic relief by preventing the potent pulmonary vasoconstriction caused by hypoxia.

Surgical interventions for pulmonary hypertension include atrial septostomy (AS) and lung transplantation. AS is a palliative procedure that involves the creation of an intraatrial right-to-left shunt to decompress the right ventricle. It is used for a select group of patients awaiting lung transplantation. Lung transplantation is indicated for patients who do not respond to drug therapy and progress to severe right-sided heart failure.

Secondary Pulmonary Arterial Hypertension

Secondary pulmonary arterial hypertension (SPAH) occurs when a primary disease causes a chronic increase in pulmonary artery pressures. SPAH can develop as a result of parenchymal lung disease, left ventricular dysfunction, intracardiac shunts, chronic pulmonary thromboembolism, or systemic connective tissue disease. The specific primary disease can result in anatomic or vascular changes causing pulmonary hypertension.

Symptoms can reflect the underlying disease, but some are directly attributable to SPAH, including dyspnea, fatigue, lethargy, and chest pain. Diagnosis of SPAH is similar to that of IPAH.

- Treatment of SPAH consists mainly of treating the underlying primary disorder. When irreversible pulmonary vascular damage has occurred, therapies used for IPAH are initiated.

PYELONEPHRITIS

Description

Pyelonephritis is an inflammation of the renal parenchyma and collecting system (including the renal pelvis). *Urosepsis* is a systemic infection arising from a urologic source. If not treated promptly, it can lead to septic shock and death (see Shock, p. 565).

Pathophysiology

Pyelonephritis usually begins with colonization and infection of the lower urinary tract via the ascending urethral route. Bacteria normally found in the intestinal tract, such as *Escherichia coli*, frequently cause pyelonephritis.

A preexisting factor is often present, such as *vesicoureteral reflux* (retrograde or backward movement of urine from lower to upper urinary tract) or dysfunction of lower urinary tract function, such as obstruction from benign prostatic hyperplasia or a urinary stone. For residents of long-term care facilities, catheter-associated urinary tract infections (CAUTIs) are common causes of pyelonephritis and urosepsis.

Acute pyelonephritis commonly starts in the renal medulla and spreads to the adjacent cortex. *Chronic pyelonephritis* usually results from recurring infections involving the upper urinary tract. However, it may also occur in the absence of an existing infection, recent infection, or history of urinary tract infections (UTIs). In chronic pyelonephritis, the kidneys become small, atrophic, and shrunken and lose function because of fibrosis (scarring). It often progresses to end-stage renal disease (ESRD) when both kidneys are involved, even if the underlying infection or problem is successfully eradicated (see Kidney Disease, Chronic, p. 370).

Clinical Manifestations

Acute manifestations of pyelonephritis vary from mild fatigue to the sudden onset of chills, fever, vomiting, malaise, flank pain, and costovertebral tenderness on the affected side. Dysuria, urinary urgency, and frequency may also be present. *Costovertebral tenderness* to percussion (costovertebral angle [CVA] pain) is typically present on the affected side. Acute manifestations generally subside within a few days even without specific therapy, although bacteriuria or pyuria persists.

Diagnostic Studies

- Urinalysis shows pyuria, bacteriuria, hematuria, and WBC casts.
- CBC count with WBC differential is done to identify leukocytosis.
- Urine and blood cultures may also be obtained.
- Ultrasound is used to identify anatomic abnormalities, hydronephrosis, renal abscesses, or stones.

Chronic pyelonephritis is diagnosed by radiologic imaging and biopsy rather than clinical features. Biopsy results indicate the loss of functioning nephrons, infiltration of the parenchyma with inflammatory cells, and fibrosis.

Interprofessional Care

Patients with severe infections or complicating factors such as nausea and vomiting with dehydration require hospital admission. Parenteral antibiotics are often given initially in the hospital to rapidly establish high serum and urinary drug levels.

The patient with mild symptoms may be treated as an outpatient with antibiotics for 14 to 21 days. Symptoms and signs typically improve or resolve within 48 to 72 hours after starting therapy. Relapses may be treated with a 6-week course of antibiotics. Antibiotic prophylaxis may also be used for recurrent infections.

Nursing Management

Goals

The patient with pyelonephritis will have normal renal function, normal body temperature, no complications, relief of pain, and no recurrence of symptoms.

Nursing Diagnoses/Collaborative Problem

- Impaired urinary elimination
- Readiness for enhanced self-health management
- Potential complication: urosepsis

Nursing Interventions

It is important that the patient receive early treatment for cystitis to prevent ascending infections. Because the patient with structural abnormalities of the urinary tract is at increased risk for infection, emphasize the need for regular medical care.

Nursing interventions vary depending on symptom severity. These interventions include teaching the patient about the disease process with emphasis on continuing medications as prescribed, having a follow-up urine culture, and recognizing manifestations of recurrence or relapse.

- In addition to antibiotic therapy, encourage the patient to drink at least eight glasses of fluid every day, even after the infection has been treated.
- The patient with frequent relapses or reinfections may be treated with long-term, low-dose antibiotics. Understanding the rationale for therapy is important to enhance patient adherence.

RAYNAUD'S PHENOMENON

Description

Raynaud's phenomenon is an episodic vasospastic disorder of the small cutaneous arteries, most frequently involving the fingers and toes. It occurs primarily in women between 15 and 40 years of age. Abnormalities in the vascular, intravascular, and neuronal mechanisms cause an imbalance between vasodilation and vasoconstriction.

Primary Raynaud's phenomenon occurs in isolation while secondary Raynaud's phenomenon occurs in association with an underlying disease (e.g., rheumatoid arthritis, scleroderma, systemic lupus erythematosus). Other contributing factors include occupation-related conditions, such as use of vibrating machinery, work in cold environments, or exposure to heavy metals (e.g., lead).

Clinical Manifestations

Exposure to cold, emotional upsets, tobacco use, and caffeine often trigger symptoms.

- The disorder is characterized by vasospasm-induced color changes (white, red, and blue) of fingers, toes, ears, and nose. Decreased perfusion results in pallor (white). The digits then become cyanotic (bluish purple). These changes are subsequently followed by rubor (red), caused by the hyperemic response when blood flow is restored.
- The patient usually describes cold and numbness in the vasoconstrictive phase, with throbbing and aching pain, tingling,

and swelling in the hyperemic phase. An episode usually lasts only minutes but may persist for several hours.

- After frequent, prolonged attacks, the skin may become thickened and the nails brittle. Complications include punctate lesions (small holes) of the fingertips and superficial gangrenous ulcers in advanced stages.
- Diagnosis is based on persistent symptoms for at least 2 years.

Nursing and Interprofessional Management

When conservative management is ineffective, drug therapy is considered.

- Sustained-release calcium channel blockers (e.g., nifedipine [Procardia]) relax smooth muscles of the arterioles by preventing the influx of calcium into the cells.
- Vasodilators (e.g., transdermal glyceryl trinitrate [Nitro-Dur]) may be given, and statins may lessen the severity of Raynaud's phenomenon.

Prompt intervention is needed for patients with digital ulceration and/or critical ischemia. Treatment options include IV prostacyclin infusion (c.g., iloprost), antibiotics, analgesics, and possibly an endothelin receptor antagonist (e.g., bosentan [Tracleer]) and surgical debridement of necrotic tissue. Sympathectomy is considered in advanced cases.

▼ Patient and Caregiver Teaching

Teaching should be directed toward preventing recurrent episodes.

- Loose, warm clothing should be worn for protection from cold, including gloves for working in a refrigerator or freezer or handling cold objects.
- Temperature extremes should be avoided. Immersing hands in warm water often decreases the spasm.
- Patients should stop using all tobacco products and avoid caffeine and other drugs with vasoconstrictive effects (e.g., pseudoephedrine).
- Provide patients with information about stress management techniques as appropriate.

REACTIVE ARTHRITIS

Reactive arthritis (Reiter's syndrome) is associated with a symptom complex that includes urethritis (in men) or cervicitis (in women), conjunctivitis, and mucocutaneous lesions. It occurs more commonly in young men than in young women.

- Although the exact etiology is unknown, reactive arthritis appears to be a reaction triggered in the body after exposure to specific genitourinary or GI tract infections. *Chlamydia tracho-matis* is most often implicated in sexually transmitted reactive arthritis.

- Reactive arthritis is also associated with GI infections with *Shigella, Salmonella, Campylobacter,* or *Yersinia* species and other microorganisms.

Individuals with inherited HLA-B27 are at increased risk for developing reactive arthritis after sexual contact or exposure to certain enteric pathogens, supporting the suggestion of a genetic predisposition.

- Urethritis develops within 1 to 2 weeks after sexual contact or GI infection. Low-grade fever, conjunctivitis, and arthritis may occur over the next several weeks.
- This arthritis tends to be asymmetric, frequently involving large joints of the lower extremities and toes. Lower back pain may occur with severe disease.
- Mucocutaneous lesions commonly occur as small, painless, superficial ulcerations on the tongue, oral mucosa, and glans penis. Soft tissue manifestations commonly include Achilles tendinitis or plantar fasciitis.
- The erythrocyte sedimentation rate (ESR) may be elevated.

Most patients recover in 2 to 16 weeks. Reactive arthritis is often associated with *C. trachomatis* infection, so treatment of patients and their sexual partners with doxycycline (Vibramycin) is widely recommended. Antibiotics have no effect on arthritis or other symptoms. Drug therapy may also include nonsteroidal antiinflammatory drugs (NSAIDs) and disease-modifying antirheumatic drugs (DMARDs) (e.g., methotrexate, sulfasalazine). Physical therapy may be helpful during recovery.

REFRACTIVE ERRORS

Refractive errors are the most common visual problem. This defect prevents light rays from converging to a single point of focus on the retina. Defects are a result of irregularities in corneal curvature, lens-focusing power, or eye length. Types of refractive errors include:

- *Myopia* (nearsightedness), the most common refractive error, is caused by light rays focusing in front of the retina, resulting in an inability to accommodate for objects at a distance.
- *Hyperopia* (farsightedness) is caused by light rays focusing behind the retina, requiring an effort such as squinting to focus the light rays on the retina for near objects.
- *Presbyopia* results in an age-related loss of accommodation with an inability to focus on near objects. The lens becomes

larger, firmer, and less elastic. The condition generally appears about the age of 40 years.

- *Astigmatism* is caused by an irregular corneal curvature bending incoming light rays unequally so that the rays do not come to a single point of focus on the retina. Astigmatism can occur in conjunction with any of the other refractive errors.

The major symptom of refractive errors is blurred vision. Additional complaints may include ocular discomfort, eye strain, or headaches. Management of refractive errors is by vision correction, which may include eyeglasses, contact lenses, refractive surgery, or surgical implantation of an artificial lens.

RESPIRATORY FAILURE, ACUTE

Description

The major function of the respiratory system is gas exchange, which involves the transfer of O_2 and CO_2 between inhaled tidal volumes and circulating blood volume within the pulmonary capillary bed. Respiratory failure results when one or both of these gas-exchanging functions are inadequate.

Respiratory failure is not a disease but a symptom of an underlying process affecting lung function. When respiratory function is insufficient, O_2 delivery, cardiac output (CO), clinical assessment findings, and/or baseline metabolic state may exhibit abnormalities specific to the affected body system(s). Respiratory failure occurs as a result of one or more diseases involving the lungs or other body systems (Table 71). Respiratory failure is classified as hypoxemic, hypercapnic, or both.

- *Hypoxemic respiratory failure* is also referred to as oxygenation failure because the primary problem is inadequate O_2 transfer between the alveoli and pulmonary capillaries. Hypoxemic respiratory failure is commonly defined as a partial pressure of O_2 in arterial blood (PaO_2) of 60 mm Hg or less when the patient is receiving an inspired O_2 concentration of at least 60%.
- *Hypercapnic respiratory failure* is also referred to as ventilatory failure because the primary problem is insufficient CO_2 removal. Hypercapnic respiratory failure is commonly defined as a partial pressure of CO_2 in arterial blood ($PaCO_2$) greater than 45 mm Hg in combination with acidemia (pH less than 7.35).

Pathophysiology

Hypoxemic Respiratory Failure

Four physiologic mechanisms may cause hypoxemia and subsequent hypoxemic respiratory failure: (1) mismatch between

TABLE 71   Causes of Hypoxemic and Hypercapnic Respiratory Failure*

Hypoxemic Respiratory Failure	Hypercapnic Respiratory Failure
Respiratory System	**Respiratory System**
• Acute respiratory distress syndrome (ARDS)	• Asthma
• Toxic inhalation (e.g., smoke inhalation)	• COPD
• Pneumonia	• Cystic fibrosis
• Hepatopulmonary syndrome (e.g., low-resistance flow state, V/Q mismatch)	**Central Nervous System**
• Massive pulmonary embolism (e.g., thrombus emboli, fat emboli)	• Brainstem injury or infarction
	• Sedative and opioid overdose
	• Spinal cord injury
• Pulmonary artery laceration and hemorrhage	• Severe head injury
• Inflammatory state and related alveolar injury	**Chest Wall**
	• Thoracic trauma (e.g., flail chest)
Cardiovascular System	• Kyphoscoliosis
• Anatomic shunt (e.g., ventricular septal defect)	• Pain
• Cardiogenic pulmonary edema	• Severe obesity
• Shock (decreasing blood flow through pulmonary vasculature)	**Neuromuscular System**
• High-cardiac-output states: diffusion limitation	• Myasthenia gravis
	• Critical illness polyneuropathy
	• Acute myopathy
	• Toxin exposure or ingestion (e.g., tree tobacco, acetylcholinesterase inhibitors, carbamate or organophosphate poisoning)
	• Amyotrophic lateral sclerosis
	• Phrenic nerve injury
	• Guillain-Barré syndrome
	• Poliomyelitis
	• Muscular dystrophy
	• Multiple sclerosis

V/Q, Ventilation-perfusion.
*This list is not all-inclusive.

ventilation (V) and perfusion (Q), commonly referred to as V/Q mismatch; (2) shunt; (3) diffusion limitation; and (4) hypoventilation. The most common causes are V/Q mismatch and shunt.

- Many diseases and conditions cause *V/Q mismatch*. The most common are those with increased airway secretions (e.g., chronic obstructive pulmonary disease [COPD]) or alveolar secretions (e.g., pneumonia) or bronchospasm (e.g., asthma). V/Q mismatch may also result when alveoli collapse (atelectasis) or as a result of pain.

- *Shunt* occurs when blood exits the heart without having participated in gas exchange. A shunt can be viewed as an extreme V/Q mismatch. There are two types of shunt: anatomic and intrapulmonary. O_2 therapy alone may be ineffective in increasing the PaO_2 if hypoxemia is caused by shunt.

- *Diffusion limitation* occurs when gas exchange across the alveolar-capillary interface is compromised by a process that thickens, damages, or destroys the alveolar membrane or affects blood flow through the pulmonary capillaries. Diffusion limitation is worsened by disease states affecting the pulmonary vascular bed, such as severe COPD or recurrent pulmonary emboli. Some diseases cause the alveolar-capillary membrane to become thicker (fibrotic), which slows gas transport. These diseases include pulmonary fibrosis, interstitial lung disease, and acute respiratory distress syndrome (ARDS). The classic sign of diffusion limitation is hypoxemia that is present during exercise but not at rest.

- *Alveolar hypoventilation* is a generalized decrease in ventilation that results in increased $PaCO_2$ and decreased PaO_2. Alveolar hypoventilation may be the result of restrictive lung disease, central nervous system (CNS) disease, chest wall dysfunction, or neuromuscular disease.

Frequently, hypoxemic respiratory failure is caused by a combination of V/Q mismatch, shunt, diffusion limitation, and alveolar hypoventilation.

Hypercapnic Respiratory Failure

Hypercapnic respiratory failure is sometimes called ventilatory failure. When CO_2 levels cannot be maintained within normal limits by the respiratory system, one of two primary problems exists: (1) an increase in CO_2 production or (2) a decrease in alveolar ventilation.

- Many conditions can limit ventilation (Table 71). They can be grouped into four categories: (1) abnormalities of the airways and alveoli, (2) abnormalities of the CNS, (3) abnormalities of the chest wall, and (4) neuromuscular conditions.

Clinical Manifestations

Respiratory failure may develop suddenly (minutes or hours) or gradually (several days or longer). A sudden decrease in PaO_2 or a rapid rise in $PaCO_2$ implies a serious condition that can quickly become a life-threatening emergency.

Manifestations are related to the extent of the change in PaO_2 and $PaCO_2$, the speed of change (acute versus chronic), and the ability to compensate. When the patient's compensatory mechanisms fail, respiratory failure occurs. It is important to monitor trends in arterial blood gas (ABG) values and/or pulse oximetry to evaluate the extent of change.

- Mental status changes such as restlessness, confusion, and combative behavior suggest inadequate O_2 delivery to the brain
- Morning headache, a slower respiratory rate, and a decreased level of consciousness may indicate issues with CO_2 removal. Tachycardia, tachypnea, and mild hypertension can be early signs of acute respiratory failure. Such changes can indicate an attempt by the heart and lungs to compensate for decreased O_2 delivery and rising CO_2 levels.
- Cyanosis is an unreliable and a late indicator of hypoxemia.
- As the PaO_2 decreases and acidosis increases, the myocardium becomes dysfunctional, resulting in angina and dysrhythmias. Cerebral and renal damage may occur if the hypoxia is severe and prolonged.

The patient may have a rapid, shallow breathing pattern or a respiratory rate that is slower than normal. A change from a rapid to a slower rate in a patient in acute respiratory distress suggests extreme progression of respiratory fatigue and increased possibility of respiratory arrest.

- Assumption of tripod position, pursed-lip breathing, and two- or three-word dyspnea indicate respiratory distress.
- There may be a change in the inspiratory (I) to expiratory (E) (I/E) ratio. Normally the I/E ratio is $1:2$. In patients in respiratory distress with airflow obstruction, the ratio may increase to $1:3$ or $1:4$.
- You may observe *retraction* (inward movement) of the intercostal spaces or the supraclavicular area and the use of accessory muscles during inspiration or expiration. Use of the accessory muscles signifies moderate distress. Paradoxic breathing indicates severe distress.

Immediately report changes in mental status, such as agitation, confusion, or a decreased level of consciousness (LOC), which may indicate rapid deterioration and the need for mechanical ventilation.

Diagnostic Studies

- ABGs determine the levels of $PaCO_2$, PaO_2, bicarbonate, and pH.
- Chest x-ray helps to identify possible causes of respiratory failure.
- A catheter may be inserted into a peripheral artery for monitoring BP and obtaining ABGs.
- Pulse oximetry monitors oxygenation status but reveals little about lung ventilation.
- Other studies may include CBC, serum electrolytes, urinalysis, and ECG.
- Sputum and blood cultures are obtained as necessary to determine sources of possible infection.
- If pulmonary embolus is suspected, a V/Q lung scan or CT scan may be done.

In severe respiratory failure requiring endotracheal intubation, end-tidal CO_2 ($ETCO_2$) may be used to help confirm correct tube placement within the airway immediately after intubation. $ETCO_2$ may also be used during ventilator management to assess trends in lung ventilation. A central venous or pulmonary artery catheter may be used to measure hemodynamic parameters.

Nursing and Interprofessional Management

Prevention of atelectasis, pneumonia, and complications of immobility, as well as optimizing hydration and nutrition, can potentially decrease the risk of respiratory failure in acutely ill patients. Consider age-related and acuity-related changes in physiology when assessing risk of acute respiratory failure.

Because many different problems can cause respiratory failure, specific care of these patients varies. Goals and related interventions to maximize O_2 delivery are essential to improving the patient's oxygenation and ventilation status. The primary goal is to treat the underlying cause of the respiratory failure. Other supportive goals include maintaining an adequate cardiac output and hemoglobin concentration.

- Interventions are directed toward reversing the process that resulted in the development of acute respiratory failure.
- Decreased cardiac output is treated by administration of IV fluids, drugs as prescribed, or both.
- If hemoglobin concentration is less than 9 g/dL (less than 90 g/L), packed RBCs may be transfused.
- Additional information on care for the patient with acute respiratory failure is presented in eNursing Care Plan 67-1 (available on the website).

Nursing Diagnoses
- Impaired gas exchange
- Ineffective airway clearance
- Ineffective breathing pattern

Respiratory Therapy

The major goals of care for acute respiratory failure include maintaining adequate oxygenation and ventilation. Interventions include O_2 therapy, mobilization of secretions, and positive pressure ventilation (PPV).

Oxygen Therapy.   The primary goal of O_2 therapy is to correct hypoxemia (see Oxygen Therapy, p. 718). If hypoxemia is secondary to V/Q mismatch, supplemental O_2 is administered at 1 to 3 L/min by nasal cannula or 24% to 32% by simple face mask or Venturi mask. Hypoxemia secondary to an intrapulmonary shunt is usually not responsive to high O_2 concentrations, and the patient usually requires PPV (see Mechanical Ventilation, p. 712).

- Patients with chronic hypercapnia should initially receive O_2 therapy through a low-flow device such as a nasal cannula at 1 to 2 L/minute or a Venturi mask at 24% to 28%. O_2 should be given with careful titration and at the lowest possible dose needed to keep arterial O_2 concentration by pulse oximetry (SpO_2) and PaO_2 within patient-specific clinical goals. Closely monitor these patients for changes in mental status, respiratory rate, and ABG results until their PaO_2 level has reached their baseline normal value.

Mobilization of Secretions.   Retained pulmonary secretions may cause or exacerbate acute respiratory failure by blocking O_2 movement into the alveoli and removal of CO_2. Secretions can be mobilized through effective coughing, adequate hydration and humidification, chest physical therapy, patient positioning, ambulation when possible, and tracheal suctioning.

Effective Coughing and Positioning.   If secretions are obstructing the airway, encourage the patient to cough. The patient with neuromuscular weakness from disease or exhaustion may not be able to generate sufficient airway pressures to produce an effective cough. *Augmented coughing (quad coughing)* may be helpful. Perform augmented coughing by placing the palm of your hand (or the palms of both hands) on the patient's abdomen below the xiphoid process. As the patient ends a deep inspiration and begins the expiration, push your hands forcefully into the abdomen, increasing abdominal pressure and facilitating the cough.

- Positioning the patient by elevating the head of the bed to at least 45 degrees or using a reclining chair bed may help maximize thoracic expansion.

- Lateral or side-lying positioning may be used in patients with disease involving only one lung, such as right-sided pneumonia. This position, termed *good lung down,* allows for improved V/Q matching in the affected lung.
- Patients should be side-lying if there is a possibility that the tongue will obstruct the airway or aspiration may occur. Keep an oral or nasal artificial airway at the bedside, ready for use.

Hydration and Humidification.   Thick and viscous secretions are difficult to expel. Adequate fluid intake (2 to 3 L/day) keeps secretions thin and easier to remove. If the patient is unable to take sufficient fluids orally, IV hydration is used. Assess for signs of fluid overload by clinical evaluation (e.g., crackles, dyspnea) and invasive monitoring (e.g., increased central venous pressure) at regular intervals.

Airway Suctioning.   If the patient is unable to expectorate secretions, nasopharyngeal, oropharyngeal, or nasotracheal suctioning is done. Suctioning through an artificial airway, such as an endotracheal tube, is performed as needed. (See Artificial Airways, p. 683.) Suction cautiously and closely monitor the patient for complications (e.g., hypoxia, increased intracranial pressure, dysrhythmias).

Positive Pressure Ventilation.   If intensive measures fail to improve ventilation and oxygenation, and the patient continues to show signs of acute respiratory failure, ventilatory assistance may be initiated (see Mechanical Ventilation, p. 712). PPV may be provided invasively using orotracheal or nasotracheal intubation or noninvasively by a nasal or face mask.

Drug Therapy

Goals of drug therapy for patients in acute respiratory failure include relief of bronchospasm, reduction of airway inflammation and pulmonary congestion, treatment of pulmonary infection, and reduction of severe anxiety and restlessness.

Relief of Bronchospasm.   Relief of bronchospasm increases alveolar ventilation. Short-acting bronchodilators, such as albuterol (Ventolin HFA) can be used with either a hand-held nebulizer or a metered-dose inhaler and spacer. In acute bronchospasm, these drugs may be given at 15- to 30-minute intervals until a response occurs.

Reduction of Airway Inflammation.   Corticosteroids (e.g., methylprednisolone [Solu-Medrol]) may be used in conjunction with bronchodilating agents when bronchospasm and inflammation are present. Inhaled corticosteroids require 4 to 5 days for optimum therapeutic effects and are not used for acute respiratory failure.

Reduction of Pulmonary Congestion. IV diuretics (e.g., furosemide [Lasix]) and nitroglycerin are used to decrease the pulmonary congestion caused by heart failure. If atrial fibrillation is also present, calcium channel blockers and β-adrenergic blockers are used to decrease heart rate and improve cardiac output.

Treatment of Pulmonary Infections. Pulmonary infections can either cause or exacerbate acute respiratory failure. IV antibiotics, such as azithromycin (Zithromax) or ceftriaxone, are often given to treat infections.

Reduction of Severe Anxiety and Restlessness. Anxiety, restlessness, and agitation result from hypoxia. In addition, fear caused by the inability to breathe and a sense of loss of control may increase anxiety. Anxiety, pain, and agitation increase O_2 consumption, which may worsen hypoxemia and increase CO_2 production. Sedation and analgesia are used to decrease anxiety, agitation, and pain. Follow an evidence-based and goal-directed protocol using only the dosing needed to meet patient-specific goals.

Nutritional Therapy

Maintenance of protein and energy stores is especially important because nutritional depletion causes a loss of respiratory muscle mass, which may prolong recovery. During acute respiratory failure, the risk of aspiration typically prevents oral intake. Enteral or parenteral nutrition should generally be started within 24 to 48 hours.

RESTLESS LEGS SYNDROME

Description

Restless legs syndrome (RLS), also known as *Willis-Ekbom disease* (WED), is characterized by unpleasant sensory (paresthesias) and motor abnormalities of one or both legs. Up to 10% of the U.S. population may have RLS.

There are two distinct types of RLS: primary (idiopathic) and secondary. A majority of cases are primary, and many patients with this type of RLS report a positive family history. Secondary RLS can be seen in metabolic abnormalities associated with iron deficiency, renal failure, polyneuropathy associated with diabetes mellitus, rheumatoid arthritis, or pregnancy. Anemia, pregnancy, and certain drugs can cause or worsen symptoms.

Pathophysiology

RLS is believed to be related to a dysfunction in the brain's basal ganglia circuits that use the neurotransmitter dopamine, which controls movements. In RLS, this dysfunction causes the urge to move the legs. Abnormal iron metabolism or brain iron deficiencies reflected by low serum ferritin may also play a role in RLS.

Clinical Manifestations

The severity of RLS sensory symptoms ranges from infrequent minor discomfort (paresthesias including numbness, tingling, "pins and needles") to severe pain. Sensory symptoms often appear first and are manifested as an annoying and uncomfortable (but usually not painful) sensation in the legs. Over time, RLS symptoms become more frequent and severe.

- Some persons compare the sensations to bugs crawling on the skin.
- The leg pain is localized within the calf muscles, although some patients also experience pain in the upper extremities and trunk.
- Pain at night can disrupt sleep, which is often relieved by physical activity such as walking, stretching, rocking, or kicking.

Diagnostic Studies

RLS is a clinical diagnosis based in large part on the patient's history or the report of the bed partner related to nighttime activities. Diagnostic criteria include (1) urge to move the legs, often accompanied by uncomfortable or unpleasant sensations in the legs; (2) any uncomfortable sensations that begin or worsen with periods of inactivity; (3) any uncomfortable sensations that are partially or totally relieved by movement, so long as the activity continues; (4) urge to move the legs and any accompanying sensations that become worse in the evening or night; and (5) occurrence of these features is not primary to another medical or behavioral condition.

- Polysomnography studies during sleep distinguish RLS from other clinical conditions (e.g., sleep apnea) that disturb sleep.
- CBC, serum ferritin levels, and renal function tests (e.g., serum creatinine) may help to exclude secondary causes of RLS.

Nursing and Interprofessional Management

The goal of interprofessional management is to reduce discomfort and distress and improve sleep quality. When RLS is secondary to uremia or iron deficiency, treatment of these conditions will decrease symptoms.

- Nondrug approaches include establishing regular sleep habits, encouraging exercise including yoga, avoiding activities that cause symptoms, and eliminating aggravating factors such as alcohol, caffeine, and certain drugs (antipsychotics, lithium, antihistamines, antidepressants).

- A vibratory counterstimulation device can compete with and diminish RLS sensations.

If nondrug measures fail to provide symptom relief, drug therapy is an option. The main drugs used in RLS are dopaminergic agents such as carbidopa-levodopa (Sinemet) and dopamine agonists (e.g., ropinirole [Requip]), pramipexole [Mirapex]) to increase the amount of dopamine in the brain. The antiseizure drug gabapentin enacarbil (Horizant) is used to decrease the sensory sensations. Iron supplementation is considered for iron deficiency or low serum ferritin levels.

Other drugs that may be used include antiseizure drugs and benzodiazepines. Low doses of opioids (e.g., oxycodone) are usually reserved for those patients with severe symptoms who fail to respond to other drug therapies.

RETINAL DETACHMENT

Description

Retinal detachment is a separation of the sensory retina and underlying pigment epithelium with fluid accumulation between the two layers. Almost all patients with an untreated, symptomatic retinal detachment become blind in the involved eye. Risk factors include increasing age, severe myopia, cataract surgery, eye trauma, and family or personal history of retinal detachment.

Pathophysiology

The most common cause is a retinal break, which is a full-thickness interruption in the retinal tissue. Retinal holes are spontaneous atrophic breaks, and retinal tears occur when the vitreous shrinks with aging and pulls on the retina.

Once there is a retinal break, liquid vitreous may leak between the sensory and retinal pigment epithelium layers, causing detachment.

Clinical Manifestations

Symptoms of a detaching retina include photopsia ("light flashes"), floaters, and a "cobweb" or ring in the vision field. Once the retina is detached, a painless loss of peripheral or central vision occurs.

Diagnostic Studies

- Direct and indirect ophthalmoscopy or slit lamp microscopy
- Ultrasound to help identify a detachment

Interprofessional Care

Some retinal breaks are not likely to progress to detachment. In these situations the ophthalmologist monitors the patient, giving precise information about warning signs and symptoms of impending detachment and instructing the patient to seek immediate evaluation if any of those signs or symptoms are recognized. The ophthalmologist usually refers the patient with a detachment to a retinal specialist.

Treatment objectives are to seal any retinal breaks and relieve inward traction on the retina. Surgical treatment to seal breaks may include laser photocoagulation and cryopexy. Management of inward retinal traction can involve a scleral buckling procedure, pneumatic retinopexy, and vitrectomy.

- Visual prognosis is dependent on the extent, length, and area of detachment.

Nursing Management

In most cases, retinal detachment is an urgent situation, and the patient is confronted suddenly with the need for surgery. The patient needs emotional support, especially during the immediate preoperative period.

- With postoperative pain, administer prescribed drugs for pain, and teach the patient to take these drugs as necessary when discharged.
- Discharge planning is important. Begin this process as early as possible because the patient may not be hospitalized long.

▼ **Patient and Caregiver Teaching**

- Instruct the patient with an increased risk of retinal detachment about the signs and symptoms of detachment and to seek immediate evaluation if any of these occur.
- Promote the use of proper protective eyewear to help avoid retinal detachment related to trauma.
- After eye surgery for retinal detachment, review the signs and symptoms of retinal detachment with the patient because the risk of detachment in the other eye is increased.

Patient and caregiver teaching after eye surgery is discussed in Table 22, p. 115.

R

RHEUMATIC FEVER AND HEART DISEASE

Description

Rheumatic fever (RF) is an acute inflammatory disease of the heart. *Rheumatic heart disease* is a chronic condition resulting from RF that is characterized by scarring and deformity of the heart valves.

Pathophysiology

RF is a complication that occurs as a delayed result (usually after 2 to 3 weeks) after a group A streptococcal pharyngitis. Symptoms of RF appear to be related to an abnormal immunologic response to group A streptococcal cell membrane antigens. RF affects the heart, skin, joints, and central nervous system (CNS).

About 40% of RF episodes are marked by pancarditis, meaning all layers of the heart (endocardium, myocardium, pericardium) are involved.

- Rheumatic endocarditis is found mainly in the valves, with swelling and erosion of the valve leaflets. Vegetations form and initially create a fibrous thickening of the valve leaflets, fusion of commissures and chordae tendineae, and fibrosis of the papillary muscle. Stenosis and regurgitation may occur in valve leaflets. The mitral and aortic valves are most commonly affected.
- Nodules, called *Aschoff's bodies,* are formed by a reaction to inflammation, with accompanying swelling and fragmentation of collagen fibers. As the Aschoff's bodies age, they become more fibrous, and scar tissue forms in the myocardium.
- Rheumatic pericarditis develops and affects both layers of the pericardium, which becomes thickened and covered with a fibrinous exudate.

The lesions of RF are systemic and involve the skin, joints, and CNS. Painless subcutaneous nodules, arthralgias or arthritis, and chorea may develop.

Clinical Manifestations

The presence of two major criteria, or one major and two minor criteria, plus evidence of a preceding group A streptococcal infection indicates a high probability of acute RF.

Major Criteria

- *Carditis* is the most important manifestation of RF and results in three signs: (1) an organic heart murmur or murmurs of mitral or aortic regurgitation, or mitral stenosis; (2) heart enlargement and heart failure (HF) occurring secondary to myocarditis; and (3) pericarditis resulting in distant heart sounds, chest pain, a pericardial friction rub, or signs of effusion.
- *Monoarthritis or polyarthritis,* the most common finding in RF, involves swelling, warmth, redness, tenderness, and limitation of motion. The larger joints (particularly the knees, ankles, elbows, and wrists) are most severely affected.
- *Sydenham's chorea* is the major CNS manifestation. It is characterized by involuntary movements (especially of the face

and limbs), muscle weakness, and disturbances of speech and gait.

■ *Erythema marginatum* lesions are a less common feature. The bright pink, nonpruritic, maplike macular lesions occur mainly on the trunk and proximal extremities and may be exacerbated by heat (e.g., warm bath).

■ *Subcutaneous nodules* are firm, small, hard, painless swellings found most commonly over extensor surfaces of the joints, especially the knees, wrists, and elbows.

Minor Criteria

Minor clinical manifestations are frequently present and helpful in diagnosing the disease. These include fever, polyarthralgia, and certain laboratory tests (e.g., elevated C-reactive protein [CRP], elevated WBC count).

Evidence of Infection

Evidence of a preceding group A streptococcal infection include a positive result on a rapid antigen test for group A streptococci, an elevated antistreptolysin-O titer, or a positive throat culture.

Diagnostic Studies

■ Chest x-ray may show an enlarged heart if HF is present.

■ Echocardiogram may show valvular insufficiency and pericardial fluid or thickening.

■ ECG reveals a prolonged PR interval with delayed atrioventricular (AV) conduction.

Interprofessional Care

Treatment consists of drug therapy and supportive measures. Antibiotic therapy eliminates residual group A streptococci remaining in the tonsils and pharynx and prevents the spread of organisms to close contacts. Salicylates, nonsteroidal antiinflammatory drugs (NSAIDs), and corticosteroids are effective in controlling the fever and joint manifestations. Corticosteroids are also used if severe carditis is present.

Nursing Management

Goals

The patient with RF or rheumatic heart disease will have normal or baseline heart function, resumption of daily activities without joint pain, and verbalization of the ability to manage the disease sequelae.

Nursing Diagnoses

■ Activity intolerance

■ Decreased cardiac output

■ Ineffective health management

Nursing Interventions

RF is preventable through the early detection and immediate treatment of group A streptococcal pharyngitis. Your role is to teach people in the community to seek medical attention for symptoms of streptococcal pharyngitis, and to emphasize the need for prompt and adequate treatment.

The primary goals of managing a patient with RF are to control and eradicate the infecting organism; prevent cardiac complications; and relieve joint pain, fever, and other symptoms.

- Administer antibiotics as ordered and teach the patient that oral antibiotics require adherence to the full course of therapy.
- Administer antipyretics, NSAIDs, and corticosteroids and monitor fluid intake.
- Promoting optimal rest is essential to reduce cardiac workload and the body's metabolic needs. After acute symptoms have subsided, the patient without carditis can ambulate.
- If the patient has carditis with HF, strict bed rest restrictions apply. Encourage nonstrenuous activities once recovery has begun.

▼ **Patient and Caregiver Teaching**

- Teach the patient with a history of previous RF about the disease process, possible sequelae, and the need for continuous prophylactic antibiotics.
- Patient and caregiver teaching should include good nutrition, hygiene practices, and adequate rest.
- Caution the patient about the possibility of developing valvular heart disease. Teach the patient to seek medical attention if excessive fatigue, dizziness, palpitations, or exertional dyspnea develops.

RHEUMATOID ARTHRITIS

Description

Rheumatoid arthritis (RA) is a chronic, systemic autoimmune disease characterized by inflammation of connective tissue in the diarthrodial (synovial) joints. RA is typically marked by periods of remission and exacerbation and frequently accompanied by extraarticular manifestations.

RA occurs globally, affecting all ethnic groups. However, incidence increases with age, peaking between the ages of 30 and 50 years. An estimated 1.5 million adult Americans are affected by RA. Almost three times as many women have the disease as men.

Pathophysiology

The exact cause of rheumatoid arthritis is unknown. However, it likely results from a combination of genetic and environmental triggers. An autoimmune etiology, which is currently the most widely accepted theory, suggests that changes associated with RA begin when a genetically susceptible person has an initial immune response to an antigen. The antigen, which is probably not the same in all patients, triggers formation of an abnormal immunoglobulin G (IgG). RA is marked by the presence of autoantibodies against this abnormal IgG. The autoantibodies, known as *rheumatoid factor* (RF), combine with IgG to form immune complexes that deposit on synovial membranes or superficial articular cartilage in the joints.

- Immune complex formation leads to complement activation and an inflammatory response. Neutrophils attracted to the site of inflammation release proteolytic enzymes that damage articular cartilage and cause the synovial lining to thicken.
- Other inflammatory cells include T helper ($CD4^+$) cells and proinflammatory cytokines, such as interleukin-1 (IL-1), interleukin-6 (IL-6), and tumor necrosis factor (TNF).
- Genetic predisposition is important in the development of RA.

Without adequate treatment, more than 60% of patients with RA may develop marked functional impairment within 20 years of diagnosis. If unarrested, the disease progresses through four stages, which are identified in Table 72.

Clinical Manifestations

RA typically develops insidiously. Nonspecific manifestations such as fatigue, anorexia, weight loss, and generalized stiffness may precede the onset of joint symptoms. The stiffness becomes more localized after weeks to months.

Joint Manifestations

Articular involvement is marked by pain, stiffness, limitation of motion, and signs of inflammation (heat, swelling, tenderness). Joint symptoms occur symmetrically and frequently affect the small joints of the hands and feet, as well as the larger peripheral joints, including wrists, elbows, shoulders, knees, hips, ankles, and jaw.

- The patient typically has joint stiffness after periods of inactivity. (See Table 60 for a comparison of the manifestations of RA and osteoarthritis [OA].)
- As RA progresses, inflammation and fibrosis of the joint capsule and supporting structures may cause deformity and disability. Muscle atrophy and tendon destruction around the joint can cause one articular surface to slip past the other *(subluxation).*

TABLE 72   Stages of Rheumatoid Arthritis

Stage	Characteristics
I	• Synovitis marked by: • Synovial membrane swelling with excess blood • Membrane containing small areas of lymphocyte infiltration • High WBC counts in synovial fluid (5000 to 60,000/µL) • X-ray results: soft tissue swelling, possible osteoporosis, but no evidence of joint destruction
II	• Increased joint inflammation, spreading across cartilage into joint cavity • Signs of gradual destruction in joint cartilage • Narrowing joint space from loss of cartilage
III	• Formation of synovial pannus • Joint cartilage becomes eroded, bone exposed • X-ray results: extensive cartilage loss, erosion at joint margins, possible deformity
IV	• End-stage: inflammatory process subsides • Loss of joint function • Formation of subcutaneous nodules

Source: Rheumatoid Arthritis.net: a Health Union Community: Understanding RA stages and progressions. Retrieved from *http://rheumatoidarthritis.net/what-is-ra/stages-and-progression.*

Typical hand distortions include "ulnar drift," "swan neck," and boutonniere deformities.

Extraarticular Manifestations

RA can affect nearly every system in the body. Extraarticular manifestations of RA are depicted in Fig. 64-5, Lewis et al, *Medical-Surgical Nursing,* ed 10, p. 1545.

Rheumatoid nodules develop in about half of all patients with RA. They appear subcutaneously as firm, nontender, granuloma-type masses and are usually found over the extensor surfaces of joints such as the fingers and elbows. Nodules at the base of the spine and back of the head are common in older adults.

Sjögren's syndrome can occur by itself or in conjunction with other arthritic disorders such as RA and systemic lupus erythematosus (SLE). Affected patients have diminished lacrimal and salivary gland secretion, leading to a dry mouth; burning, itchy eyes with decreased tearing; and photosensitivity. (See Sjögren's syndrome, p. 583.)

Felty syndrome is rare but can occur in patients with long-standing RA. It is characterized by an enlarged spleen and low white blood cell (WBC) count. Patients with Felty syndrome are at increased risk for infection and lymphoma.

Flexion contractures and hand deformities cause diminished grasp strength, affecting the patient's ability to perform self-care tasks. Cataract development and loss of vision can result from scleral nodules. Depression may also occur.

Diagnostic Studies

A diagnosis is often made based on history and physical findings. Some laboratory tests are useful to confirm the diagnosis and to monitor disease progression.

- Erythrocyte sedimentation rate (ESR) and C-reactive protein (CRP) are general indicators of active inflammation.
- RF assay is positive in 80% of adults with RA, and titers rise during active disease.
- Antinuclear antibody (ANA) titers may increase.
- High levels of antibodies to citrullinated peptide (anti-CCP) are more specific than RF for RA. In some cases, testing may allow an early, accurate diagnosis.
- Synovial fluid analysis in early disease often shows a straw-colored fluid with many fibrin flecks. The WBC count of synovial fluid is elevated (up to 25,000/μL).
- Tissue biopsy can confirm inflammatory changes in the synovium.
- X-rays alone are not diagnostic of RA. They may show only soft tissue swelling and possible bone demineralization in early disease. A narrowed joint space, articular cartilage destruction, erosion, subluxation, and deformity are seen in later disease. Malalignment and ankylosis may be noted in advanced disease.

Interprofessional Care

Care of the patient with RA begins with a thorough program of education and drug therapy. Teach the patient and caregivers about the disease process and home management strategies. Include information on correct drug administration, the need to report side effects, and importance of medical and laboratory follow-up visits. The physical therapist helps the patient maintain joint motion and muscle strength. An occupational therapist helps the patient maintain upper extremity function and encourages use of splints or other assistive devices for joint protection. A balance of rest and activity is also encouraged.

Drug Therapy

Drugs remain the cornerstone of RA treatment. Because irreversible joint changes can occur as early as the first year of RA, HCPs aggressively prescribe disease-modifying antirheumatic drugs (DMARDs). These drugs may slow disease progression and lessen risk of joint erosion and deformity. The choice of drug is based on disease activity, the patient's functional level, and lifestyle considerations, such as the desire to become pregnant.

- Treatment of early RA often involves methotrexate (Rheumatrex) because it reduces clinical symptoms in days to weeks, is inexpensive, and has a lower toxicity compared with other drugs. Methotrexate therapy requires frequent laboratory monitoring.
- Sulfasalazine (Azulfidine) and the antimalarial drug hydroxychloroquine (Plaquenil) may be effective DMARDs for mild to moderate disease.
- Leflunomide (Arava) is a synthetic DMARD that blocks immune cell overproduction and has efficacy similar to that of methotrexate and sulfasalazine.
- Tofacitinib (Xeljanz), a JAK (Janus kinase) inhibitor, is used to treat moderate to severe active RA. The drug interferes with JAK enzymes that contribute to joint inflammation in RA.

Biologic response modifiers (BRMs) (also called biologics or immunotherapy agents) are also used to slow disease progression in RA. They can be used alone or in combination therapy with a DMARD to treat patients with moderate to severe disease who have not responded to DMARDs.

- Tumor necrosis factor inhibitors include etanercept (Enbrel), infliximab (Remicade), adalimumab (Humira), certolizumab (Cimzia), and golimumab (Simponi). Other biologic and targeted inhibitors that may be used include anakinra (Kineret), tocilizumab (Actemra), abatacept (Orencia), and rituximab (Rituxan).

Additional drugs used infrequently for treating RA include antibiotics (minocycline [Minocin]), immunosuppressants (azathioprine [Imuran]), penicillamine (Cuprimine), and gold compounds (auranofin [Ridaura] or gold sodium thiomalate [Myochrysine]) may be used to manage symptoms during disease flare-ups. Intraarticular injections may temporarily reduce acute pain and inflammation.

Various NSAIDs and salicylates such as enteric-coated aspirin are included in the drug regimen to treat arthritis pain and inflammation. Celecoxib (Celebrex), the only available cyclooxygenase (COX)-2 inhibitor, is effective in RA as well as OA.

Nursing Management

Goals

The patient with RA will have satisfactory pain relief and minimal loss of joint function, participate in planning and implementing the therapeutic regimen, maintain a positive self-image, and perform self-care to the maximum amount possible.

Nursing Diagnoses

- Chronic pain
- Impaired physical mobility
- Disturbed body image

Nursing Interventions

Prevention of RA is not possible at this time. Community education should focus on symptom recognition to promote early diagnosis and treatment.

Interventions begin with a careful physical assessment (joint pain, swelling, range of motion, general health status), psychosocial assessment (family support, sexual satisfaction, emotional stress, financial constraints, vocation and career limitations), and environmental assessment (transportation, home, and work modifications).

- Inflammation may be effectively managed through the administration of NSAIDs, DMARDs, and biologic/targeted therapy agents. Discuss the action and side effects of each drug and the necessary laboratory monitoring. Make the drug regimen as understandable as possible.
- Nondrug management may include the use of therapeutic heat and cold, rest, relaxation techniques, joint protection, biofeedback, transcutaneous electrical nerve stimulation (TENS), and hypnosis.
- Lightweight splints may be prescribed to rest an inflamed joint and prevent deformity from muscle spasms and contractures. Remove splints regularly to assess, give skin care, and perform range-of-motion (ROM) exercises. Reapply splints as prescribed.
- Plan care and procedures around the patient's morning stiffness. Sitting or standing in a warm shower, sitting in a tub with warm towels around the shoulders, or soaking the hands in a basin of warm water may relieve joint stiffness and allow the patient to perform activities of daily living comfortably.
- Alternating scheduled rest periods with activity helps relieve fatigue and pain. Help the patient identify activity modifications to avoid overexertion.
- Good body alignment while resting can be maintained with a firm mattress or bed board. Encourage positions of extension and teach the patient to avoid positions of flexion. Avoid pillows

R

under the knees. A small, flat pillow may be used under the head and shoulders.

Sample activities that protect small joints from stress are listed in Table 64-10, Lewis et al, *Medical-Surgical Nursing,* ed 10, p. 1531.

- Assistive devices such as built-up utensils, button hooks, and raised toilet seats simplify tasks. A cane or a walker offers support and relief of pain when walking.
- Heat and cold therapy helps to relieve stiffness, pain, and muscle spasm. Application of ice may help during periods of disease exacerbation. Moist heat appears to offer better relief of chronic stiffness.
- Reinforce participation in an exercise program and ensure correct performance of the exercises. Gentle ROM exercises are usually done daily to keep the joints functional.

▼ **Patient and Caregiver Teaching**
- Self-management and adherence to an individualized home program requires the patient's thorough understanding the nature and course of RA, and the goals of therapy. Consider the patient's value system and perception of the disease.
- Help the patient recognize fears and concerns faced by all people living with a chronic illness.
- Evaluate the family support system. Financial planning may be necessary. Community resources such as home care nurse visits, homemaker services, vocational rehabilitation, and self-help groups may provide support.

SCLERODERMA

Description

Scleroderma (systemic sclerosis) is a disorder of the connective tissue characterized by fibrotic, degenerative, and occasionally inflammatory changes in the skin, blood vessels, synovium, skeletal muscle, and internal organs. Two types of disease exist: *localized scleroderma,* which is the more common form, and *diffuse systemic scleroderma.*

Skin changes of localized disease are usually limited to the face, fingers, and distal extremities without involvement of the trunk or internal organs. The prognosis for patients with limited disease is generally better than for those with diffuse disease. Most cases occur in women. The usual age at onset is between 30 and 50 years.

Pathophysiology

The exact cause of scleroderma is unknown. Immunologic dysfunction and vascular abnormalities are believed to play a role in the development of widespread systemic disease. Excessive collagen production leads to progressive tissue fibrosis and blood vessel occlusion, which affects the functioning of organs such as the lungs, kidney, heart, and GI tract.

- Vascular alterations, primarily involving the small arteries and arterioles, are almost always present and are some of the earliest changes in scleroderma.
- Other risk factors associated with skin thickening include exposure to coal, plastics, and silica dust.

Clinical Manifestations

Manifestations range from a diffuse skin thickening with rapidly progressive and widespread organ involvement to the more benign limited cutaneous form. Symmetric painless swelling or thickening of the skin of the fingers and hands may progress to diffuse scleroderma of the trunk. In *limited disease*, skin thickening generally does not extend above the elbow or knee, although the face can be affected. In more *diffuse disease,* the skin loses elasticity and becomes taut and shiny, producing an expressionless face with tightly pursed lips.

Clinical manifestations can be described by the acronym *CREST*: *c*alcinosis (painful calcium deposits in skin), *R*aynaud's phenomenon, *e*sophageal dysfunction (difficulty swallowing), *s*clerodactyly (tightening of the skin on the fingers), and *t*elangiectasia (red spots from capillary dilation on hands, face, and lips).

- Raynaud's phenomenon (paroxysmal vasospasm of digits in response to cold or stress) is the most common initial complaint in limited systemic sclerosis. Raynaud's phenomenon may precede the onset of systemic disease by decades (see Raynaud's Phenomenon, p. 530).
- About 20% of people with scleroderma develop secondary Sjögren's syndrome, a condition associated with dry eyes and dry mouth (see Sjögren's Syndrome, p. 583). Dysphagia, gum disease, and dental decay can result.
- Gastric acid reflux can occur as a result of esophageal fibrosis. Additional GI effects include constipation from colonic hypomotility and diarrhea due to malabsorption from bacterial overgrowth.
- Lung involvement includes pleural thickening, pulmonary fibrosis, pulmonary artery hypertension, and abnormal pulmonary function.
- Primary heart disease consists of pericarditis, pericardial effusion, and dysrhythmias. Myocardial fibrosis resulting in heart failure occurs with diffuse scleroderma.

S

- Renal disease was previously a major cause of death in diffuse scleroderma. Recent improvements in dialysis, bilateral nephrectomy in patients with uncontrollable hypertension, and kidney transplantation have offered hope to patients with renal failure. In particular, the use of angiotensin-converting enzyme (ACE) inhibitors (e.g., lisinopril [Prinivil]) has had a marked impact on the treatment of renal disease.

Diagnostic Studies

- Blood studies may reveal mild hemolytic anemia.
- Anticentromere antibodies related to CREST syndrome are found in about 60% to 80% of people with localized scleroderma. Antibodies to topoisomerase-1 are present in about 30% of people with diffuse disease. Presence of either antibody is highly specific for diagnosis.
- If renal involvement is present, urinalysis may show proteinuria, microscopic hematuria, and casts.
- X-rays show evidence of subcutaneous calcification, distal esophageal hypomotility, and/or bilateral pulmonary fibrosis.
- Pulmonary function studies reveal decreased vital capacity and lung compliance.

Interprofessional Care

No specific treatment is available for scleroderma. Supportive care is directed to preventing or treating the secondary complications of involved organs. Physical therapy helps maintain joint mobility and preserve muscle strength. Occupational therapy assists the patient in maintaining functional abilities.

Drug Therapy

No specific drug or combination of drugs has proven effective for treatment of scleroderma. Vasoactive agents are often prescribed in early disease. Calcium channel blockers (nifedipine [Procardia], diltiazem [Cardizem]) and the angiotensin II blocker losartan (Cozaar) are common treatments for Raynaud's phenomenon. Reserpine, an α-adrenergic blocking agent, increases blood flow to the fingers. Bosentan (Tracleer), an endothelin receptor antagonist, and the vasodilator epoprostenol (Flolan) may help prevent and treat digital ulcers. They also improve exercise capacity and heart and lung dynamics.

Corticosteroids may have little effect on scleroderma and may cause a renal crisis. Topical agents may provide some relief from joint pain. Capsaicin cream may be useful as a local analgesic and as a vasodilator.

Other therapies prescribed to treat specific systemic problems include (1) tetracycline for diarrhea caused by bacterial overgrowth, (2) histamine (H_2)-receptor blockers (e.g., cimetidine) and proton pump inhibitors (e.g., omeprazole [Prilosec]) for esophageal symptoms, (3) antihypertensive agent (e.g., captopril, propranolol [Inderal], methyldopa) for hypertension with renal involvement, and (4) immunosuppressive drugs (e.g., cyclophosphamide, mycophenolate mofetil).

Nursing Management

Because prevention is not possible, nursing interventions often begin during hospitalization for diagnostic purposes. Emotional stress and cold ambient temperatures may aggravate Raynaud's phenomenon.

Teach the patient to protect the hands and feet from cold exposure and possible burns or cuts that might heal slowly. Encourage the patient to avoid smoking because of its vasoconstricting effect. Alcohol-free lotions may help to alleviate skin dryness and cracking but must be rubbed in for a long time because of skin thickness.

- A consultation with a dietitian is beneficial. Dysphagia may be reduced by eating small, frequent meals, chewing carefully and slowly, and drinking fluids. Heartburn may be minimized by taking antacids 45 to 60 minutes after each meal and by sitting upright for at least 2 hours after eating. The head of the bed may be elevated on blocks to reduce nighttime reflux.
- Job modifications are often necessary because stair climbing, typing, writing, and cold exposure may pose problems.
- Emphasize daily oral hygiene because neglect of the narrowed mouth may lead to increased tooth and gum disease.

Teach the patient to actively carry out therapeutic exercises. Reinforce the use of moist heat applications and assistive devices and the organization of activities to preserve strength and reduce disability. Sexual dysfunction from body changes, pain, muscle weakness, limited mobility, decreased self-esteem, and decreased vaginal secretions may require sensitive counseling.

SEIZURE DISORDERS

Description

A *seizure* is a transient, uncontrolled electrical discharge of neurons in the brain that interrupts normal function. Seizures may accompany a variety of disorders, or they may occur spontaneously without any apparent cause.

- Metabolic disturbances that cause seizures include acidosis, electrolyte imbalances, hypoglycemia, hypoxia, alcohol and barbiturate withdrawal, dehydration, and water intoxication.

- Extracranial disorders that can cause seizures include heart, lung, liver, and kidney disease; systemic lupus erythematosus; diabetes mellitus (DM); hypertension; and septicemia.

Epilepsy is a disease marked by a continuing predisposition to seizures, with neurobiologic, cognitive, psychologic, and social consequences. The incidence of epilepsy is higher in young children and older adults.

Pathophysiology

The most common causes of seizure during the first 6 months of life are severe birth injury, congenital defects involving the central nervous system (CNS), infections, and inborn errors of metabolism.

In people between 20 and 30 years of age, a seizure disorder usually occurs as a result of structural lesions such as trauma, brain tumors, or vascular disease. After the age of 50 years, primary causes of seizure are stroke and metastatic brain tumors. Nearly 30% of all epilepsy cases are idiopathic. Some types of epilepsy tend to run in families, suggesting a genetic influence.

The etiology of recurring seizures (epilepsy) has long been attributed to a group of abnormal neurons *(seizure focus)* that undergo spontaneous firing. This firing spreads by physiologic pathways to involve adjacent or distant areas of the brain. The factor that causes this abnormal firing is not clear. Any stimulus that causes the cell membrane of the neuron to depolarize induces a tendency to spontaneous firing. Often the brain area from which epileptic activity arises is found to have scar tissue *(gliosis)*. Scarring is believed to interfere with the normal chemical and structural environment of brain neurons, making them more likely to fire abnormally.

In addition to neuronal alterations, changes in the function of astrocytes may play several key roles in recurring seizures. Activation of astrocytes by hyperactive neurons is one of the crucial factors that predisposes nearby neurons to generate an epileptic discharge.

Clinical Manifestations

Clinical manifestations are determined by the site of the electrical disturbance. The preferred method of classifying epileptic seizures is presented in Table 58-5, in Lewis et al, *Medical-Surgical Nursing,* ed 10, p. 1375. This system is based on the clinical and electroencephalographic (EEG) manifestations of seizures and divides seizures into two major classes: *generalized* and *focal.*

Depending on the type, a seizure may progress through several phases: (1) the *prodromal phase,* with sensations or behavior changes that precede a seizure; (2) the *aural phase,* with a sensory warning that is similar each time a seizure occurs; (3) the *ictal phase,* from first symptoms to the end of seizure activity; and (4) the *postictal phase,* the recovery period after the seizure.

Generalized Seizures

Generalized seizures involve both sides of the brain and are characterized by bilateral synchronous epileptic discharge in the brain. In most cases the patient loses consciousness for a few seconds to several minutes.

- *Tonic-clonic* (formerly known as grand mal) seizures are the most common generalized seizures. This type of seizure is characterized by a loss of consciousness and falling to the ground if the patient is upright, followed by stiffening of the body (tonic phase) for 10 to 20 seconds and subsequent jerking of the extremities (clonic phase) for another 30 to 40 seconds. Cyanosis, excessive salivation, tongue or cheek biting, and incontinence may accompany the seizure. In the postictal phase the patient usually has muscle soreness, feels tired, and may sleep for several hours. The patient has no memory of the seizure activity.

- *Typical absence* (petit mal) seizures usually occur only in children and rarely continue beyond adolescence. This type of seizure may cease altogether as the child ages, or it may evolve into another type of seizure. The typical clinical manifestation of a simple absence seizure is a brief staring spell resembling "daydreaming" that lasts only a few seconds. In complex absence seizures, the blank stare is accompanied by some type of movement (e.g., blinking, chewing, hand gestures) and can last up to 20 seconds. When untreated, the seizures may occur up to 100 times each day. The EEG demonstrates a 3-Hz (cycles per second) spike-and-wave pattern that is unique to this type of seizure. Hyperventilation and flashing lights can precipitate absence seizures.

- *Atypical absence* seizures are another type of generalized seizure characterized by a staring spell. A brief warning phase (aura), peculiar behavior during the seizure, and confusion after the seizure are also common.

- Other types of generalized seizures include myoclonic, atonic, tonic, and clonic seizures.

Focal Seizures

Focal seizures (formerly called partial seizures) begin in one hemisphere of the brain in a specific region of the cortex, as indicated

S

by the EEG. They produce sensory, motor, cognitive, or emotional manifestations based on the function of the area of the brain involved. For example, if the discharging focus is located in the medial aspect of the postcentral gyrus, the patient may experience paresthesias and tingling or numbness in the leg on the side opposite the focus.

Focal seizures are divided according to their clinical expressions into *simple* focal seizures (person remains conscious and alert) and *complex* focal seizures (person has a change in or loss of consciousness).

Focal seizures may be confined to one side of the brain and remain focal in nature, or they may spread to involve the entire brain, culminating in a generalized tonic-clonic seizure.

Complications

Status epilepticus is a state of continuous seizure activity or a condition in which seizures recur in rapid succession without return to consciousness between seizures. It can occur with any type of seizure. Status epilepticus is the most serious complication of epilepsy and represents a neurologic emergency.

- During repeated seizures, the brain uses more energy than can be supplied. As neurons become exhausted and cease to function, permanent brain damage may result.
- Convulsive status epilepticus is the most dangerous because it can cause potentially fatal ventilatory insufficiency, hypoxemia, cardiac dysrhythmias, and systemic acidosis.
- Severe injury can result from physical trauma during a seizure. Patients who lose consciousness during a seizure are at greatest risk.

Perhaps the most common complication of seizure disorder is the effect it has on the patient's lifestyle. Antiseizure medications and the continued need to manage a chronic disease can contribute to depression. Although attitudes have improved in recent years, epilepsy still carries a social stigma that can lead to discrimination in employment and educational opportunities. Transportation may also be difficult because of legal sanctions against driving.

Diagnostic Studies

- Most important in diagnosis are accurate and comprehensive descriptions of the seizures and the patient's health history.
- EEG is useful only if it shows abnormalities. Some patients who do not have seizure disorders have abnormal EEG patterns, whereas many patients with seizure disorders have normal EEGs between seizures.

- CBC, serum chemistry panel,, studies of liver and kidney function, and urinalysis can rule out metabolic disorders.
- CT scan and MRI can rule out a structural lesion.
- Cerebral angiography, single-photon emission computed tomography (SPECT), magnetic resonance spectroscopy (MRS), magnetic resonance angiography (MRA), and positron emission tomography (PET) may be used.

Interprofessional Care

Most seizures are self-limiting and do not cause body injury. However, in cases of status epilepticus, significant body harm, or first-time seizure, medical care should be sought immediately. Table 58-7, Lewis et al, *Medical-Surgical Nursing,* ed 10, p. 1378, summarizes the emergency care of the patient with a generalized tonic-clonic seizure.

Drug Therapy

Seizure disorders are treated primarily with antiseizure drugs (see Table 58-8, Lewis et al, *Medical-Surgical Nursing,* ed 10, p. 1378). Medications generally act by stabilizing the nerve cell membranes and preventing the spread of the epileptic discharge.

The principle of drug therapy is to begin with a single drug based on the patient's age and weight with consideration of the type, frequency, and cause of seizure. Then the dosage is increased until the seizures are controlled or toxic side effects occur. If seizure control is not achieved with a single drug, the drug dosage and timing or administration may be changed or a second drug may be added.

- Primary drugs to treat generalized tonic-clonic and focal seizures are phenytoin (Dilantin), carbamazepine (Tegretol), phenobarbital, divalproex (Depakote), and primidone (Mysoline). The drugs used to treat absence and myoclonic seizures include ethosuximide (Zarontin), divalproex (Depakote), and clonazepam (Klonopin).
- Other antiseizure drugs include gabapentin (Neurontin), lamotrigine (Lamictal), topiramate (Topamax), tiagabine (Gabitril), levetiracetam (Keppra), and zonisamide (Zonegran). Some drugs are effective for multiple seizure types.
- Treatment of status epilepticus requires initiation of a rapid-acting antiseizure medication given IV. Drugs most commonly used are lorazepam (Ativan) and diazepam.
- Antiseizure drugs should not be discontinued abruptly after long-term use because this can precipitate seizures.

Surgical interventions for patients whose epilepsy cannot be controlled with drug therapy include anterior temporal lobe resection; extratemporal resection and lesionectomies; hemispherectomies; multilobar resections; and corpus callosum sections. These

S

surgeries remove the epileptic focus or prevent spread of epileptic activity in the brain.
- Alternative therapies, such as vagal nerve stimulation and biofeedback, may also be used.

Nursing Management

Goals

The patient with seizures will be free from injury during a seizure, have optimal mental and physical functioning while taking antiseizure drugs, and have satisfactory psychosocial functioning.

Nursing Diagnoses

- Ineffective breathing pattern
- Risk for injury
- Ineffective health management

Nursing Interventions

The patient with a seizure disorder should practice good general health habits (e.g., maintaining a proper diet, getting adequate rest, exercising). Help the patient to identify and avoid events or situations that precipitate the seizures such as excessive alcohol intake, fatigue, and loss of sleep.

Nursing care for a hospitalized patient or for a person who has had seizures as a result of metabolic factors should focus on observation and treatment of the seizure, teaching, and psychosocial intervention.

- Carefully observe and record all aspects of a seizure event to support an accurate diagnosis and subsequent treatment. The description should include the exact onset of the seizure (which body part was affected first, and how); the course and nature of the seizure activity (loss of consciousness, tongue biting, automatisms, stiffening, jerking, total lack of muscle tone); the body parts involved and their sequence of involvement; and the presence of autonomic signs (dilated pupils, excessive salivation, altered breathing, cyanosis, flushing, diaphoresis, or incontinence).
- Assessment of the postictal period should include a detailed description of the level of consciousness (LOC), vital signs, memory loss, muscle soreness, speech disorders (aphasia, dysarthria), weakness or paralysis, sleep period, and the duration of each sign or symptom.
- During the seizure, you should do the following: Maintain a patent airway for the patient, protect the patient's head, turn the patient to the side, loosen constrictive clothing, and ease the patient to the floor if seated. After the seizure, the patient may require suctioning and oxygen.

- A seizure can be a frightening experience for the patient and family. Assess the level of their understanding and provide information about how and why the event occurred.

▼ **Patient and Caregiver Teaching**

Prevention of recurring seizures is the major goal in the treatment of epilepsy. Drugs must be taken regularly and continually, often for a lifetime. You have an important role in teaching the patient and caregivers. Guidelines for teaching are shown in Table 73.

TABLE 73   Patient & Caregiver Teaching

Seizure Disorders

Include the following information in the teaching plan for the patient with a seizure disorder.

1. Take antiseizure medications as prescribed. Report any and all drug side effects to the HCP. When necessary, blood is drawn to ensure maintenance of therapeutic drug levels. Schedule regular communication with the HCP to explore additional treatment options.
2. Use nondrug techniques, such as relaxation therapy, to potentially reduce the number of seizures.
3. Be aware of community and online resources for education and help with tracking and explaining seizure activity.
4. Wear a medical alert bracelet or necklace, and carry an identification card.
5. Avoid excessive alcohol intake, fatigue, and loss of sleep.
6. Eat regular meals and snacks in between if feeling shaky, faint, or hungry.
7. For women of childbearing age, be knowledgeable regarding antiseizure medications and contraceptive use.

Caregivers should receive the following information.

Focal Seizures

1. Stay calm. Guide patient to safety to prevent injury, but do not restrain.
2. Observe for asymmetry of activity and focus on specific actions, such as lip smacking and abnormal movements.
3. Assess patient's level of consciousness and ability to converse and respond appropriately
4. Observe the time the event started and stopped. Pay attention to the time of return to baseline.

Continued

TABLE 73   Patient & Caregiver Teaching

Seizure Disorders—cont'd

Generalized Tonic-Clonic Seizures

1. When seizure occurs outside the hospital setting, activate ERS if (1) the duration is greater than 5 minutes; (2) events recur without the patient's recovering to baseline status; (3) the patient is unable to establish a normal breathing pattern or is injured or pregnant; or (4) you do not know if this is a first-time seizure event.
2. Maintain patient safety. Lower the patient to the floor or bed, remove eyeglasses if on, and loosen restrictive clothing.
3. Do not place anything in the patient's mouth. Patient's teeth/dentures may be damaged, and the caregiver may be bitten.
4. Position patient on side (if possible) to improve ability to release oral secretions.
5. Observe the time event started and stopped. Pay attention to the time of return to baseline.
6. Assess for possible injury or any lingering motor weakness.

ERS, Emergency response services.

SEXUALLY TRANSMITTED INFECTIONS

Sexually transmitted infections (STIs) are diseases that spread through sexual contact with the penis, vagina, anus, mouth, or body fluids of an infected person. Mucosal tissues in the genitals (urethra in men, vagina in women), rectum, and mouth are especially susceptible to the bacteria and viruses that cause STIs. Common infections that are transmitted sexually are listed in Table 74.

Infections that are associated with sexual transmission can also be contracted by other routes, such as through blood or blood products or by autoinoculation. See Gonorrhea, p. 250; Syphilis, p. 613; Herpes, Genital, p. 303; Warts, Genital, p. 677; and Chlamydial Infection, p. 122.

An estimated 110 million people in the United States are currently infected with one or more STIs. In the United States, all cases of gonorrhea and syphilis and, in most states, chlamydial infection must be reported to the state or local public health authorities for purposes of surveillance and partner notification. Surveillance and partner notification are a major part of the effort to prevent and control the spread of STIs. Nurses play an important role in STI reporting and are mandated to report these STIs to public health authorities.

TABLE 74 Causes of Sexually Transmitted Infections (STIs)

Sexually Transmitted Infection	Cause
Bacteria	
Chlamydia	*Chlamydia trachomatis*
Gonorrhea	*Neisseria gonorrhoeae*
Syphilis	*Treponema pallidum*
Viruses	
Genital herpes	Herpes simplex virus (HSV 1 or 2)
Genital warts (condylomata acuminata)	Human papillomavirus (HPV)
Human immunodeficiency virus (HIV) infection/acquired immunodeficiency syndrome (AIDS)	HIV
Hepatitis B and C	Hepatitis B and C viruses
Molluscum contagiosum	Poxvirus (molluscum contagiosum virus)
Parasites/Protozoa	
Trichomoniasis	*Trichomonas vaginalis*

Many factors are related to the high rates of STIs (Table 75). Earlier reproductive maturity and increased longevity have resulted in a longer sexual life span.

- Other factors include greater sexual freedom, lack of barrier methods (e.g., condoms) during sexual activity, and an increased emphasis on sexuality in the media.
- Urbanization and easier travel are some of the global changes that contribute to increased opportunities for exposure to all infectious diseases, including STIs.
- Youth under age 25 and those who are socially and economically disadvantaged are disproportionately affected by STIs.
- The male condom is considered to be the best form of protection (other than abstinence) against STIs. However, condoms are not frequently used in the general population for contraception.

S

TABLE 75 Risk Factors for Sexually Transmitted Infections (STIs)

High-Risk Populations
- Women
- Men who have sex with men
- Adolescents and young adults (age <25 years)
- Men and women in correctional facilities
- Victims of sexual assault

High-Risk Behaviors
- Having new or multiple sexual partners
- Having more than one sexual partner
- Having sexual partners who have had multiple partners
- Sharing needles used to inject drugs
- Alcohol or drug dependence or abuse (inhibits judgment)
- Inconsistent or incorrect use of condoms or other barrier methods

High-Risk Medical History
- Not being vaccinated for STIs for which vaccines are available
- Previous STI.

Nursing Management

Goals

The patient with an STI will demonstrate understanding of the mode of transmission and the risk posed by STIs, complete treatment and return for appropriate follow-up care, notify or assist in notification of sexual contacts about their need for testing and treatment, abstain from intercourse until infection is resolved, and demonstrate knowledge of safer sex practices.

Nursing Diagnoses

- Risk for infection
- Ineffective health maintenance
- Anxiety

Nursing Interventions

The diagnosis of an STI may be met with a variety of emotions such as shame, guilt, anger, and a desire for vengeance. Provide counseling and encourage the patient to verbalize feelings. A referral for professional counseling to explore ramifications of having an STI may be indicated.

All patients should return to the treatment center for a repeat culture from infected sites or serologic testing at designated times to determine effectiveness of treatment.

- Explain to the patient that cures are not always obtained on the first treatment, to reinforce the need for a follow-up visit.
- Advise the patient to inform sexual partners of the need for treatment, regardless of whether they are free of symptoms or experiencing symptoms.

Emphasize hygiene measures to the patient with an STI. An important measure is frequent hand washing and bathing.

- Bathing and cleaning of involved areas can provide local comfort and prevent secondary infection.
- Teach patients that douching after sex is never recommended because it can push bacteria higher into the reproductive tract.
- Sexual abstinence is indicated during the communicable phase of the infection. If sexual activity occurs before the patient has completed treatment, the use of condoms or other barrier methods may prevent spread of infection and reinfection.

▼ **Patient Teaching**
Be prepared to discuss "safe" sex practices with all patients, not only those who are perceived to be at risk. These practices include abstinence, monogamy with an uninfected partner, avoidance of certain high-risk sexual practices, and the use of condoms and other barriers to limit contact with potentially infectious body fluids or lesions. See Table 76 for a patient teaching guide regarding STIs.

SHOCK

Description
Shock is a syndrome characterized by decreased tissue perfusion and impaired cellular metabolism. The four main categories of shock are cardiogenic, hypovolemic, distributive, and obstructive.

- Although the cause, initial presentation, and management strategies vary for each type of shock, the physiologic responses of the cells to hypoperfusion are similar.

Cardiogenic Shock
Cardiogenic shock occurs when either systolic or diastolic dysfunction of the pumping action of the heart results in reduced cardiac output (CO). The heart's inability to pump the blood forward is classified as systolic dysfunction. The most common

TABLE 76   Patient Teaching

Sexually Transmitted Infections (STIs)

When teaching the patient with sexually transmitted infections:

1. Explain precautions to take such as
   - Using condoms and other barrier methods with every sexual encounter
   - Voiding and washing genitalia and surrounding area after sex to flush out some organisms and potentially reduce exposure to infection
   - Being monogamous
   - Asking potential partners about sexual history
   - Asking potential partners if they have been tested for STIs
   - Avoiding sex with partners who use IV drugs or who have visible oral, inguinal, genital, perineal, or anal lesions
2. Explain the importance of taking all antibiotics and/or antiviral agents as prescribed. Symptoms will improve after 1-2 days of therapy, but organisms may still be present.
3. Teach patients about the need for treatment of sexual partners to prevent transmission and reinfection.
4. Instruct patients to abstain from sexual intercourse during treatment, and to use condoms or other barrier methods when sexual activity is resumed, to prevent spread of infection and reinfection.
5. Explain the importance of follow-up examination and retesting at least once after treatment, if appropriate, to confirm complete cure and prevent relapse.
6. Allow patients and partners to verbalize concerns to clarify areas that need explanation.
7. Instruct patient about symptoms of complications and need to report problems to ensure proper follow-up and early treatment of reinfection.
8. Inform patient regarding state of infectivity to prevent a false sense of security, which might result in careless sexual practices and poor personal hygiene.
9. Inform patients about health department requirements for reporting certain STIs.

cause of systolic dysfunction is acute myocardial infarction (MI). Cardiogenic shock is the leading cause of death from acute MI. The patient experiences impaired tissue perfusion and cellular metabolism because of cardiogenic shock.

- The patient presents with tachycardia, hypotension, and a narrowed pulse pressure. A low CO (less than 4 L/min) and *cardiac index* (less than 2.5 L/min/m^2) result when systolic dysfunction is present.

- Tachypnea and pulmonary congestion are evident by the presence of crackles. An increase in the pulmonary artery wedge pressure (PAWP) and pulmonary vascular resistance is also noted.
- Signs of peripheral hypoperfusion (e.g., cyanosis, pallor, diaphoresis, diminished pulses, decreased capillary refill time) are apparent.
- Decreased renal blood flow results in sodium and water retention and decreased urine output.
- Anxiety, confusion, and agitation may develop as cerebral perfusion is impaired.

Studies helpful in diagnosing cardiogenic shock include laboratory studies (e.g., cardiac biomarkers, b-type natriuretic peptide [BNP]), electrocardiogram (ECG), chest x-ray, and echocardiogram.

Hypovolemic Shock

Hypovolemic shock occurs when there is a loss of intravascular fluid volume. The loss may be either an absolute or a relative volume loss.

- *Absolute hypovolemia* results when fluid is lost through hemorrhage, GI loss (e.g., vomiting, diarrhea), fistula drainage, diabetes insipidus, or diuresis.
- In *relative hypovolemia,* fluid volume moves out of the vascular space into the extravascular space (e.g., intracavity space). This fluid shift is called *third spacing.* One example of relative volume loss is leakage of fluid from the vascular space to the interstitial space occurring with increased capillary permeability, as seen in burns.

In hypovolemic shock, the size of the vascular compartment remains unchanged while the volume of blood or plasma decreases. A reduction in intravascular volume results in decreased venous return to the heart, decreased preload, decreased stroke volume, and decreased CO. A cascade of events results in decreased tissue perfusion and impaired cellular metabolism, the hallmarks of shock (Fig. 20). A total blood loss of 15% to 30% results in a sympathetic nervous system (SNS)–mediated response that causes an increase in heart rate, CO, and respiratory rate and depth. If hypovolemia is corrected at this time, tissue dysfunction is generally reversible.

- If volume loss is greater than 30%, blood volume must be immediately replaced with blood products. A loss of more than 40% of the total blood volume results in irreversible tissue destruction.

S

PATHOPHYSIOLOGY MAP

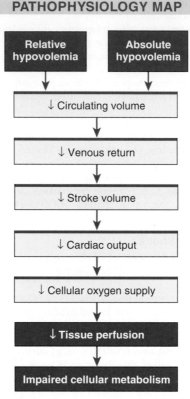

Fig. 20 The pathophysiology of hypovolemic shock. (Modified from Urden LD, Stacy KM, Lough ME: *Critical care nursing: diagnosis and management,* ed 6, St Louis, 2010, Mosby.)

Laboratory studies include serial measurements of hemoglobin and hematocrit levels, electrolytes, lactate, blood gases, and central venous oxygenation (ScvO$_2$), as well as hourly urine outputs.

Distributive Shock (Neurogenic, Anaphylactic, Septic)
Neurogenic Shock
Neurogenic shock is a hemodynamic phenomenon that can occur within 30 minutes and last up to 6 weeks after a spinal cord injury. The injury results in massive vasodilation without compensation because of the loss of SNS vasoconstrictor tone. This leads to a

pooling of blood in the blood vessels, tissue hypoperfusion, and ultimately impaired cellular metabolism.

Spinal anesthesia can also temporarily block transmission of impulses from the SNS. Depression of the vasomotor center of the medulla from drugs (e.g., opioids, benzodiazepines) may result in decreased vasoconstrictor tone of the peripheral blood vessels and neurogenic shock.

- Clinical manifestations are hypotension (from massive vasodilation) and bradycardia (from unopposed parasympathetic stimulation).

The patient in neurogenic shock may not be able to regulate body temperature. The inability to regulate temperature, combined with massive vasodilation, promotes heat loss. Initially, the patient's skin will be warm because of the massive dilation. As the heat disperses, the patient is at risk for hypothermia.

The pathophysiology of neurogenic shock is described in Fig. 66-4, Lewis et al, *Medical-Surgical Nursing,* ed 10, p. 1592.

Anaphylactic Shock
Anaphylactic shock is an acute and life-threatening hypersensitivity (allergic) reaction to a sensitizing substance, such as a drug, chemical, vaccine, food, or insect venom. The reaction quickly causes massive vasodilation, release of vasoactive mediators, and an increase in capillary permeability.

- As capillary permeability increases, fluid leaks from the vascular space into the interstitial space. Anaphylactic shock can lead to respiratory distress as a result of laryngeal edema or severe bronchospasm, and to circulatory failure consequent to massive vasodilation.
- Patients present with a sudden onset of dizziness, chest pain, incontinence, swelling of the lips and tongue, wheezing, and stridor. Skin changes include flushing, pruritus, urticaria, and angioedema.
- A patient can develop a severe allergic reaction leading to anaphylactic shock after contact with, inhalation or ingestion of, or injection with an antigen (allergen) to which the person has previously been sensitized.

Septic Shock
Septic shock is the presence of *sepsis* (systemic inflammatory response to infection) with hypotension despite fluid resuscitation, along with inadequate tissue perfusion, resulting in tissue hypoxia. The main organisms that cause sepsis are gram-negative and gram-positive bacteria. Parasites, fungi, and viruses can also lead to the development of sepsis and septic shock. The pathophysiology of septic shock is described in Fig. 66-5, Lewis et al, *Medical-Surgical Nursing,* ed 10, p. 1593.

- When a microorganism enters the body, the normal immune/inflammatory cascade responses start. However, in severe sepsis and septic shock, the body's response to the microorganism is exaggerated. There is an increase in inflammation and coagulation along with a decrease in fibrinolysis. Endotoxins from the microorganism cell wall stimulate the release of cytokines and other proinflammatory mediators. The combined effects of the mediators result in damage to the endothelium, vasodilation, increased capillary permeability, and neutrophil and platelet aggregation and adhesion to the endothelium.
- Clinical manifestations include an initial decreased ejection fraction with the ventricles dilating to maintain stroke volume. The ejection fraction typically improves and the ventricular dilation resolves over 7 to 10 days. Persistence of a high CO and a low systemic vascular resistance (SVR) beyond 24 hours is an ominous finding often associated with development of severe hypotension and multiple organ dysfunction syndrome (MODS) (see Systemic Inflammatory Response Syndrome (SIRS) and MODS, p. 617).
- Respiratory failure is common. The patient initially hyperventilates, resulting in respiratory alkalosis. Once the patient can no longer compensate, respiratory acidosis develops.
- Other clinical signs include decreased urine output, alteration in neurologic status, and GI dysfunction, such as GI bleeding and paralytic ileus.

Obstructive Shock

Obstructive shock develops when a physical obstruction to blood flow occurs with a decreased CO. This can be caused from a restriction to diastolic filling of the right ventricle secondary to compression (e.g., cardiac tamponade, tension pneumothorax, pulmonary embolism, superior vena cava syndrome). The pathophysiology of obstructive shock is described in Fig. 66-6, Lewis et al, *Medical-Surgical Nursing,* ed 10, p. 1593.

- Patients experience a decreased CO, increased afterload, and variable left ventricular filling pressures, depending on the obstruction. Other clinical signs include jugular venous distention and pulsus paradoxus. Rapid assessment and immediate treatment are important to prevent further hemodynamic compromise and possibly cardiac arrest.

Stages of Shock

Shock is categorized into four overlapping stages: (1) initial stage, (2) compensatory stage, (3) progressive stage, and (4) refractory stage.

Initial Stage

The *initial stage* of shock begins at the cellular level. This stage is usually not clinically apparent. Metabolism changes at the cellular level from aerobic to anaerobic, causing lactic acid buildup. Lactic acid is a waste product that is removed by the liver. However, this removal process requires oxygen, which is unavailable because of the decrease in tissue perfusion.

Compensatory Stage

In the *compensatory stage,* the body activates neural, hormonal, and biochemical mechanisms to overcome the increasing consequences of anaerobic metabolism and maintain homeostasis.

- One of the classic signs of shock is a drop in BP. The SNS stimulates vasoconstriction and the release of the potent vasoconstrictors epinephrine and norepinephrine. Blood flow to the most essential organs, the heart and brain, is maintained. Blood flow to the kidneys, GI tract, and lungs is diverted.
- The myocardium responds to SNS stimulation and the increase in oxygen demand by increasing heart rate and contractility.
- Shunting blood from the lungs has an important effect on the patient in shock. Areas of the lungs participating in ventilation are not perfused because of decreased blood flow to the lungs. The patient has a compensatory increase in the rate and depth of respirations.
- Decreased blood flow to the kidneys activates the renin-angiotensin-aldosterone system, resulting in vasoconstriction and sodium and water reabsorption.

If the cause of shock is corrected at this stage, the patient recovers with few or no residual effects. If the cause of shock is not corrected and the body is unable to compensate, the patient goes on to the progressive stage of shock.

Progressive Stage

The *progressive stage* of shock begins as compensatory mechanisms fail. Continued decreased cellular perfusion and altered capillary permeability are distinguishing features of this stage. The patient may have diffuse and profound edema *(anasarca).* In this stage, aggressive interventions are necessary to prevent the development of MODS.

- CO begins to fall, with a resultant decrease in BP and peripheral perfusion, including a decrease in coronary artery, cerebral, and peripheral perfusion. Myocardial dysfunction from decreased perfusion results in dysrhythmias, myocardial ischemia, and possibly myocardial infarction.
- The combined effects of pulmonary vasoconstriction and bronchoconstriction are impaired gas exchange, decreased

S

compliance, and worsening ventilation-perfusion mismatch. The patient presents with tachypnea, crackles, and an overall increased work of breathing.

- As the blood supply to the GI tract is decreased, the normally protective mucosal barrier becomes ischemic, which predisposes the patient to ulcers and GI bleeding.
- The patient has a decreased urine output and an elevated blood urea nitrogen (BUN) and serum creatinine. Metabolic acidosis occurs from an inability to excrete acids and reabsorb bicarbonate.
- Loss of the functional ability of the liver leads to a failure to metabolize drugs and waste products such as ammonia and lactate. Jaundice results from an accumulation of bilirubin.
- Dysfunction of the hematologic system places the patient at risk for the development of disseminated intravascular coagulation (DIC) (see Disseminated Intravascular Coagulation, p. 191).

Refractory Stage

In the final stage of shock, the *refractory stage,* decreased perfusion from peripheral vasoconstriction and decreased cardiac output exacerbate anaerobic metabolism. The loss of intravascular volume worsens hypotension and tachycardia and decreases coronary blood flow. Cerebral blood flow cannot be maintained and cerebral ischemia results.

- The patient demonstrates profound hypotension and hypoxemia. In this final stage, recovery is unlikely. The organs are in failure, and the body's compensatory mechanisms are overwhelmed.

Diagnostic Studies

- Obtaining a thorough medical and surgical history and a history of recent events (e.g., surgery, chest pain, trauma) provides valuable data.
- Blood studies may include CBC, DIC screen, cardiac enzymes, BUN, glucose, electrolytes, arterial blood gases (ABGs), lactate, blood cultures, and liver enzymes.
- Twelve-lead ECG, continuous cardiac monitoring, and chest x-ray.
- Continuous pulse oximetry, invasive and non-invasive hemodynamic monitoring.

See Table 66-2, Lewis et al, *Medical-Surgical Nursing,* ed 10, p. 1590, for further information.

Interprofessional Care: General Measures

Critical factors in management are early recognition and treatment. Prompt intervention in the early stages may prevent the decline to the progressive or irreversible stage. Successful management includes (1) identification of patients at risk for shock; (2) integration of the patient's history, physical examination, and clinical findings to establish a diagnosis; (3) interventions to control or eliminate the cause of the decreased perfusion; (4) protection of target and distal organs from dysfunction; and (5) provision of multisystem supportive care.

Emergency care of the patient in shock is presented in Table 77. General management strategies begin with ensuring that the patient is responsive and has a patent airway. Once the airway is established, with either a natural airway or an endotracheal tube, O_2 delivery must be optimized.

- Supplemental O_2 and mechanical ventilation may be necessary to support the delivery of oxygen to maintain an arterial oxygen saturation of at least 90% (arterial partial pressure of O_2 [PaO_2] greater than 60 mm Hg) to avoid hypoxemia (see Artificial Airways: Endotracheal Tubes, p. 683, Oxygen Therapy, p. 718, and Mechanical Ventilation, p. 712). The mean arterial pressure and circulating blood volume are optimized with fluid replacement and drug therapy (see Tables 66-7 and 66-8 in Lewis et al, *Medical-Surgical Nursing,* ed 10, pp. 1597 and 1599).

Interprofessional Care: Specific Measures
In addition to general management of shock, there are specific interventions for different types of shock (Table 78).

Nursing Management
Goals
The patient with shock will have evidence of adequate tissue perfusion, restoration of normal or baseline BP, return/recovery of organ function, avoidance of complications from prolonged states of hypoperfusion, and prevention of health care–acquired complications of disease management and care.

Nursing Diagnoses
- Ineffective peripheral tissue perfusion
- Risk for decreased cardiac tissue perfusion
- Ineffective cerebral tissue perfusion and ineffective renal perfusion
- Anxiety

Nursing Interventions
You have an important role in the prevention of shock, beginning with the identification of patients at risk. In general, patients who are older or immunocompromised or have chronic illnesses are at

Text continued on p. 579

TABLE 77 Emergency Management

Shock

Etiology*	Assessment Findings	Interventions
Surgical	• Restlessness	**Initial**
• Postoperative bleeding	• Confusion	• If unresponsive, assess circulation, airway, and breathing (CAB).
• Ruptured organ or vessel	• Anxiety	• If responsive, monitor airway, breathing, and circulation (ABC).
• Gastrointestinal bleeding	• Feeling of impending doom	• Stabilize cervical spine as appropriate.
• Aortic dissection	• Decreased level of consciousness	• Control any external bleeding with direct pressure or pressure dressing.
• Vaginal bleeding	• Weakness	• Give high-flow O_2 (100%) by non-rebreather mask or bag-valve-mask.
• Ruptured ectopic pregnancy or ovarian cyst	• Rapid, weak, thready pulses	• Anticipate need for intubation and mechanical ventilation.
	• Dysrhythmias	• Establish IV access with two large-bore catheters (14 to 16 gauge) or an intraosseous access device, or assist with insertion of central line.
	• Hypotension	• Begin fluid resuscitation with crystalloids (e.g., 30 mL/kg, repeated until hemodynamic improvement is noted).
	• Narrowed pulse pressure	

Medical
- Myocardial infarction
- Dehydration
- Addisonian crisis
- Diabetes insipidus
- Sepsis
- Diabetes mellitus
- Pulmonary embolus

Trauma
- Ruptured or lacerated vessel or organ (e.g., spleen)
- Fractures, spinal injury
- Multiorgan injury

- Cool, clammy skin (warm skin in early onset of septic and neurogenic shock)
- Tachypnea, dyspnea, or shallow, irregular respirations
- Decreased O_2 saturation
- Extreme thirst
- Nausea and vomiting
- Chills
- Pallor
- Cyanosis
- Obvious hemorrhage or injury
- Temperature dysregulation

- Draw blood for laboratory studies (e.g., blood cultures, lactate, WBCs). Assess for life-threatening injuries (e.g., cardiac tamponade, liver laceration, tension pneumothorax).
- Consider vasopressor therapy if hypotension persists after fluid resuscitation.
- Insert an indwelling bladder catheter and nasogastric tube.
- Start antibiotic therapy after blood cultures if sepsis is suspected.
- Obtain 12-lead ECG and treat dysrhythmias.

Ongoing Monitoring
- ABCs
- Level of consciousness
- Vital signs, including pulse oximetry; peripheral pulses, capillary refill, skin color and temperature
- Respiratory status
- Heart rate and rhythm
- Urine output

*See Table 66-1 in Lewis, et al, *Medical-Surgical Nursing*, ed 10, p. 1588, for additional etiologies of shock.

S

TABLE 78 Interprofessional Care

Shock

Oxygenation	Circulation	Drug Therapies	Supportive Therapies
Cardiogenic Shock			
• Provide supplemental O_2 (e.g., nasal cannula, non-rebreather mask) • Intubation and mechanical ventilation, if necessary • Monitor $ScvO_2/SvO_2$	• Restore blood flow with thrombolytics, angioplasty with stenting, emergent coronary revascularization • Reduce workload of heart with circulatory assist devices: IABP, VAD	• Nitrates (e.g., nitroglycerin) • Inotropes (e.g., dobutamine) • Diuretics (e.g., furosemide) • β-Adrenergic blockers (contraindicated with ↓ ejection fraction)	• Treat dysrhythmias.
Hypovolemic Shock			

• Provide supplemental O_2
• Monitor $ScvO_2/SvO_2$
	• Rapid fluid replacement using two large-bore (14 to 16 gauge) peripheral IV lines, an intraosseous access device, or central venous catheter
	• Restore fluid volume (e.g., blood or blood products, crystalloids)
	• End points of fluid resuscitation:
	  • CVP 15 mm Hg
	  • PAWP 10-12 mm Hg
		• No specific drug therapy	• Correct the cause (e.g., stop bleeding, GI losses).
			• Use warmed IV fluids, including blood products (if appropriate).

Septic Shock

- Provide supplemental O_2
- Intubation and mechanical ventilation, if necessary
- Monitor $ScvO_2/SvO_2$

- Aggressive fluid resuscitation (e.g., 30 mL/kg of crystalloids, repeated as long as hemodynamic improvement is noted)
- End points of fluid resuscitation:
  - CVP 8-12 mm Hg and/or focused physical exam
  - MAP ≥65 mm Hg
  - Urine output ≥0.5 mL/kg/hr
  - Normalized lactate levels

- Antibiotics as ordered
- Vasopressors (e.g., norepinephrine)
- Inotropes (e.g., dobutamine)
- Anticoagulants (e.g., low-molecular-weight heparin)

- Obtain cultures (e.g., blood, wound) before beginning antibiotics.
- Monitor temperature.
- Control blood glucose.
- Stress ulcer prophylaxis

Neurogenic Shock

- Maintain patent airway
- Provide supplemental O_2
- Intubation and mechanical ventilation (if necessary)

- Cautious administration of fluids

- Vasopressors (e.g., phenylephrine)
- Atropine (for bradycardia)

- Minimize spinal cord trauma with stabilization.
- Monitor temperature.

Continued

S

TABLE 78 Interprofessional Care

Shock—cont'd

Oxygenation	Circulation	Drug Therapies	Supportive Therapies
Anaphylactic Shock			
• Maintain patent airway • Optimize oxygenation with supplemental O_2 • Intubation and mechanical ventilation, if necessary	• Aggressive fluid resuscitation with colloids	• Epinephrine (IM or IV) • Antihistamines (e.g., diphenhydramine) • Histamine (H_2)-receptor blockers (e.g., ranitidine [Zantac]) • Bronchodilators: nebulized (e.g., albuterol) • Corticosteroids (if hypotension persists)	• Identify and remove offending cause. • Prevent via avoidance of known allergens. • Premedicate with history of prior sensitivity (e.g., contrast media).
Obstructive Shock			
• Maintain patent airway • Provide supplemental O_2 • Intubation and mechanical ventilation, if necessary	• Restore circulation by treating cause of obstruction • Fluid resuscitation may provide temporary improvement in CO and BP	• No specific drug therapy	• Treat cause of obstruction (e.g., pericardiocentesis for cardiac tamponade, needle decompression or chest tube insertion for tension pneumothorax, embolectomy for pulmonary embolism).

CO, Cardiac output; CVP, central venous pressure; IABP, intraaortic balloon pump; MAP, mean arterial pressure; PAWP, pulmonary artery wedge pressure; ScvO₂/SvO₂, central venous oxygenation/mixed venous oxygenation; VAD, ventricular assist device.

an increased risk. Any person who has surgery or trauma is at risk for shock resulting from conditions such as hemorrhage, spinal cord injury, and sepsis.

Your role in shock involves (1) monitoring the patient's ongoing physical and emotional status, (2) identifying trends to detect changes in the patient's condition, (3) planning and implementing nursing interventions and therapy, (4) evaluating the patient's response to therapy, (5) providing emotional support to the patient and caregiver, and (6) collaborating with other members of the interprofessional team to coordinate care.

Do not overlook or underestimate the effects of fear and anxiety on the patient and caregiver when faced with a critical, life-threatening situation. Fear, anxiety, and pain may aggravate respiratory distress and increase the release of catecholamines.

- Monitor the patient's mental state and level of pain using valid assessment tools. Provide drugs to decrease anxiety and pain as appropriate.
- Talk to the patient and encourage the caregiver to talk to the patient, even if the patient is intubated, sedated, or appears comatose. Hearing is often the last sense to decrease. Even patients who cannot respond may still be able to hear. If the intubated patient is capable of writing, provide a "magic slate" or a pencil and paper.
- Do not overlook the patient's spiritual needs. Offer to call a member of the clergy rather than wait for the patient or caregiver to express a wish for spiritual counseling.

Caregivers can have a therapeutic effect on the patient. To perform this role, they need to be supportive and comforting. Encourage caregivers to perform simple comfort measures if desired. Provide privacy and assure the patient and caregivers that assistance is readily available.

Rehabilitation of the patient who has experienced critical illness necessitates correction of the precipitating cause, prevention or early treatment of complications, and education focused on disease management and/or prevention of recurrence based on the initial cause of shock.

- Continue to monitor the patient for indications of complications throughout recovery, including decreased range of motion, decreased physical endurance, renal failure after acute tubular necrosis, and the development of fibrotic lung disease secondary to acute respiratory distress syndrome (ARDS).
- Patients recovering from shock may require diverse services after discharge. These can include admission to transitional care units (e.g., for mechanical ventilation weaning) or rehabilitation centers (inpatient or outpatient), or management by home health

S

care agencies. Start planning a safe transition from the hospital to home as soon as the patient is admitted to the hospital.
- See also eNursing Care Plan 66-1: Patient in Shock, on the website.

SICKLE CELL DISEASE

Description

Sickle cell disease (SCD) is a group of inherited, autosomal recessive disorders characterized by an abnormal form of hemoglobin (Hgb) in the erythrocyte. This abnormal hemoglobin, *hemoglobin S* (Hgb S), causes the erythrocyte to stiffen and elongate, taking on a sickle shape in response to low O_2 levels.

SCD is usually diagnosed during routine neonatal screening. It is an incurable disease that is often fatal by middle age from renal or pulmonary failure and/or stroke.

Pathophysiology

Types of SCD include sickle cell anemia, sickle cell-thalassemia, sickle cell Hgb C disease, and sickle cell trait. *Sickle cell anemia,* the most severe of the SCD syndromes, occurs when a person is homozygous for hemoglobin S (Hgb SS). The person has inherited Hgb S from both parents.

Sickle cell-thalassemia and *sickle cell Hgb C* occur when a person inherits Hgb S from one parent and another type of abnormal hemoglobin (e.g., thalassemia or hemoglobin C) from the other parent. Both of these forms of SCD are less common and less severe than sickle cell anemia.

Sickle cell trait occurs when a person is heterozygous for hemoglobin S (Hgb AS). The person has inherited hemoglobin S from one parent and normal hemoglobin (hemoglobin A) from the other parent. Sickle cell trait is typically a mild to asymptomatic condition.

The major pathophysiologic event of SCD is sickling of erythrocytes. Sickling episodes are most commonly triggered by low O_2 tension in the blood. Hypoxia or deoxygenation of the RBCs can be caused by viral or bacterial infection (most common factor), high altitude, emotional stress, surgery, and blood loss. Other triggering events include dehydration, increased hydrogen ion concentration (acidosis), decreased plasma volume, and low body temperature. A sickling episode can also occur without an obvious cause.
- Sickled RBCs become rigid and take on an elongated, crescent shape. Sickled cells cannot easily pass through capillaries or

other small vessels and can cause vascular occlusion, leading to acute or chronic tissue injury. The resulting hemostasis promotes a self-perpetuating cycle of local hypoxia, deoxygenation of more erythrocytes, and more sickling.

- Circulating sickled cells are hemolyzed by the spleen, leading to anemia. Initially the sickling of cells is reversible with reoxygenation, but eventually the condition becomes irreversible because of cell membrane damage from recurrent sickling.

Sickle cell crisis is a severe, painful, acute exacerbation of erythrocyte sickling causing a vaso-occlusive crisis. As blood flow is impaired by sickled cells, vasospasm occurs, further restricting blood flow. Tissue ischemia, infarction, and necrosis eventually occur from lack of oxygen. Shock is a possible life-threatening consequence because of severe oxygen depletion of the tissues and a reduction of the circulating fluid volume. Sickle cell crisis can begin suddenly and persist for days to weeks.

- The frequency, extent, and severity of sickling episodes are highly variable and unpredictable but largely depend on the percentage of Hgb S present. Individuals with sickle cell anemia have the most severe form because erythrocytes contain a high percentage of Hgb S.

Clinical Manifestations

The manifestations of SCD vary greatly from person to person. Many people with sickle cell anemia are in reasonably good health most of the time. However, they may have chronic health problems and pain because of organ tissue hypoxia and damage (e.g., involving the kidneys or liver). The typical patient is anemic but asymptomatic except during sickling episodes.

- Because most individuals with sickle cell anemia have dark skin, pallor is more readily detected by examining the mucous membranes. The skin may have a grayish cast. Because of the hemolysis, jaundice is common, and patients are prone to gallstones (cholelithiasis).
- The primary symptom associated with sickling is pain. During sickle cell crisis the pain is quite severe as a result of tissue ischemia. The back, chest, extremities, and abdomen are most commonly affected. Pain episodes are accompanied by fever, swelling, tenderness, tachypnea, hypertension, and nausea and vomiting.

Complications

With repeated episodes of sickling there is gradual involvement of all body systems, especially the spleen, lungs, kidneys, and brain.

S

- Infection is a major contributor to morbidity and mortality in patients with sickle cell disease. Pneumonia is the most common infection.
- The spleen becomes infarcted, dysfunctional, and small because of repeated scarring.
- *Acute chest syndrome* is a pulmonary complication that includes pneumonia, tissue infarction, and fat embolism, resulting in pulmonary hypertension, myocardial infarction (MI), and ultimately cor pulmonale.
- The kidneys may be injured from the lack of oxygen, resulting in renal failure.
- Stroke can result from thrombosis and infarction of cerebral blood vessels.
- The heart may become ischemic and enlarged, leading to heart failure.
- Retinal vessel obstruction may result in hemorrhage, scarring, retinal detachment, and blindness.
- Bone changes may include osteoporosis and osteosclerosis after infarction. Chronic leg ulcers can result from hypoxia.

Diagnostic Studies

- Peripheral blood smear may reveal sickled cells and abnormal reticulocytes.
- Hgb S can be identified by the sickling test, which uses erythrocytes (in vitro) and exposes them to a deoxygenation agent.
- Findings of hemolysis (jaundice, elevated serum bilirubin levels) and abnormal laboratory test results (see Table 8, p. 33) may be present.
- Skeletal x-rays, MRI, and Doppler studies may be indicated to assess for bone and joint deformities, stroke, and deep vein thromboses, respectively.

Nursing and Interprofessional Management

Care is directed toward preventing and alleviating symptoms from complications of the disease, minimizing end-organ damage, and promptly treating serious sequelae such as acute chest syndrome. Teach patients with SCD to avoid high altitudes, maintain adequate fluid intake, and treat infections promptly.

- Immunizations for pneumococcus, *Haemophilus influenzae,* influenza, and hepatitis should be administered.
- Chronic leg ulcers may be treated with bed rest, antibiotics, warm saline soaks, mechanical or enzyme debridement, and grafting if necessary.
- Sickle cell crises may require hospitalization. O_2 may be administered to treat hypoxia and control sickling. Rest may be

instituted to reduce metabolic requirements, and fluids and electrolytes are administered to reduce blood viscosity and maintain renal function.

- Transfusion therapy is indicated when an aplastic crisis occurs. These patients, like those with thalassemia major, may require chelation therapy to reduce transfusion-produced iron overload.
- During an acute crisis, optimal pain control usually includes large doses of continuous (rather than as-needed [prn]) opioid analgesics along with breakthrough analgesia, often in the form of patient-controlled analgesia (PCA).
- Infection must be treated. Patients with acute chest syndrome are treated with broad-spectrum antibiotics, O_2 therapy, and fluid therapy.
- Although many antisickling agents have been tried, hydroxyurea (Hydrea) is the only one shown to be clinically beneficial. This drug increases the production of hemoglobin F (fetal hemoglobin), which is accompanied by a reduction in hemolysis, an increase in hemoglobin concentration, and a decrease in sickled cells and painful crises.
- Hematopoietic stem cell transplantation (HSCT) is the only available treatment that can cure some patients with SCD.

▼ **Patient and Caregiver Teaching**

Patient teaching and support are important in long-term care of the patient. The patient and caregivers need to understand the basis of the disease and the reasons for supportive care.

- Teach the patient ways to avoid crises, including taking steps to avoid dehydration and hypoxia, such as avoiding high altitudes and seeking medical attention quickly to counteract problems including upper respiratory tract infections.
- Also teach about pain control, because the pain during a crisis may be severe and often requires considerable analgesia.

SJÖGREN'S SYNDROME

Sjögren's syndrome is a relatively common autoimmune disease that targets moisture-producing glands, leading to the common symptoms of *xerostomia* (dry mouth) and *keratoconjunctivitis sicca* (dry eyes). The nose, throat, airways, and skin can become dry. The disease can also affect the stomach, pancreas, and intestines. Women are 10 times more likely than men to have Sjögren's syndrome.

In *primary Sjögren's syndrome,* symptoms are related to problems with the lacrimal and salivary glands. About one half of the cases of Sjögren's syndrome develop as primary disease. The patient with *secondary Sjögren's syndrome* has another autoimmune disease (e.g., rheumatoid arthritis, systemic lupus erythematosus) before Sjögren's develops.

- Sjögren's syndrome appears to be caused by genetic and environmental factors. The trigger may be a viral or bacterial infection that stimulates the immune system, causing lymphocytes to attack and damage the lacrimal and salivary glands.

Decreased tearing leads to a "gritty" sensation in the eyes, burning, blurred vision, and photosensitivity. Dry mouth produces buccal membrane fissures, altered sense of taste, dysphagia, mouth infections, and dental caries.

- Dry skin and rashes, joint and muscle pain, and thyroid problems may be present. Other exocrine glands can be affected. For example, vaginal dryness may lead to *dyspareunia* (painful intercourse).
- Autoimmune thyroid disorders are common, including Graves' disease and Hashimoto's thyroiditis.
- The disease may become more generalized and involve the lymph nodes, bone marrow, and visceral organs (pseudolymphoma). People with Sjögren's syndrome have an increased risk of developing non-Hodgkin's lymphoma.

Ophthalmologic examination (Schirmer's test), salivary flow rates, and lower lip biopsy of minor salivary glands confirm the diagnosis.

Treatment is symptomatic, including instillation of artificial tears (e.g., cyclosporine [Restasis]) as necessary to maintain adequate hydration and lubrication, surgical occlusion of the puncta lacrimalia, and increasing fluids with meals.

- Pilocarpine (Salagen) and cevimeline (Evoxac) can be used to treat symptoms of dry mouth.
- Increased humidity at home may reduce respiratory infections. Vaginal lubrication with a water-soluble jelly may increase comfort during intercourse.

SPINAL CORD INJURY

Description

Spinal cord injury (SCI) can result in temporary or permanent alteration in spinal cord function. Some 276,000 persons in the United States are living with SCI.

- SCIs are usually due to trauma, including motor vehicle collisions, falls, violence, and sports injuries. Young adult men ages 16 to 30 years have the greatest risk for SCI.

Pathophysiology

The extent of the neurologic damage caused by an SCI results from both *primary injury* (initial disruption of axons) and *secondary injury* (processes such as ischemia, hypoxia, hemorrhage, and edema).

Primary Injury

Primary SCI can be due to cord compression by bone displacement, interruption of blood supply to the cord, or traction from pulling on the cord. Penetrating trauma, such as gunshot and stab wounds, causes tearing and transection.

Secondary Injury

Secondary injury refers to ongoing, progressive damage after the primary injury. Possible causes include vascular changes due to hemorrhage, vasospasm, thrombosis, loss of autoregulation, breakdown of the blood-brain barrier, and infiltration of inflammatory cells that cause ischemia, edema, and cellular necrosis.

- *Apoptosis* (programmed cell death) may continue for weeks after injury and may contribute to postinjury demyelination. These processes lead to scar tissue formation, irreversible nerve damage, and permanent neurologic deficit. This ongoing destructive process makes it critical to initiate care and management of the patient with an SCI as soon as possible, to limit the damage.
- Because secondary injury processes occur over time, the extent of injury and prognosis for recovery are most accurately determined at 72 hours or more after injury. Figure 21 illustrates the cascade of events causing secondary injury after traumatic SCI.

Spinal and Neurogenic Shock

Spinal shock may occur after acute SCI. This temporary shock is characterized by decreased reflexes, loss of sensation, absent thermoregulation, and flaccid paralysis below the level of injury. This syndrome lasts days to weeks and may mask postinjury neurologic function.

Neurogenic shock results from the loss of vasomotor tone caused by injury and is characterized by hypotension and bradycardia. Loss of sympathetic innervation causes peripheral vasodilation, venous pooling, and decreased cardiac output. These effects are generally associated with a cervical or high thoracic injury.

Classification

SCIs are classified by the mechanism of injury, level of injury, and degree of injury. The major mechanisms of injury are flexion, hyperextension, flexion-rotation, extension-rotation, and compression. The level of injury may be cervical, thoracic, lumbar, or

PATHOPHYSIOLOGY MAP

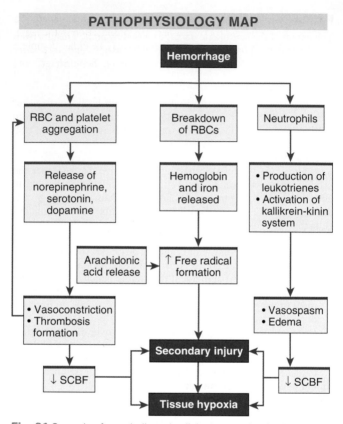

Fig. 21 Cascade of metabolic and cellular events that leads to spinal cord ischemia and hypoxia of secondary injury. *RBCs,* Red blood cells; *SCBF,* spinal cord blood flow.

sacral. Cervical and lumbar injuries are the most common because these levels are associated with the greatest flexibility and movement. The degree of spinal cord involvement may be either complete or incomplete (partial).

■ If the cervical cord is involved, paralysis of all four extremities occurs, resulting in *tetraplegia* (formerly termed *quadriplegia*). The lower the level of injury, the more function is retained in the arms.

- If the thoracic, lumbar, or sacral spinal cord is damaged, the result is *paraplegia* (paralysis and loss of sensation in the legs). The degree of spinal cord involvement may be either complete or incomplete (partial).
- *Complete cord involvement* results in total loss of sensory and motor function below the level of the injury.
- *Incomplete cord involvement* (partial transection) results in a mixed loss of voluntary motor activity and sensation and leaves some tracts intact. The degree of sensory and motor loss varies depending on the level of the injury and reflects the specific nerve tracts damaged.

Clinical Manifestations

Manifestations of SCI are related to the level and degree of injury. The patient with an incomplete lesion may demonstrate a mixture of symptoms—the higher the injury, the more serious the effects because of the proximity of the cervical cord to the medulla and brainstem.

Movement and rehabilitation potential related to specific locations of the SCI are described in Table 60-2, Lewis et al, *Medical-Surgical Nursing,* ed 10, p. 1421. In general, sensory function closely parallels motor function at all levels.

Complications

Respiratory System

Cervical injuries above the level of C4 vertebra manifest with a total loss of respiratory muscle function. Injury or fracture below the level of C4 can result in diaphragmatic breathing with respiratory insufficiency and hypoventilation.

Cardiovascular System

Any cord injury above the level of T6 leads to dysfunction of the sympathetic nervous system. The result is bradycardia, peripheral vasodilation, and hypotension (neurogenic shock).

Urinary System

Urinary retention is common in acute SCI and spinal shock. While the patient is in spinal shock, the bladder is atonic, and fails to empty (urinary retention). In the postacute phase, the bladder may become hyperirritable, with reflex emptying (urinary incontinence).

Gastrointestinal System

Decreased GI motor activity contributes to gastric distention and development of paralytic ileus. Gastric emptying may be delayed, especially in patients with higher-level SCI. Excessive release of HCl acid in the stomach may cause stress ulcers. Loss of voluntary control of the bowel after SCI results in neurogenic bowel.

S

- SCI above the level of the conus medullaris causes the anal sphincter to remain tight, and the ability to sense a full rectum is lost. Bowel movement occurs on a reflex basis when the rectum is full (incontinence).
- SCI at or below the conus medullaris causes the bowel to be areflexic. Peristalsis is impaired and stool propulsion is slow. The defecation reflex may be damaged and anal sphincter tone relaxed (retention). This leads to constipation, increased risk of incontinence, and possible impaction, ileus, or megacolon.

Integumentary System

A major consequence of lack of movement is the potential for skin breakdown over bony prominences in areas of decreased sensation. Pressure ulcers can occur quickly, leading to major infection or sepsis.

Thermoregulation

Poikilothermism (adjustment of body temperature to the room temperature) occurs because the interruption of the sympathetic nervous system prevents peripheral temperature sensations from reaching the hypothalamus. With SCI, there is decreased ability to sweat or shiver below the level of injury, which also affects the ability to regulate body temperature.

Peripheral Vascular Problems

Venous thromboembolism (VTE) is a common problem accompanying SCI in the first 3 months. Pulmonary embolism is a leading cause of death in patients with SCI.

Pain

Pain after SCI can be nociceptive or neuropathic.

- *Nociceptive pain* in SCI can develop from musculoskeletal, visceral, and/or other types of injury (e.g., skin ulceration, headache). Patients often describe musculoskeletal pain as dull or aching. It starts or worsens with movement. Visceral pain is located in the thorax, abdomen, and/or pelvis and may be dull, tender, or cramping.
- *Neuropathic pain* in SCI occurs from damage to the spinal cord or nerve roots. The pain can be located at or below the level of injury. Patients often identify neuropathic pain as hot, burning, tingling, "pins and needles," cold, and/or shooting. Even light touch can cause significant pain.

Autonomic Hyperreflexia

Autonomic hyperreflexia (also known as *dysreflexia*) is a massive uncompensated cardiovascular reaction mediated by the sympathetic nervous system. It involves stimulation of sensory receptors below the level of the SCI. The intact sympathetic nervous system below the SCI responds to the stimulation by increasing BP, but the parasympathetic nervous system is unable to directly counteract these responses via the injured spinal cord. Baroreceptors in the carotid sinus and aorta sense the hypertension and stimulate the parasympathetic system. This results in a decreased heart rate, but visceral and peripheral vessels do not dilate because efferent impulses cannot pass through the injured spinal cord.

- *Autonomic hyperreflexia* is a life-threatening situation requiring immediate resolution to prevent status epilepticus, myocardial infarction, stroke, and even death.
- The most common precipitating cause is a distended bladder or rectum, although any sensory stimulation may cause autonomic hyperreflexia.
- Manifestations include hypertension (up to 300 mm Hg systolic), blurred vision, throbbing headache, marked diaphoresis above the level of the lesion, bradycardia (30 to 40 beats/minute), piloerection, nasal congestion, and nausea. Measure BP when the patient with an SCI complains of a headache.
- Elevate the head of the bed 45 degrees or sit the patient upright, notify the HCP, and determine the cause. If symptoms persist after the source has been relieved, a rapid onset and short duration agent such as nitroglycerin, nitroprusside, or hydralazine is administered.
- Teach the patient and caregivers the causes and symptoms of autonomic hyperreflexia (see Table 60-7, Lewis et al, *Medical-Surgical Nursing,* ed 10, p. 1431). They must understand the life-threatening nature of this dysfunction, know how to relieve the cause, and be prepared to call for emergency care.

Diagnostic Studies

- CT scan is the preferred imaging study to diagnose the location and degree of injury and degree of spinal canal compromise. Cervical x-rays are obtained when CT scan is not readily available.
- MRI is used to assess soft tissue and neurologic changes and for neurologic deficits or worsening of neurologic status.
- Comprehensive neurologic examination is done along with assessment of the head, chest, and abdomen for additional injuries or trauma.
- Patients with cervical injuries who demonstrate altered mental status may need vertebral angiography to rule out vertebral artery damage.

Interprofessional Care

After stabilization at the injury scene, the person is transferred to a health care facility. A thorough assessment is done to evaluate the specific degree of deficit and establish the level and degree

of injury. The patient may go directly to surgery after initial immobilization and assessment or to the ICU for monitoring and
management.

Nonoperative Stabilization

Nonoperative treatments are focused on stabilization of the injured
spinal segment and decompression, through either traction or
realignment, to prevent secondary spinal cord damage caused by
repeated contusion or compression.

Surgical Therapy

When cord compression is certain or the neurologic disorder progresses, immediate surgery may stabilize the spinal column. Early
cord decompression may result in reduced secondary injury to the
spinal cord.

- A fusion procedure involves attaching metal screws, plates, or
  other devices to the bones of the spine to help keep them
  aligned. This is usually done when two or more vertebrae have
  been injured. Small pieces of bone may be attached to the
  injured area to help the bones fuse into one solid piece.

Drug Therapy

Methylprednisolone is no longer approved by the U.S. Food and
Drug Administration (FDA) for treatment in acute SCI. There is
no evidence of clinical benefit of methylprednisolone to treat
acute SCI, and the drug has been associated with harmful side
effects.

- Low-molecular-weight heparin (e.g., enoxaparin [Lovenox]) is
  used to prevent VTE unless contraindicated.
- Vasopressor agents such as phenylephrine or norepinephrine
  (Levophed) are used in the acute phase to maintain mean arterial pressure at a level greater than 90 mm Hg so that perfusion
  to the spinal cord is improved.

Nursing Management

Goals

The patient with an SCI will maintain an optimal level of neurologic functioning; have minimal or no complications of immobility; learn new skills, gain new knowledge, and acquire new
behaviors to be able to care for self or successfully direct others to
do so; and return to home and the community at an optimal level
of functioning.

Nursing Diagnoses

- Ineffective breathing pattern
- Ineffective peripheral tissue perfusion
- Constipation
- Impaired urinary elimination
- Risk for autonomic hyperreflexia (dysreflexia)

Nursing Interventions

High cervical injury resulting from flexion-rotation is the most complex SCI and is discussed in this section. Interventions for this type of injury can be modified for patients with less severe problems.

Immobilization. Proper immobilization of the neck involves maintenance of a neutral position. For cervical injuries, skeletal traction is now used less frequently, with the development of better surgical stabilization. When skeletal traction is used, realignment or reduction of the injury is usually provided by Crutchfield, Vinke, Gardner-Wells, or other types of skull tongs.

- Infection at the sites of tong insertion is a potential problem. Preventive care is determined by individual hospital protocols. A common protocol involves cleansing the sites twice a day with half-strength peroxide and normal saline solution and applying an antibiotic ointment, which acts as a mechanical barrier to the entrance of bacteria.

- Special beds are often used to provide frequent turning to prevent pressure sores.

After cervical fusion or other stabilization surgery, a hard cervical collar or sternal-occipital-mandibular immobilizer brace can be worn. In a stable injury for which surgery is not done, a halo fixation apparatus may be applied.

Respiratory Dysfunction. If the patient is exhausted from labored breathing or arterial blood gases (ABGs) deteriorate (indicating inadequate oxygenation or ventilation), endotracheal intubation or tracheostomy and mechanical ventilation are needed. (See Artificial Airways: Endotracheal Tubes, p. 683, Tracheostomy, p. 735, and Mechanical Ventilation, p. 712.) The possibility of respiratory arrest requires careful monitoring and readiness for prompt action. Pneumonia and atelectasis may occur due to reduced vital capacity and the loss of intercostal and abdominal muscle function, resulting in diaphragmatic breathing, pooled secretions, and an ineffective cough.

- Regularly assess breath sounds, ABGs, tidal volume, vital capacity, skin color, breathing patterns (especially the use of accessory muscles), subjective comments about the ability to breathe, and the amount and color of sputum.

- In addition to monitoring, you can support ventilation by the administration of O_2, chest physiotherapy and assisted coughing, incentive spirometry, and tracheal suctioning.

Cardiovascular Instability. If bradycardia is symptomatic, an anticholinergic medication such as atropine is administered. A pacemaker may be inserted (see Pacemakers, p. 727). Hypotension is managed with fluid replacement and a vasopressor agent, such

S

as phenylephrine or norepinephrine (Levophed). Monitor the patient for indications of hypovolemic shock secondary to hemorrhage, which may require blood transfusion.

- Sequential compression devices or compression gradient stockings are used to prevent formation of thromboemboli and to promote venous return.
- Perform range-of-motion (ROM) exercises and stretching regularly. Assess the thighs and calves of the legs for the signs of deep vein thrombosis (DVT) every shift (e.g., deep reddish color, edema).

Fluid and Nutritional Maintenance.   If the GI tract stops functioning (paralytic ileus) during the first 48 to 72 hours after the injury, a nasogastric (NG) tube must be inserted.

- Once bowel sounds are present or flatus is passed, and the patient is not receiving mechanical ventilation, a formal swallow evaluation should be done. If no risk of aspiration is identified, gradually introduce oral food and fluids.
- If the patient fails the swallow evaluation or is unable to eat because of presence of an endotracheal tube or tracheostomy, a more secure feeding tube may be placed in the stomach or jejunum.

Bowel and Bladder Management.   An indwelling catheter is usually inserted as soon as possible after injury. Strict aseptic technique for catheter care is essential to avoid introducing infection.

- *Catheter-acquired urinary tract infection* (CAUTI) is a common problem. The best method for preventing CAUTI is regular and complete bladder drainage.
- A bowel program should be started during acute care. This consists of a rectal stimulant (suppository or mini-enema) inserted daily at a regular time of day, followed by gentle digital stimulation or manual evacuation.

Temperature Control.   Because there is no vasoconstriction, piloerection, or heat loss through perspiration below the level of injury, temperature control is largely external to the patient. Monitor the environment and body temperature regularly.

Stress Ulcers.   Stress ulcers can occur because of the physiologic response to severe trauma and psychologic stress. Peak incidence is 6 to 14 days after injury. Test stool and gastric contents daily for blood, and monitor hematocrit for a slow drop. Histamine (H_2)-receptor blockers (e.g., ranitidine [Zantac], famotidine [Pepcid]) or proton pump inhibitors (e.g., pantoprazole [Protonix], omeprazole [Prilosec]) may be given prophylactically to decrease HCl acid secretion.

Sensory Deprivation.   To prevent sensory deprivation, compensate for the patient's absence of sensations by stimulating the patient above the level of injury. Conversation, music, and interesting foods can be a part of the nursing care plan. If the head of the bed must remain flat, provide prism glasses to help the patient read and watch television. Make every effort to prevent the patient from withdrawing from the environment.

Reflexes. Once spinal shock is resolved, reflexes often return with hyperactive and exaggerated responses. Penile erections can occur from a variety of stimuli, causing embarrassment and discomfort. Spasms ranging from mild twitches to convulsive movements below the level of the lesion may also occur. Reflex activity may be interpreted by the patient or caregiver as a return of function. Tactfully explain the reason for the activity. Spasms may be controlled with antispasmodic medications, such as baclofen, dantrolene (Dantrium), or tizanidine (Zanaflex).

Rehabilitation. Physiologic and psychologic rehabilitation is complex. Many of the problems identified in the acute period become chronic and continue throughout life. Rehabilitation focuses on refined retraining of physiologic processes and extensive patient, caregiver, and family teaching about how to manage the physiologic and life changes resulting from injury.

Rehabilitation and long-term management of the SCI patient are further described in Chapter 60 of Lewis et al, *Medical-Surgical Nursing,* ed 10.

SPINAL CORD TUMORS

Description

Spinal cord tumors account for 0.5% to 1% of all neoplasms. These tumors are classified as *primary* (arising from some component of cord, dura, nerves, or vessels) or *secondary* (from primary growths that have metastasized to the spinal cord).

Spinal cord tumors are further classified as *extradural* (outside the dura), *intradural-extramedullary* (between the spinal cord and dura), and *intramedullary* (within the substance of spinal cord itself) (see Fig. 60-11 and Table 60-13, Lewis et al, *Medical-Surgical Nursing,* ed 10, p. 1436).

Symptoms associated with spinal cord tumors are due to the mechanical effects of slow compression and irritation of nerve roots, displacement of the spinal cord, or gradual obstruction of the vascular supply. The slow growth does not cause autodestruction as in traumatic spinal cord injury (SCI), so complete functional restoration may be possible after the tumor is removed.

Clinical Manifestations

A common early symptom of a spinal cord tumor is back pain, with the location of the pain depending on the level of compression. The pain worsens with activity, coughing, straining, and lying down.

- Motor weakness accompanies sensory disturbances and consists of slowly increasing clumsiness, weakness, and spasticity. Paralysis can develop.
- Sensory disruption is later marked by coldness, numbness, and tingling in an extremity or extremities.
- Bladder disturbances are marked by urgency, with difficulty in starting the flow and progressing to retention with overflow incontinence.

Diagnostic Studies

Extradural tumors can be seen on routine spinal x-rays, whereas intradural and intramedullary tumors require MRI or CT scans or CT myelogram for detection. Cerebrospinal fluid (CSF) analysis may reveal tumor cells.

Nursing and Interprofessional Management

Compression of the spinal cord is an emergency. Relief of the ischemia related to the compression is the goal of therapy. Corticosteroids, usually dexamethasone in large doses, are prescribed immediately to relieve tumor-related edema.

Indications for surgery vary depending on the type of tumor. Emergency surgery may be needed to decompress the spinal cord, obtain tissue for pathology, and help to determine appropriate adjunctive treatment. Primary spinal tumors may be removed with the goal of cure. In patients with metastatic tumors, treatment is primarily palliative, with the goal of restoring or preserving neurologic function, stabilizing the spine, and alleviating pain.

Radiation therapy and/or chemotherapy may be used to treat the tumor.

- Relief of pain and return of function are the goals of treatment. Ensure that the patient receives pain medication as needed. Assess the patient's neurologic status before and after treatment.
- Depending on the neurologic dysfunction, the patient may require care as for recovery from an SCI. Rehabilitation of patients with spinal cord tumors is similar to SCI rehabilitation. See Spinal Cord Injury, p. 584.

SPLEEN DISORDERS

The spleen can be affected by many illnesses, most of which can cause some degree of *splenomegaly* (enlarged spleen). However, an enlarged spleen may be present in certain individuals without any evidence of disease.

- The degree of splenic enlargement varies with the disease. Massive splenic enlargement occurs with chronic myelogenous leukemia and thalassemia major, whereas mild splenic enlargement occurs with heart failure and systemic lupus erythematosus. When the spleen enlarges, its normal blood cell filtering and sequestering capacity increases. Consequently, there is often a reduction in the number of circulating blood cells.

A slight to moderate enlargement of the spleen is usually asymptomatic and found during routine examination of the abdomen. Massive splenomegaly can be well tolerated, but patients may complain of abdominal discomfort and early satiety. In addition to physical examination, other techniques to assess spleen size include radionuclide colloid liver-spleen scan, CT or positron emission tomography (PET) scan, MRI, and ultrasound scan.

Occasionally splenectomy is done either via laparoscopy or open laparotomy as part of the evaluation or treatment of splenomegaly. Another indication for splenectomy is splenic rupture. The spleen may rupture from trauma, inadvertent tearing during other surgical procedures, and diseases such as mononucleosis, malaria, and lymphoid neoplasms. After a splenectomy, peripheral RBC, WBC, and platelet counts can increase dramatically.

Nursing responsibilities for patients with spleen disorders vary depending on the problem.

- Splenomegaly may be painful and require analgesic administration; care in moving, turning, and positioning; and evaluation of lung expansion, because spleen enlargement may impair diaphragmatic excursion.
- If anemia, thrombocytopenia, or leukopenia develops from splenic enlargement, institute nursing measures to support the patient and prevent life-threatening complications.
- If splenectomy was performed, observe the patient for hemorrhage and shock.
- Postsplenectomy patients may develop immunologic deficiencies and be at lifelong risk for infection from encapsulated organisms such as pneumococcus. This risk is reduced by immunization with pneumococcal vaccine.

S

STOMACH CANCER

Description

Stomach (gastric) cancer is an adenocarcinoma of the stomach wall. Stomach cancer mostly affects older people. The average age at diagnosis is 69 years. More than 50% of people have advanced metastatic disease at the time of diagnosis. The 5-year survival rate is less than 30% in those with advanced disease and 71% in patients with early-stage cancer confined to the stomach.

Pathophysiology

Many factors have been implicated in stomach cancer. Stomach cancer probably begins with a nonspecific mucosal injury as a result of infection (with *Helicobacter pylori*) or repeated exposure to irritants such as bile, antiinflammatory agents, or tobacco. Stomach cancer has also been associated with diets containing smoked foods, salted fish and meat, and pickled vegetables. Other predisposing factors are obesity, family history, atrophic gastritis, pernicious anemia, adenomatous and hyperplastic polyps, and achlorhydria. Consumption of whole grains and fresh fruits and vegetables is associated with reduced rates of stomach cancer.

Stomach cancer spreads by direct extension and typically infiltrates rapidly to the surrounding tissue and liver. Seeding of tumor cells into the peritoneal cavity occurs later in the disease.

Clinical Manifestations

Stomach cancers often spread to adjacent organs before any distressing symptoms occur. Clinical manifestations include unexplained weight loss, early satiety, indigestion, abdominal discomfort or pain, and signs and symptoms of anemia.

- Anemia occurs with chronic blood loss as the lesion erodes the stomach mucosa. The patient appears pale and weak with fatigue, dizziness, weakness, and positive occult stools.
- Supraclavicular lymph nodes that are hard and enlarged suggest metastasis via the thoracic duct. The presence of ascites is a poor prognostic sign.

Diagnostic Studies

- Upper GI endoscopy is the best diagnostic tool.
- Endoscopic ultrasound and CT and positron emission tomography (PET) scans can be used to stage the disease.
- Laparoscopy can be done to determine peritoneal spread.

- Blood studies detect anemia and also elevations in liver enzymes and serum amylase, which may indicate liver and pancreatic involvement.
- Stool examination provides evidence of occult or gross bleeding.

Interprofessional Care

Treatment of choice is surgical removal of the tumor. Surgical procedures used are similar to those used for peptic ulcer disease (see Peptic Ulcer Disease, p. 484).

- Preoperative management focuses on correcting nutritional deficits and transfusing RBCs to treat anemia. Gastric decompression may be necessary if gastric outlet obstruction is present. Special preparation of the bowel is needed if the tumor has involved the colon.
- Therapy for localized stomach cancer is surgical resection followed by chemotherapy agents used in combination including 5-FU (fluorouracil) (often given with leucovorin [folinic acid]), capecitabine (Xeloda), carboplatin, cisplatin, docetaxel (Taxotere), epirubicin (Ellence), irinotecan (Camptosar), oxaliplatin (Eloxatin), and paclitaxel (Taxol) (see Chemotherapy, p. 694).
- Trastuzumab (Herceptin) and ramucirumab (Cyramza) are targeted therapy agents used to treat stomach cancer. Ramucirumab (Cyramza) binds to the receptor for vascular endothelial growth factor (VEGF) and prevents VEGF from binding to the receptor, thus preventing the growth and spread of cancer.
- The surgical aim is to remove the tumor and a margin of normal tissue. When the lesion is located in the fundus, a total gastrectomy with esophagojejunostomy is performed. Lesions located in the antrum or the pyloric region generally are treated by either a Billroth I or II procedure. When metastasis has occurred to adjacent organs, such as the spleen, ovaries, or bowel, the surgical procedure is modified and extended as necessary.

Radiation therapy may be used as a palliative measure to decrease tumor mass and provide temporary relief of obstruction (see Radiation Therapy, p. 733).

Nursing Management

Goals

The patient with stomach cancer will experience minimal discomfort, achieve optimal nutritional status, and maintain a degree of spiritual and psychologic well-being appropriate to the disease stage.

Nursing Diagnoses
- Imbalanced nutrition: less than body requirements
- Anxiety
- Acute pain
- Grieving

Nursing Interventions
Your role in the early detection of stomach cancer focuses on identifying patients at risk such as those with *H. pylori* infection, pernicious anemia, or achlorhydria. Encourage patients with a positive family history of stomach cancer to undergo diagnostic evaluation if manifestations of anemia, peptic ulcer disease, or vague epigastric distress are present.

When diagnostic tests confirm a malignancy, offer emotional and physical support, provide information, and clarify test results. Patient teaching is similar to that for peptic ulcer disease surgery (see p. 491 under Peptic Ulcer Disease).

Postoperative care is also similar to that after a Billroth I or II procedure for peptic ulcer disease. When a total gastrectomy is done, closely observe the patient for signs of fluid leakage at the site of anastomosis, as evidenced by an elevation in temperature and increasing dyspnea. Dumping syndrome may also occur with this procedure (see pp. 488-489 under Peptic Ulcer Disease).
- Postoperative wound healing may be impaired because of poor nutritional intake. This necessitates IV or oral replacement of vitamins C, D, and K; the B complex vitamins; and cobalamin. These vitamins (with the exception of cobalamin) need to be replaced because they are normally absorbed in the duodenum.

▼ Patient and Caregiver Teaching
Before discharge, instruct the patient and caregivers about comfort measures and the use of analgesics. Additional considerations include:
- Teach wound care, if needed, to the primary caregiver in the home setting.
- Dressings, special equipment, or special services may be required for the patient's continued care at home.
- Provide a list of community resources.

STROKE

Description

Stroke occurs when there is ischemia to a part of the brain or hemorrhage into the brain that results in brain cell death. Movement, sensation, or emotions controlled by the affected brain area are lost or impaired. Severity of the stroke varies according to the location and extent of the brain damage.

- The terms *brain attack* and *cerebrovascular accident* (CVA) are also used to describe stroke. The term *brain attack* communicates the urgency of recognizing the warning signs of a stroke and treating it as a medical emergency, as would be done with a heart attack (Table 79).
- Stroke is the fifth most common cause of death in the United States. An estimated 800,000 people experience strokes annually, and 15% to 30% will live with permanent disability.

TABLE 79 Patient & Caregiver Teaching

FAST for Warning Signs of Stroke

FAST is an easy way to remember the signs of stroke. Include the following information in the teaching plan for a patient at risk for stroke and the patient's caregiver.

F	Face drooping	Does one side of the face droop or is it numb? Ask the person to smile. Is the smile uneven?
A	Arm weakness	Is one arm weak or numb? Ask the person to raise both arms. Does one arm drift downward?
S	Speech difficulties	Is speech slurred? Is the person unable to speak or hard to understand? Ask the person to repeat a simple sentence like "The sky is blue." Is the sentence repeated correctly?
T	Time	Time is CRITICAL! If someone shows any of these signs (even if they go away), call 911 and get the person to the hospital. Note the time when the signs first appeared.

In addition, the following should be reported:
- Sudden trouble seeing in one or both eyes
- Sudden trouble walking, dizziness, loss of balance or coordination
- Sudden, severe headache with no known cause

S

Source: American Stroke Association: FAST. Retrieved from *www.strokeassociation.org/STROKEORG/WarningSigns/Stroke-Warning-Signs -and-Symptoms_UCM_308528_SubHomePage.jsp.*

Risk factors associated with stroke can be divided into nonmodifiable and modifiable. Stroke risk increases with multiple risk factors.

Nonmodifiable risk factors include age, ethnicity or race, and family history or heredity. Two thirds of all strokes occur in individuals older than 65 years, but stroke can occur at any age. Strokes are more common in men, but more women die from stroke than men.

- African Americans have a higher incidence of stroke and a higher death rate from stroke than any other ethnic group, which may be related in part to an increased incidence of hypertension, obesity, and diabetes mellitus (DM).
- People with a family history of stroke are also at higher risk for stroke.

Modifiable risk factors include hypertension, heart disease, diabetes mellitus, smoking, obesity, sleep apnea, metabolic syndrome, lack of physical exercise, poor diet, and drug and alcohol abuse. Hypertension is the single most important modifiable risk factor, and its treatment can reduce the risk of stroke by up to 50%.

Transient Ischemic Attack

A *transient ischemic attack* (TIA) is a transient episode of neurologic dysfunction caused by focal brain, spinal cord, or retinal ischemia, but without acute brain infarction. Clinical symptoms typically last less than 1 hour. TIAs may be caused by microemboli that temporarily block the blood flow and are a warning sign of progressive cerebrovascular disease.

Most TIAs resolve. However, it is important to teach the patient to seek treatment for any stroke symptoms because there is no way to predict if a TIA will resolve. In general, one third of individuals who experience a TIA will not experience another event, one third will have additional TIAs, and one third will progress to stroke.

TIA signs and symptoms depend on the blood vessel involved and the brain area that is ischemic.

- If the carotid system is involved, patients may have a temporary loss of vision in one eye, transient hemiparesis, numbness or loss of sensation, or a sudden inability to speak.
- Signs and symptoms of a TIA involving the vertebrobasilar system may include tinnitus, vertigo, darkened or blurred vision, ptosis, dysphagia, ataxia, and unilateral or bilateral numbness or weakness.

TIAs should be treated as medical emergencies. Teach people at risk for TIA to seek medical attention immediately with any stroke-like symptom and to identify the time of symptom onset.

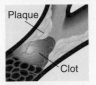 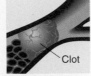 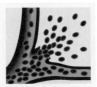

A Thrombotic stroke.
The process of clot formation (thrombosis) results in a narrowing of the lumen, which blocks the passage of the blood through the artery.

B Embolic stroke.
An embolus is a blood clot or other debris circulating the blood. When it reaches an artery in the brain that is too narrow to pass through, it lodges there and blocks the flow of blood.

C Hemorrhagic stroke.
A burst blood vessel may allow blood to seep into and damage brain tissues until clotting shuts off the leak.

Fig. 22 Major causes of stroke.

Pathophysiology

Strokes are classified as ischemic or hemorrhagic, based on the cause and underlying pathophysiology (Fig. 22 and Table 80).

Ischemic Stroke

An *ischemic stroke* results from inadequate blood flow to the brain from partial or complete occlusion of an artery. Ischemic strokes may be either thrombotic or embolic.

Thrombotic Stroke. A *thrombotic stroke* occurs from injury to a blood vessel wall and formation of a blood clot. The lumen of the blood vessel becomes narrowed, and if it becomes occluded, infarction occurs. It is the most common cause of stroke.

- Thrombotic strokes are more common in older individuals. A majority of thrombotic strokes are associated with hypertension or DM. The extent of the stroke depends on speed of onset, size of the lesion, and presence of collateral circulation.
- Most patients do not have a decreased level of consciousness in the first 24 hours unless it is caused by a brainstem stroke or other conditions, such as seizures, increased intracranial pressure (ICP), or hemorrhage.
- Ischemic stroke symptoms may progress in the first 72 hours as infarction and cerebral edema increase.

Embolic Stroke. *Embolic stroke* occurs when an embolus lodges in and occludes a cerebral artery, resulting in infarction and edema of the area supplied by the involved vessel. Embolism is the second most common cause of stroke.

S

TABLE 80 Types of Stroke

Gender and Age	Warning and Onset	Prognosis
Ischemic		
Incidence: Accounts for 87% of strokes		
Thrombotic		
Men more than women Oldest median age	*Warning:* TIA (30%-50% of cases) *Onset:* Often during or after sleep	Stepwise progression, signs and symptoms develop slowly, usually some improvement, recurrence in 20%-25% of survivors
Embolic		
Men more than women	*Warning:* TIA (uncommon) *Onset:* Sudden onset, most likely to occur during activity	Single event, signs and symptoms develop quickly, usually some improvement, recurrence common without aggressive treatment of underlying disease
Hemorrhagic		
Incidence: Accounts for 13% of strokes		
Intracerebral		
Slightly higher in women	*Warning:* Headache (25% of cases) *Onset:* With activity (often)	Progression over 24 hr Poor prognosis, fatality more likely with presence of coma
Subarachnoid		
Slightly higher in women Youngest median age	*Warning:* Headache (common) *Onset:* With activity (often), sudden onset, most commonly related to head trauma	Usually single sudden event, fatality more likely with presence of coma

TIA, Transient ischemic attack

Most emboli originate in the heart. The embolus travels to the cerebral circulation and lodges where a vessel narrows. Heart conditions associated with emboli are atrial fibrillation, myocardial infarction (MI), and inflammatory and valvular heart conditions.

- The embolic stroke often occurs rapidly, giving little time to accommodate by developing collateral circulation. The patient usually remains conscious, although a headache may develop.
- Recurrence is common unless the underlying cause is aggressively treated.

Hemorrhagic Stroke

A *hemorrhagic stroke* results from bleeding into the brain tissue itself (intracerebral or intraparenchymal hemorrhage) or into the subarachnoid space or ventricles (subarachnoid hemorrhage).

Intracerebral Hemorrhage. *Intracerebral hemorrhage* is bleeding within the brain caused by a rupture of a blood vessel. Hypertension is the most important cause of intracerebral hemorrhage. Other causes include vascular malformations, coagulation disorders, anticoagulant drugs, trauma, and ruptured aneurysm.

- Hemorrhage commonly occurs during periods of activity. Most often there is a sudden onset of symptoms, and progression occurs over minutes to hours as a result of ongoing bleeding.
- Manifestations include neurologic deficits, headache, nausea, vomiting, decreased level of consciousness, and hypertension. Extent of the symptoms varies depending on the amount, location, and duration of bleeding.
- Prognosis of patients with intracerebral hemorrhage is poor, with 40% to 80% of patients dying within 30 days, and 50% of the deaths occurring within the first 48 hours.

Subarachnoid Hemorrhage. *Subarachnoid hemorrhage* occurs when there is intracranial bleeding into the cerebrospinal fluid (CSF)–filled space between the arachnoid and pia mater membranes on the surface of the brain. Subarachnoid hemorrhage is commonly caused by rupture of a cerebral aneurysm (a lesion of congenital or acquired weakness with ballooning of vessels). Other causes of subarachnoid hemorrhage include arteriovenous malformations (AVMs), trauma, and cocaine use.

- The patient may have warning symptoms if the ballooning artery applies pressure to brain tissue, or minor warning symptoms may result from leaking of an aneurysm before major rupture. Sudden onset of a severe headache that is different from a previous headache and typically the "worst headache of one's life" is a characteristic symptom of a ruptured aneurysm.
- Loss of consciousness may or may not occur, and the patient's level of consciousness may range from alert to comatose, depending on the severity of the bleeding.

- Other manifestations include focal neurologic deficits (including cranial nerve deficits), nausea, vomiting, seizures, and stiff neck.
- Despite improvements in surgical techniques and management, many patients with subarachnoid hemorrhage die or are left with significant disability.

Clinical Manifestations

Neurologic manifestations do not significantly differ between ischemic and hemorrhagic stroke, because destruction of neural tissue is the basis of manifestations for both types of stroke. Clinical manifestations are related to the location of the stroke. Manifestations seen with specific cerebral artery involvement are listed in Table 81. Figure 23 illustrates manifestations of right- and left-sided stroke.

Motor Function

Motor deficits are the most obvious effect of stroke. Motor deficits include impairment of (1) mobility, (2) respiratory function, (3) swallowing and speech, (4) gag reflex, and (5) self-care abilities. Symptoms are caused by the destruction of motor neurons in the pyramidal pathway (nerve fibers from the brain that pass through the spinal cord to the motor cells). Because the pyramidal pathway crosses at the level of the medulla, a lesion on one side of the brain affects motor function on the opposite side of the brain

TABLE 81 Stroke Manifestations Related to Artery Involvement	
Artery	**Manifestations**
Anterior cerebral	Motor and/or sensory deficit (contralateral), sucking or rooting reflex, rigidity, gait problems, loss of proprioception and fine touch
Middle cerebral	*Dominant side:* Aphasia, motor and sensory deficit, hemianopsia *Nondominant side:* Neglect, motor and sensory deficit, hemianopsia
Posterior cerebral	Hemianopsia, visual hallucination, spontaneous pain, motor deficit
Vertebral	Cranial nerve deficits, diplopia, dizziness, nausea, vomiting, dysarthria, dysphagia, and/or coma

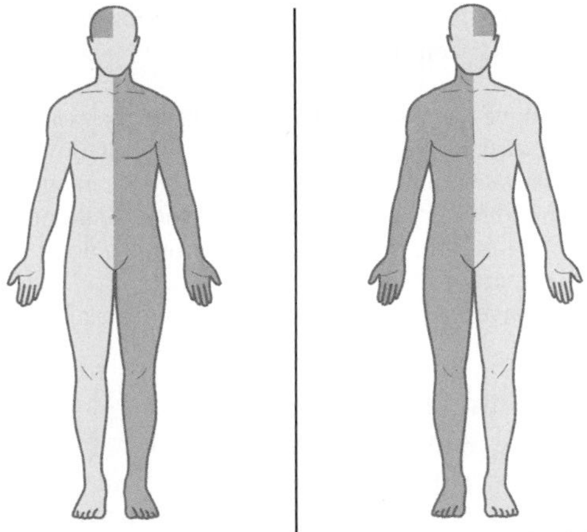

Right-brain damage (stroke on right side of the brain)	Left-brain damage (stroke on left side of the brain)
• Paralyzed left side: hemiplegia	• Paralyzed right side: hemiplegia
• Left-sided neglect	• Impaired speech/language aphasias
• Spatial-perceptual deficits	• Impaired right/left discrimination
• Tends to deny or minimize problems	• Slow performance, cautious
• Rapid performance, short attention span	• Aware of deficits: depression, anxiety
• Impulsive, safety problems	• Impaired comprehension related to language, math
• Impaired judgment	
• Impaired time concepts	

Fig. 23 Manifestations of right- and left-brain stroke.

(contralateral). Impaired spatial-perceptual orientation may further affect mobility.

■ The initial *hyporeflexia* (depressed reflexes) progresses to *hyperreflexia* (hyperactive reflexes) for most patients.

Communication

The left hemisphere is dominant for language skills in all right-handed people and most left-handed people.

■ Language disorders involve the expression and comprehension of written or spoken words. *Aphasia* (loss of comprehension and use of language) occurs when a stroke damages the dominant hemisphere of the brain.

- Many stroke patients also experience *dysarthria,* a disturbance in the muscular control of speech.

Affect

Patients who have had a stroke may have difficulty expressing their emotions. Emotional responses may be exaggerated or unpredictable. Depression and feelings associated with changes in body image and loss of function can make this worse. Patients may also be frustrated by mobility and communication problems.

Intellectual Function

Patients who have had a stroke may show impaired memory and judgment.

Diagnostic Studies

Diagnostic study results confirm manifestations of a stroke, identify likely causes, and guide decisions about therapy.

- MRI is more effective in identifying ischemic stroke than CT scans. However, CT scan is a rapid tool to rule out hemorrhage.
- CT angiography (CTA) provides visualization of cerebral blood vessels and an estimate of perfusion. CTA also detects filling defects in the cerebral arteries.
- Magnetic resonance angiography (MRA) can detect vascular lesions and blockages similar to CTA.
- Angiography can identify cervical and cerebrovascular occlusion, atherosclerotic plaques, and malformation of vessels.
- Intraarterial digital subtraction angiography (DSA) involves injection of a contrast agent to visualize vessels in the neck and Circle of Willis.
- Transcranial Doppler (TCD) ultrasonography has been effective in detecting microemboli and vasospasm in the major cerebral arteries.
- If the suspected cause of the stroke includes emboli from the heart, diagnostic cardiac tests should be done.

Interprofessional Care

Prevention

The goals of stroke prevention include management of modifiable risk factors to prevent a stroke. Health promotion focuses on (1) healthy diet, (2) weight control, (3) regular exercise, (4) not smoking, (5) limiting alcohol consumption, (6) BP management, and (7) routine health assessments. Patients with known risk factors such as DM, hypertension, obesity, high serum lipids, or cardiac dysfunction require close management.

- Measures to prevent the development of a thrombus or embolus are used in patients with TIAs because they are at high risk for stroke. Antiplatelet drugs are usually the chosen treatment to prevent stroke in patients who have had a TIA. Aspirin at a dose of 81 to 325 mg/day is the most frequently used antiplatelet agent. Other drugs include ticlopidine, clopidogrel (Plavix), dipyridamole (Persantine), and combined dipyridamole and aspirin (Aggrenox). For patients who have atrial fibrillation, oral anticoagulation can include warfarin (Coumadin) and the direct factor Xa inhibitors: rivaroxaban (Xarelto), dabigatran (Pradaxa), and apixaban (Eliquis). Statins (simvastatin [Zocor], lovastatin) have also been shown to be effective in the prevention of stroke for individuals who have experienced a TIA in the past.

- Surgical therapy for the patient with TIA from carotid disease includes carotid endarterectomy, transluminal angioplasty, and stenting.

Acute Care: Ischemic Stroke

The goals of acute care are preserving life, preventing further brain damage, and reducing disability. In the unresponsive person, acute care begins with managing the airway, breathing, and circulation. O_2 administration, artificial airway insertion, intubation, and mechanical ventilation may be required. Table 57-7, Lewis et al, *Medical-Surgical Nursing*, ed 10, p. 1354, outlines emergency management of the patient with a stroke.

- After baseline neurologic assessment, patients are monitored closely for signs of increasing neurologic deficit.
- Elevated BP is common immediately after a stroke and may be a protective response to maintain cerebral perfusion. Immediately after ischemic stroke in those patients who do not receive fibrinolytic therapy, the use of drugs to lower BP is recommended only if BP is markedly increased (systolic BP greater than 220 mm Hg or diastolic greater than 120 mm Hg).
- Fluid and electrolyte balance must be controlled carefully. Adequate fluid intake is a priority. Although the goal is to maintain perfusion to the brain, overhydration may compromise perfusion by increasing cerebral edema. Management of increased ICP includes practices that improve venous drainage such as elevating the head of the bed, maintaining head and neck in alignment, and avoiding hip flexion. For additional measures that reduce ICP, see Increased Intracranial Pressure, p. 342.

Drug Therapy.   Recombinant tissue plasminogen activator (tPA) is administered IV to reestablish blood flow and prevent cell death for patients with acute onset of ischemic stroke. This drug must be administered within 3 to 4.5 hours of the onset of clinical signs. Patients are screened carefully before tPA can be given, including a CT or MRI scan to rule out hemorrhagic stroke, blood tests for

S

coagulation disorders, and screening for recent history of GI bleeding, head trauma, or major surgery.

- During infusion, closely monitor the patient's vital signs to assess for improvement or deterioration related to intracerebral hemorrhage.
- Control of BP is critical during and for 24 hours after treatment.
- Aspirin may be initiated within 24 to 48 hours of an ischemic stroke. Other platelet inhibitors including ticlopidine, clopidogrel (Plavix), and dipyridamole (Persantine) or anticoagulants may also be used to prevent further clot formation.

Surgical Therapy. Stent retrievers (e.g., Solitaire FR, Trevo) are a way of opening blocked arteries in the brain by using a removable stent system. Stent retrievers are becoming the most effective way of managing ischemic stroke.

Acute Care: Hemorrhagic Stroke

Drug Therapy. Anticoagulants and platelet inhibitors are contraindicated in patients with hemorrhagic stroke. The main drug therapy for patients with hemorrhagic stroke is that for management of hypertension. Oral and IV agents may be used to maintain BP within a normal to high-normal range (systolic BP less than 160 mm Hg).

- Seizure prophylaxis in the acute period after intracerebral and subarachnoid hemorrhages is situation specific.

Surgical Therapy. Surgical interventions for hemorrhagic stroke include immediate evacuation of aneurysm-induced hematomas or cerebellar hematomas larger than 3 cm. Individuals who have an AVM may experience a hemorrhagic stroke if the AVM ruptures.

- Treatment of AVM is with surgical resection and/or radiosurgery (i.e., Gamma Knife). Both may be preceded by interventional neuroradiology procedures to embolize the blood vessels that supply the AVM.

Subarachnoid hemorrhage is usually caused by a ruptured aneurysm. Approximately 20% of patients will have multiple aneurysms. Treatment of an aneurysm involves clipping or coiling the aneurysm to prevent rebleeding.

- After aneurysmal occlusion via clipping or coiling, hyperdynamic therapy (hemodilution-induced hypertension achieved using vasoconstricting agents such as phenylephrine or dopamine and hypervolemia) may be instituted in an effort to increase the mean arterial pressure and increase cerebral perfusion. Volume expansion is achieved using crystalloid or colloid solution.
- The calcium channel blocker nimodipine is given to patients with subarachnoid hemorrhage to decrease the effects of vasospasm and to minimize cerebral damage.

- Subarachnoid and intracerebral hemorrhage can involve bleeding into the ventricles of the brain. Insertion of a ventriculostomy can dramatically improve CSF drainage.

Rehabilitation Care

After the stroke has stabilized for 12 to 24 hours, care shifts from preserving life to lessening disability and achieving optimal function. Many of the interventions discussed in the acute phase are maintained during this phase.

Nursing Management

Goals

Establish the goals of nursing care together with the patient, caregiver, and family. Typical goals are that the patient will (1) maintain a stable or improved level of consciousness, (2) achieve maximum physical functioning, (3) attain maximum self-care abilities and skills, (4) maintain stable body functions (e.g., bladder control), (5) maximize communication abilities, (6) maintain adequate nutrition, (7) avoid complications of stroke, and (8) maintain effective personal and family coping.

See eNursing Care Plan 57-1 for the patient with stroke on the website.

Nursing Diagnoses

- Decreased intracranial adaptive capacity
- Risk for aspiration
- Impaired physical mobility
- Impaired verbal communication
- Unilateral neglect
- Impaired urinary elimination
- Impaired swallowing
- Situational low self-esteem

Nursing Interventions

Respiratory System. During the acute phase after a stroke, management of respiratory function is a nursing priority. An oropharyngeal airway may be used in comatose patients to prevent the tongue from falling back and obstructing the airway and to provide access for suctioning. Alternatively, a nasopharyngeal airway may be used to provide airway protection and access. Interventions include frequently assessing airway patency and function, providing oxygenation, suctioning, promoting patient mobility, positioning the patient to prevent aspiration, and encouraging deep breathing.

Neurologic System. The primary clinical assessment tool to evaluate and document neurologic status in acute stroke patients is the National Institutes of Health (NIH) Stroke Scale (NIHSS), which measures stroke severity (see NIHSS in Table 57-10, Lewis et al, *Medical-Surgical Nursing,* ed 10, p. 1358). A decreasing level of consciousness may indicate increasing ICP.

Cardiovascular System. Nursing goals for the cardiovascular system are aimed at maintaining homeostasis. Interventions include (1) monitoring vital signs frequently; (2) monitoring cardiac rhythms; (3) calculating intake and output, noting imbalances; (4) regulating IV infusions; (5) adjusting fluid intake to the individual needs of the patient; (6) monitoring lung sounds for crackles and rhonchi indicating pulmonary congestion; and (7) monitoring heart sounds for murmurs or for S_3 or S_4 heart sounds.

- After a stroke, the patient is at risk for venous thromboembolism (VTE), especially in a weak or paralyzed lower extremity. The most effective prevention is to keep the patient moving. Teach active range-of-motion (ROM) exercises if the patient has voluntary movement in the affected extremity. For the patient with hemiplegia, perform passive ROM exercises several times each day.

- Other measures to prevent VTE include positioning to minimize the effects of dependent edema and the use of sequential compression devices.

Musculoskeletal System. The goal for the musculoskeletal system is to maintain optimal function, which is accomplished by prevention of joint contractures and muscle atrophy.

- In the acute phase, ROM exercises and positioning are important interventions. Passive ROM exercise is begun on the first day of hospitalization. Muscle atrophy secondary to lack of innervation and inactivity can develop after a stroke, so exercise is an important intervention for rehabilitation and recovery.

Interventions to optimize musculoskeletal function include (1) trochanter roll at the hip to prevent external rotation; (2) hand cones (not rolled washcloths) to prevent hand contractures; (3) arm supports with slings and lap boards to prevent shoulder displacement; (4) avoidance of pulling the patient by the arm to avoid shoulder displacement; (5) posterior leg splints, footboards, or high-top tennis shoes to prevent footdrop; and (6) hand splints to reduce spasticity.

Integumentary System. Interventions for prevention of skin breakdown include (1) pressure relief by position changes, special mattresses, or wheelchair cushions; (2) good skin hygiene; (3) emollients applied to dry skin; and (4) early mobility. An example of a position change schedule is side-back-side, with a maximum duration of 2 hours for any position.

- Position the patient on the weak or paralyzed side for only 30 minutes. If an area of redness develops and does not return to normal color within 15 minutes of pressure relief, the epidermis and dermis are damaged.

- Do not massage the damaged area, because this may cause additional damage. Control of pressure is the single most important factor in both the prevention and treatment of skin breakdown.

Gastrointestinal System. The most common bowel problem is constipation. Physical activity also promotes bowel function. Laxatives, suppositories, or additional stool softeners may be ordered if the patient does not respond to increased fluid and fiber. Bowel retraining may be needed and continues into the rehabilitation phase.

Urinary System. In the acute stage of stroke, the primary urinary problem is poor bladder control, resulting in incontinence.

- Take steps to promote normal bladder function and avoid the use of an indwelling catheter.
- Long-term use of an indwelling catheter is associated with urinary tract infections and delayed bladder retraining. An intermittent catheterization program may be used for patients with urinary retention.

Nutrition. The patient may initially receive IV infusions to maintain fluid and electrolyte balance and to administer drugs. Patients with severe impairment may require enteral or parenteral nutrition support. Patients should have their nutritional needs addressed in the first 72 hours of admission to the hospital, because nutrition is important for recovery and healing.

- To assess swallowing ability, elevate the head of the bed to an upright position (unless contraindicated) and give the patient a small amount of crushed ice or ice water to swallow. If the gag reflex is present and the patient is able to swallow safely, you may proceed with feeding.
- Place food on the unaffected side of the mouth. Feedings must be followed by scrupulous oral hygiene because food may collect on the affected side of the mouth.

Communication. During the acute stage, your role in meeting the psychologic needs of the patient is primarily supportive.

- An alert patient is usually anxious because of a lack of understanding of what has happened and the inability to communicate. Give the patient extra time to comprehend and respond to communication.

Sensory-Perceptual Alterations. *Homonymous hemianopsia* (blindness in the same half of each visual field) is a common problem after a stroke.

- Initially help the patient to compensate by arranging the environment within the patient's perceptual field, such as arranging

S

the food tray so that all food is on the right side or the left side to accommodate for field of vision.

- Later the patient learns to compensate for the visual defect by consciously attending to or scanning the neglected side. The weak or paralyzed extremities are carefully checked for adequacy of dressing, hygiene, and trauma.

Other visual problems may include diplopia, loss of the corneal reflex, and ptosis, especially if the stroke is in the vertebrobasilar arterial distribution. Diplopia is often treated with an eye patch. If the corneal reflex is absent, the patient is at risk for a corneal abrasion and should be observed closely for and protected against eye injuries.

Coping.   A stroke is usually a sudden, extremely stressful event for the patient, caregiver, and significant others.

- Reactions vary considerably but may involve fear, apprehension, denial of severity of the stroke, depression, anger, and sorrow.
- During the acute phase of caring for the patient and family, nursing interventions designed to facilitate coping involve providing information and emotional support.
- Explanations to the patient should be clear and understandable. Decision making and upholding the patient's wishes during this challenging time are of utmost importance.

Home Care and Rehabilitation.   The patient is usually discharged from the acute care setting to home, an intermediate or long-term care facility, or a rehabilitation facility. You have an excellent opportunity to prepare the patient and family for hospital discharge through teaching, demonstration and return demonstration, practice, and evaluation of self-care skills before discharge. Total care is considered in discharge planning in relation to medications, nutrition, mobility, exercises, hygiene, and toileting.

Follow-up care is carefully planned to permit continuing nursing, physical, occupational, and speech therapy, as well as medical care.

Rehabilitation requires an interprofessional approach so that patient and caregiver can benefit from the combined, expert care of a stroke team. The team must communicate and coordinate care to achieve the patient's goals. You are in a good position to facilitate this process and are often the key to successful rehabilitation efforts.

The rehabilitation nurse assesses the patient, caregiver, and family with attention to (1) rehabilitation potential of the patient, (2) physical status of all body systems, (3) presence of complications caused by the stroke or other chronic conditions, (4) cognitive status of the patient, (5) family resources and support, and (6) expectations of the patient and caregiver related to the rehabilitation program.

Rehabilitation and long-term management of the stroke patient are further described in Chapter 57 of Lewis et al, *Medical-Surgical Nursing,* ed 10.

▼ **Patient and Caregiver Teaching**

- Provide the caregiver with instruction and practice in home care while the patient is hospitalized. This allows for support and encouragement as well as opportunities for feedback. Adjustments in the home environment, such as the removal of a door to accommodate a wheelchair, can be made before discharge.
- Your instruction related to home care should include exercise and ambulation techniques; dietary requirements; recognition of signs indicating the possibility of another stroke (e.g., headache, vertigo, numbness, visual disturbances); understanding of emotional lability and the possibility of depression; medication routine; and time, place, and frequency of follow-up activities, such as occupational therapy and physical therapy.
- Assist the caregiver to stay healthy after the patient is discharged. Emphasize the importance of planning for respite or rest from caregiving activities on a regular basis.

SYPHILIS

Description

Syphilis is a sexually transmitted bacterial infection that can have serious long-term complications if not treated effectively. There has been a shift in the population most affected by syphilis, with rates highest among men 20 to 29 years old and 75% of new cases reported among men who have sex with men.

Pathophysiology

Syphilis is caused by *Treponema pallidum,* a bacterial spirochete. It is transmitted through direct contact with a syphilitic lesion called a chancre, which can occur externally on the genitals, anus, or lips or internally in the vagina, rectum, mouth, or tongue.

- The incubation period for syphilis can range from 10 to 90 days (average, 21 days).
- An infected pregnant woman can transmit syphilis to her fetus during her pregnancy and is at high risk for stillbirth or having babies that develop complications after birth including seizures and death.

Clinical Manifestations

Signs and symptoms of syphilis can mimic those of other infections. Consequently, compared with other STIs, it is more difficult

S

to recognize syphilis. Without treatment, the infection progresses to the next stage.

- In the *primary stage, chancres* (painless indurated lesions found on the penis, vulva, and lips and in the mouth, vagina, and rectum) occur 10 to 90 days after inoculation. The draining of the microorganisms into the lymph nodes causes regional lymphadenopathy.
- In the *secondary stage,* syphilis is systemic. Bacteria spread to all major organ systems. Manifestations include flu-like symptoms and generalized adenopathy. Cutaneous lesions include a bilateral, symmetric nonpruritic rash usually involving the trunk, palms, and soles; mucous patches in the mouth, tongue, or cervix; and condylomata lata (moist, weeping papules) in the anal and genital area.
- *Latent* syphilis follows the secondary stage and is a period during which the immune system is able to suppress the infection. There are no signs or symptoms of syphilis during this time.
- The *late* or *tertiary stage* of syphilis is the most severe, which appears 1 to 20 years after initial infection. Because antibiotics can cure syphilis, manifestations of late syphilis are rare. When late syphilis occurs, it is responsible for significant morbidity and mortality.

Complications

Complications mostly occur in late syphilis. The *gummas* (destructive lesions) of late syphilis may produce irreparable damage to bone, liver, or skin.

- In cardiovascular syphilis, the resulting aneurysm may press on structures such as the intercostal nerves, causing pain. Scarring of the aortic valve results in aortic valve insufficiency and heart failure.
- Neurosyphilis causes degeneration of the brain with mental deterioration. Problems related to sensory nerve involvement are a result of *tabes dorsalis* (progressive locomotor ataxia). Loss of vision and position sense in the feet and legs can also occur. Walking becomes more difficult as joint stability is lost. There may be sudden attacks of pain anywhere in the body.

Diagnostic Studies

- Detailed and accurate sexual history is important.
- Darkfield microscopy and direct fluorescent antibody tests of lesion exudate or tissue can confirm the diagnosis.
- To screen for syphilis, Venereal Disease Research Laboratory (VDRL) and rapid plasma reagin (RPR) testing can detect

nonspecific antitreponemal antibodies, which are usually positive 10 to 14 days after chancre appearance.

- To confirm a diagnosis of syphilis, the fluorescent treponemal antibody absorption (FTA-ABS) test and the *T. pallidum* particle agglutination (TP-PA) test can detect specific antitreponemal antibodies.

Interprofessional Care

Management is aimed at initiating treatment early and eradicating all syphilitic organisms. However, treatment cannot reverse damage that is already present in the late stage of the disease.

- Penicillin G benzathine is the recommended treatment for all stages of syphilis. When penicillin is contraindicated, doxycycline or tetracycline may be used. Aqueous procaine penicillin G is the treatment of choice for neurosyphilis.
- It is important that all sexual contacts in the last 90 days be treated.
- Reexamination and follow-up testing are recommended every 6 months for up to 2 years.

Nursing Management: Syphilis

See Nursing Management: Sexually Transmitted Infections, pp. 564-565.

SYSTEMIC EXERTION INTOLERANCE DISEASE

Description

Systemic exertion intolerance disease (SEID), formerly known as chronic fatigue syndrome, is a serious, complex, multisystem disease where individual exertion (physical, emotional, cognitive) can adversely affect multiple organs. SEID is a poorly understood disease that can have a devastating impact on patients and their families.

SEID affects at least 83,000 to 2.5 million people in the United States, with the true prevalence unknown. Women are affected more often than men. SEID occurs in all ethnic and socioeconomic groups.

Pathophysiology

The precise mechanisms of SEID remain unknown, with many theories about the etiology.

- Neuroendocrine abnormalities have been implicated involving a hypofunction of the hypothalamic-pituitary-adrenal (HPA) axis and hypothalamic-pituitary-gonadal axis, which together regulate the stress response and reproductive hormone levels.

- Several microorganisms have been investigated as etiologic agents, including herpesviruses (e.g., Epstein-Barr virus [EBV], cytomegalovirus [CMV]), retroviruses, enteroviruses, *Candida albicans, Mycoplasma.*
- Because of cognitive deficits such as decreased memory, attention, and concentration, it has been proposed that SEID is caused by changes in the central nervous system.

Clinical Manifestations and Diagnostic Studies

It is often difficult to distinguish between SEID and fibromyalgia because many clinical features are similar (Table 82). In about half of cases, SEID develops insidiously, or intermittent episodes gradually become chronic. A diagnosis of SEID requires the patient have three symptoms: (1) profound fatigue lasting at least 6 months, (2) postexertional malaise, total exhaustion after minor physical or mental exertion that patients sometimes describe as a "crash," and

TABLE 82 Common Features of Fibromyalgia and Systemic Exertion Intolerance Disease (SEID)	
Common Feature	**Description**
Occurrence	Affects previously healthy young and middle-aged women.
Etiology (theories)	Infectious trigger, dysfunction in HPA axis, alteration in CNS
Clinical manifestations	Generalized musculoskeletal pain, malaise and fatigue, cognitive dysfunction, headaches, sleep disturbances, depression, anxiety, fever
Disease course	Variable intensity of symptoms, fluctuates over time
Diagnosis	No definitive laboratory tests or joint and muscle examinations. Mainly a diagnosis of exclusion
Therapy	Symptomatic treatment may include antidepressant drugs such as amitriptyline and fluoxetine (Prozac). Other measures are heat, massage, regular stretching, biofeedback, stress management, and relaxation training. Patient and caregiver teaching is essential.

HPA, Hypothalamic-pituitary-adrenal.

(3) unrefreshing sleep. The presence of either cognitive impairment or *orthostatic intolerance* (worsening of symptoms upon standing) is also required for diagnosis.

- The patient may become angry and frustrated with the inability of HCPs to diagnose the problem. The disorder may have a major impact on work and family responsibilities.

Physical examination and diagnostic studies can rule out other possible causes of the patient's symptoms. No laboratory test can diagnose SEID or measure its severity.

Nursing and Interprofessional Management

Because no definitive treatment exists for SEID, supportive management is essential. Tell the patient what is known about the disease. Take complaints seriously.

- Nonsteroidal antiinflammatory drugs (NSAIDs) can be used to treat headaches, muscle and joint aches, and fever. Antihistamines and decongestants can be used to treat allergic symptoms. Tricyclic antidepressants (e.g., doxepin, amitriptyline) and selective serotonin reuptake inhibitors (e.g., fluoxetine [Prozac], paroxetine [Paxil]) can improve mood and sleep disorders. Clonazepam (Klonopin) can also be used to treat sleep disturbances and panic disorders.
- Total rest can potentiate the self-image of being an invalid, whereas strenuous exertion can exacerbate the exhaustion. Therefore it is important to plan a carefully graduated exercise program.
- Behavioral therapy may be used to promote a positive outlook, as well as to lessen overall disability, fatigue, and other symptoms.
- One of the major problems facing many patients with SEID is economic security. When the illness strikes, they cannot work or must decrease work time.

SEID does not appear to progress. Although most patients recover or at least gradually improve over time, some do not show substantial improvement. Recovery is more common in individuals with a sudden onset of SEID.

SYSTEMIC INFLAMMATORY RESPONSE SYNDROME (SIRS) AND MULTIPLE ORGAN DYSFUNCTION SYNDROME (MODS)

Description

Systemic inflammatory response syndrome (SIRS) is a systemic inflammatory response to a variety of insults, including infection (referred to as sepsis), ischemia, infarction, and injury. Generalized inflammation in organs remote from the initial insult characterizes SIRS. Many mechanisms can trigger a systemic inflammatory response, including:

- *Mechanical tissue trauma*: burns, crush injuries, surgical procedures
- *Abscess formation*: intraabdominal, extremities
- *Ischemic or necrotic tissue*: pancreatitis, vascular disease, myocardial infarction
- *Microbial invasion*: bacteria, viruses, fungi, parasites
- *Endotoxin release*: gram-negative and gram-positive bacteria
- *Global perfusion deficits*: post–cardiac resuscitation, shock states
- *Regional perfusion deficits*: distal perfusion deficits

Multiple organ dysfunction syndrome (MODS) is failure of two or more organ systems in an acutely ill patient such that homeostasis cannot be maintained without intervention. MODS results from SIRS, but the transition from SIRS to MODS does not occur in a clear-cut manner.

- Prognosis for the patient with MODS is poor, with mortality rates at 70% to 80% when three or more organ systems fail.

Pathophysiology and Clinical Manifestations

When the inflammatory response is activated, consequences occur, including activation of inflammatory cells and release of mediators, direct damage to the endothelium, and hypermetabolism.

- An increase in vascular permeability allows mediators and protein to leak out of the endothelium and into the interstitial space.
- WBCs begin to digest the foreign debris, and the coagulation cascade is activated.
- Hypotension, decreased perfusion, microemboli, and redistributed or shunted blood flow eventually compromise organ perfusion.

The respiratory system is often the first system to show signs of dysfunction in SIRS and MODS. Inflammatory mediators have a direct effect on the pulmonary vasculature. Endothelial damage from the release of inflammatory mediators results in increased capillary permeability. Fluid then moves to the alveoli, causing alveolar edema. Alveoli collapse, and the end result is acute respiratory distress syndrome (ARDS) (see p. 13).

Cardiovascular changes include myocardial depression and massive vasodilation in response to increasing tissue demands. To compensate for hypotension, heart rate and stroke volume increase, but increased capillary permeability diminishes venous return and thus preload. Eventually, either perfusion of vital organs becomes insufficient or the cells are unable to use oxygen, and their function is further compromised.

Neurologic dysfunction commonly manifests as mental status changes, which can be an early sign of SIRS or MODS. Confusion, agitation, disorientation, lethargy, or coma may occur. These changes may be caused by hypoxemia or may be the direct effect of inflammatory mediators or impaired perfusion.

Acute kidney injury is frequently seen in SIRS and MODS. Hypoperfusion and the effects of the mediators can cause acute kidney injury. Antibiotics commonly used to treat gram-negative bacteria (e.g., aminoglycosides) can be nephrotoxic. Careful monitoring of drug levels is essential to avoid the nephrotoxic effects.

In the early stages of SIRS and MODS, blood is shunted away from the GI mucosa, making it highly vulnerable to ischemic injury. Decreased perfusion leads to a breakdown of the mucosal barrier, thereby increasing the risk for ulceration and GI bleeding.

- Breakdown of the mucosal barrier of the gut also results in the potential for bacterial movement from the GI tract into the circulation.

Metabolic changes are pronounced in SIRS and MODS. Both syndromes trigger a hypermetabolic response. The net result is a catabolic state, and lean body mass (muscle) is lost.

- The hypermetabolism may last for days and results in liver dysfunction.
- The liver is unable to synthesize albumin that is necessary to maintain plasma oncotic pressure, adding to the loss of intravascular fluid to the interstitial space.
- As the state of hypermetabolism persists, the patient is unable to convert lactate to glucose, and lactate accumulates (lactic acidosis). Eventually the liver is unable to maintain a glucose level, and the patient becomes hypoglycemic.

Disseminated intravascular coagulation (DIC) may result from dysfunction of the coagulation system. DIC results in simultaneous microvascular clotting and bleeding because of the depletion of clotting factors and platelets in addition to excessive fibrinolysis (see Disseminated Intravascular Coagulation, p. 191).

Electrolyte imbalances are common and result from hormonal and metabolic changes and fluid shifts. These changes exacerbate mental status changes, neuromuscular dysfunction, and dysrhythmias.

- Release of antidiuretic hormone and aldosterone results in sodium and water retention; aldosterone increases urinary potassium loss, and catecholamines cause potassium to move into the cells, resulting in hypokalemia.

- Metabolic acidosis results from impaired tissue perfusion, hypoxia, a shift to anaerobic metabolism, and progressive renal dysfunction.
- Hypocalcemia, hypomagnesemia, and hypophosphatemia are common.

The clinical manifestations of SIRS and MODS are presented in Table 66-10, Lewis et al, *Medical-Surgical Nursing,* ed 10, p. 1606.

Nursing and Interprofessional Management

The most important goal in the management of SIRS and MODS is to prevent the progression of SIRS to MODS. A critical component of the nursing role is vigilant assessment and ongoing monitoring to detect early signs of deterioration or organ dysfunction.

Interprofessional care of patients with MODS focuses on prevention and treatment of infection, maintenance of tissue oxygenation, nutritional and metabolic support, and appropriate support for individual failing organs.

- Aggressive infection control is essential to decrease the risk for health care–associated infections (HAIs). Early, aggressive surgery is recommended to remove necrotic tissue (e.g., early debridement of burn tissue), which can provide a culture medium for microorganisms. Aggressive pulmonary management, including early ambulation, can reduce the risk of infection. Strict asepsis can decrease infections related to intraarterial lines, endotracheal tubes, urinary catheters, IV lines, and other invasive devices or procedures.
- Hypoxemia frequently occurs in patients with SIRS or MODS. Interventions to decrease oxygen demand and increase oxygen delivery are essential. Sedation, mechanical ventilation, analgesia, and rest may decrease oxygen demand and should be considered.
- Hypermetabolism in SIRS or MODS can result in profound weight loss, cachexia, and further organ failure. Nutritional support is vital to preserve organ function. Providing early and adequate nutrition decreases morbidity and mortality. The use of the enteral route is preferred to parenteral nutrition.

Support of any failing organ is a primary goal of therapy. For example, the patient with ARDS requires aggressive oxygen therapy and mechanical ventilation. Renal failure may require dialysis or continuous renal replacement therapy.

A final consideration may be that further interventions are futile. It is important to maintain communication between the health care team and the patient's family and caregivers regarding realistic goals and likely outcomes for the patient with MODS. Withdrawal of life support and providing end-of-life care may be the best option for the patient.

SYSTEMIC LUPUS ERYTHEMATOSUS

Description

Systemic lupus erythematosus (SLE) is a multisystem inflammatory autoimmune disease. It typically affects the skin, joints, serous membranes (pleura, pericardium), and renal, hematologic, and neurologic systems. SLE is marked by a chronic unpredictable course, with alternating exacerbations and remissions. Women are 6 to 10 times more likely to develop SLE than men. It is observed more often in African Americans, Asian Americans, and Native Americans than in whites.

Pathophysiology

The etiology of the abnormal immune response in SLE is unknown. Based on the high prevalence of SLE among family members, a genetic influence is suspected.

- Hormones are also known to play a role in the etiology of SLE. Onset or worsening of disease symptoms sometimes occurs after menarche, with the use of oral contraceptives, and during or after pregnancy. SLE symptoms worsen in the immediate postpartum period.

- Environmental factors believed to contribute to the occurrence of SLE include sun or ultraviolet light exposure, stress, and exposure to some chemicals and toxins. Infectious agents such as viruses also may stimulate immune hyperactivity. In addition, at least 40 medications currently in use may trigger SLE. Frequently identified drugs are procainamide, hydralazine, and quinidine.

SLE is characterized by the production of various autoantibodies against nucleic acids (e.g., single- and double-stranded deoxyribonucleic acid [DNA]), erythrocytes, coagulation proteins, lymphocytes, and platelets. Autoimmune reactions are directed against constituents of the cell nucleus (antinuclear antibodies [ANA]), particularly DNA.

Circulating immune complexes containing antibody against DNA are deposited in the basement membranes of capillaries in the kidneys, heart, skin, brain, and joints. These complexes trigger inflammation that causes tissue destruction. An overaggressive autoimmune response is also related to activation of B and

S

T cells. Specific disease effects depend on the involved cell types or organs.

Clinical Manifestations and Complications

No characteristic pattern occurs in the progressive organ involvement. General complaints, including fever, weight loss, joint pain *(arthralgia),* and excessive fatigue, may precede an exacerbation of disease activity.

Dermatologic Manifestations

Vascular skin lesions can appear in any location but are most likely to develop in sun-exposed areas. Severe skin reactions can occur in people who are photosensitive. The classic butterfly rash over the cheeks and bridge of the nose occurs in 55% to 85% of patients at some time during the disease.

- Oral or nasopharyngeal membrane ulcers can occur.
- Alopecia is common, and the scalp becomes dry, scaly, and atrophied.

Musculoskeletal Problems

Polyarthralgia, pain in multiple joints, with morning stiffness is often the patient's first complaint. Arthritis occurs in 95% of patients with SLE. Diffuse swelling is accompanied by joint and muscle pain.

- Lupus-related arthritis is generally nonerosive, but it may cause deformities such as swan neck, ulnar deviation, and subluxation with hyperlaxity of the joints.

Cardiopulmonary Problems

Tachypnea and cough in patients with SLE suggest restrictive lung disease. Cardiac involvement including dysrhythmias resulting from fibrosis of the sinoatrial (SA) and atrioventricular (AV) nodes indicates advanced disease.

- Hypertension and hypercholesterolemia require aggressive treatment and careful monitoring.

Renal Problems

About 75% of persons with SLE experience kidney damage. Renal involvement varies from mild proteinuria to rapid, progressive glomerulonephritis. Treatment typically includes corticosteroids, cytotoxic agents (cyclophosphamide), and immunosuppressive agents (azathioprine [Imuran], cyclosporine, and mycophenolate mofetil [CellCept]).

Nervous System Problems

Seizures are the most common neurologic manifestation. They are generally controlled by corticosteroids or antiseizure drugs.

- Cognitive dysfunction may result from the deposition of immune complexes within the brain tissue. It is marked by disordered thinking, disorientation, and memory deficits. Various psychiatric disorders reported in SLE include depression, mood disorders, anxiety, and psychosis, although they may be related to the stress of having a major illness or to associated drug therapies. Occasionally a stroke or aseptic meningitis may be attributable to SLE. Headaches are common and can become severe during a flare (exacerbation).

Hematologic Problems

Abnormal blood conditions are common in SLE due to the formation of antibodies against blood cells. Anemia, leukopenia, thrombocytopenia, and coagulation disorders (excessive bleeding or clotting) are often present. Many patients with SLE benefit from high-intensity treatment with warfarin.

Infections

Patients with SLE appear to have increased susceptibility to infections, possibly related to defects in the ability to phagocytize invading bacteria, deficiencies in the production of antibodies, and the immunosuppressive effect of many antiinflammatory drugs. Infection, most commonly pneumonia, is a major cause of death.

Diagnostic Studies

- Diagnosis of SLE is based on distinct criteria. No specific test is diagnostic for SLE, but a variety of abnormalities may be present in the blood. SLE is marked by the presence of ANA in 97% of persons with the disease.
- Anti-DNA antibodies are found in one half of the persons with SLE, but lupus can still be present if these antibodies are not identified.
- Anti-Smith (Sm) antibodies are found in 30% to 40% of persons with SLE and are almost always considered diagnostic.
- Nearly 30% of people with SLE have antiphospholipid antibodies. Antibodies to histone are most often seen in people with drug-induced SLE.
- Elevated erythrocyte sedimentation rate (ESR) and C-reactive protein (CRP) levels are not diagnostic of SLE but may be used to monitor disease activity.

Interprofessional Care

A major challenge in SLE treatment is to manage the active phase of the disease while preventing complications of treatment. The prognosis of SLE can be improved with early diagnosis, prompt recognition of serious organ involvement, and effective therapeutic regimens.

Drug Therapy

Nonsteroidal antiinflammatory drugs (NSAIDs) are an important intervention, especially for patients with mild polyarthralgia or polyarthritis. Antimalarial agents such as hydroxychloroquine (Plaquenil) are also often used to treat fatigue and moderate skin and joint problems, as well as to prevent flares.

Corticosteroid therapy should be limited, but tapering doses of IV methylprednisolone may control exacerbations of polyarthritis. Steroid-sparing immunosuppressants (e.g., methotrexate) can serve as an alternate treatment.

Immunosuppressive drugs such as azathioprine (Imuran) and cyclophosphamide may be prescribed to reduce the need for long-term corticosteroid therapy or to treat severe organ-system disease, such as lupus nephritis.

- Topical immunomodulators are an alternative to corticosteroids for treating serious skin conditions. Tacrolimus (Protopic) and pimecrolimus (Elidel) suppress immune activity in the skin, including the butterfly rash and possibly discoid (round, coin-shaped) lesions.

Nursing Management
Goals
The patient with SLE will have satisfactory pain relief, adhere to the therapeutic regimen to achieve maximum symptom management, demonstrate awareness of and avoid activities that induce disease exacerbation, and maintain optimal role function and a positive self-image.

Nursing Diagnoses
- Fatigue
- Impaired comfort
- Impaired skin integrity

Nursing Interventions
During an exacerbation, patients may become abruptly and dramatically ill. Nursing interventions include accurately recording the severity of symptoms and documenting response to therapy. Specifically assess fever pattern, joint inflammation, limitation of motion, location and degree of discomfort, and fatigue.

- Monitor the patient's weight and fluid intake and output if corticosteroids are prescribed, because of the fluid-retention effect of these drugs and the possibility of renal failure. Collection of 24-hour urine for protein and creatinine clearance may be ordered.
- Observe for signs of bleeding that result from drug therapy, such as pallor, skin bruising, petechiae, or tarry stools.
- Carefully assess the patient's neurologic status. Assess for visual disturbances, headaches, personality changes, and forgetfulness. Psychosis may indicate central nervous system

disease or may be the effect of corticosteroid therapy. Nerve irritation of the extremities (peripheral neuropathy) may produce numbness, tingling, and weakness of the hands and feet.

- Explain the nature of the disease, therapy, and diagnostic procedures. Emotional support for the patient and family is essential.

▼ Patient and Caregiver Teaching

Help the patient understand that even strong adherence to the treatment plan is not a guarantee against exacerbation, because the course of the disease is unpredictable. Help the patient and caregivers to eliminate or reduce exposure to precipitating factors such as fatigue, sun exposure, emotional stress, infection, drugs, and surgery. Patient and caregiver teaching is outlined in Table 83. Counsel the patient and caregivers that SLE generally has a good prognosis.

- Many couples require pregnancy and sexual counseling. For the best outcome, pregnancy should be planned at a point when the disease activity is minimal.
- Pain and fatigue may interfere with quality of life. Pacing techniques and relaxation therapy can help the patient remain involved in day-to-day activities.

TABLE 83 Patient & Caregiver Teaching

Systemic Lupus Erythematosus

Include the following information in the teaching plan for a patient with systemic lupus erythematosus and the patient's caregiver.

- Disease process
- Names of drugs, actions, side effects, dosage, administration
- Pain management strategies
- Energy conservation and pacing techniques
- Therapeutic exercise, use of heat therapy (for arthralgia)
- Relaxation therapy
- Avoidance of physical and emotional stress
- Avoidance of exposure to individuals with infection
- Avoidance of drying soaps, powders, household chemicals
- Use of sunscreen protection (at least SPF 15) and protective clothing, with minimal sun exposure from 11:00 AM to 3:00 PM
- Regular medical and laboratory evaluations
- Sexual and pregnancy counseling as needed
- Community resources and health care agencies

SPF, Sun protection factor.

S

TESTICULAR CANCER

Description

Testicular cancer is rare, but it is the most common type of cancer in men between 15 and 35 years of age. Testicular tumors are more common in men with undescended testicles (cryptorchidism) in infancy or with a family history of testicular cancer or anomalies. Most testicular cancers develop from two types of embryonic germ cells: seminomas and nonseminomas.

Clinical Manifestations

Testicular cancer may have a slow or rapid onset.

- The patient may notice a painless lump in his scrotum, as well as scrotal swelling. The scrotal mass is usually nontender and very firm.
- Some patients report a dull ache or heavy sensation in the lower abdomen, perianal area, or scrotum.
- Manifestations associated with metastasis include lower back and/or chest pain, cough, and dyspnea.

Diagnostic Studies

- Palpation of scrotal contents is used to assess for masses and swelling.
- Ultrasound of the testes is indicated when testicular cancer is suspected.
- Blood serum levels of α-fetoprotein (AFP), lactate dehydrogenase (LDH), and human chorionic gonadotropin (hCG) are done if testicular cancer is suspected.
- Chest x-ray and CT scan of the abdomen and pelvis are used to detect metastasis.

Nursing and Interprofessional Management

Testicular cancer is one of the most curable types of cancer. Management generally involves a radical orchiectomy (surgical removal of the affected testis, spermatic cord, and regional lymph nodes). Retroperitoneal lymph node dissection and removal may also be done.

- Testicular germ cell tumors are more sensitive to systemic chemotherapy than any other adult solid tumor. Chemotherapy protocols use a combination of agents, including bleomycin, etoposide, ifosfamide (Ifex), and cisplatin.

The prognosis for patients with testicular cancer has improved, and 95% of all patients obtain complete remission if the disease is detected in the early stages. All patients with testicular cancer, regardless of pathology or stage, require meticulous follow-up monitoring and regular physical examinations, chest x-ray, CT scan, and assessment of hCG and AFP. The goal is to detect relapse when tumor burden is minimal.

- Because of the high risk for infertility after chemotherapy and/ or pelvic radiation, the cryopreservation of sperm in a sperm bank before treatment begins should be sensitively discussed.

THALASSEMIA

Description

Thalassemia is a group of diseases involving inadequate production of normal hemoglobin (Hgb) and therefore decreased erythrocyte production. Hemolysis also occurs in thalassemia.

- Thalassemia is commonly found in members of ethnic groups whose origins are near the Mediterranean Sea and equatorial or near-equatorial regions of Asia, the Middle East, and Africa.

Pathophysiology

Thalassemia has an autosomal recessive genetic basis that results in a decreased or absent globulin protein. α-Globin chains are absent or reduced in α-thalassemia, and β-globin chains are absent or reduced in β-thalassemia. An individual with thalassemia may have a heterozygous or homozygous form of the disease.

- In *thalassemia minor (thalassemic trait),* the person is heterozygous, with one thalassemic gene and one normal gene. Thalassemia minor is a mild form of the disease.
- In *thalassemia major,* the person is homozygous, with two thalassemic genes. Thalassemia major is a severe form of the disease.

Clinical Manifestations

- The patient with thalassemia minor is frequently asymptomatic, with mild to moderate anemia, microcytosis (small cells) and hypochromia (pale cells).
- The patient who has thalassemia major is pale and displays other general manifestations of anemia (see Anemia, p. 29). In addition, the person has marked splenomegaly, hepatomegaly, and jaundice from hemolysis of red blood cells (RBCs). Chronic bone marrow hyperplasia leads to expansion of the marrow space. This may cause thickening of the cranium and the maxillary cavity walls.
- Thalassemia major is a life-threatening disease in which growth, both physical and mental, is often retarded.

T

Interprofessional Care

The laboratory findings in thalassemia major are summarized in Table 8, p. 33.

- Thalassemia minor requires no treatment because the body adapts to the reduction in normal Hgb.
- Thalassemia major is managed with blood transfusions or exchange transfusions in conjunction with chelating agents that bind to iron: oral deferasirox (Exjade) or deferiprone (Ferriprox) or IV or subQ deferoxamine (Desferal). These agents reduce the iron overloading (hemochromatosis) that occurs with chronic transfusion therapy.
- Because RBCs are sequestered in the enlarged spleen, thalassemia may be treated by splenectomy.
- Although hematopoietic stem cell transplantation remains the only cure for patients with thalassemia, the risks associated with this procedure may outweigh its benefits. With proper iron chelation therapy, patients are living longer.

THROMBOANGIITIS OBLITERANS

Thromboangiitis obliterans (Buerger's disease) is a nonatherosclerotic, segmental, recurrent inflammatory vaso-occlusive disorder of the small and medium-sized arteries and veins of the upper and lower extremities. The disorder occurs predominantly in men younger than 45 years of age with a long history of tobacco use, but without other cardiovascular disease (CVD) risk factors (e.g., hypertension, hyperlipidemia, diabetes).

In the acute phase of Buerger's disease, an inflammatory thrombus forms and blocks the vessel. Over time, the thrombus becomes more organized, and the vessel wall inflammation subsides.

During the chronic phase, thrombosis and fibrosis in the vessel cause tissue ischemia. The symptom complex of Buerger's disease is often confused with peripheral artery disease (PAD) and other autoimmune diseases (e.g., scleroderma).

- Patients may have intermittent claudication of the feet, hands, or arms. As the disease progresses, rest pain and ischemic ulcerations develop.
- Other signs and symptoms may include color and temperature changes of the limbs, paresthesia, superficial vein thrombosis, and cold sensitivity.

There are no laboratory or diagnostic tests specific to Buerger's disease. Diagnosis is based on the age at onset, history of tobacco use, clinical symptoms, involvement of distal vessels, presence of ischemic ulcerations, and exclusion of disorders, including diabetes, autoimmune disease, thrombophilia, and other source of emboli.

Treatment is the complete cessation of tobacco and marijuana use in any form. Conservative management includes avoiding limb exposure to cold temperatures, a supervised walking program, antibiotics to treat any infected ulcers, and analgesics to manage the ischemic pain.

Teach patients to avoid trauma to the extremities. Painful ulcerations may require finger or toe amputations. The amputation rate in patients who continue tobacco use after diagnosis is much higher than in those who stop.

THROMBOCYTOPENIA

Description

Thrombocytopenia is a reduction of platelets below 150,000/µL (150 × 10^9/L). Acute, severe, or prolonged decreases from this normal range can result in abnormal hemostasis that manifests as prolonged bleeding from minor trauma or spontaneous bleeding without injury.

Platelet disorders can be inherited (e.g., Wiskott-Aldrich syndrome), but the vast majority are acquired. A common cause of acquired disorders is the ingestion of drugs such as quinine, aspirin, or myelosuppressive chemotherapy agents.

Immune Thrombocytopenic Purpura

Immune thrombocytopenic purpura (ITP), the most common acquired thrombocytopenia, is an autoimmune syndrome of the abnormal destruction of circulating platelets. Antibody-coated platelets, mistakenly identified as foreign, are destroyed by macrophages in the spleen. ITP generally manifests as an acute condition in children and a chronic condition in adults.

Thrombotic Thrombocytopenic Purpura

Thrombotic thrombocytopenic purpura (TTP) is an uncommon syndrome characterized by hemolytic anemia, thrombocytopenia, neurologic abnormalities, fever (in the absence of infection), and renal abnormalities. TTP is almost always associated with hemolytic-uremic syndrome (HUS).

- The disease is associated with enhanced agglutination of platelets, which form microthrombi that deposit in arterioles and capillaries.
- In most cases, the syndrome is caused by the deficiency of a plasma enzyme (ADAMTS13) that usually breaks down the von Willebrand (vWF) clotting factor into normal size.
- TTP is seen primarily in previously healthy adults.

T

- The syndrome may be idiopathic (autoimmune disorder with antibodies against ADAMTS13), caused by certain drug toxicities (e.g., chemotherapy, cyclosporine, quinine, oral contraceptives, valacyclovir [Valtrex], clopidogrel [Plavix]), pregnancy or preeclampsia, infection, or known autoimmune disorder such as systemic lupus erythematosus or scleroderma.
- TTP is a medical emergency because bleeding and clotting occur simultaneously

Heparin-Induced Thrombocytopenia

Heparin-induced thrombocytopenia (HIT), also called *heparin-induced thrombocytopenia and thrombosis syndrome* (HITTS), may develop 5 to 10 days after heparin therapy is initiated. In HIT, an immune-mediated response to heparin causes platelet destruction and vascular endothelial injury.

- Antibodies are created against a heparin-platelet complex, and platelets are removed prematurely from circulation, leading to thrombocytopenia and formation of platelet-fibrin thrombi.
- HIT leads to venous or arterial thrombosis. Deep vein thromboses and pulmonary emboli are common complications. Additional complications may include arterial vascular infarcts resulting in skin necrosis, stroke, and end-organ damage (e.g., kidneys).
- As many as 3% of patients on heparin therapy develop HIT. HIT should be suspected if the platelet count drops by more than 50% from baseline or if a thrombus forms while the patient is on heparin therapy.
- Symptoms of bleeding are unusual because the platelet count rarely drops below 20,000/μL.

Clinical Manifestations

Many patients with thrombocytopenia are asymptomatic.

- The most common symptom is bleeding, usually mucosal or cutaneous. Mucosal bleeding may manifest as epistaxis and gingival bleeding, and large bullous hemorrhages may appear on the buccal mucosa. Bleeding into the skin is manifested as petechiae, purpura, or superficial ecchymoses.
- Prolonged bleeding after routine procedures such as venipuncture or IM injection may indicate thrombocytopenia. Be aware of manifestations that reflect internal blood loss, including weakness, fainting, dizziness, tachycardia, abdominal pain, and hypotension.

The major complication of thrombocytopenia is hemorrhage in any area of the body, including the joints, retina, and brain. Cerebral hemorrhage may be fatal.

Diagnostic Studies

- For comparison of laboratory results in various types of thrombocytopenia, see Table 30-12, Lewis et al, *Medical-Surgical Nursing,* ed 10, p. 623.
- Platelet count is decreased below 150,000/μL (150 $\times$ 10^9/L). Spontaneous life-threatening hemorrhages (e.g., intracranial bleeding) may occur with counts below 20,000/μL (20 $\times$ 10^9/L).
- Specific assays for antigens help differentiate ITP from other types of thrombocytopenia.
- Bone marrow analysis may show normal or increased megakaryocytes (precursors of platelets). It is done to rule out leukemia, aplastic anemia, and other myeloproliferative disorders.
- Flow cytometry can be used to detect antiplatelet antibodies.

Interprofessional Care

Immune Thrombocytopenic Purpura

Multiple therapies are used to manage the patient with ITP. If the patient is asymptomatic, therapy may not be used unless the platelet count is below 10,000/μL. Corticosteroids (e.g., prednisone) are used initially to suppress the phagocytic response of splenic macrophages.

Splenectomy may be indicated if the patient is not responding to the conservative treatments. Approximately 60% to 70% of patients benefit from splenectomy, resulting in a complete or partial remission. High doses of IV immunoglobulin (IVIG) and a component of IVIG, anti-Rh$_0$(D) (anti-D, WinRho), may be used in the patient who is unresponsive to corticosteroids or splenectomy, or for whom splenectomy is not an option.

- Romiplostim (Nplate) and eltrombopag (Promacta) are used for patients with chronic ITP who have had an insufficient response to the other treatments or have a contraindication to splenectomy. These drugs are thrombopoietin receptor agonists and increase platelet production.
- Immunosuppressive therapy may be used in refractory cases including rituximab (Rituxan), cyclophosphamide, azathioprine (Imuran), and mycophenolate mofetil (CellCept).
- Platelet transfusions are not indicated until the count is less than 10,000/μL (10 $\times$ 10^9/L) or if there is anticipated bleeding before a scheduled procedure.

Thrombotic Thrombocytopenic Purpura

TTP may be managed in a variety of ways. The first step is to treat the underlying disorder (e.g., infection) or remove the causative agent, if identified. If untreated, TTP usually results in irreversible renal failure and death. Plasma exchange (plasmapheresis) may be needed to aggressively reverse the process. Treatment should be continued daily until the patient's platelet counts normalize and hemolysis has ceased.

Corticosteroids may be added to this treatment. Rituximab has been used for patients who are refractory to plasma exchange. Other immunosuppressants such as cyclosporine or cyclophosphamide may also be used. Splenectomy may be considered for patients in whom the disease is refractory to plasma exchange or immunosuppression. Administration of platelets is generally contraindicated because it may lead to new vWF-platelet complexes and increased clotting.

Heparin-Induced Thrombocytopenia

Heparin must be discontinued when HIT is first recognized. Heparin flushes for vascular catheters should also be stopped.

To maintain anticoagulation, fondaparinux (Arixtra), a factor Xa inhibitor (indirect thrombin inhibitor), may be used. Warfarin should be started only when the platelet count has reached at least 150,000/μL. If the clotting is severe, the most commonly used treatment modalities are plasmapheresis to clear the platelet-aggregating IgG from the blood, protamine sulfate to interrupt the circulating heparin, thrombolytic agents to treat the thromboembolic events, and surgery to remove clots. Platelet transfusions are not effective because they may enhance thromboembolic events.

Patients who have had HIT should never be given heparin or low-molecular-weight heparin (LMWH). This should be clearly indicated in the patient's health record.

Nursing Management

Goals

The patient with thrombocytopenia will have no gross or occult bleeding, maintain vascular integrity, and manage home care to prevent any complications related to an increased risk for bleeding.

See eNursing Care Plan 30-2 for the patient with thrombocytopenia, available on the website for Lewis et al, *Medical-Surgical Nursing*, ed 10.

Nursing Diagnoses

- Risk for bleeding
- Impaired oral mucous membrane
- Deficient knowledge

Nursing Interventions

Discourage excessive use of over-the-counter (OTC) medications known to be possible causes of acquired thrombocytopenia. Many medications contain aspirin as an ingredient. Aspirin reduces platelet adhesiveness, thus potentially contributing to bleeding.

Encourage people to have a complete medical evaluation if manifestations of bleeding tendencies (e.g., prolonged epistaxis, petechiae) develop. Observe for early signs of thrombocytopenia in patients receiving cancer chemotherapy drugs.

The goal during acute episodes of thrombocytopenia is to prevent or control hemorrhage. In the patient with thrombocytopenia, bleeding is usually from superficial sites. Deep bleeding (into the muscles, joints, and abdomen) usually occurs only when clotting factors are diminished. Emphasize that a seemingly minor nosebleed or new petechiae may indicate potential hemorrhage and that the HCP should be notified.

- In a woman with thrombocytopenia, menstrual blood loss may exceed the usual amount and duration. Counting sanitary napkins used during menses is an important intervention to detect excess blood loss.
- Proper administration of platelet transfusions is an important nursing responsibility.
- Monitor patients with ITP for response to therapy.

▼ Patient and Caregiver Teaching
Teach the person with acquired thrombocytopenia to avoid causative agents when possible. If causative agents cannot be avoided (e.g., chemotherapy), the patient should learn to avoid injury or trauma during these periods and to detect the clinical signs and symptoms of bleeding caused by thrombocytopenia.

- Patients with either ITP or acquired thrombocytopenia should plan periodic medical evaluations to assess their status and to treat situations in which exacerbations and bleeding are likely to occur.
- The impact of either an acute or chronic condition on the patient's quality of life should also be addressed.

For a more complete listing of precautions that patients should take when their platelet count is low, see Table 30-15, Lewis et al, *Medical-Surgical Nursing,* ed 10, p. 626.

THYROID CANCER

Description
Thyroid cancer is the most common type of cancer of the endocrine system. The incidence of thyroid cancer has risen significantly in the past 25 years. Thyroid cancer affects more women than men, and the incidence is higher in whites and Asian Americans. Adults at increased risk include those who had head and neck radiation therapy during childhood, were exposed to radioactive fallout, or have a personal or family history of goiter.

T

Four main types of thyroid cancer are papillary, follicular, medullary, and anaplastic.

- *Papillary thyroid cancer* is the most common type, accounting for about 70% to 80% of all thyroid cancers. Papillary cancer tends to grow slowly and spreads initially to lymph nodes in the neck.
- *Follicular thyroid cancer* makes up about 10% to 15% of all thyroid cancers and tends to occur in older patients. Follicular cancer first grows into the cervical lymph nodes and then spreads to the lungs and bones.
- *Medullary thyroid cancer,* which accounts for up to 10% of all thyroid cancers, is more likely to occur in families and to be associated with other endocrine problems. It is diagnosed by genetic testing for a *protooncogene* called *RET.* Medullary thyroid cancer is a type of multiple endocrine neoplasia. This type of cancer is often poorly differentiated and associated with early metastasis.
- *Anaplastic thyroid cancer,* found in less than 2% of patients with thyroid cancer, is the most advanced and aggressive thyroid cancer. It is the least likely to respond to treatment and has a poor prognosis.

Clinical Manifestations

The primary sign of thyroid cancer is a painless, palpable nodule or nodules in an enlarged thyroid gland. Patients or HCPs discover most of these nodules during palpation of the neck. Some patients may have difficulty swallowing or breathing because of tumor growth invading the trachea or esophagus.

Diagnostic Studies

Nodular thyroid gland enlargement or palpation of a mass requires further evaluation.

- Ultrasound is often the first diagnostic test used. CT, MRI, positron emission tomography (PET), and ultrasound-guided fine-needle aspiration (FNA) are other options.
- A thyroid scan may be done to evaluate for a malignancy. A nodule that does not take up radioactive iodine has a higher risk of being malignant.
- Elevations in serum calcitonin are associated with medullary thyroid cancer. In papillary and follicular cancers, serum thyroglobulin is elevated.

Nursing and Interprofessional Management

Surgical removal of the tumor is the primary treatment for thyroid cancer. Surgical procedures may range from unilateral total lobectomy with removal of the isthmus to near-total thyroidectomy with bilateral lobectomy.

Radioactive iodine (RAI) may be given to some patients to destroy any remaining cancer cells after surgery. External beam radiation therapy may be given as palliative treatment for patients with metastatic thyroid cancer.

Many thyroid cancers are thyroid-stimulating hormone (TSH)-dependent, and thyroid hormone therapy in high doses is often prescribed to inhibit pituitary secretion of TSH. Chemotherapy, including doxorubicin, may be used for advanced disease. Vandetanib (Caprelsa), lenvatinib (Lenvima), sorafenib tosylate (Nexavar), and cabozantinib (Cometriq) are targeted therapy agents used for treatment of metastatic thyroid cancer. These drugs inhibit tyrosine kinases, which are enzymes that are involved in growth of cancer cells.

Nursing care for the patient with thyroid cancer is similar to that for the patient undergoing thyroidectomy (see Surgical Therapy section in Hyperthyroidism, p. 334). Because of the surgical site location and the potential for hypocalcemia, the patient requires frequent postoperative assessment. Assess the patient for airway obstruction, bleeding, and tetany, because a parathyroid gland may have been disturbed or removed during surgery.

TRIGEMINAL NEURALGIA

Description

Trigeminal neuralgia (TN) (tic douloureux) is characterized by sudden, usually unilateral, brief, recurrent episodes of severe stabbing pain in the distribution of the trigeminal nerve. It is seen twice as often in women as in men. The majority of cases are in people older than 40 years.

- Risk factors are multiple sclerosis and hypertension. Other factors that may cause neuralgia include herpesvirus infection, infection of the teeth and jaw, and a brainstem infarct.

Pathophysiology

The trigeminal nerve is the fifth cranial nerve (CN V) and has both motor and sensory branches. The sensory branches, primarily the maxillary and mandibular branches, are involved in TN.

- The majority of TN cases result from vascular compression of the trigeminal nerve root by an abnormal loop of the superior cerebellar artery. Constant compression appears to lead to chronic injury, causing demyelination of the nerve and impairment of the nociceptive system. TN also may be secondary to

T

underlying pathology, such as multiple sclerosis, shingles, or masses in the cerebellum or brainstem.

Clinical Manifestations

TN is classified as classic (TN 1) or atypical (TN 2). Patients may experience both types.

The *classic* form, *TN 1,* manifests with an abrupt onset of paroxysms of excruciating pain described as burning or knifelike, or a lightning-like shock, in the lips, upper or lower gums, cheek, forehead, or side of the nose.

- Intense pain, twitching, grimacing, and frequent blinking and tearing of the eye occur during the acute attack (giving rise to the term *tic*). Some patients may also experience facial sensory loss.
- The attacks are usually brief, lasting seconds to 2 or 3 minutes, and are generally unilateral.
- Recurrences are unpredictable. Attacks may occur several times each day or weeks or months apart.
- After the refractory (pain-free) period, a phenomenon known as *clustering* can occur. It is characterized by a cycle of pain and refractoriness that continues for hours.

The *atypical* form, *TN 2,* is distinguished by constant aching, burning, crushing, or stabbing pain. The pain has a lower intensity and does not subside completely.

- Painful episodes are usually initiated by a triggering mechanism of light touch at a specific point (trigger zones) along the distribution of the nerve branches.
- Precipitating stimuli include chewing, toothbrushing, feeling a hot or cold blast of air on the face, washing the face, yawning, or even talking.
- As a result, the patient may not eat properly, neglect hygienic practices, wear a cloth over the face, and withdraw from interaction with other individuals. The patient may sleep excessively as a means of coping with the pain.

Diagnostic Studies

- The first episode of TN is sudden with a memorable onset. Diagnosis is based almost entirely on history.
- Neurologic assessment and CT scan or MRI of the brain are used to rule out any lesions, tumors, or vascular abnormalities.

Interprofessional Care

The goal of treatment is relief of pain.

Drug Therapy

Antiseizure drug therapy may reduce pain by stabilizing the neuronal membrane and blocking nerve firing. These drugs are usually effective in treating TN 1 but less effective for TN 2. First-line drugs include carbamazepine (Tegretol) and oxcarbazepine (Trileptal). Topiramate (Topamax), clonazepam (Klonopin), phenytoin (Dilantin), lamotrigine (Lamictal), divalproex (Depakote), gabapentin, and baclofen may be used. Tricyclic antidepressants such as amitriptyline or nortriptyline (Pamelor) can be used to treat constant burning or aching pain. Analgesics or opioids are usually not effective in controlling pain in TN1 but may help with pain in TN2.

Surgical Therapy

If a conservative approach is ineffective or the patient is unable to tolerate adverse effects of prescribed drugs, surgical therapy is available.

- In percutaneous procedures, affected nerve fibers are damaged to eliminate pain. Although most patients are pain-free after such procedures, pain relief lasts longer with microvascular decompression.

Nursing Management

Monitor the patient's response to drug therapy and note any side effects. Discuss alternative pain management measures, such as acupuncture, biofeedback, and yoga.

Environmental management is essential during an acute period to decrease triggering stimuli. Keep the room at an even, moderate temperature and free of drafts.

Teach the patient about the importance of nutrition, hygiene, and oral care. Convey a nonjudgmental attitude if previous neglect is apparent.

- A small, soft-bristled toothbrush or a warm mouthwash assists in promoting oral care.
- Hygiene activities are best carried out when analgesia is at its peak.
- Food that is high in protein and calories and easily chewed should be served lukewarm and offered frequently. If oral intake is sharply reduced and the patient's nutritional status is compromised, a nasogastric (NG) tube can be inserted on the unaffected side for enteral feedings.

For the patient who has had surgery, compare the postoperative pain level with the preoperative level. Frequently evaluate the corneal reflex, extraocular muscle function, hearing, sensation, and facial nerve function. General postoperative nursing care

T

for a craniotomy is appropriate if intracranial surgery has been performed.

- After a percutaneous radiofrequency procedure, apply an ice pack to the jaw on the operative side for 3 to 5 hours. To avoid injuring the mouth, the patient should not chew on the operative side until sensation has returned.

▼ **Patient and Caregiver Teaching**

Plan for regular follow-up care and instruct the patient regarding the dosage and side effects of prescribed drugs. Encourage the patient to manage environmental stimuli and to use stress reduction methods.

Long-term management after surgical intervention depends on the residual effects of the procedure used. If anesthesia is present or the corneal reflex is altered, teach the patient to (1) chew on the unaffected side, (2) avoid hot foods or beverages that can burn the mucous membranes, (3) check the oral cavity after meals to remove food particles, (4) practice meticulous oral hygiene and continue with semiannual dental visits, (5) protect the face against extremes of temperature, (6) use an electric razor, (7) wear a protective eye shield and avoid rubbing the eyes, and (8) examine eye regularly for symptoms of infection or irritation.

TUBERCULOSIS

Description

Tuberculosis (TB) is an infectious disease caused by *Mycobacterium tuberculosis*. It usually involves the lungs, but any organ can be infected, including brain, kidneys, and bones. More than 2 billion people (one third of the world's population) are infected with TB. It is the leading cause of death in patients with human immunodeficiency virus (HIV) infection/acquired immunodeficiency syndrome (AIDS). Although the prevalence of TB has increased in Europe, in the United States it has steadily declined since reaching a resurgence peak in 1992.

In the United States, people at higher risk include the homeless, residents of inner-city neighborhoods, foreign-born individuals, those living or working in institutions (long-term care facilities, prisons), IV drug users, and those with limited income or access to health care.

- *M. tuberculosis* that develops resistance to isoniazid and rifampin is defined as *multidrug-resistant tuberculosis* (MDR-TB). Resistance results from incorrect prescribing, lack of public health case management, and patient nonadherence to the prescribed regimen.

Pathophysiology

M. tuberculosis is a gram-positive, acid-fast bacillus that is usually spread from person to person via airborne droplets produced by speaking, breathing, sneezing, and coughing.

- TB is not highly infectious because transmission usually requires close, frequent, or prolonged exposure. The disease cannot be spread by touching, sharing food utensils, kissing, or any other type of physical contact.
- Once inhaled, small particles lodge in bronchiole and alveolus.
- The organisms find favorable environments for growth primarily in the lungs, kidneys, epiphyses of bone, cerebral cortex, and adrenal glands.

Classification

Several systems can be used to classify TB. The American Thoracic Society classifies TB based on development of the disease (Table 84). TB can also be classified according to (1) its presentation—primary, latent, or reactivated—and (2) whether it is pulmonary or extrapulmonary.

Primary infection occurs when the bacteria are inhaled but there is an effective immune response and the bacteria become inactive. Most people have an effective immune response to encapsulate these organisms for the rest of their lives.

Latent TB infection (LTBI) occurs in a person who does not have active TB. People with LTBI have a positive skin test but are asymptomatic. Although they cannot transmit TB, they may develop active TB disease at some point in their lives. Therefore treatment of LTBI is important.

Active TB disease results if the initial immune response is not adequate, the body cannot contain the organisms, and the bacteria replicate. When active disease develops within the first 2 years of infection, it is termed *primary TB*. Postprimary TB, or *reactivation TB,* is defined as TB disease occurring 2 or more years after the initial infection.

Clinical Manifestations

- Active TB disease may initially manifest with fatigue, malaise, anorexia, unexplained weight loss, low-grade fevers, and night sweats.
- Sometimes TB has a more acute, sudden presentation. The patient may have a high fever, chills, generalized flu-like symptoms, pleuritic pain, and a productive cough.
- In patients with HIV infection, classic manifestations of TB such as fever, cough, and weight loss may be incorrectly

T

Class	Exposure or Infection	Description
0	No TB exposure	No TB exposure, not infected (no history of exposure, negative tuberculin skin test)
1	TB exposure, no infection	TB exposure, no evidence of infection (history of exposure, negative tuberculin skin test)
2	Latent TB infection, no disease	TB infection without disease (significant reaction to tuberculin skin test, negative bacteriologic studies, no x-ray findings compatible with TB, no clinical evidence of TB)
3	TB, clinically active	TB infection with clinically active disease (positive bacteriologic studies, or both a significant reaction to tuberculin skin test and clinical or x-ray evidence of current disease)
4	TB, but not clinically active	No current disease (history of previous episode of TB or abnormal, stable x-ray findings in a person with a significant reaction to tuberculin skin test. Negative bacteriologic studies if done. No clinical or x-ray evidence of current disease)
5	TB suspect	TB suspect (diagnosis pending). Person should not be in this classification for >3 mo.

TABLE 84　Classification of Tuberculosis (TB)

Source: American Thoracic Society.

attributed to pneumonia caused by *Pneumocystis jiroveci* or other HIV-associated opportunistic diseases.

- The clinical manifestations of extrapulmonary TB depend on the organs infected. For example, renal TB can cause dysuria and hematuria. Bone and joint TB may cause severe pain. Headaches, vomiting, and lymphadenopathy may be present with TB meningitis.

Complications

Miliary TB results from widespread dissemination of the mycobacterium. The infection is characterized by a large amount of TB bacilli and may be fatal if left untreated.

- Clinical manifestations may slowly progress over a period of days, weeks, or months. Symptoms vary depending on which organs are infected.
- Hepatomegaly, splenomegaly, and generalized lymphadenopathy may also be present.

Pleural TB can result from either primary disease or reactivation of a latent infection. *Empyema* is less common than effusion but may occur with large numbers of tubercular organisms in the pleural space.

Diagnostic Studies

- Tuberculin skin test (TST): Induration (not redness) at the injection site means that the person has been exposed to TB and has developed antibodies. See Chapter 26, Lewis et al, *Medical-Surgical Nursing,* ed 10, for guidelines in performing and interpreting TSTs.
- Interferon (INF)-gamma release assays (IGRAs)
- Blood test to detect response to mycobacterial antigens
- Chest x-ray: Diagnosis cannot be based solely on x-ray because other diseases may mimic TB.
- Bacteriologic studies: Stained sputum smears for acid-fast bacilli (AFB test) can identify tubercle bacilli; cultures to grow tubercle bacilli confirm diagnosis.

Interprofessional Care

Most patients with TB are treated on an outpatient basis and continue to work and maintain their lifestyles with few changes. Hospitalization may be needed for severely ill or debilitated patients.

Drug Therapy

The mainstay of TB treatment is drug therapy.

Active Tuberculosis Disease. Because of the growing prevalence of MDR-TB, it is important to manage the patient with active TB aggressively. Drug therapy is divided into two phases: initial and continuation (see Tables 27-11 and 27-12, Lewis et al, *Medical-Surgical Nursing,* ed 10, p. 509). In most circumstances the treatment regimen for patients with previously untreated TB consists of a 2-month initial phase with four-drug therapy—isoniazid, rifampin, pyrazinamide, and ethambutol.

- Nonadherence is a major factor in the emergence of multidrug resistance and treatment failures. Many individuals do not

T

adhere to the treatment program despite understanding that nonadherence can lead to reactivation of TB and multidrug-resistant TB.

- *Directly observed therapy* (DOT) involves providing the anti-tuberculous drugs directly to patients and watching as they swallow the medications.

Latent Tuberculosis Infection.   In people with LTBI, drug therapy helps prevent a TB infection from developing into active TB disease. The standard treatment regimen for LTBI is 9 months of daily INH.

Bacille Calmette-Guérin (BCG) vaccine is given to infants in parts of the world with a high prevalence of TB. The BCG vaccine should be considered for individuals who meet specific criteria (e.g., health care workers who are continually exposed to patients with MDR-TB and when infection control precautions are not successful).

Nursing Management

Goals
The patient with tuberculosis will comply with the therapeutic regimen, have no recurrence of disease, have normal pulmonary function, and take appropriate measures to prevent the spread of the disease.

Nursing Diagnoses
- Ineffective breathing pattern
- Ineffective airway clearance
- Risk for infection (spread to others)

Nursing Interventions
The ultimate goal is to eradicate TB worldwide.

- Screening programs in known high-risk groups are of value in detecting people with TB.
- Chest x-rays to assess for the presence of TB in people with a positive TST result should be encouraged.
- Reducing prevalence of HIV infection, poverty, overcrowded living conditions, malnutrition, smoking, and drug and alcohol abuse can help minimize TB infection rates.

If hospitalization is needed for patients suspected of having TB, special measures should be taken.

- Airborne infection isolation is indicated for the patient with pulmonary or laryngeal TB until the patient is noninfectious (defined as effective drug therapy, clinical improvement, and three negative AFB smears).
- High-efficiency particulate air (HEPA) masks are worn by those entering the patient's room. Health care professionals should be

"fit tested" each time a different brand or model of mask is used, to ensure proper mask size.

▼ **Patient and Caregiver Teaching**

- Teach hospitalized patients to cover the nose and mouth with paper tissues every time they cough, sneeze, or produce sputum.
- Teach the patient and caregivers about adherence to the prescribed regimen. Strategies to improve adherence include teaching and counseling, reminder systems, incentives or rewards, contracts, and DOT.
- Because about 5% of individuals experience relapses, teach the patient to recognize symptoms that indicate the recurrence of TB. If these symptoms occur, immediate medical attention should be sought.
- Also teach the patient about factors that could reactivate TB, such as immunosuppression or malignancy.

ULCERATIVE COLITIS

Ulcerative colitis is an autoimmune disorder that, along with Crohn's disease, is referred to as *inflammatory bowel disease* (IBD). See Inflammatory Bowel Disease, p. 348, for a discussion of the disorder.

URETHRITIS

Description

Urethritis is an inflammation of the urethra. Causes of urethritis include a bacterial or viral infection, trichomonal and monilial infection (especially in women), chlamydial infection, and gonorrhea (especially in men).

In *men,* purulent discharge usually indicates a gonococcal urethritis. A clear discharge typically signifies a nongonococcal urethritis. Urethritis also produces bothersome lower urinary tract symptoms (LUTS), including dysuria, urgency, and frequent urination, similar to those seen with cystitis.

In *women,* urethritis is difficult to diagnose. It frequently produces bothersome LUTS, but urethral discharge may not be present.

Nursing and Interprofessional Management

Treatment is based on identifying and treating the cause and providing symptomatic relief.

- Drugs used to treat bacterial infections include trimethoprim/sulfamethoxazole, doxycycline (Vibramycin), ceftriaxone, and nitrofurantoin. Metronidazole (Flagyl) and clotrimazole may be

used to treat *Trichomonas* infection. Drugs such as nystatin or fluconazole may be used for monilial infections. For chlamydial infections, doxycycline may be used.
- Warm sitz baths may temporarily relieve bothersome symptoms.

Teach female patients to avoid using vaginal deodorant sprays and to properly cleanse the perineal area after bowel movement or urination. Teach all patients to avoid sexual intercourse until symptoms subside. Teach patients with sexually transmitted urethritis to refer their sex partners for evaluation and testing if they had sexual contact in the 60 days preceding onset of the symptoms or diagnosis.

URINARY INCONTINENCE

Description

Urinary incontinence (UI) is an involuntary leakage of urine. Although it is more prevalent among older women and men, it is not a natural consequence of aging. Often, UI can be significantly improved with proper management.

Pathophysiology

UI can result from anything that interferes with bladder or urethral sphincter control.
- Using the acronym *DRIP,* the causes include *D: d*elirium, *d*ehydration, *d*epression; *R: r*estricted mobility, *r*ectal impaction; *I: i*nfection, *i*nflammation, *i*mpaction; and *P: p*olyuria, *p*olypharmacy.
- UI disorders include stress, urge, overflow, and reflex incontinence. Patients may have more than one type of incontinence. (For a complete description of UI, see Table 45-16, Lewis et al, *Medical-Surgical Nursing,* ed 10, p. 1056.)

Diagnostic Studies

- A focused history, physical assessment, and a voiding record provide information about the onset of UI, factors that provoke urinary leakage, and associated conditions.
- Pelvic examination assesses for organ prolapse and evaluates pelvic floor muscle strength.
- Urinalysis identifies possible factors contributing to transient incontinence or urinary retention (e.g., urinary infection, diabetes mellitus).
- Measure postvoid residual (PVR) urine in the patient undergoing evaluation for UI. The PVR volume is obtained by asking

the patient to urinate, followed by catheterization or use of bladder ultrasound within a relatively brief period (preferably 10 to 20 minutes).
- Urodynamic testing is indicated in selected cases of UI.
- Imaging studies of the upper urinary tract (e.g., ultrasound) are obtained when incontinence is associated with urinary tract infections or there is evidence of upper urinary tract involvement.

Interprofessional Care

Transient, reversible factors are corrected initially, followed by management of the type of UI. In general, less invasive treatments are attempted before more invasive methods (e.g., surgery) are used.

Several behavioral therapies may be used, including (1) pelvic floor muscle training (Kegel exercises) to help some patients manage stress, urge, or mixed UI and (2) biofeedback to assist the patient to identify, isolate, contract, and relax the pelvic muscles.

Drug Therapy

Drug therapy varies according to UI type.
- In *stress UI,* drugs have a limited role in management. α-Adrenergic agonists can be used to increase bladder sphincter tone and urethral resistance but have limited benefit.
- In *urge* and *reflex UI,* drugs play a key management role. Anticholinergic drugs (muscarinic receptor blockers) block the action of acetylcholine at muscarinic receptors. They relax the bladder muscle and inhibit overactive detrusor contractions. These preparations include immediate- and extended-release tolterodine (Detrol, Detrol LA); immediate- and extended-release and transdermal oxybutynin (Ditropan XL, Oxytrol Transdermal System); twice-daily trospium chloride; extended-release solifenacin (VESIcare); and darifenacin (Enablex).
- Botox (onabotulinumtoxin A) can be used in the treatment of UI as a result of detrusor overactivity. Botox is injected into the bladder, resulting in relaxation of the bladder, an increase in its storage capacity, and a decrease in UI.

For a list of additional drugs used in various types of incontinence, see Table 45-19 in Lewis et al, *Medical-Surgical Nursing,* ed 10, p. 1059.

Surgical Therapy

Surgical techniques also vary according to the type of UI.
- Surgical correction of stress UI may reposition the urethra and/or create a backboard of support, or otherwise stabilize the urethra and bladder neck and make them better able to adapt to changes in intraabdominal pressure.

- Another technique for stress UI augments the urethral resistance of the intrinsic sphincter unit with a sling or periurethral injectable.
- Retropubic colposuspension and pubovaginal sling placement appear to be most effective. Typically, both procedures are performed through low transverse incisions.
- Placement of a suburethral sling, using autologous fascia, cadaveric fascia, or a synthetic material, is also used to correct stress UI in women.
- An artificial urethral sphincter can be used in men with intrinsic sphincter deficiency and severe stress UI.
- Bulking agents can be injected underneath the mucosa of the urethra to correct stress UI in women or men.

Nursing Management

Recognize both the physical and emotional problems associated with incontinence. Maintain and enhance the patient's dignity, privacy, and feelings of self-worth.

- Take a two-step approach involving containment devices to manage existing urinary leakage and a definitive plan to reduce or resolve the factors leading to incontinence.
- Emphasize consuming an adequate volume of fluids and reducing or eliminating bladder irritants (particularly caffeine and alcohol) from the diet.
- Advise the patient to maintain a regular, flexible schedule of urination (usually every 2 to 3 hours while awake).
- Advise patients to quit smoking, because it increases the risk of stress UI.
- Aggressive management of constipation is recommended, beginning with ensuring adequate fluid intake, increasing dietary fiber, lightly exercising, and judiciously using stool softeners.
- Behavioral treatments include bladder retraining and pelvic floor muscle training. (A patient teaching guide for pelvic floor muscle exercises is found in Table 45-18, Lewis et al, *Medical-Surgical Nursing,* ed 10, p. 1058.)
- Assess patient strategies and share information on products designed to contain urine.
- In inpatient or long-term care facilities, nursing management of UI includes maximizing toilet access. This assistance may be offering the urinal or bedpan or assisting the patient to the bathroom every 2 to 3 hours or at scheduled times. Ensure that toilets with adequate privacy are accessible to patients.

URINARY RETENTION

Description

Urinary retention is the inability to empty the bladder despite micturition or the accumulation of urine in the bladder because of an inability to urinate. In certain cases, it is associated with urinary leakage or postvoid dribbling, called overflow urinary incontinence (UI).

- Acute urinary retention, which is the total inability to pass urine via micturition, is a medical emergency. Chronic urinary retention is defined as incomplete bladder emptying despite urination.

Pathophysiology

Urinary retention is caused by two different dysfunctions of the urinary system: bladder outlet obstruction and deficient detrusor (bladder wall muscle) contraction strength.

- *Bladder outlet obstruction* leads to urinary retention when the blockage is so severe that the bladder can no longer evacuate its contents despite detrusor contraction. A common cause of obstruction in men is an enlarged prostate.
- Common causes of *deficient detrusor contraction strength* are neurologic diseases affecting the sacral vertebral segments 2, 3, and 4; long-standing diabetes mellitus; overdistention; long-term alcoholism; and drugs (e.g., anticholinergic drugs).

Diagnostic Studies

The diagnostic studies for urinary retention are the same as those for UI (see Urinary Incontinence, p. 644).

Interprofessional Care

Behavioral therapies that were described for UI also may be used in the management of urinary retention. Scheduled toileting and double voiding may be effective in chronic urinary retention associated with moderate postvoid residual volumes.

- Double voiding is an attempt to maximize bladder evacuation by having the patient urinate, sit on the toilet for 3 to 4 minutes, and urinate again before exiting the bathroom.
- If catheterization is required for acute or chronic urinary retention, intermittent catheterization is preferred, to decrease the risk of catheter-associated urinary tract infections (CAUTIs) and urethral irritation.

Drug Therapy

Several drugs may be administered to promote bladder evacuation. For patients with obstruction at the bladder neck, an α-adrenergic antagonist may be prescribed to relax the bladder neck muscle, prostatic urethra, and possibly dual-innervated rhabdosphincter, diminishing urethral resistance.

Surgical Therapy

Surgical interventions are used to manage urinary retention caused by obstruction. Transurethral or open surgical techniques are used to treat benign or malignant prostatic enlargement, bladder neck contracture, urethral strictures, or dyssynergia of the bladder neck.

- Pelvic reconstruction using an abdominal or transvaginal approach can correct bladder outlet obstruction in women with severe pelvic organ prolapse.

Nursing Management

Acute urinary retention is a medical emergency that requires prompt recognition and bladder drainage. Insert a catheter (as ordered) unless otherwise directed. See Urinary Catheterization, p. 739.

- Teach the patient with acute urinary retention to minimize risk, including avoiding intake of large volumes of fluid over a brief period.
- Advise the patient who is unable to urinate to drink a cup of coffee or brewed caffeinated tea to maximize urinary urgency, and then attempt to urinate while in a tub of warm water or a warm shower.
- If these measures do not lead to successful urination, advise the patient to seek immediate care.

Patients with chronic urinary retention may be managed by behavioral methods or with an indwelling catheter or by intermittent catheterization, surgery, or drugs. Scheduled toileting and double voiding are the primary behavioral interventions used for chronic retention.

URINARY TRACT CALCULI

Description

Each year an estimated 1 to 2 million people in the United States have *nephrolithiasis* (kidney stone disease). Except for struvite stones, associated with urinary tract infection (UTI), stone disorders are more common in men than in women. A majority of patients are between 20 and 55 years of age.

- The incidence is also higher in people with a family history of stone formation. Stones can recur in up to 50% of patients.

- Stone formation occurs more often in the summer months, supporting a role for dehydration in this process.
- The term *calculus* refers to the stone, and *lithiasis* refers to stone formation.

Pathophysiology

Many factors are involved in the incidence and type of stone formation, including metabolic, dietary, genetic, climatic, lifestyle, and occupational influences. Many theories have been proposed to explain the formation of stones in the urinary tract.

- Crystals, when in a supersaturated concentration, can precipitate and unite to form a stone. Keeping urine dilute and free-flowing reduces the risk of recurrent stone formation in many individuals.
- Urinary pH, solute load, and inhibitors in the urine affect the formation of stones. The higher the pH, the less soluble are calcium and phosphate. The lower the pH, the less soluble are uric acid and cystine.

Other important factors in stone development include obstruction with associated urinary stasis and UTI with urea-splitting bacteria (e.g., *Proteus, Klebsiella, Pseudomonas,* and some species of staphylococci). These bacteria cause the urine to become alkaline, contributing to the formation of struvite (calcium-magnesium-ammonium phosphate) stones.

- Infected stones, entrapped in the kidney, may assume a staghorn configuration as they enlarge. These stones can lead to hydronephrosis, renal infection, and loss of kidney function.
- There are five major categories of stones: calcium phosphate, calcium oxalate, uric acid, cystine, and struvite. Stone composition may be mixed, although calcium stones are the most common.

Clinical Manifestations

The first symptom is usually sudden, severe pain. Typically, a person feels sharp pain in the flank area, back, or lower abdomen. People describe the pain as excruciating.

- *Renal colic* is the term used for the sharp, severe pain, which results from the stretching, dilation, and spasm of the ureter in response to the obstructing stone. Nausea and vomiting may also occur.
- Urinary stones cause manifestations when they obstruct urinary flow. The type of pain is determined by the location of the stone. If the stone is nonobstructing, pain may be absent. If it produces obstruction in a calyx or at the ureteropelvic junction (UPJ), the patient may experience dull costovertebral flank pain or even

colic. Pain resulting from the passage of a calculus down the ureter is intense and colicky. The patient may be in mild shock, with cool, moist skin. As a stone nears the ureterovesical junction (UVJ), pain will be felt in the lateral flank and sometimes down into the testicles or labia or groin.

- Manifestations may also include those of a UTI, with dysuria, fever, and chills.

Diagnostic Studies

- Noncontrast helical (spiral) CT scan, ultrasound, and intravenous pyelogram (IVP) may be used.
- Urinalysis is used to assess for hematuria, crystalluria, and urine pH. Urine pH checks for struvite stones and renal tubular necrosis (tendency to alkaline pH) and uric acid stones (tendency to acidic pH).
- Retrieval and analysis of the stones are important in the diagnosis of the underlying problem contributing to stone formation.
- Serum calcium, phosphorus, sodium, potassium, bicarbonate, uric acid, and creatinine levels and blood urea nitrogen (BUN) are also measured.

Interprofessional Care

Evaluation and management of the patient with renal lithiasis consist of two concurrent approaches. The *first approach* is directed toward management of the acute attack by treating the pain, infection, or obstruction. Administer opioids to relieve renal colic pain. Many stones are 4 mm or less in size and will pass spontaneously. However, such a stone may take weeks to pass. Tamsulosin (Flomax) or terazosin, α-adrenergic blockers that relax the smooth muscle in the ureter, can be used to facilitate stone passage.

The *second approach* is evaluation for the cause of stone formation and prevention of further stone development. Information obtained from the patient includes family history of stone formation, geographic location of residence, nutritional assessment (including intake of vitamins A and D), activity pattern (active or sedentary), history of periods of prolonged illness with immobilization or dehydration, and history of disease or surgery involving the GI or genitourinary (GU) tract.

Adequate hydration, dietary sodium restrictions, dietary changes, and drugs minimize urinary stone formation.

- Various drugs are prescribed that prevent stone formation by altering urine pH, preventing excessive urinary excretion of a substance, or correcting a primary disease (e.g., hyperparathyroidism).

U

Treatment of struvite stones requires control of infection. Acetohydroxamic acid inhibits the chemical action caused by persistent bacteria and thus retards struvite stone formation. If infection cannot be controlled, the stone may have to be surgically removed.

Indications for open surgical, endourology, or lithotripsy stone removal include:

- Stones too large for spontaneous passage (usually larger than 7 mm), associated with bacteriuria or symptomatic infection, or causing impaired renal function, persistent pain, nausea, or paralytic ileus
- Medical treatment not successful
- Patient with only one kidney

Endourologic procedures include the use of endoscopes to reach stones in the urinary tract. *Cystoscopy* can remove small stones in the bladder. For large stones, a *cystolitholapaxy* is performed using a lithotrite to crush stones. A *cystoscopic lithotripsy* uses an ultrasonic lithotrite to pulverize stones. Complications with these cystoscopic procedures include hemorrhage, retained stone fragments, and infection. Flexible *ureteroscopes* can be used in removing stones from the renal pelvis and upper urinary tract by means of ultrasonic, laser, or electrohydraulic lithotripsy. The same types of lithotripsy can be used during a percutaneous nephrolithotomy by way of a nephroscope inserted through the skin into the kidney pelvis.

Lithotripsy is a procedure for eliminating calculi from the urinary tract. Specific lithotripsy techniques include percutaneous ultrasonic lithotripsy, electrohydraulic lithotripsy, laser lithotripsy, and extracorporeal shock wave lithotripsy. Extracorporeal shock wave lithotripsy and laser lithotripsy are the most common.

Hematuria is common after lithotripsy procedures. A self-retaining ureteral stent is often placed after this outpatient procedure to promote passage of sand (shattered stone) and to prevent obstruction caused by sand buildup in the ureter. The stent is often removed 2 weeks after lithotripsy.

- If a stone is large or positioned in the mid or distal ureter, additional treatment such as surgery may be necessary.

A small group of patients require open surgical procedures including patients with pain, obstruction, and infection. The type of open surgery (e.g., *nephrolithotomy, pyelolithotomy, ureterolithotomy*) depends on location of the stone. For open surgery on the kidney or ureter, a flank incision directly below the diaphragm and across the side is usually the preferred approach.

Nutritional Therapy

A high fluid intake (at least 3 L/day) is recommended after an episode of urolithiasis to produce urine output of at least 2 L/day and prevent recurrent stone formation.

- Limit consumption of colas, coffee, and tea, because high intake of these beverages tends to increase the risk of recurring urinary calculi.
- A low-sodium diet is recommended, because high sodium intake increases calcium excretion in the urine. Foods high in calcium, oxalate, and purines are listed in Table 45-12, Lewis et al, *Medical-Surgical Nursing,* ed 10, p. 1049.

Nursing Management

Goals
The patient with urinary tract calculi will have relief of pain, no urinary tract obstruction, and an understanding of measures to prevent recurrence of stones.

Nursing Diagnoses
- Acute pain
- Impaired urinary elimination
- Deficient knowledge

Nursing Interventions
Preventive measures related to the person who is on bed rest or is relatively immobile for a prolonged period include maintaining an adequate fluid intake, turning the patient every 2 hours, and helping the patient sit or stand if possible to maximize urinary flow.

Pain management and patient comfort are primary nursing responsibilities in managing a person with an obstructing stone and renal colic.

- To ensure that any spontaneously passed stones are retrieved, strain all urine voided by the patient, using gauze or a urine strainer.
- Encourage ambulation to promote movement of the stone from the upper to the lower urinary tract. To ensure safety, tell the patient who is experiencing acute renal colic to ask for assistance when ambulating, particularly if opioid analgesics are being given.

▼ Patient and Caregiver Teaching
- Prevention of stone recurrence includes adequate fluid intake to produce a urine output of approximately 2 L/day.
- Dietary restriction of purines may be helpful for the patient at risk for developing uric acid stones.
- Teach the patient the dosage, scheduling, and potential side effects of drugs used to reduce the risk of stone formation.
- Selected patients may be taught to self-monitor urinary pH or urinary output.

URINARY TRACT INFECTIONS

Description

Urinary tract infections (UTIs) are the most common bacterial infection in women. *Escherichia coli (E. coli)* is the most common pathogen causing a UTI.

- Bacterial counts in the urine of 10^5 colony-forming units per milliliter (CFU/mL) or higher typically indicate a UTI. However, bacterial counts as low as 10^2 to 10^3 CFU/mL in a person with symptoms are also indicative of UTI.
- Fungal and parasitic UTIs are uncommon and are seen most frequently in the patient who is immunosuppressed, has kidney disorders or diabetes mellitus (DM) or has taken multiple courses of antibiotics.

Classification

A UTI can be broadly classified as an upper or a lower UTI according to its location within the urinary system. Infection of the upper urinary tract (involving the renal parenchyma, pelvis, and ureters) typically causes fever, chills, and flank pain, whereas a lower-urinary-tract infection does not usually have systemic manifestations.

Specific terms are used to further delineate UTI location. For example, *pyelonephritis* implies inflammation usually caused by infection of the renal parenchyma and collecting system, *cystitis* indicates inflammation of the bladder wall, and *urethritis* is inflammation of the urethra. *Urosepsis* is a UTI that has spread systemically and is a life-threatening condition requiring emergency treatment.

Classifying a UTI as uncomplicated or complicated is also useful.

- *Uncomplicated UTIs* are those that occur in an otherwise normal urinary tract and usually involve only the bladder.
- *Complicated UTIs* are those associated with coexisting obstruction, stones, or catheters; abnormal genitourinary (GU) tract; DM or neurologic diseases; immunosuppression; pregnancy-induced changes; recurrent infection; or antibiotic resistance. The individual with a complicated infection is at risk for pyelonephritis, urosepsis, and renal damage.

Pathophysiology

The urinary tract above the urethra is normally sterile, and organisms that cause UTIs are usually introduced by way of the ascending route from the urethra. Most infections are caused by gram-negative aerobic bacilli normally found in the GI tract. Table 85 lists risk factors for UTIs.

- A common factor contributing to ascending infection is urologic instrumentation (e.g., catheterization, cystoscopic examinations). Instrumentation allows bacteria that are normally present at the opening of the urethra to enter the urethra or bladder.
- Sexual intercourse promotes "milking" of bacteria from the vagina and perineum and may cause minor urethral trauma that predisposes women to UTIs.
- UTIs rarely result from hematogenous spread, whereby blood-borne bacteria secondarily invade the kidneys, ureters, or bladder from elsewhere in the body.

Catheter-associated urinary tract infections (CAUTIs) are the most common health care–associated infection (HAI). The cause of CAUTIs is often *E. coli* and, less frequently, *Pseudomonas* organisms. Most often these infections are underrecognized and undertreated, leading to extended hospital stays, higher health care costs, and increased rates of patient morbidity and mortality.

Clinical Manifestations

Lower urinary tract symptoms (LUTS) are seen in UTIs of both the upper and lower urinary tracts.

- Symptoms include dysuria, frequent urination (more often than every 2 hours), urgency, and suprapubic discomfort or pressure. Older adults tend to experience generalized abdominal discomfort, rather than dysuria and suprapubic pain.
- The urine may contain visible blood (hematuria) or sediment, giving it a cloudy appearance.
- Flank pain, chills, and fever indicate an infection involving the upper urinary tract (pyelonephritis).

Multiple factors may produce LUTS similar to those associated with UTI. For example, patients with bladder tumors or those receiving intravesical chemotherapy or pelvic radiation therapy usually experience urinary frequency, urgency, and dysuria. Interstitial cystitis also produces urinary symptoms that are similar to those of UTI and is sometimes confused with UTI (see Interstitial Cystitis/Painful Bladder Syndrome, p. 356).

Diagnostic Studies

- Dipstick urinalysis is done initially to identify presence of nitrites (indicating bacteriuria), WBCs, and leukocyte esterase (an enzyme present in WBCs indicating pyuria).
- After confirmation of bacteriuria and pyuria, a urine culture with sensitivity may be obtained.

TABLE 85 Risk Factors for Urinary Tract Infections

Factors Increasing Urinary Stasis
- Intrinsic obstruction (stone, tumor of urinary tract, urethral stricture, BPH)
- Extrinsic obstruction (tumor, fibrosis with compression of urinary tract)
- Urinary retention (e.g., neurogenic bladder)
- Renal impairment

Foreign Bodies
- Urinary tract calculi
- Catheters (indwelling, external condom catheter, ureteral stent, nephrostomy tube, intermittent catheterization)
- Urinary tract instrumentation (cystoscopy)

Anatomic Factors
- Congenital defects leading to obstruction or urinary stasis
- Fistula (abnormal opening) exposing urinary stream to skin, vagina, or feces
- Shorter female urethra and colonization from normal vaginal flora
- Obesity

Factors Compromising Immune Response
- Aging
- Human immunodeficiency virus infection
- Diabetes mellitus

Functional Disorders
- Constipation
- Voiding dysfunction with detrusor sphincter dyssynergia

Other Factors
- Pregnancy
- Menopause
- Multiple sex partners (women)
- Use of spermicidal agents, contraceptive diaphragm (women), bubble baths, feminine hygiene sprays
- Poor personal hygiene
- Habitual delay of urination ("nurse's bladder," "teacher's bladder")

BPH, Benign prostatic hyperplasia.

- A CT urogram or ultrasound may be obtained when obstruction of the urinary system is suspected.

Interprofessional Care
Drug Therapy
Uncomplicated cystitis can be treated using a short-term course of antibiotics, typically for 3 days. By contrast, complicated UTIs require treatment for a longer period of time, lasting 7 to 14 days or more.

- First-choice drugs for empirical treatment of uncomplicated or initial UTIs are trimethoprim/sulfamethoxazole, nitrofurantoin (Macrodantin), and fosfomycin (Monurol).
- Other antibiotics that may be used to treat uncomplicated UTI include ampicillin, amoxicillin, and cephalosporins. The fluoroquinolones [ciprofloxacin (Cipro), levofloxacin (Levaquin), ofloxacin, and gatifloxacin are used to treat complicated UTIs.
- In patients with UTIs caused by fungi, amphotericin or fluconazole (Diflucan) is the preferred therapy.
- Prophylactic or suppressive antibiotics are sometimes given to patients who have repeated UTIs.
- A urinary analgesic such as oral phenazopyridine may be used to relieve discomfort caused by severe dysuria.

Nursing Management
Goals
The patient with a UTI will have relief from bothersome LUTS, prevention of upper urinary tract involvement, and prevention of recurrence. See eNursing Care Plan 45-1 for the patient with a UTI on the website for Lewis et al, *Medical-Surgical Nursing,* ed 10.

Nursing Diagnoses
- Impaired urinary elimination
- Readiness for enhanced self-health management

Nursing Interventions
Health promotion activities, especially for individuals who are at an increased risk for UTI, include teaching preventive measures such as (1) emptying the bladder regularly and completely, (2) evacuating the bowel regularly, (3) wiping the perineal area from front to back after urination and defecation, and (4) drinking an adequate amount of liquid each day. Daily intake of cranberry or cranberry tablets may reduce the number of UTIs.

- All patients undergoing instrumentation of the urinary tract are at risk for developing CAUTI. You have a major role in the prevention of these infections. Avoidance of unnecessary catheterization and early removal of indwelling catheters are the most effective measures for reducing CAUTI. Always follow aseptic technique during these procedures.

- Wash your hands before and after contact with each patient. Wear gloves for care of urinary catheters. The American Nurses Association offers an evidence-based clinical tool for decreasing CAUTI (*http://nursingworld.org/CAUTI-Tool*).
- Acute intervention for the patient with a UTI includes adequate fluid intake. Fluid flushes out bacteria before they have a chance to colonize in the bladder. Caffeine, alcohol, citrus juice, chocolate, and highly spiced foods or beverages should be avoided because they may irritate the bladder.
- Application of local heat to the suprapubic area or lower back may relieve the discomfort associated with a UTI. A warm shower or sitting in a tub of warm water filled to above the waist can also provide temporary relief.

▼ **Patient and Caregiver Teaching**

Instruct the patient about the prescribed drug therapy and side effects. Emphasize the importance of taking the full course of antibiotics.

- Instruct the patient to monitor for signs of improvement (e.g., cloudy urine becomes clear) and a decrease in symptoms.
- Teach patients to promptly report any of the following to their HCP: (1) persistence of bothersome LUTS beyond the antibiotic treatment course, (2) onset of flank pain, or (3) fever.
- Teach the patient and caregiver about the need for ongoing care, including taking antimicrobial drugs as ordered, maintaining adequate daily fluid intake, voiding regularly (approximately every 3 to 4 hours), urinating before and after intercourse, and temporarily discontinuing the use of a diaphragm.

If treatment is complete and symptoms are still present, instruct the patient to get follow-up care. Recurrent symptoms associated with bacterial persistence or inadequate treatment typically occur within 1 to 2 weeks after completion of therapy.

VAGINAL, CERVICAL, AND VULVAR INFECTIONS

Definition

Infection and inflammation of the vagina, cervix, and vulva occur when the natural defenses of the acid vaginal secretions (maintained by a sufficient estrogen level) and the presence of *Lactobacillus* are disrupted. Aging, poor nutrition, and drugs (e.g., antibiotics, oral contraceptives, corticosteroids) can affect the bacterial flora or mucosa, leading to alterations in the pH balance of the genital tract.

Pathophysiology

Organisms gain entrance to the lower genital tract through sexual intercourse, contact with contaminated hands or clothing, or douching. Table 86 presents the causes, manifestations and interprofessional care of common infections of the female lower genital tract.

- Oral contraceptives, antibiotics, and corticosteroids may change the vaginal pH and trigger an overgrowth of the organisms present. For example, *Candida albicans* may be present in small numbers in the vagina. An overgrowth of this organism causes vulvovaginitis.
- Vulvar infections, such as herpes and genital warts, can be sexually transmitted when no visible lesions are present (see Herpes, Genital, p. 303, and Warts, Genital, p. 677).

Clinical Manifestations

Abnormal vaginal discharge is a common sign of infection. See Table 86 for additional manifestations of lower genital tract infections.

Diagnostic Studies

Evaluation of genital problems includes a history, physical examination, and appropriate laboratory and diagnostic studies. Because many problems relate to sexual activity, a sexual history is essential.

- Ulcerative lesions are cultured for herpesvirus.
- Vulvar dystrophies are examined by colposcope, with biopsy specimens taken.
- Vaginal discharge is evaluated by examining the discharge under a microscope and obtaining cultures.
- With cervicitis, endocervical cultures are obtained for chlamydia and gonorrhea.
- Sexually transmitted infections (STIs) are discussed on p. 562.

Interprofessional Care

Antibiotics taken as directed will cure bacterial infections. Women with vaginal conditions or cervical infection should abstain from intercourse for at least 1 week. Douching should be avoided. Sexual partners must be evaluated and treated if the patient is diagnosed with trichomoniasis, chlamydial infection, gonorrhea, syphilis, or HIV infection.

TABLE 86 Infections of the Lower Genital Tract

Infection and Etiology	Manifestations	Drug Therapy
Vulvovaginal Candidiasis		
Candida albicans (fungus)	Pruritus, thick white curd-like discharge	Antifungal agents (e.g., miconazole [Monistat 7], clotrimazole [Gyne-Lotrimin, Mycelex] [available over the counter, as cream or suppository]) Fluconazole (Diflucan) Butoconazole 2% vaginal cream (Gynazole-1) Terconazole (Terazol 3) vaginal creams and suppositories
Trichomonas Vaginitis		
Trichomonas vaginalis (protozoan)	Sexually transmitted Pruritus, frothy greenish or gray discharge Hemorrhagic spots on cervix or vaginal walls	Metronidazole (Flagyl) or tinidazole (Tindamax) for patient and partner

Continued

TABLE 86 Infections of the Lower Genital Tract—cont'd

Infection and Etiology	Manifestations	Drug Therapy
Bacterial Vaginosis		
Gardnerella vaginalis *Corynebacterium vaginale*	Watery discharge with fish-like odor May or may not have other symptoms	Oral or vaginal metronidazole (Flagyl), vaginal clindamycin (Clindesse), or oral tinidazole (Tindamax) Symptomatic female partners need to be treated. Lactobacillus acidophilus taken orally by diet (e.g., yogurt, fermented soy products) or supplements can decrease unwanted vaginal bacteria.
Cervicitis		
Chlamydia trachomatis or *Neisseria gonorrhoeae* (most often)	Sexually transmitted Mucopurulent discharge with postcoital spotting from cervical inflammation	Based on cause Common treatment includes azithromycin (Zithromax) and ceftriaxone. Treat patient and partner.
Severe Recurrent Vaginitis (more than four episodes per year)		
C. albicans (most often) or non-albicans strains	May be indication of HIV infection All women who are unresponsive to first-line treatment should be offered HIV testing.	Drug appropriate to opportunistic organism

KOH, Potassium hydroxide.

Treatment of vulvar skin conditions is symptomatic, controlling the itching and hence the scratching. High-potency topical cortico-steroid ointment such as clobetasol helps relieve itching. Interrupting the "itch-scratch cycle" prevents further secondary damage to the skin.

Nursing Management

Teach women about common genital conditions and how to reduce their risks. Recognize symptoms that indicate a problem and help women seek care in a timely manner.

When a woman is diagnosed with a genital condition, ensure that she fully understands the directions for treatment. Teach patients how to properly take prescribed drugs and to get follow-up care. Partners should be treated so that reinfection does not occur. When a woman is using a vaginal medication such as an antifungal cream for the first time, show her the applicator and how to fill it. Also teach where and how the applicator should be inserted by using visual aids or models. Vaginal creams should be inserted before going to bed so that the medication will remain in the vagina for a long period of time. Women using vaginal creams or supposi-tories may wish to use panty liners during the day, when the residual medication drains out.

VALVULAR HEART DISEASE

Description

Valvular heart disease is defined according to the affected valve or valves (mitral, aortic, tricuspid, pulmonary) and the type of dys-function: *stenosis* or *regurgitation.*

- The pressures on either side of an open valve normally are equal. However, in *stenosis,* the valve opening is smaller, impeding the forward flow of blood and creating a pressure difference on the two sides of the open valve. The degree of stenosis (constric-tion or narrowing) is reflected in the pressure differences (i.e., the higher the gradient, the greater the stenosis).
- In *regurgitation* (also called *incompetence* or *insufficiency*), incomplete closure of valve leaflets results in a backward flow of blood.

Congenital heart conditions are the most common cause of valve disorders in children and adolescents. Aortic stenosis and mitral regurgitation are the common valve disorders in older adults. Other causes of valve disease in adults include disorders related to acquired immunodeficiency syndrome (AIDS) and the use of some antiparkinsonian drugs.

TABLE 87 Manifestations of Valvular Heart Disease

Type	Manifestations
Mitral valve stenosis	Dyspnea on exertion, hemoptysis, fatigue. Atrial fibrillation on ECG. Palpitations. Loud, accentuated S_1. Low-pitched, diastolic murmur.
Mitral valve regurgitation	*Acute:* Generally poorly tolerated. New systolic murmur with rapid development of pulmonary edema and cardiogenic shock. *Chronic:* Weakness, fatigue, exertional dyspnea, palpitations, S_3 gallop, holosystolic murmur.
Mitral valve prolapse	Palpitations, dyspnea, chest pain, activity intolerance, syncope, holosystolic murmur.
Aortic valve stenosis	Angina, syncope, dyspnea on exertion, heart failure, normal or soft S_1, diminished or absent S_2, systolic murmur, prominent S_4.
Aortic valve regurgitation	*Acute:* Abrupt onset of profound dyspnea, chest pain, left ventricular failure, and cardiogenic shock. *Chronic:* Fatigue, exertional dyspnea, orthopnea, PND. Water-hammer pulse, heaving precordial impulse, diminished or absent S_1, S_3, or S_4. Soft high-pitched diastolic murmur, Austin Flint murmur.
Tricuspid and pulmonic stenosis	*Tricuspid:* Peripheral edema, ascites, hepatomegaly. Diastolic low-pitched murmur with increased intensity during inspiration. *Pulmonic:* Fatigue, loud midsystolic murmur.

PND, Paroxysmal nocturnal dyspnea.

Clinical manifestations of valvular heart disease are presented in Table 87.

Mitral Valve Stenosis

Pathophysiology

Most cases of adult mitral valve stenosis result from rheumatic heart disease. Less common causes include congenital mitral stenosis, rheumatoid arthritis, and systemic lupus erythematosus (SLE).

- Rheumatic endocarditis causes scarring of valve leaflets and chordae tendineae. Contractures and adhesions develop between the commissures (the junctional areas).

- The stenotic mitral valve takes on a "fish mouth" shape because of the thickening and shortening of mitral valve structures. Flow obstruction increases left atrial pressure and volume, resulting in higher pulmonary vasculature pressure and eventually involving the right ventricle.

Clinical Manifestations

The primary symptom is exertional dyspnea due to reduced lung compliance. Fatigue and palpitations from atrial fibrillation may also occur. Heart sounds include a loud first heart sound and a low-pitched, rumbling diastolic murmur (best heard at the apex with the stethoscope bell).

Other clinical manifestations are identified in Table 87.

Mitral Valve Regurgitation

Pathophysiology

Mitral valve function depends on the integrity of mitral leaflets, chordae tendineae, papillary muscles, left atrium (LA), and left ventricle (LV). A defect in any of these structures can result in regurgitation. Myocardial infarction with left ventricular failure increases the risk for rupture of the chordae tendineae and acute mitral regurgitation (MR).

- Most cases of MR are caused by myocardial infarction, chronic rheumatic heart disease, mitral valve prolapse, ischemic papillary muscle dysfunction, and infective endocarditis.
- MR allows blood to flow backward from the LV to the LA because of incomplete valve closure during systole. Both chambers of the left side of the heart must work harder to preserve an adequate cardiac output (CO).
- In acute MR, abrupt dilation of the LA or LV does not occur. The sudden increase in pressure and volume is transmitted to the pulmonary bed, resulting in pulmonary edema and, if not treated, cardiogenic shock.
- In chronic MR, the additional volume load results in left atrial enlargement and left ventricular dilation and hypertrophy, and finally a decrease in CO.

Clinical Manifestations

Patients with acute MR have thready peripheral pulses and cool, clammy extremities. A low CO may mask a new systolic murmur. Rapid assessment (e.g., cardiac catheterization) and intervention (e.g., valve repair or replacement) are critical for a positive outcome.

Patients with chronic MR may remain asymptomatic for many years until the development of some degree of left ventricular failure. Manifestations are identified in Table 87.

Mitral Valve Prolapse

Pathophysiology

Mitral valve prolapse (MVP) is an abnormality of the mitral valve leaflets and papillary muscles or chordae that allows the leaflets to prolapse, or "buckle," back into the left atrium during systole. It is the most common form of valvular heart disease in the United States.

- MVP is usually benign, but serious complications can occur, including mitral regurgitation, infective endocarditis, sudden cardiac death, and cerebral ischemia.
- There is an increased familial incidence in some patients resulting from a connective tissue defect affecting only the valve, or as part of Marfan's syndrome or other hereditary conditions that influence the structure of collagen in the body.

Clinical Manifestations

MVP encompasses a broad spectrum of severity. Most patients are asymptomatic and remain so for their entire lives. Clinical manifestations may include those identified in Table 87.

- Patients may or may not have chest pain. If chest pain occurs, episodes tend to occur in clusters, especially during periods of emotional stress. Chest pain may occasionally be accompanied by dyspnea, palpitations, and syncope and does not respond to antianginal treatment (e.g., nitrates).

Patients with MVP generally have a benign, manageable course unless problems related to MR develop. Table 88 provides a teaching plan for patients with MVP.

Aortic Valve Stenosis

Pathophysiology

Congenital aortic stenosis is generally found in childhood, adolescence, or young adulthood. In older patients, *aortic stenosis* is a result of rheumatic fever or degeneration similar to that in coronary artery disease.

- In rheumatic valve disease, fusion of the commissures and secondary calcification cause the valve leaflets to stiffen and retract, resulting in stenosis. Isolated aortic valve stenosis is usually nonrheumatic in origin.
- Aortic stenosis causes obstruction of flow from the left ventricle to the aorta during systole. The effect is left ventricular hypertrophy and increased myocardial oxygen consumption secondary to the increased myocardial mass.
- As the disease progresses and compensatory mechanisms fail, reduced CO leads to pulmonary hypertension and heart failure.

TABLE 88 Patient & Caregiver Teaching

Mitral Valve Prolapse

Include the following information in the teaching plan for a patient with mitral valve prolapse (MVP) and the patient's caregiver.

- Take drugs as prescribed (e.g., β-adrenergic blockers to control palpitations, chest pain).
- Adopt healthy eating habits.
- Avoid caffeine because it is a stimulant and may exacerbate symptoms.
- If you use diet pills or other over-the-counter drugs, check for common ingredients that are stimulants (e.g., caffeine, ephedrine) because these can exacerbate symptoms.
- Begin (or maintain) an exercise program to achieve optimal health.
- Contact the HCP or emergency medical services if symptoms develop or worsen (e.g., palpitations, fatigue, shortness of breath, anxiety).

Clinical Manifestations

Symptoms of aortic stenosis (AS) develop when the valve orifice becomes about one third of its normal size. Symptoms include the classic triad of angina, syncope, and exertional dyspnea, reflecting left ventricular failure. Common manifestations are presented in Table 87. Left untreated, severe AS has an approximately 50% mortality rate at 1 year.

Aortic Valve Regurgitation

Pathophysiology

Aortic regurgitation may be the result of primary disease of the aortic valve leaflets, the aortic root, or both.

- Acute aortic regurgitation is caused by infective endocarditis, trauma, or aortic dissection and constitutes a life-threatening emergency.
- Chronic aortic regurgitation is generally the result of rheumatic heart disease, a congenital bicuspid aortic valve, syphilis, or chronic arthritic conditions such as ankylosing spondylitis or reactive arthritis.
- Aortic regurgitation causes retrograde blood flow from the ascending aorta into the LV, resulting in volume overload.
- Myocardial contractility eventually declines, and blood volume increases in the LA and pulmonary bed. This leads to pulmonary hypertension and right ventricular failure.

Clinical Manifestations

Clinical manifestations of acute and chronic aortic valve regurgitation are presented in Table 87.

Tricuspid and Pulmonic Valve Disease

Diseases of the tricuspid and pulmonic valves are uncommon, with stenosis occurring more frequently than regurgitation. Tricuspid stenosis results in right atrial enlargement and elevated systemic venous pressures. Pulmonic stenosis results in right ventricular hypertension and hypertrophy. Table 87 presents clinical manifestations of these valve diseases.

Diagnostic Studies: Valvular Heart Disease

- CT scan of the chest with contrast is the gold standard for evaluating aortic disorders.
- ECG shows variations in heart rate (HR), rhythm, and possible ischemia or chamber enlargement.
- Echocardiogram reveals valve structure, function, and heart chamber size.
- Transesophageal echocardiography and Doppler color-flow imaging help diagnose and monitor valvular heart disease progression.
- Real-time 3-D echocardiography helps assess mitral valve and congenital heart disease.
- Chest x-ray reveals heart size, altered pulmonary circulation, and valve calcification.
- Cardiac catheterization detects chamber pressure changes and pressure gradients (differences) across the valves.

Interprofessional Care: Valvular Heart Disease

An important aspect of conservative therapy is the prevention of recurrent rheumatic fever and infective endocarditis. Treatment depends on the valve involved and the severity of disease. It focuses on preventing exacerbations of heart failure, acute pulmonary edema, thromboembolism, and recurrent endocarditis. Heart failure is treated with vasodilators, positive inotropes, β-adrenergic blockers, diuretics, and a low-sodium diet.

- Anticoagulant therapy is used to prevent and treat systemic or pulmonary emboli, and it is also used as a prophylactic measure in patients with atrial fibrillation.
- Atrial dysrhythmias are common and treated with calcium channel blockers, β-adrenergic blockers, digoxin, antidysrhythmic drugs, or electrical cardioversion.
- An alternative treatment for some patients with valvular heart disease is the *percutaneous transluminal balloon valvuloplasty*

(PTBV) procedure. Balloon valvuloplasty is used more often for pulmonic, aortic, and mitral stenosis. PTBV is done in the heart catheterization laboratory. It involves threading a balloon-tipped catheter from the femoral artery to the stenotic valve so that the balloon may be inflated in an attempt to separate valve leaflets.

- The PTBV procedure is generally indicated for older patients and those who are poor surgical candidates.

Surgical Therapy

The type of surgery used depends on the valves involved, pathology and severity of the disease, and patient's clinical condition.

- Valve repair is usually the surgical procedure of choice. It is often used in mitral or tricuspid valvular heart disease.

Mitral *commissurotomy* (valvulotomy) is the procedure of choice for patients with pure mitral stenosis. The open method of commissurotomy (which has largely replaced the older, less precise closed method) requires the use of cardiopulmonary bypass, removal of thrombi from the atrium, and a commissure incision. Next the fused chordae are separated by splitting the papillary muscle and debriding the calcified valve.

- Open surgical *valvuloplasty* involves repairing the valve by suturing the torn leaflets, chordae tendineae, and papillary muscles. It is primarily used to treat mitral regurgitation or tricuspid regurgitation.
- Further repair or reconstruction of the valve may be necessary and can be achieved by *annuloplasty,* a procedure also used in cases of mitral or tricuspid regurgitation. Annuloplasty involves reconstruction of the annulus, with or without the aid of prosthetic rings.

Valve Replacement. Valve replacement may be required for mitral, aortic, tricuspid, and, occasionally, pulmonic valvular disease.

- Prosthetic valves are categorized as *mechanical* or *biologic* (tissue) *valves.* Mechanical valves are made of combinations of metal alloys, pyrolite carbon, and Dacron. Biologic valves are constructed from bovine, porcine, and human (cadaver) cardiac tissue. Mechanical prosthetic valves are more durable and last longer than biologic tissue valves, but they carry an increased risk of thromboembolism and require long-term anticoagulant therapy. Biologic valves do not require anticoagulant therapy because of their low thrombogenicity. However, they are less durable and tend to develop early calcification, tissue degeneration, and stiffening of leaflets.
- Long-term anticoagulation is needed for those patients with biologic valves who have atrial fibrillation. Some patients

with biologic valves or annuloplasty with prosthetic rings may need anticoagulation the first few months after surgery, until the suture lines are covered by endothelial cells (endothelialized).

- The choice of valves depends on many factors. For example, if the patient cannot take anticoagulants (e.g., women of child-bearing age), a biologic valve is considered. A mechanical valve may be best for a younger patient because it is more durable. For patients older than 65 years, durability is less important than avoiding the risks of bleeding from anticoagulants, so most receive a biologic valve.

Nursing Management: Valvular Heart Disease
Goals
The patient with valvular heart disease will have normal cardiac function, improved activity tolerance, and an understanding of the disease process and maintenance measures.

Nursing Diagnoses
- Decreased cardiac output
- Activity intolerance
- Excess fluid volume

Nursing Interventions
Diagnosing and treating streptococcal infection and providing prophylactic antibiotics for patients with a history of rheumatic fever are critical to prevent acquired rheumatic valve disease. Patients at risk for endocarditis and any patients with certain high-risk heart conditions must also receive prophylactic antibiotics.

- The patient must adhere to recommended therapies. The individual with a history of rheumatic fever, endocarditis, and congenital heart disease should know the symptoms of valvular heart disease so that early medical treatment may begin. Your role is to implement and evaluate the effectiveness of therapeutic interventions.
- Design activities considering the patient's limitations. An appropriate exercise plan can increase cardiac tolerance. Activities that cause fatigue and dyspnea should be restricted.
- Develop your patient's activities of daily living plan to emphasize conserving energy, setting priorities, and taking planned rest periods.
- Consider referral to a vocational counselor if the patient has a physically or emotionally demanding job.
- Perform ongoing cardiac assessments to monitor the effectiveness of medications. Teach the actions and side effects of drugs to improve adherence.

- The patient on anticoagulation therapy (e.g., with warfarin [Coumadin]) after surgery for valve replacement must have the international normalized ratio (INR) checked regularly to determine adequacy of therapy. INR values of 2.5 to 3.5 are therapeutic for patients with mechanical valves.

▼ **Patient and Caregiver Teaching**
- Teach the patient to notify the HCP about any manifestations of infection or heart failure or signs of bleeding.
- Encourage patients to wear a medical identification (Medic Alert) device.

VARICOSE VEINS

Description
Varicose veins (varicosities) are dilated (to 3 mm or larger in diameter), tortuous superficial veins, commonly found in the saphenous vein system. They may be small and innocuous or large and bulging.

- *Primary* varicose veins (idiopathic), caused by weakness of the vein walls, are more common in women.
- *Secondary* varicosities typically result from result from direct injury, a previous venous thromboembolism (VTE), or excessive vein distention. Secondary varicose veins may also occur in the esophagus (esophageal varices), vulva, spermatic cords (varicoceles), and anorectal area (hemorrhoids), and as abnormal arteriovenous (AV) connections.

Pathophysiology
The etiology of varicose veins is multifactorial. Risk factors include family history of chronic venous disease, weakness of the vein structure, female gender, Hispanic ethnicity, tobacco use, increasing age, obesity, multiparity, history of VTE, venous obstruction resulting from extrinsic pressure by tumors, phlebitis, previous leg injury, and occupations that require prolonged standing or sitting.

- In primary varicose veins, weak vein walls allow the vein valve ring to enlarge so that the leaflets no longer fit together properly (incompetent). Incompetent vein valves allow backward blood flow, particularly when the patient is standing. This results in increased venous pressure and further venous distention.

Clinical Manifestations
Discomfort from varicose veins varies dramatically and tends to be worse after episodes of superficial thrombophlebitis. The most

common varicose vein symptoms include a heavy, achy pain after prolonged standing or sitting, which is relieved by walking or limb elevation. Some patients feel pressure or a cramplike, burning sensation. Swelling and/or nocturnal leg cramps may also occur.

Superficial venous thrombosis is the most frequent complication of varicose veins and may occur spontaneously or after trauma, surgical procedures, or pregnancy.

Diagnostic Studies

- Superficial varicose veins can be diagnosed by appearance.
- Duplex ultrasound detects obstruction and reflux in the venous system.

Interprofessional Care

Conservative treatment involves rest with limb elevation, graduated compression stockings, leg-strengthening exercise such as walking, and weight loss if indicated.

Venoactive drugs (e.g., diosmin, hesperidin, rutosides [Venoruton]) have been used to treat varicose veins and advanced chronic venous disease. Therapeutic benefits of venoactive drugs include pain relief, edema reduction, and decreased leg cramping and restless legs symptoms. These drugs have been widely used in Europe. They are not approved by the U.S. Food and Drug Administration (FDA); however, many are available over the counter as dietary or herbal supplements (e.g., rutosides [e.g., horse chestnut seed extract], gotu kola, pine bark).

Sclerotherapy involves the injection of a substance that obliterates venous telangiectasias (i.e., spider veins) and small superficial varicose veins. Direct IV injection of a sclerosing agent such as hypertonic saline induces inflammation and results in eventual thrombosis of the vein. After injection, a graduated compression stocking or compression bandage is recommended. Patients should not travel long distances during the first week after sclerotherapy to minimize the risk of a VTE.

- Other noninvasive options include transcutaneous laser therapy for telangiectasias and high-intensity pulsed-light therapy for reticular veins.

Surgical intervention is indicated for recurrent superficial vein thrombosis or when chronic venous insufficiency cannot be controlled with conservative therapy. Traditional surgical intervention involves ligation of the entire vein (usually the greater saphenous) and removal of its incompetent branches. An alternative but time-consuming technique is ambulatory phlebectomy, which involves pulling the varicosity through a "stab" incision, followed by excision of the vein.

Nursing Management

Prevention is a key factor related to varicose veins. Instruct the patient to avoid sitting or standing for long periods, maintain ideal body weight, take precautions against injury to the extremities, avoid wearing constrictive clothing, and walk daily.

After vein ligation surgery, check extremities regularly for color, movement, sensation, temperature, presence of edema, and pedal pulses. Some bruising and discoloration are considered normal.

- Elevate the patient's legs 15 degrees to decrease edema.
- Apply graduated compression stockings or bandages. Remove them every 8 hours for a short period and then reapply them.

Long-term management of varicose veins is directed toward improving circulation, relieving discomfort, improving cosmetic appearance, and avoiding complications such as superficial thrombophlebitis and ulceration. Varicose veins can recur in other veins after surgery.

▼ Patient and Caregiver Teaching

- Teach the patient the proper use and care of custom-fitted graduated compression stockings. The patient should apply the stockings in bed, before rising in the morning.
- Stress the importance of periodically positioning the legs above heart level.
- The overweight patient may need assistance with weight loss.
- Patients with a job that requires long periods of standing or sitting need to frequently flex and extend their hips, legs, and ankles and change positions.

VENOUS THROMBOSIS

Description

Venous thrombosis involves the formation of a thrombus (blood clot) in association with inflammation of the vein. It is the most common disorder of the veins and is classified as either superficial vein thrombosis or deep vein thrombosis.

Superficial vein thrombosis is the formation of a thrombus in a superficial vein, usually the greater or lesser saphenous vein.

Deep vein thrombosis (DVT) is a disorder involving a thrombus in a deep vein, most commonly the iliac or femoral vein. *Venous thromboembolism* (VTE) is the preferred term and represents the spectrum of pathology from DVT to pulmonary embolism (PE). Table 89 compares superficial vein thrombosis and VTE.

	SVT	VTE
TABLE 89 Comparison of Superficial Vein Thrombosis (SVT) and Venous Thromboembolism (VTE)		
Usual Location	Typically, superficial leg veins (e.g., varicosities) Occasionally, superficial arm veins	Deep veins of arms (e.g., axillary, subclavian), legs (e.g., femoral), pelvis (e.g., iliac, inferior or superior vena cava), and pulmonary system
Clinical Findings	Tenderness, itchiness, redness, warmth, pain, inflammation, and induration along the course of the superficial vein Vein appears as a palpable cord. Edema rarely occurs.	Tenderness to pressure over involved vein, induration of overlying muscle, venous distention Edema of affected extremity May have mild to moderate pain, deep reddish color to area caused by venous congestion *Note:* Some patients may have no obvious physical changes in the affected extremity.
Sequelae	If untreated, clot may extend to deeper veins, and VTE may occur.	Embolization to lungs (pulmonary embolism) may occur and may result in death.* Pulmonary hypertension and post-thrombotic syndrome with or without venous leg ulceration may develop.

*See Pulmonary Embolism, p. 523.

Pathophysiology

Three important factors *(Virchow's triad)* in the etiology of venous thrombosis are venous stasis, damage of the endothelium (inner lining of the vein), and hypercoagulability of the blood. The patient at risk for the development of VTE usually has a predisposing condition to these three disorders.

Venous stasis occurs when the valves are dysfunctional or the muscles of the extremities are inactive. Venous stasis occurs more frequently in people who are obese, have chronic heart failure or atrial fibrillation, have been on long trips without regular exercise, undergo a prolonged surgical procedure, or are immobile for long periods (e.g., with spinal cord injury or hip fracture).

Damage to the endothelium of the vein may be caused by direct (e.g., surgery, intravascular catheterization, trauma, fracture, burns, prior VTE) or indirect (chemotherapy, vasculitis, sepsis, diabetes) injury to the vessel. Damaged endothelium has decreased fibrinolytic properties, which predispose the patient to thrombus development.

Hypercoagulability of the blood occurs in many disorders, including severe anemias, polycythemia, malignancies (e.g., cancers of the breast, brain, pancreas, and gastrointestinal tract), nephrotic syndrome, hyperhomocysteinemia, and protein C, protein S, and antithrombin deficiency.

- Women who use tobacco, take oral contraceptives or hormone therapy, are older than 35 years of age, or have a family history of VTE are at extremely high risk for a thrombotic event.

Localized platelet aggregation and fibrin entrap RBCs, WBCs, and more platelets to form a thrombus. A frequent site of thrombus formation is the valve cusps of veins.

- As the thrombus enlarges, blood cells and fibrin collect behind it, producing a larger clot with a "tail" that eventually occludes the lumen of the vein.
- If a thrombus only partially blocks the vein, the thrombus becomes covered by endothelial cells and the thrombotic process stops.
- If the thrombus does not detach, it undergoes lysis or becomes firmly organized and adherent within 5 to 7 days.
- The organized thrombus may detach and result in an embolus that flows through the venous circulation to the heart and lodges in the pulmonary circulation, resulting in PE.

Superficial Vein Thrombosis

Clinical Manifestations and Diagnosis

The patient may have a palpable, firm, subcutaneous cordlike vein. The surrounding area may be itchy, tender to the touch, reddened, and warm. A mild temperature elevation and leukocytosis may be present. Edema of the extremity may occur.

Duplex ultrasound is used to confirm the diagnosis (5 cm or larger clot) and to rule out clot extension to a deep vein.

Interprofessional Care

For patients with a lower leg superficial vein thrombosis, subcutaneous fondaparinux (Arixtra) reduces symptomatic VTE, and superficial vein thrombosis extension and recurrence without causing major bleeding problems.

If the superficial vein thrombosis affects a very short vein segment (less than 5 cm) and is not near the saphenofemoral junction, anticoagulants may not be necessary, and oral nonsteroidal antiinflammatory drugs (NSAIDs) can ease symptoms.

- Additional interventions to relieve SVT symptoms include telling the patient to wear graduated compression stockings or bandages, elevate the affected limb above level of heart, apply topical NSAIDs, and perform mild exercise such as walking.

Venous Thromboembolism
Clinical Manifestations and Diagnosis
The patient with lower extremity VTE may have unilateral leg edema, pain, tenderness with palpation, dilated superficial veins, a sense of fullness in the thigh or the calf, paresthesias, warm skin, erythema, or a systemic temperature greater than 100.4° F (38° C).

- If the inferior vena cava is involved, both legs may be edematous and cyanotic. If the superior vena cava is involved, similar symptoms may occur in the arms, neck, back, and face.

Diagnosis of an initial VTE is based on clinical assessment combined with D-dimer testing and duplex ultrasound.

Complications
The most serious complications of VTE are PE, chronic thromboembolic pulmonary hypertension, post-thrombotic syndrome, and phlegmasia cerulea dolens.

- *Post-thrombotic syndrome* (PTS) can result from chronic venous hypertension caused by valvular destruction (from inflammation and scarring), stiff noncompliant vein walls, and persistent venous obstruction. Symptoms include pain, aching, sensation of heaviness, cramps, itching, and tingling. Clinical signs include persistent edema, increased pigmentation, eczema, secondary varicosities, and lipodermatosclerosis.
- *Phlegmasia cerulea dolens* (swollen, blue, painful leg), a rare complication, may develop in a patient in the advanced stages of cancer. It results from severe lower extremity VTE(s) that involve the major leg veins, causing near-total occlusion of venous outflow. Patients typically experience sudden massive swelling, deep pain, and intense cyanosis of the extremity.

Diagnostic Studies
- Platelet count, hemoglobin (Hgb), hematocrit (Hct), D-dimer testing, and coagulation tests (bleeding time, prothrombin time [PT], and partial thromboplastin time [PTT]) may be altered if underlying blood dyscrasias are present.

- Venous compression ultrasound evaluates deep femoral, popliteal, and posterior tibial veins.
- Duplex ultrasound and color-flow Doppler determine the location and extent of venous thrombi.
- Venogram (phlebogram) can determine the extent and location of the clot.

V

Interprofessional Care

In patients at risk for VTE, a variety of interventions are used. Patients on bed rest should change position every 2 hours. Unless contraindicated, teach patients to flex and extend their feet, knees, and hips at least every 2 to 4 hours while awake. Patients who can get out of bed should be in a chair for meals and ambulate at least four to six times per day as able. Tell the patient and the caregiver about the importance of these measures.

- Graduated compression stockings, when fitted correctly (for both size and length) and worn properly and consistently from hospital admission until discharge or full mobility, decrease VTE risk in surgical patients.
- *Intermittent pneumatic compression devices* (IPCs) use inflatable sleeves or boots to compress the calf and thigh and/or foot and ankle to improve venous return. IPCs may be used with elastic compression stockings. IPCs are not worn when a patient has an active VTE because of the risk of PE.

Anticoagulants are used routinely for VTE prevention and treatment. The goal of anticoagulant therapy for VTE prophylaxis is to prevent clot formation. The goals for treatment of a confirmed VTE are to prevent new clot development, spread of the clot, and embolization.

Three major classes of anticoagulants are available: (1) vitamin K antagonists, (2) thrombin inhibitors (both indirect and direct), and (3) factor Xa inhibitors. Anticoagulant therapy does not dissolve the clot. Clot lysis begins naturally through the body's intrinsic fibrinolytic system (see Table 37-10 on anticoagulant therapy, Lewis et al, *Medical-Surgical Nursing,* ed 10, p. 820).

Although most patients with VTE are managed medically, a small number of select patients with extensive, acute, proximal VTE who are not candidates for catheter-directed thrombolysis and/or interventional radiology therapies (because of high bleeding risk) may undergo surgery.

- Vena cava interruption devices (e.g., Greenfield, Vena Tech, TrapEase filters) can be inserted percutaneously through the right femoral or right internal jugular vein. The filters act as a sieve, permitting filtration of clots without interruption of blood flow.
- The interventional radiology procedures for an occluded vein are similar to those used in the treatment of lower extremity

peripheral arterial disease (PAD). Such procedures include mechanical thrombectomy, placement of a pharmacomechanical device, and post-thrombus extraction, angioplasty, and/or stenting.

Nursing Management

Goals. The patient with VTE will have pain relief, decreased edema, no skin ulceration, no bleeding complications, and no evidence of PE.

Nursing Diagnoses/Collaborative Problems

- Acute pain
- Ineffective health maintenance
- Risk for impaired skin integrity
- Potential complication: bleeding related to anticoagulant therapy
- Potential complication: PE

Nursing Interventions

Focus your nursing care for the patient with VTE on the prevention of embolus formation and reduction of inflammation. Review with the patient any drugs, vitamins, minerals, and dietary and herbal supplements being taken that may interfere with anticoagulant therapy.

- Check the results of appropriate tests before initiating, administering, or adjusting anticoagulant therapy.
- Monitor for and reduce the risk of bleeding that may occur with anticoagulant therapy.
- Bed rest with limb elevation may be prescribed for patients with acute VTE. Early ambulation after VTE results in a more rapid decrease in edema and limb pain. Teach the patient and the caregiver the importance of exercise, and assist the patient in ambulating several times a day.

▼ Patient and Caregiver Teaching

- Focus discharge teaching on modification of VTE risk factors, use of elastic compression stockings, importance of monitoring laboratory values, dietary and medication instructions, and guidelines for follow-up care. Once the edema is resolved, measure the patient for custom-fitted elastic compression stockings. Use of such stockings (or sleeves in the case of upper extremity VTE) is recommended for at least 2 years after VTE.
- Advise the patient to avoid all nicotine products.
- Instruct the patient to avoid constrictive clothing.
- Teach patients to avoid standing or sitting in a motionless, leg-dependent position. Encourage frequent exercise of the calf muscles, active walking, avoiding caffeinated beverages, and sitting in an aisle seat during long flights. For those at high risk for VTE who are planning a long trip, recommend properly

fitted, knee-high graduated compression stockings during travel to decrease edema and VTE risk.

- Teach the patient and caregiver about signs and symptoms of PE, such as sudden onset of dyspnea, tachypnea, and pleuritic chest pain.
- Instruct the patient and caregiver about drug dosage, actions, and side effects; the need for routine blood tests; and what symptoms need immediate medical attention.
- Teach patients taking low-molecular-weight heparin (LMWH) or fondaparinux and their caregivers how to give the drug subcutaneously.
- Teach patients taking warfarin (Coumadin) to follow a consistent diet of foods containing vitamin K (e.g., dark green leafy vegetables) and to avoid any supplements containing vitamin K. Encourage proper hydration to prevent additional hypercoagulability of the blood, which may occur with dehydration.
- Active patients need to avoid contact sports and high-risk (for trauma) activities (e.g., skiing). Teach older patients about safety precautions to prevent falls (e.g., avoid use of throw rugs).
- Help the patient develop an exercise program with an emphasis on leg strength training and aerobic activity.

WARTS, GENITAL

Description

Genital warts (condylomata acuminata) are caused by the human papillomavirus (HPV). There are approximately 150 papillomavirus types. More than 40 types can be sexually transmitted. Some of these can cause warts on the skin, whereas others can cause cancers of the genital tract or oropharynx.

Pathophysiology

Ninety percent of genital warts are caused by HPV types 6 and 11. HPV is transmitted by skin-to-skin contact, most commonly during vaginal, anal, or oral sex, but it can be transmitted during nonpenetrative sexual activity. The basal epithelial cells infected with HPV undergo transformation and proliferation to form a warty growth. The incubation period of the virus can range from weeks to months to years. Infection with one type of HPV does not prevent infection with another type.

Clinical Manifestations

Most individuals who have HPV do not know they are infected, because symptoms are often not present. Genital warts are discrete, single, or multiple papillary growths that are white to gray and pink flesh–colored. They may grow and coalesce to form large, cauliflower-like masses.

- In men, the warts may occur on the penis and scrotum, around the anus, or in the urethra.
- In women, the warts may be located on the vulva, vagina, and cervix and in the perianal area.
- Itching or bleeding on defecation may occur with anal warts.

Diagnostic Studies

- A diagnosis can be made based on the characteristic appearance of the lesions.
- Biopsy provides a definitive diagnosis. Serologic and cytologic testing can be used to rule out carcinomas, secondary syphilis, or benign neoplasms.

Interprofessional Care

Genital warts are difficult to treat and often require multiple office visits. The primary goal is the removal of symptomatic warts.

- A common treatment is 80% to 90% trichloroacetic acid (TCA) or bichloroacetic acid (BCA) applied directly to the wart surface.
- Podophyllin resin (10% to 25%), a cytotoxic agent, is recommended for small external genital warts.
- Podofilox (Condylox) liquid or gel can be applied by the patient for 3 successive days.
- Imiquimod cream (Aldara), an immune response modifier, can be applied three times per week for up to 16 weeks.

If the warts do not regress with any of these therapies, treatments such as cryotherapy with liquid nitrogen, electrocautery, laser therapy, intralesional use of α-interferon, and surgical excision may be indicated. Because treatment does not destroy the virus, merely the infected tissue, recurrence and reinfection are possible, and careful long-term follow-up is advised.

Three vaccines are available to protect against certain strains of HPV. Ideally, individuals should receive a vaccine before the start of sexual activity, but even those who are infected with HPV can still get protection against HPV types not already acquired. The HPV vaccine reduces the risk of anal cancer and may protect against oropharyngeal cancer.

Nursing Management: Genital Warts

See Nursing Management: Sexually Transmitted Infections, pp. 564-565.

PART TWO

Treatments and Procedures

AMPUTATION

Description

An *amputation* is the removal of a body extremity by trauma or surgery. An estimated 2 million people in the United States are living with limb loss. Middle-aged and older people have the highest incidence of amputation because of the effects of peripheral vascular disease (most common), atherosclerosis, and vascular changes related to diabetes mellitus. Amputation in young people is usually secondary to trauma (e.g., from motor vehicle crashes, land mine explosions, or farming-related accidents).

- The goal of amputation surgery is to preserve extremity length and function while removing all infected, pathologic, or ischemic tissue. (For the levels of amputation of the upper and lower extremities, see Fig. 62-22 in Lewis et al, *Medical-Surgical Nursing,* ed 10, p. 1488.)

Nursing Management

Control of causative illnesses such as peripheral vascular disease, diabetes mellitus, chronic osteomyelitis, and skin ulcers can prevent or delay the need for amputation.

- Teach patients with these conditions to carefully examine the lower extremities daily for signs of skin infection or breakdown. Teach the patient to report problems to the HCP such as changes in skin color or temperature, decrease or absence of sensation, tingling, burning pain, or the presence of a lesion.
- Instruct people in safety precautions in recreational activities and the performance of potentially hazardous work. It is important for you to recognize the tremendous psychologic and social implications of an amputation. The disruption in body image caused by an amputation often results in the patient going through the grieving process. Use therapeutic communication to assist the patient and caregiver during this process to develop a realistic attitude about the future.

Preoperative Care

Before surgery, reinforce information that the patient and caregiver have received about the reasons for the amputation, proposed prosthesis, and mobility-training program.

- Teach the patient upper extremity exercises such as push-ups in bed or the wheelchair to promote arm strength, which is essential for crutch walking and gait training.
- If a compression bandage is to be used after surgery, instruct the patient about its purpose and how it will be applied. If an

immediate prosthesis is planned, discuss general ambulation expectations.

Tell the patient that it may feel as if the amputated limb is still present after surgery. This phenomenon, termed *phantom limb sensation,* occurs in many amputees.

- As recovery and ambulation progress, phantom limb sensation and pain usually subside, although the pain can become chronic.
- The patient may also complain of shooting, burning, or crushing pain and feelings of coldness, heaviness, and cramping.

Postoperative Care

Prevention and detection of complications are important during the postoperative period. Carefully monitor the patient's vital signs and dressing for hemorrhage at the operative site. Careful attention to sterile technique during dressing changes reduces the potential for wound infection.

- If an immediate postoperative prosthesis has been applied, careful surveillance of the surgical site is required. A surgical tourniquet must always be available for emergency use. If excessive bleeding occurs, notify the surgeon immediately.
- Not all patients are candidates for prostheses. The seriously ill or debilitated patient may not have the upper body strength or energy required to use a prosthesis. Mobility with a wheelchair may be the most realistic goal in this situation.

Flexion contractures may delay the rehabilitation process. The most common and debilitating contracture is hip flexion. Patients should avoid sitting in a chair for more than 1 hour with hips flexed or with pillows under the surgical extremity.

▼ Patient and Caregiver Teaching

As the patient's overall condition improves, an exercise regimen is normally started under supervision of the HCP and physical therapist.

- Active range-of-motion exercises of all joints should be started as soon after surgery as the patient's pain level and medical status permit.
- Crutch walking is started as soon as the patient is physically able. After an immediate postsurgical fitting, orders related to weight bearing must be carefully followed to avoid disruption of the skin flap and delay of the healing process.
- Before discharge, instruct the patient and the caregiver about residual limb care, ambulation, prevention of contractures, recognition of complications, exercise, and follow-up care. Table 90 outlines patient and caregiver teaching after an amputation.

TABLE 90 Patient & Caregiver Teaching

A

After an Amputation

After an amputation, include the following instructions when teaching the patient and the caregiver.

- Inspect the residual limb daily for signs of skin irritation, especially erythema, excoriation, and odor. Pay particular attention to areas prone to pressure.
- Discontinue use of the prosthesis if irritation develops. Have the area checked before resuming use of the prosthesis.
- Wash the residual limb thoroughly each night with warm water and a bacteriostatic soap. Rinse thoroughly and dry gently. Expose the residual limb to air for 20 minutes.
- Do not use any substance such as lotions, alcohol, powders, or oil on residual limb unless prescribed by the health care provider.
- Wear only a residual limb sock that is in good condition and supplied by the prosthetist.
- Change residual limb sock daily. Launder in a mild soap, squeeze, and lay flat to dry.
- Use prescribed pain management techniques.
- Perform range of motion (ROM) to all joints daily. Perform general strengthening exercises, including the upper extremities, daily.
- Do not elevate the residual limb on a pillow.
- Lie prone with hip in extension for 30 minutes three or four times daily.

ARTIFICIAL AIRWAYS: ENDOTRACHEAL TUBES

Description

An artificial airway is created by inserting a tube into the trachea, bypassing upper airway and laryngeal structures. The tube is placed into the trachea through the mouth or nose past the larynx *(endotracheal [ET] intubation)* or through a stoma in the neck *(tracheostomy)*. ET intubation is more common than tracheostomy in the ICU. Fig. 24 shows the parts of an ET tube.

- Indications for ET intubation include upper airway obstruction, apnea, high risk of aspiration, ineffective clearance of secretions, and respiratory distress. It is performed quickly and safely at the bedside.

In *oral ET intubation,* the ET tube is passed through the mouth and between the vocal cords and into the trachea with the aid of a

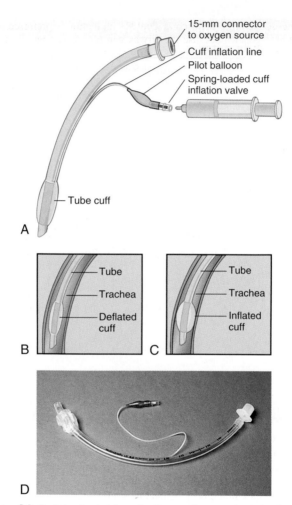

Fig. 24 Endotracheal tube. **A,** Parts of an endotracheal tube. **B,** Tube in place with cuff deflated. **C,** Tube in place with the cuff inflated. **D,** Photo of tube before placement.

laryngoscope or bronchoscope. Oral ET intubation is preferred for most emergencies because the airway can be secured rapidly and a larger-diameter tube is used. A larger-bore ET tube provides less airway resistance and allows easier performance of suctioning and fiberoptic bronchoscopy if needed.

- There are risks associated with oral ET intubation. It is difficult to place an oral tube if head and neck mobility is limited (e.g., with suspected spinal cord injury). Teeth can be chipped or accidentally removed during the procedure. Salivation is increased and swallowing is difficult. The patient can obstruct the ET tube by biting down on it. Sedation along with a bite block or oropharyngeal airway can be used to avoid this. The ET tube and bite block (if used) should be secured (separately) to the face. Mouth care is a challenge.

In *nasal ET intubation,* the ET is placed blindly (i.e., without seeing the larynx) through the nose and nasopharynx and past the vocal cords.

- Nasal intubation is contraindicated in patients with facial fractures or suspected fractures at the base of the skull and postoperatively after cranial surgery.

Nasal ET tubes are more likely to kink than oral tubes. The work of breathing is greater because the longer, narrower tube offers more airflow resistance; suctioning and secretion removal are more difficult. Nasal tubes have been linked with increased incidence of sinus infection and ventilator-associated pneumonia (VAP).

Nursing and Interprofessional Management

Unless ET intubation is emergent, consent is obtained. Tell the patient and caregiver the reason for ET intubation, steps that will occur, and the patient's role. Explain that while intubated, the patient will not be able to speak, but that you will provide other means of communication. Also explain that the patient may have removable mitts placed as a reminder not to move the tube.

- Have a self-inflating bag-valve-mask (BVM) device (e.g., Ambu bag) available and attached to O_2; have suctioning equipment ready at the bedside; and establish IV access. ET intubation is described in Lewis et al, *Medical-Surgical Nursing,* ed 10, p. 1570.

Management of a patient with an artificial airway is often a shared responsibility between you and a respiratory therapist, with specific management tasks determined by agency policy. Nursing responsibilities for the patient with an artificial airway may include some or all of the following: (1) maintaining correct tube placement, (2) maintaining proper cuff inflation, (3) monitoring oxygenation and ventilation, (4) maintaining tube patency, (5) assessing for complications, (6) providing oral care and maintaining skin integrity, and (7) fostering comfort and communication.

Continuously monitor the patient with an ET tube for proper tube placement. Observe for symmetric chest wall movement, and auscultate to confirm bilateral breath sounds.

- It is an emergency if the ET tube is not positioned properly. If malpositioning occurs, stay with the patient, maintain the airway, support ventilation, and secure appropriate assistance to immediately reposition the tube. It may be necessary to ventilate the patient with a BVM device (Ambu bag) and 100% O_2. If a malpositioned tube is not repositioned, no oxygen will be delivered to the lungs, or the entire tidal volume will be delivered to one lung, placing the patient at risk for pneumothorax.

The cuff is an inflatable, pliable sleeve encircling the lower, outer wall of the ET tube. The cuff stabilizes and seals the ET tube within the trachea and prevents the escape of ventilating gases.

Excess volume in the ET tube cuff can cause tracheal damage. To avoid this, inflate the cuff with air, and measure and monitor the cuff pressure. Normal arterial tracheal perfusion is estimated at 30 mm Hg. To ensure adequate tracheal perfusion, maintain cuff pressure at 20 to 25 cm H_2O. Measure and record cuff pressure after intubation and on a routine basis (e.g., every 8 hours) using the *minimal occluding volume* (MOV) *technique* or the *minimal leak technique* (MLT).

- The steps in the MOV technique for cuff inflation are as follows: (1) for the mechanically ventilated patient, place a stethoscope over the trachea and inflate the cuff to MOV by adding air until no air leak is heard at peak inspiratory pressure (end of ventilator inspiration); (2) for the spontaneously breathing patient, inflate until no sound is heard after a deep breath or after inhalation with a BVM; (3) use a manometer to verify that cuff pressure is between 20 and 25 mm Hg; and (4) record cuff pressure in the chart.
- If adequate cuff pressure cannot be maintained or larger volumes of air are needed to keep the cuff inflated, the cuff could be leaking or there could be tracheal dilation at the cuff site. In such situations, notify the HCP.

The procedure for MLT is similar with one exception. Remove a small amount of air from the cuff until a slight air leak is auscultated at peak inflation. Both techniques aim to prevent the risks of tracheal damage resulting from high cuff pressures.

- Closely monitor the patient with an ET tube for adequate oxygenation and ventilation by assessing clinical findings, arterial blood gases (ABGs), SpO_2, and other indicators of oxygenation status.

- Do not routinely suction a patient. Regularly assess the patient to determine the need for suctioning. Indications for suctioning include (1) visible secretions in the ET tube, (2) sudden onset of respiratory distress, (3) suspected aspiration of secretions, (4) increase in respiratory rate with or without sustained coughing, and (5) sudden decrease in SpO_2. Other signs that may indicate the patient needs suctioning include an increase in peak airway pressure and auscultation of adventitious breath sounds over the trachea or bronchi. See Table 91 for open and closed suctioning techniques.
- With an oral ET tube in place, the patient's mouth is always open. Moisten the lips, tongue, and gums with saline or water swabs to prevent mucosal drying. Proper oral care provides

---

TABLE 91 Suctioning Procedures for Patient on Mechanical Ventilator

General Measures for Open- and Closed-Suction Techniques

1. Gather all supplies and equipment.
2. Wash hands and don personal protective equipment.
3. Explain procedure and patient's role in assisting with secretion removal by coughing.
4. Monitor patient's cardiopulmonary status (e.g., vital signs, SpO_2, SvO_2 or $ScvO_2$, ECG, level of consciousness) before, during, and after the procedure.
5. Turn on suction and set vacuum to 100-120 mm Hg.
6. Pause ventilator alarms.

Open-Suction Technique

7. Open sterile catheter package using the inside of the package as a sterile field. NOTE: Suction catheter should be no wider than one-half the diameter of the ET tube (e.g., for a 7-mm ET tube, select a 10F suction catheter).
8. Fill the sterile solution container with sterile normal saline or water.
9. Don sterile gloves.
10. Pick up sterile suction catheter with dominant hand. Using nondominant hand, secure the connecting tube (to suction) to the suction catheter.
11. Check equipment for proper functioning by suctioning a small volume of sterile saline solution from the container. *(Go to step 13.)*

Continued

TABLE 91   Suctioning Procedures for Patient on Mechanical Ventilator—cont'd

Closed-Suction Technique

12. Connect the suction tubing to the closed suction port.
13. Hyperoxygenate the patient for 30 seconds using one of the following methods:
    - Activate the suction hyperoxygenation setting on the ventilator using nondominant hand.
    - Increase FIO_2 to 100%. NOTE: Remember to return FIO_2 to baseline level at the completion of the procedure if not done automatically after preset time by ventilator.
    - Disconnect the ventilator tubing from the ET tube and manually ventilate the patient with 100% O_2 using a BVM device.* Administer five or six breaths over 30 seconds. NOTE: Use of a second person to deliver the manual breaths significantly increases the V_T delivered.
14. With suction off, gently and quickly insert the catheter using the dominant hand. When you meet resistance, pull back ½ inch.
15. Apply continuous or intermittent suction using the nondominant thumb. Withdraw the catheter over 10 seconds or less.
16. Hyperoxygenate for 30 seconds as described in step 13.
17. If secretions remain and the patient has tolerated the procedure, perform two or three suction passes as described in steps 14 and 15. NOTE: Rinse the suction catheter with sterile saline solution between suctioning passes as needed.
18. Reconnect patient to ventilator (open-suction technique).
19. At the completion of ET tube suctioning, rinse the catheter and connecting tubing with the sterile saline solution.
20. Suction oral pharynx. NOTE: Use a separate catheter for this step when using the closed-suction technique.
21. Discard the suction catheter and rinse the connecting tubing with the sterile saline solution (open-suction technique).
22. Reset FIO_2 (if necessary) and ventilator alarms.
23. Reassess patient for signs of effective suctioning.

Adapted from Seckel MA: Suctioning: endotracheal or tracheostomy tube. In Wiegand DL, editor: *AACN procedure manual for critical care*, ed 7. In press.
BVM, Bag-valve-mask; *ECG,* electrocardiogram; *ET,* endotracheal; *FIO₂,* fraction of inspired oxygen; *PEEP,* positive end-expiratory pressure; *SpO₂,* arterial oxygen saturation by pulse oximetry; *SvO₂,* mixed venous oxygen saturation; *ScvO₂,* central venous oxygen saturation; *V_T,* tidal volume.
*Attach a PEEP valve to the BVM for patients on >5 cm H_2O PEEP.

comfort and prevents injury to the gums and dental plaque formation.

- Meticulous care is required to prevent skin breakdown on the face, lips, tongue, and/or nares because of pressure from the ET tube and/or bite block or from the method used to secure the ET tube to the patient's face. Reposition and resecure or retape the ET tube every 24 hours and as needed.

For the nasally intubated patient, remove the old tape and clean the skin around the ET tube with saline-soaked gauze or cotton swabs. For the orally intubated patient, remove the bite block (if present) and the old tape. Provide oral hygiene and then reposition the ET tube to the opposite side of the mouth. Replace the bite block (if appropriate) and reconfirm proper cuff inflation and tube placement. Secure the ET tube again per agency policy.

- Use of two staff members to perform the repositioning procedure is recommended to prevent accidental dislodgement. Monitor the patient for signs of respiratory distress throughout the procedure.

BASIC LIFE SUPPORT FOR HEALTH CARE PROVIDERS

Description

Basic life support (BLS) consists of a series of actions and skills performed by the rescuer(s) based on assessment findings.

- The first actions the rescuer performs on finding an adult victim are to simultaneously assess for responsiveness and look for signs of breathing. This is done by tapping or shaking the victim's shoulder and asking, "Are you all right?" and scanning the victim's chest for signs of breathing. If the victim does not respond and if there is no breathing or abnormal breathing is present (e.g., agonal gasps), and the rescuer is alone, the rescuer shouts for help.
- If someone responds, the rescuer asks him or her to activate the emergency response system (ERS) (e.g., through the use of a mobile phone) and to get an *automatic external defibrillator* (AED) (if available).
- If no one responds, the rescuer activates the ERS (e.g., through the use of a mobile phone), gets an AED (if available), returns to the victim, and begins *cardiopulmonary resuscitation* (CPR), with defibrillation if necessary.

Cardiopulmonary Resuscitation (CPR)

Cardiac arrest is characterized by the absence of a pulse and breathing in an unconscious victim. The current approach for CPR is the chest *compressions–airway–breathing* (CAB) sequence.

- The first step in CPR is to perform a pulse check by palpating the carotid pulse for at least 5 but no more than 10 seconds. While maintaining a head-tilt position with one hand on the forehead, locate the victim's trachea using two or three fingers of the other hand. If a pulse is felt, give one rescue breath every 5 to 6 seconds (10 to 12 breaths per minute) and recheck the pulse every 2 minutes. If no pulse is felt, initiate CAB.

- Chest compression technique consists of fast and deep applications of pressure on the sternum. The victim must be in the supine position when the compressions are performed. Chest compressions are combined with rescue breathing for an effective resuscitation effort of a victim of cardiac arrest. The compression-ventilation ratio for one- or two-rescuer CPR is 30 compressions to 2 breaths (Table 92). To maintain the quality and rate of compressions, rescuers should change roles every 2 minutes. Mechanical chest compression devices may be used to provide chest compressions during prehospital care and in the emergency department.

TABLE 92   Adult One- and Two-Rescuer Basic Life Support With Automatic External Defibrillator (AED)

Assess

- Determine unresponsiveness: tap or shake victim's shoulder; shout, "Are you all right?"
- Check for no breathing or abnormal breathing (e.g., gasping).

Activate Emergency Response System (ERS)

- Activate ERS (e.g., call 911) and get the AED (if available) (outside of hospital).
- Call a code and ask for the AED or crash cart (in hospital).

Check for Pulse

- Feel for carotid pulse (5-10 seconds).
- If victim has a pulse but is not breathing or not breathing adequately, begin rescue breathing at a rate of 1 breath every 5-6 seconds (see Fig. A-1, Lewis et al, *Medical-Surgical Nursing*, ed 10, p. 1650), and recheck circulation every 2 minutes.

TABLE 92   Adult One- and Two-Rescuer Basic Life Support With Automatic External Defibrillator (AED)—cont'd

Begin High-Quality CPR

- If there is no pulse, expose the victim's chest and immediately begin chest compressions (see Fig. A-2, Lewis et al, *Medical-Surgical Nursing*, ed 10, p. 1651).
- Deliver compressions at a rate of 100-120 per minute.
- Compress the chest at least 2 inches but not greater than 2.4 inches.
- Allow for complete chest recoil after each compression.
- Deliver a compression-ventilation ratio of 30 compressions to 2 breaths.*
- Minimize interruptions in compressions by delivering the 2 breaths in <10 seconds.

Deliver Effective Breaths

- Open airway adequately (see Fig. A-1, *A*, Lewis et al, *Medical-Surgical Nursing*, ed 10, p. 1650).
- Deliver breath to produce a visible chest rise (see Fig. A-1, *B* and *C*, Lewis et al, *Medical-Surgical Nursing*, ed 10, p. 1650).
- Avoid excessive ventilation.

Integrate Prompt Use of the AED

- Use AED as soon as possible.
- If rhythm is shockable, deliver one shock and then resume chest compressions immediately after delivery of shock.
- If the rhythm is not shockable, resume CPR and recheck rhythm every five cycles.

Continue CPR

- Continue CPR between rhythm checks and shocks, and until ACLS providers arrive or the victim shows signs of movement.

*For patients with ongoing CPR and an advanced airway in place, a ventilation rate of 1 breath every 6 seconds (10 breaths per minute) is recommended.
ACLS, Advanced cardiovascular life support; *CPR,* cardiopulmonary resuscitation.
Sources: American Heart Association: *BLS for healthcare providers—student manual,* Dallas, 2011, The Association; and American Heart Association: *Highlights of the 2015 American Heart Association guidelines update for CPR and ECC,* Dallas, 2015, The Association.

B

- When the AED or advanced cardiovascular life support (ACLS) team arrives, assess the victim's rhythm. If the victim has a shockable rhythm (e.g., ventricular tachycardia, ventricular fibrillation), deliver one shock followed by five cycles of CPR before checking the rhythm. If the rhythm is not a shockable rhythm, resume CPR and recheck the rhythm every five cycles.
- If the victim has a pulse but is gasping (e.g., agonal breathing) or not breathing, establish an open airway and begin rescue breathing. Open an adult's airway by hyperextending the head. Use the *head tilt–chin lift maneuver.* This involves tilting the head back with one hand and lifting the chin forward with the fingers of the other hand. Use the *jaw-thrust maneuver* if you suspect a cervical spine injury. Attempt to ventilate the victim using a mouth-to-barrier (recommended) device (e.g., face mask, bag-valve-mask) or by mouth-to-mouth resuscitation. Give ventilations with the victim's nostrils pinched. Take a regular (not deep) breath and tightly seal your lips around the victim's mouth. Give one breath and watch for a rise in the victim's chest. Continue rescue breaths at a rate of 10 to 12 per minute.
- If the victim cannot be ventilated, proceed with CPR. When providing the next rescue breaths, look for and remove any visible objects from the victim's mouth (Table 93 and Fig. 25).

TABLE 93   Management of the Adult Choking Victim

Conscious Adult Choking Victim
Assess Victim for Severe Airway Obstruction
Look for any of the following signs:
- Poor or no air exchange
- Clutching the neck with the hands, making the universal choking sign
- Weak, ineffective cough or no cough at all
- High-pitched noise while inhaling or no noise at all
- Increased respiratory difficulty
- Possible cyanosis

Ask the victim if he or she is choking. If the victim nods yes and cannot talk or has any of the symptoms noted above, severe airway obstruction is present and you must take immediate action.

TABLE 93 Management of the Adult Choking Victim—cont'd

Abdominal Thrusts (Heimlich Maneuver) With Standing or Sitting Victim

1. Stand or kneel behind victim and wrap arms around the victim's waist.
2. Make fist with one hand.
3. Place thumb side of fist against victim's abdomen. Position fist midline, slightly above navel and well below breastbone.
4. Grasp fist with other hand and press fist into victim's abdomen with a quick, forceful upward thrust.
5. Give each new thrust with a separate, distinct movement to relieve the obstruction. CAUTION: If victim is pregnant or obese, give chest thrusts instead of abdominal thrusts. Position hands (as described) over lower portion of the breastbone and apply quick backward thrusts.
6. Repeat thrusts until object is expelled or victim becomes unresponsive.

Unconscious Adult Choking Victim

If you see a choking victim collapse and become unresponsive:

1. Activate the emergency response system (ERS).
2. Lower the victim to the ground and begin CPR, starting with compressions (do not check for a pulse).
3. Open the victim's mouth wide each time you prepare to give breaths. Look for the object. If you see the object and can easily remove it, do so with your fingers. If you do not see the object, continue with CPR using the chest compression–airway–breathing sequence.
4. If efforts to ventilate are unsuccessful, continue with CPR.

Source: American Heart Association: *BLS for healthcare providers—student manual*, Dallas, 2011, The Association.
NOTE: BLS guidelines are expected to be updated on an ongoing basis and are available in a Web-based format at *https://eccguidelines.heart.org/index.php/circulation/cpr-ecc-guidelines-2*.
BLS, Basic life support; *CPR,* cardiopulmonary resuscitation.

Hands-Only CPR

Hands-only CPR can be used to help adult victims who suddenly collapse from cardiac arrest outside of a health care setting. If you witness this event (as a bystander), you can choose to provide chest compressions only (push fast and deep in the center of the chest) or conventional CPR (described previously). Both methods are effective when done in the first few minutes of an out-of-hospital cardiac arrest.

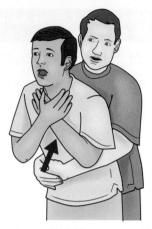

Fig. 25 Abdominal thrusts *(Heimlich maneuver)* administered to a conscious (standing) choking victim.

CHEMOTHERAPY

Description
Chemotherapy (antineoplastic therapy) is the use of chemicals as a systemic therapy for cancer. It is a primary cancer treatment for most solid tumors and hematologic malignancies (e.g., leukemias, lymphomas). The goal of chemotherapy is to eliminate or reduce the number of cancer cells present in the primary tumor and at metastatic tumor site(s).

- The two major categories of chemotherapeutic drugs are *cell cycle phase–nonspecific* and *cell cycle phase–specific*. These agents are often administered in combination to maximize effectiveness by using drugs that function by different mechanisms and throughout the cell cycle.

Classification of Chemotherapeutic Drugs
Chemotherapy drugs are generally classified according to their molecular structure and mechanisms of action (Table 94).

Methods of Administration
The IV route is the most common route for chemotherapy administration. Major concerns associated with the IV administration of antineoplastic drugs include venous access difficulties, device- or catheter-related infection, and *extravasation* (infiltration of drugs into tissues surrounding the infusion site). Many chemotherapy drugs are either irritants or vesicants.

TABLE 94 Drug Therapy

Chemotherapy

Mechanism(s) of Action	Example(s)

Alkylating Agents
Cell Cycle Phase–Nonspecific Agents

Damage DNA by causing breaks in the double-stranded helix. If repair does not occur, cells will die immediately (cytocidal) or when they attempt to divide (cytostatic).

bendamustine (Treanda), busulfan (Myleran), chlorambucil (Leukeran), cyclophosphamide, dacarbazine (DTIC-Dome), ifosfamide (Ifex), mechloretha-mine (Mustargen), melphalan (Alkeran), temozolomide (Temodar), thiotepa

Nitrosoureas
Cell Cycle Phase–Nonspecific Agents

Like alkylating agents, break DNA helix, interfering with DNA replication. Cross blood-brain barrier.

carmustine (Gliadel), lomustine (Gleostine), streptozocin (Zanosar)

Platinum Drugs
Cell Cycle Phase–Nonspecific Agents

Bind to DNA and RNA, miscoding information and/or inhibiting DNA replication, so that cells die.

carboplatin, cisplatin (Platinol-AQ), oxaliplatin (Eloxatin)

Antimetabolites
Cell Cycle Phase–Specific Agents

Mimic naturally occurring substances, thereby interfering with enzyme function or DNA synthesis. Primarily act during S phase. Purine and pyrimidine are building blocks of nucleic acids needed for DNA and RNA synthesis.

- Interfere with purine metabolism.

  cladribine, clofarabine (Clolar), fludarabine, mercaptopurine, nelarabine (Arranon), pentostatin (Nipent), thioguanine

- Interfere with pyrimidine metabolism.

  capecitabine (Xeloda); cytarabine (Cytosar-U, DepoCyt), floxuridine, 5-fluorouracil (5-FU), gemcitabine (Gemzar)

C

Continued

TABLE 94 Drug Therapy

Chemotherapy—cont'd

Mechanism(s) of Action	Example(s)
• Interfere with folic acid metabolism.	methotrexate (Trexall), pemetrexed (Alimta)
• Interfere with DNA synthesis.	hydroxyurea (Hydrea, Droxia)

Antitumor Antibiotics

Cell Cycle Phase–Nonspecific Agents

Bind directly to DNA. Inhibit DNA synthesis and interfere with transcription of RNA.	bleomycin, dactinomycin (Cosmegen), daunorubicin (Cerubidine, DaunoXome), doxorubicin (Doxil), epirubicin (Ellence), idarubicin, mitomycin, mitoxantrone, valrubicin (Valstar)

Mitotic Inhibitors

Cell Cycle Phase–Specific Agents

Taxanes

Antimicrotubule agents that interfere with mitosis. Act during late G_2 phase and mitosis to stabilize microtubules. Inhibit cell division.	albumin-bound paclitaxel (Abraxane), docetaxel (Taxotere), paclitaxel (Taxol)

Vinca Alkaloids

Act in M phase to inhibit mitosis.	vinblastine, vincristine, vinorelbine (Navelbine)

Others

Microtubular inhibitors.	estramustine (Emcyt), ixabepilone (Ixempra), eribulin (Halaven)

Topoisomerase Inhibitors

Cell Cycle Phase–Specific Agents

Inhibit topoisomerases (normal enzymes) that make reversible breaks and repairs in DNA that allow for flexibility of DNA in replication.	etoposide, irinotecan (Camptosar), teniposide (Vumon), topotecan (Hycamtin)

TABLE 94 Drug Therapy

Chemotherapy—cont'd

Mechanism(s) of Action	Example(s)
Miscellaneous	
Enzyme derived from the yeast *Erwinia*. Depletes the supply of asparagine (amino acid) for leukemic cells that are dependent on exogenous source of this amino acid. Inhibits protein synthesis.	Erwinia asparaginase, L-asparaginase (Elspar)
Causes changes in DNA in leukemia cells, leading to cell death.	arsenic trioxide (Trisenox)
Suppresses mitosis. Appears to alter DNA, RNA, and protein.	procarbazine (Matulane)

NOTE: Many of these drugs are irritants or vesicants that require special attention during administration to avoid extravasation. It is important to know this information about a drug before administering it.

- *Irritants* will damage the intima of the vein, causing phlebitis and sclerosis and limiting future peripheral venous access.
- *Vesicants* may cause severe local tissue breakdown and necrosis if inadvertently infiltrated into the skin.

To minimize these problems, a central vascular access device may be placed in large blood vessels to permit frequent, continuous, or intermittent administration of chemotherapy, thus avoiding multiple venipunctures. (See Central Venous Access Devices, Chapter 16, p. 294, Lewis et al, *Medical-Surgical Nursing,* ed 10.)

Regional chemotherapy delivers the drug directly to the tumor site. Examples of this type of administration include intraarterial, intraperitoneal, intrathecal (intraventricular), and intravesical bladder chemotherapy.

Effects of Chemotherapy

Chemotherapy agents cannot selectively distinguish between normal cells and cancer cells. Chemotherapy-induced side effects are caused by the destruction of normal cells that are rapidly proliferating such as those in the bone marrow, lining of the gastrointestinal system, and integumentary system (skin, hair, and nails).

Effects of chemotherapy are caused by general cytotoxicity and organ-specific drug toxicities.

The adverse effects of these drugs can be classified as acute, delayed, or chronic.

- *Acute toxicity* includes anaphylactic and hypersensitivity reactions, extravasation or a flare reaction, anticipatory nausea and vomiting, and dysrhythmias.
- *Delayed effects* are numerous and include delayed nausea and vomiting, mucositis, alopecia, skin rashes, bone marrow depression, altered bowel function, and a variety of neurotoxicities.
- *Chronic toxicities* involve damage to organs such as the heart, liver, kidneys, and lungs.

Nursing management of side effects and problems caused by chemotherapy and radiation therapy is provided in Table 15-11, Lewis et al, *Medical-Surgical Nursing,* ed 10, pp. 251 to 252.

Nursing Management: Chemotherapy and Radiation Therapy

You have an important role in helping patients deal with the side effects of chemotherapy and radiation therapy.

- Myelosuppression is one of the most common effects of chemotherapy, and to a lesser extent, it can also occur with radiation therapy. It can result in life-threatening and distressing effects, including infection, hemorrhage, and overwhelming fatigue. Monitor the CBC, particularly the neutrophil, platelet, and RBC counts.
- Fatigue is a nearly universal symptom, affecting most patients with cancer. You can help patients recognize that fatigue is a common effect of therapy. Ignoring fatigue may lead to an increase in symptoms. However, maintaining exercise and activity within tolerable limits is often helpful in managing fatigue. Guidelines for the evaluation and management of cancer-related fatigue are available online at *www.nccn.org*.

The intestinal mucosa is one of the tissues that are most sensitive to chemotherapy and radiation therapy, resulting in nausea and vomiting, diarrhea, mucositis, and anorexia. These problems can affect the patient's hydration and nutritional status and sense of well-being.

- Assess patients with nausea and vomiting for signs and symptoms of dehydration and metabolic alkalosis. Nausea and vomiting can be successfully managed with antiemetic regimens, dietary modification, and other nondrug interventions.
- Both radiation therapy– and chemotherapy-induced diarrhea are best managed with diet modification, antidiarrheals,

antimotility agents, and antispasmodics (see Table 42-2, Lewis et al, *Medical-Surgical Nursing,* ed 10, p. 931).

■ Mucositis can be alleviated with systemic and/or topical analgesics and antibiotics if infection is present. Monitor and get prompt treatment for oral candidiasis (which often occurs with mucositis). Frequent cleansing with saline and water and topical application of anesthetic gels directly to the lesions are standard care measures.

■ Monitor the patient with anorexia during and after treatment to ensure that weight loss does not become excessive. Also observe for dehydration. Small, frequent meals of high-protein, high-calorie bland foods are better tolerated than large meals.

Skin changes with chemotherapy range from mild erythema and hyperpigmentation to more distressing effects such as acral erythema. Alopecia caused by chemotherapy is usually reversible. Hair generally begins to grow back 3 to 4 weeks after the drugs are discontinued.

■ With radiation therapy, skin effects occur only locally, in the treatment field. Basic skin care instructions are presented in Table 15-12, Lewis et al, *Medical-Surgical Nursing,* ed 10, p. 255. Verify these guidelines with your institution's radiation oncology department before using.

▼ **Patient and Caregiver Teaching**
Teaching is an important part of your role related to chemotherapy and radiation therapy.

■ Explore the patient's attitude about treatment so that misconceptions or fear can be discussed.

■ To decrease the fear and anxiety often associated with chemotherapy and radiation therapy, tell the patient what to expect during a course of treatment. Good nursing judgment is essential to determine the amount of information that the patient and caregiver can assimilate.

CHEST TUBES AND PLEURAL DRAINAGE

Description
Whenever fluid or air accumulates in the pleural space, the pressure becomes positive instead of negative, and the lungs collapse. Chest tubes are inserted to drain the pleural space and to reestablish negative pressure, allowing for proper lung expansion. Tubes may also be inserted in the mediastinal space postoperatively to remove air and fluid.

Chest Tube Insertion

Chest tube insertion can be performed in the emergency department (ED), in the operating room, or at the patient's bedside. The patient is positioned with the arm raised above the head on the affected side to expose the midaxillary area, the standard site for insertion.

- The area is cleansed with antiseptic solution and the chest wall is infiltrated with a local anesthetic. A small incision is made over a rib. The chest tube is then advanced up and over the top of the rib, to avoid the intercostal nerves and blood vessels (Fig. 26).

- Once inserted, the tube is connected to a pleural drainage system. Two tubes may be connected to the same drainage unit with a Y-connector.

- The incision is closed with sutures and the chest tube is secured. The wound is covered with an occlusive dressing.

- Insertion of a chest tube and its presence in the pleural space are painful. Monitor the patient's comfort at frequent intervals and use appropriate pain-relieving interventions.

Pleural Drainage

There are two types of pleural drainage systems (Fig. 27). The *first type* is a *flutter valve,* which consists of a one-way rubber valve within a rigid plastic tube. It is attached to the external end of the chest tube. During inspiration, when pressure in the chest is greater than atmospheric pressure, the valve opens. During expiration, when intrathoracic pressure is less than atmospheric pressure, the valve closes. The flutter valve can be used during emergency transport and for management of a small to moderate-sized pneumothorax.

The *second type* of pleural drainage system is larger and has three basic compartments (chambers). A variety of commercial, disposable plastic chest drainage systems are available.

- The first compartment, or collection chamber, receives fluid and air from the pleural space. The drained fluid stays in this chamber while the air vents to the second chamber, called the water-seal chamber. This chamber contains 2 cm of water and acts as a one-way valve. Air enters from the collection chamber and bubbles up through the water. The water prevents backflow of air into the patient from the system.

- A third compartment, the suction control chamber, applies suction to the chest drainage.

- Initially, brisk bubbling of air occurs in this chamber when a pneumothorax is evacuated. During normal use, there will be

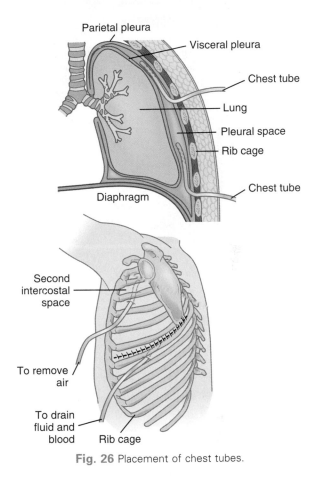

Parietal pleura
Visceral pleura
Chest tube
Lung
Pleural space
Rib cage
Chest tube
Diaphragm

Second intercostal space

To remove air

To drain fluid and blood
Rib cage

Fig. 26 Placement of chest tubes.

intermittent bubbling because of an increase in intrathoracic pressure during exhalation, coughing, or sneezing. Eventually, the air leak seals and the lung fully expands.

Nursing Management: Chest Drainage

General guidelines for nursing care of the patient with chest tubes and water-seal drainage systems are presented in Table 27-21, Lewis et al, *Medical-Surgical Nursing,* ed 10, p. 525.

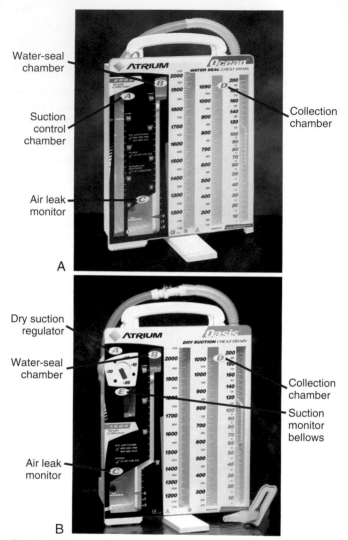

Fig. 27 Chest drainage units. Both units have three chambers: (1) collection chamber, (2) water-seal chamber, and (3) suction control chamber. Suction control chamber requires a connection to a wall suction source that is dialed up higher than the prescribed level. **A,** Water suction. This unit uses water in the suction control chamber to control the wall suction pressure. **B,** Dry suction. This unit controls wall suction by using a regulator control dial. (Courtesy Atrium Medical Corporation, Hudson, New Hampshire.)

Drainage System

- Keep all tubing coiled loosely below chest level without kinking or compression.
- Keep all connections among the chest tubes, drainage tubing, and drainage collector tight, and tape at connections.
- Observe for air fluctuations (tidaling) and bubbling in the water-seal chamber.
- Mark the time of measurement and fluid level on the chamber according to the unit standards. Changes in the quantity or characteristics of drainage should be reported to the HCP.
- Observe for air fluctuations and bubbling in the water-seal chamber. If tidaling is not observed, the drainage system is blocked, the lungs are reexpanded, or the system is attached to suction. If bubbling increases, there may be an air leak.
- Suspect a leak when bubbling is continuous. Retape tubing connections and ensure that the dressing is air occlusive. If a leak persists, briefly clamp the chest tube at the patient's chest. If the leak stops, then the air leak is coming from the patient.
- High fluid levels in the water seal indicate residual negative pressure. The chest system may need to be vented by using the high-negativity release valve available on the drainage system to release residual pressure from the system.
- Never elevate the drainage system to the level of the patient's chest because this will cause fluid to drain back into the lungs.
- If the drainage system unit is overturned and the water seal is disrupted, return it to an upright position and encourage the patient to take a few deep breaths, followed by forced exhalations and cough maneuvers.
- Milking or stripping chest tubes is no longer recommended because these practices can dangerously increase intrapleural pressures and damage lung tissue. Position tubing so that drainage flows freely to negate the need for milking or stripping.

Patient's Clinical Status

- Monitor the patient's clinical status. Assess vital signs, lung sounds, and pain level.
- Assess for and notify HCP about manifestations of reaccumulation of air and fluid in the chest (decreased or absent breath sounds), significant bleeding (>100 mL/hr), chest drainage site infection (drainage, erythema, fever, increased WBC count), poor wound healing, or. Evaluate for subcutaneous emphysema at the chest tube site.
- Encourage the patient to periodically cough and breathe deeply to facilitate lung expansion, and encourage range-of-motion exercises to the shoulder on the affected side. Encourage

incentive spirometry every hour while the patient is awake, to prevent atelectasis or pneumonia.

- If the chest tube becomes disconnected, immediately reestablish the water-seal system and attach a new drainage system as soon as possible.
- Use meticulous sterile technique during dressing changes to reduce the incidence of infection.

Chest Tube Removal

Chest tubes are removed when the lungs are reexpanded and fluid drainage has ceased or is minimal. Suction is usually discontinued and gravity drainage is used for 24 hours before tube removal.

- To remove the tube (1) cut the suture; (2) have the patient take a deep breath, exhale, and bear down (Valsalva maneuver); and (3) remove the tube.
- The site is immediately covered with an airtight dressing, and the pleura will seal off. The wound heals in several days.
- A chest x-ray is done to evaluate for pneumothorax or fluid reaccumulation.

DIALYSIS

Dialysis is a technique in which substances move from the blood through a semipermeable membrane and into a dialysis solution (dialysate). It is used to correct fluid and electrolyte imbalances and remove waste products in renal failure. It can also be used to treat drug overdoses.

The two methods of dialysis are *peritoneal dialysis* (PD) and *hemodialysis* (HD) (Table 95).

- In PD the peritoneal membrane acts as the semipermeable membrane.
- In HD an artificial membrane (usually made of cellulose-based or synthetic materials) is used as the semipermeable membrane and is in contact with the patient's blood.

Dialysis is begun when the patient's uremia can no longer be adequately treated with conservative medical management. Generally dialysis is initiated when the glomerular filtration rate (GFR) (or creatinine clearance) of the patient with kidney disease is <15 mL/min. This criterion can vary widely in different clinical situations, and the nephrologist determines when to start dialysis on the basis of the patient's clinical status. Certain uremic complications, including encephalopathy, neuropathies, uncontrollable hyperkalemia, pericarditis, and accelerated hypertension, indicate the need for immediate dialysis.

TABLE 95 Comparison of Peritoneal Dialysis and Hemodialysis

Advantages	Disadvantages
Peritoneal Dialysis	
• Immediate initiation in almost any hospital	• Bacterial or chemical peritonitis
• Less complicated than hemodialysis	• Protein loss into dialysate
• Portable system with CAPD	• Exit site and tunnel infections
• Fewer dietary restrictions	• Self-image problems with catheter placement
• Relatively short training time	• Hyperglycemia
• Usable in patient with vascular access problems	• Surgery for catheter placement
• Less cardiovascular stress	• Contraindicated in patients with multiple abdominal surgeries, traumatic injury, unrepaired hernia
• Home dialysis possible	• Requires completion of education program
• Preferable for diabetic patient	• Catheter can migrate
	• Best instituted with willing partner
Hemodialysis	
• Rapid fluid removal	• Vascular access problems
• Rapid removal of urea and creatinine	• Dietary and fluid restrictions
• Effective potassium removal	• Heparinization may be necessary
• Less protein loss	• Extensive equipment necessary
• Lowering of serum triglycerides	• Hypotension during dialysis
• Home dialysis possible	• Added blood loss that contributes to anemia
• Temporary access can be placed at bedside	• Specially trained personnel necessary
	• Surgery for permanent access placement
	• Self-image problems with permanent access

CAPD, Continuous ambulatory peritoneal dialysis.

D

Most patients with end-stage renal disease (ESRD) are treated with dialysis because (1) there is a lack of donated organs, (2) some patients are physically or mentally unsuitable for transplantation, or (3) some patients do not want transplants.

■ An increasing number of individuals, including older adults and those with complex medical problems, receive maintenance dialysis. Chronologic age is not a factor in determining candidacy for dialysis. Factors that are important are the patient's ability to cope and the existing support system.

Dialysis is discussed in Chapter 46 of Lewis et al, *Medical-Surgical Nursing*, ed 10, pp. 1084 to 1085.

ENTERAL NUTRITION

Enteral nutrition (EN, also known as *tube feeding*) is nutrition (e.g., liquefied food or formula) delivered into the GI tract distal to the oral cavity through a tube, catheter, or stoma. EN is used for the patient who has a functioning GI tract but is unable to take any or enough oral nourishment, or when it is unsafe to do so.

EN is easily administered, safer, more physiologically efficient, and typically less expensive than parenteral nutrition. Fig. 28 shows the location of commonly used enteral feeding tubes.

- Nasally and orally placed tubes (orogastric, nasogastric [NG], nasoduodenal, or nasojejunal) are most commonly used for short-term feeding (<4 weeks).
- Nasoduodenal and nasojejunal tubes are transpyloric tubes. These tubes are used when pathophysiologic conditions such as risk of aspiration warrant delivering the feeding below the patient's pyloric sphincter.

If the feedings are necessary for an extended time, other tubes are placed in the stomach or small bowel by surgical, endoscopic, or fluoroscopic procedures.

Common delivery options are continuous infusion by pump, intermittent infusion by gravity, intermittent bolus by syringe, and cyclic feedings by infusion pump. Continuous infusion is most often used for critically ill patients. Intermittent feeding may be preferred as the patient improves or at home.

Tube Feedings and Safety

Aspiration and dislodged tubes are two important safety concerns. You have a critical role to ensure that tube feedings are safely administered.

Patient Position

Elevate head of bed to a minimum of 30 degrees, but preferably 45 degrees, to prevent aspiration. Check institution policy for suspending feeding while the patient is supine. If intermittent delivery is used, the head of the bed should remain elevated for 30 to 60 minutes after feeding.

Aspiration Risk

Evaluate enterally fed patients for risk of aspiration. Before starting tube feedings, ensure that the tube is in the proper position.

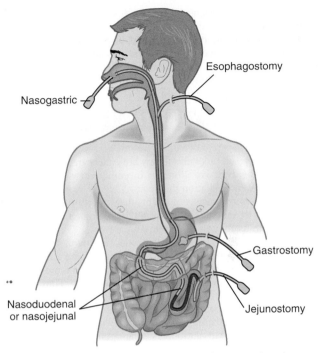

Fig. 28 Common enteral feeding tube placement locations.

Maintain head-of-bed elevation as described. With increased residual volume, there is increased risk for aspiration of formula into the lungs.

- Check gastric residual volumes every 4 hours during the first 48 hours of gastric feeding. After the enteral feeding goal rate is achieved, gastric residual monitoring may be decreased to every 6 to 8 hours in non–critically ill patients or continued every 4 hours in critically ill patients.

Tube Position

Obtain x-ray confirmation of newly inserted nasal or orogastric tubes before feeding or administering medications. Maintain proper placement of tube after feedings are started.

- To determine if a feeding tube has maintained the proper position, mark the exit site of the feeding tube at the time of the initial x-ray, and observe for a change in the external tube length during feedings. Recheck the tube insertion length at regular intervals.

The types of problems encountered in patients receiving tube feedings and corrective measures are presented in Table 39-12, Lewis et al, *Medical-Surgical Nursing,* ed, 10, p. 867.

Patient teaching includes skin care, tube care, feeding administration, and potential complications.

IMMUNOTHERAPY AND TARGETED THERAPY

Description

Immunotherapy and targeted therapy are cancer treatment modalities that can be effective alone or in combination with surgery, chemotherapy, and radiation therapy.

- *Immunotherapy* consists of agents that modify the relationship between host and tumor by altering the biologic response of the host to the tumor cell (Table 96).
- *Targeted therapy* interferes with cancer growth by targeting specific cellular receptors and pathways that are important in tumor growth (Table 96). Targeted therapies are more selective for specific molecular targets than chemotherapy. Thus targeted therapy agents are able to kill cancer cells with less damage to normal cells compared with chemotherapy agents.

Types of targeted therapy agents include various tyrosine kinase inhibitors, monoclonal antibodies, angiogenesis inhibitors, and proteasome inhibitors.

- *Tyrosine kinase inhibitors* block an important enzyme that activates the signaling pathways that regulate cell proliferation and survival.
- *Monoclonal antibodies* bind to specific target cells and inhibit the internalization of receptor-antibody complexes and signaling pathways. They may also stimulate an immunologic response in the patient.
- *Angiogenesis inhibitors* work by preventing the mechanisms necessary for vascularization of tumors.
- *Proteasome inhibitors* promote an accumulation of proteins because they interfere with proteasomes (intracellular multienzyme complexes that degrade proteins). Thus they cause altered cell function.

Indications for and side effects of immunotherapy and targeted therapy agents are included in Table 96.

Nursing Management

The effects of immunotherapy and targeted therapy are acute and dose-limited. Capillary leak syndrome and pulmonary edema are

TABLE 96 Immunotherapy and Targeted Therapy*

Mechanism(s) of Action	Example(s)
Cytokines	
Inhibits DNA and protein synthesis. Suppresses cell proliferation. Increases cytotoxic effects of natural killer (NK) cells.	α-interferon (Intron A)
Stimulates proliferation of T and B cells. Activates NK cells.	interleukin-2 (aldesleukin [Proleukin])
Vaccines	
Live attenuated strain of *Mycobacterium bovis* induces immune response. Used intravesically to treat bladder cancer (see Lewis et al, *Medical-Surgical Nursing*, ed, 10, Chapter 45).	BCG vaccine
Vaccine against prostate cancer that stimulates the immune system against the cancer (see Lewis et al, *Medical-Surgical Nursing*, ed, 10, Chapter 54).	sipuleucel-T (Provenge)
Kinase Inhibitors	
Epidermal Growth Factor Receptor Tyrosine Kinase Inhibitors	
Inhibit epidermal growth factor receptor (EGFR) tyrosine kinase(TK).	cetuximab (Erbitux) panitumumab (Vectibix) erlotinib (Tarceva) gefitinib (Iressa)
Inhibits EGFR TK and binds HER-2.	lapatinib (Tykerb)
BCR-ABL Tyrosine Kinase Inhibitors	
Inhibit BCR-ABL TK. Primarily used in chronic myeloid leukemia.	dasatinib (Sprycel) imatinib (Gleevec) nilotinib (Tasigna) bosutinib (Bosulif)

I

Continued

TABLE 96 Immunotherapy and Targeted Therapy—cont'd

Mechanism(s) of Action	Example(s)
Multi-Tyrosine Kinase Inhibitors	
Inhibit multiple TKs.	sorafenib (Nexavar)
	sunitinib (Sutent)
	axitinib (Inlyta)
	regorafenib (Stivarga)
	vandetanib (Caprelsa)
	pazopanib (Votrient)
	cabozantinib (Cometriq)
Anaplastic Lymphoma Kinase Inhibitors	
Inhibit anaplastic lymphoma kinase (ALK).	crizotinib (Xalkori)
	ceritinib (Zykadia)
BRAF and MEK Kinase Inhibitors	
Inhibit BRAF and MEK enzymes.	vemurafenib (Zelboraf)
	dabrafenib (Tafinlar)
	trametinib (Mekinist)
mTOR Kinase Inhibitors	
Inhibit a specific protein known as the mechanistic target of rapamycin (mTOR).	everolimus (Afinitor) temsirolimus (Torisel)
Human Epidermal Growth Factor Receptor-2	
Monoclonal antibody to human epidermal growth factor receptor-2 (HER-2) that attaches to the antigen, then is taken into the cells and eventually kills them.	pertuzumab (Perjeta) trastuzumab (Herceptin)
Trastuzumab connected to a chemotherapy drug called DM1.	ado-trastuzumab emtansine (Kadcyla)
CD20 Monoclonal Antibodies	
Bind CD20 antigen, causing cytotoxicity and radiation injury.	ibritumomab tiuxetan/ yttrium-90 (Zevalin)
Bind CD20 antigen, causing cytotoxicity.	ofatumumab (Arzerra) rituximab (Rituxan)
CD52 Monoclonal Antibody	
Binds CD52 antigen (found on T and B cells, monocytes, NK cells, neutrophils).	alemtuzumab (Campath)

TABLE 96 Immunotherapy and Targeted Therapy—cont'd	
Mechanism(s) of Action	**Example(s)**
Angiogenesis Inhibitors	
Bind vascular endothelial growth factor (VEGF), thereby inhibiting angiogenesis.	bevacizumab (Avastin) pazopanib (Votrient) ramucirumab (Cyramza)
Proteasome Inhibitors	
Inhibits proteasome activity, which functions to regulate cell growth.	bortezomib (Velcade) carfilzomib (Kyprolis)
Immunomodulatory Drugs (IMiDs)	
Inhibit production of TNF, IL-6, and VEGF (which leads to its antiangiogenic effects). Stimulate T and NK cells and increase interferon gamma and IL-2 production.	thalidomide (Thalomid) lenalidomide (Revlimid) pomalidomide (Pomalyst) apremilast (Otezla)
Programmed Death Receptor (PD)-1 Blockers	
Block PD-1, a protein on T cells that normally helps keep these cells from attacking other cells, thus boosting immune response against cancer cells.	nivolumab (Opdivo) pembrolizumab (Keytruda)

*This list is not all-inclusive.
BCG, Bacille Calmette-Guérin; *BRAF,* B-Raf; *IL,* interleukin; *TNF,* tumor necrosis factor.

problems that require critical care nursing. Bone marrow depression that occurs with immunotherapy is usually more transient and less severe than that observed with chemotherapy.

- Fatigue associated with immunotherapy can be so severe that it can constitute a dose-limiting toxicity. As these agents are combined with chemotherapy, therapy-related effects increase.
- Acetaminophen administered before treatment and every 4 hours after treatment can help relieve the flulike syndrome associated with immunotherapy. IV meperidine (Demerol) has been used to control the severe chills associated with some immunotherapy.

Other nursing measures include monitoring vital signs and temperature, planning for periods of rest for the patient, assisting with activities of daily living (ADLs), and monitoring for adequate oral intake.

MECHANICAL VENTILATION

Description

Mechanical ventilation is the process by which room air or oxygen-enriched air is moved into and out of the lungs by a mechanical ventilator. Mechanical ventilation is not curative. It is a means of supporting patients until they recover the ability to breathe independently or until a decision is made to withdraw ventilatory support. Indications for mechanical ventilation include (1) apnea or an impending inability to breathe, (2) acute respiratory failure, (3) severe hypoxia, and (4) respiratory muscle fatigue.

Types of Mechanical Ventilation

The two major types of mechanical ventilation are negative pressure ventilation and positive pressure ventilation (PPV).

- *Negative pressure ventilation* involves the use of chambers that encase the chest or body and surround it with intermittent subatmospheric or negative pressure. Intermittent negative pressure around the chest wall causes the chest to be pulled outward. This reduces intrathoracic pressure. Air rushes in through the upper airway, which is outside the sealed chamber. Expiration is passive; the machine cycles off, allowing chest retraction. This type of ventilation is similar to normal ventilation in that decreased intrathoracic pressures produce inspiration and expiration is passive. Negative pressure ventilation is noninvasive and does not require an artificial airway.

- Several portable negative pressure ventilators are available for home use for patients with neuromuscular diseases, central nervous system disorders, diseases and injuries of the spinal cord, or severe chronic obstructive pulmonary disease (COPD). Negative pressure ventilators are not used extensively for acutely ill patients.

- *Positive pressure ventilation* (PPV) is the primary method used with acutely ill patients. During inspiration, the ventilator pushes air into the lungs under positive pressure. Intrathoracic pressure is raised during lung inflation rather than lowered as occurs in spontaneous ventilation. Expiration occurs passively, as in normal expiration. PPV units are categorized as either volume or pressure ventilators.

Nursing Management

For nursing management of the patient receiving mechanical ventilation, see eNursing Care Plan 65-1, available on the website for Lewis et al, *Medical-Surgical Nursing,* ed 10.

OSTOMIES

Description

An *ostomy* is a surgically created opening on the abdomen that allows for the discharge of body waste. The outermost portion that is visible is a *stoma*. The stoma is the result of the large or small bowel being brought to the outside of the abdomen and sutured in place. When a stoma is created as a fecal diversion, feces will drain through the stoma instead of the anus.

An ostomy is necessary when the normal elimination route is no longer possible. For example, if the person has stage III transverse colon cancer, the diseased portion of the colon is surgically removed with a margin of healthy tissue. Sometimes the tumor can be resected, leaving enough healthy tissue to immediately *anastomose* (reconnect) the two remaining ends of healthy bowel, and no ostomy is necessary. If the tumor involves the rectum and is large enough to necessitate the removal of the anal sphincters, the anus is sutured shut and a permanent ostomy is created.

Types of Ostomies

Ostomies are named according to location and type (Fig. 29). An ostomy in the ileum is called an *ileostomy* and an ostomy in the colon is called a *colostomy*. The ostomy is further characterized by its anatomic site (e.g., sigmoid or transverse colostomy). The more distal the ostomy, the more the intestinal contents resemble feces that is eliminated from an intact colon and rectum. A comparison of colostomies and ileostomies is shown in Table 97.

The major types of ostomies are end stoma, loop, and double-barrel ostomies.

- An *end stoma* is created by dividing the bowel and bringing the proximal end as a single stoma. The distal portion of the GI tract is surgically removed, or the distal segment is oversewn and left in the abdominal cavity. If the distal bowel is removed, then the stoma is permanent.
- A *loop stoma* is constructed by bringing a loop of bowel to the abdominal surface and then opening the anterior part of the bowel to provide fecal diversion. This results in one stoma with a proximal and distal opening and an intact posterior bowel

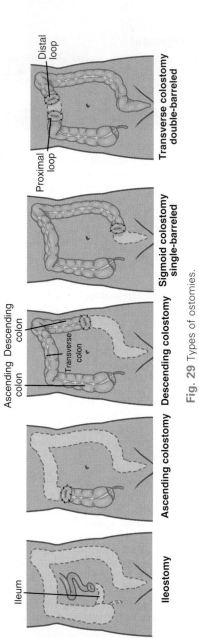

Fig. 29 Types of ostomies.

TABLE 97 Comparison of Ileostomy and Colostomy

Characteristic	Ileostomy	COLOSTOMY		
		Ascending	Transverse	Sigmoid
Stool consistency	Liquid to semiliquid	Semiliquid	Semiliquid to semiformed	Formed
Fluid requirement	Increased	Increased	Possibly increased	No change
Bowel regulation	No	No	No	Yes (if there is a history of a regular bowel pattern)
Pouch and skin barriers	Yes	Yes	Yes	Dependent on regulation
Irrigation	No	No	No	Possibly every 24-48 hr (if patient meets criteria)
Indications for surgery	Ulcerative colitis, Crohn's disease, diseased or injured colon, familial polyposis, trauma, cancer	Perforating diverticulum in lower colon, trauma, rectovaginal fistula, inoperable tumors of colon, rectum, or pelvis	Same as for ascending	Cancer of the rectum or rectosigmoidal area, perforating diverticulum, trauma

wall that separates the two openings. A loop stoma is usually temporary.

- In a *double-barrel stoma,* the bowel is divided, and both the proximal and distal ends are brought through the abdominal wall as two separate stomas. The proximal one is the functioning stoma; the distal, nonfunctioning stoma is referred to as the mucus fistula. The double-barreled stoma is usually temporary.

The procedures used to perform ostomy surgeries are further discussed in Chapter 42 in Lewis et al, *Medical-Surgical Nursing,* ed 10, pp. 958 to 959.

Nursing Management

Preoperative Care

Psychologic preparation and emotional support are important as the person copes with the change in body image and a loss of control over elimination and its odors.

- A wound, ostomy, and continence nurse (WOCN) should select the site where the ostomy will be positioned and mark the abdomen preoperatively. Stomas placed outside the rectus muscle increase the chance of developing a hernia. A flat site makes it much easier to create a good seal and avoid leakage from the bag.

Postoperative Care

Postoperative nursing care includes assessment of the stoma and provision of an appropriate pouching system that protects the skin and contains drainage and odor. The stoma should be dark pink to red. A dusky blue stoma indicates ischemia, and a brown-black stoma indicates necrosis. Assess and document stoma color every 4 hours. Teach the patient that the stoma will be mildly to moderately swollen the first 2 to 3 weeks after surgery.

Nursing care for the patient with an ostomy is presented in eNursing Care Plan 42-3 on the website.

Colostomy Care

A colostomy in the ascending and transverse colon produces semiliquid stools. Instruct the patient to use a drainable pouch. A colostomy in the sigmoid or descending colon produces semi-formed or formed stools and sometimes can be regulated by the irrigation method. The patient may or may not wear a drainage pouch. A well-balanced diet and adequate fluid intake are important.

Colostomy irrigations may be used to stimulate emptying of the colon. Regularity is possible only when the stoma is in the distal colon or rectum. If bowel control is achieved, there should be little or no spillage between irrigations, and the patient may need to wear only a pad or cover over the stoma.

▼ **Patient and Caregiver Teaching**

Colostomy

- Pouching systems consist of an adhesive skin barrier and a bag or pouch to collect the feces. The skin barrier is a piece of pectin-based or karaya wafer that has a measurable thickness and hydrocolloid adhesive properties. Teach the patient to perform a pouch change, provide appropriate skin care, control odor, care for the stoma, and identify signs and symptoms of complications.
- Instruct the patient about the importance of adequate fluids and a healthy diet and when to seek health care.
- Home care and outpatient follow-up by a WOCN are highly recommended. Patients should be discharged with written information about their particular ostomy, instructions for pouch changes, a list of supplies and where to purchase them (including names and phone numbers of retailers), and outpatient follow-up appointments with the surgeon and the WOC nurse.
- Emotional support, interventions from skillful WOCNs, and visits from people who have successfully learned to manage their ostomies will help patients learn to cope with and manage the new stoma. Resources such as the United Ostomy Associations of America (*www.ostomy.org*) may also be helpful.
- For ostomy teaching guidelines, see Table 42-28, Lewis et al, *Medical-Surgical Nursing*, ed 10, p. 961.

Ileostomy Care

- Because regularity cannot be established, a pouch must be worn at all times. An open-ended, drainable pouch is preferable so drainage can be easily emptied. The drainable pouch is usually worn for 4 to 7 days before being changed unless leakage occurs.
- In the first 24 to 48 hours after surgery, the amount of drainage from the stoma may be negligible. Once peristalsis returns, the patient may experience a period of high-volume output of 1500 to 1800 mL/day. Later, the average amount can be 500 mL/day.

▼ **Patient and Caregiver Teaching**

Ileostomy

- Instruct the patient to drink at least 2 to 3 L/day when there are excessive fluid losses from heat and sweating. Patients must learn signs and symptoms of fluid and electrolyte imbalance so they can take appropriate action.

- A low-fiber diet is ordered initially. Fiber-containing foods are reintroduced gradually. A return to a normal presurgical diet is the goal.
- A stoma bleeds easily when it is touched because it has a high vascular supply. Tell the patient that minimal oozing of blood is normal.
- Encourage the patient to share concerns and ask questions. Provide information in a manner that is easily understood, recommend support services, and assist patients to develop confidence and competence in managing the stoma.
- Help the patient understand that sexual function or sexual activity may be affected.

OXYGEN THERAPY

Description

O_2 therapy is frequently used in the treatment of chronic obstructive pulmonary disease (COPD) and other problems associated with hypoxemia. Long-term continuous O_2 therapy (LTOT) increases survival and improves exercise capacity and mental status in hypoxemic patients.

Goals for O_2 therapy are to keep the SaO_2 above 90% during rest, sleep, and exertion, or PaO_2 greater than 60 mm Hg. O_2 is administered to treat hypoxemia caused by a variety of problems such as COPD, shock, pulmonary emboli, and many others.

Methods of Administration

Various methods of O_2 administration are used (Table 98). The method selected depends on factors such as the fraction of inspired O_2 concentration (FIO_2), the patient's mobility and cooperation, humidification, comfort, and cost.

- O_2 obtained from cylinders or wall systems is dry. Dry O_2 has an irritating effect on the mucous membranes and dries secretions. Therefore it is important that a high flow of O_2 delivering greater than 35% to 50% oxygen be humidified when administered.

Complications

O_2 supports combustion and increases the rate of burning, so it is important to prohibit smoking or open flames in the area in which O_2 is being used. A "No Smoking" sign should be prominently displayed on the patient's door. Also caution the patient against smoking cigarettes with an O_2 cannula in place because it can cause significant burns.

Text continued on p. 726

TABLE 98 Methods of Oxygen Administration

Description	Nursing Interventions
Low-Flow Delivery Devices *Nasal Cannula* • Most commonly used device • O_2 delivered via plastic nasal prongs. • Safe and simple method that allows some freedom of movement. Patient can eat, talk, or cough while wearing device. • Useful for a patient requiring low O_2 concentrations. • O_2 concentrations of 24% (at 1 L/min) to 44% (at 6 L/min) can be obtained.	• Stabilize nasal cannula when caring for a restless patient. • Amount of O_2 inhaled depends on room air and patient's breathing pattern. • Most patients with COPD can tolerate 2 L/min delivered by cannula. • Assess patient's nares and ears for skin breakdown. May need to pad cannula where it sits on ears. • If flow rates are >5 L/min, nasal and sinus membranes may dry, causing pain.

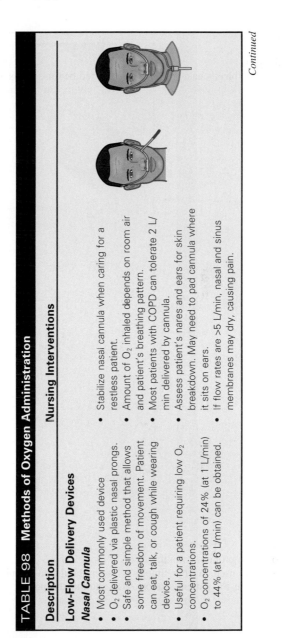

Continued

0

TABLE 98 Methods of Oxygen Administration—cont'd

Description	Nursing Interventions
Simple Face Mask	
• Covers patient's nose and mouth. • Used only for short periods, especially when transporting patients. • Longer use is typically not tolerated because of tight seal and heat generated around nose and mouth from mask. • O_2 concentrations of 35%–50% can be achieved with flow rates of 6-12 L/min. • Mask provides adequate humidification of inspired air.	• Wash and dry under mask q2hr. • Mask must fit snugly. • Nasal cannula may be provided while patient is eating. • Watch for pressure necrosis at top of ears from elastic straps if patient wears for a longer time. (Gauze or other padding may alleviate this problem.)

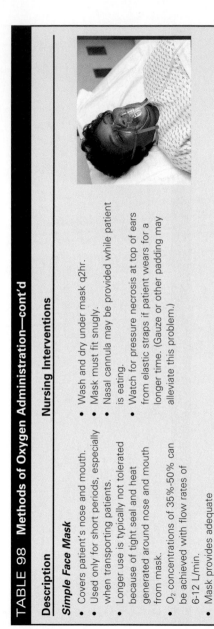

Partial and Non-Rebreather Masks

- Useful for short-term (24 hr) therapy for patients needing higher O_2 concentrations (60%-90% at 10-15 L/min).
- O_2 flows into reservoir bag and mask during inhalation.
- This bag allows patient to rebreathe about first third of exhaled air (rich in O_2) in conjunction with flowing O_2.
- Vents remain open on partial mask only. Some facilities prefer this over non-rebreather as a safety issue.

- O_2 flow rate must be sufficient to keep bag from collapsing during inspiration to avoid CO_2 buildup.
- If deflation occurs, increase liter flow to keep bag inflated.
- Mask should fit snugly.
- With non-rebreather masks, make sure valves are open during expiration and closed during inhalation, to prevent drastic decrease in FIO_2.
- Monitor patient closely because more advanced interventions may be required, such as CPAP, BiPAP, or intubation with mechanical ventilation.

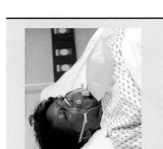

Continued

O

TABLE 98   Methods of Oxygen Administration—cont'd

Description	Nursing Interventions
Oxygen-Conserving Cannula • Generally indicated for long-term O_2 therapy at home vs. during hospitalization (e.g., pulmonary fibrosis, pulmonary hypertension). • May be "moustache" (Oxymizer) or "pendant" type. • Cannula has a built-in reservoir that ↑ O_2 concentration and allows patient to use lower flow, usually 30%-50%, which increases comfort, lowers cost, and can be increased with activities. • Can deliver up to 8 L/min O_2.	• May cause necrosis over tops of ears. Can be padded • Cannula cannot be cleaned. Manufacturer recommends changing cannula every week. • It is more expensive than standard cannulas and requires evaluation with ABGs and oximetry to determine correct flow for patient. • Cannula is highly visible.

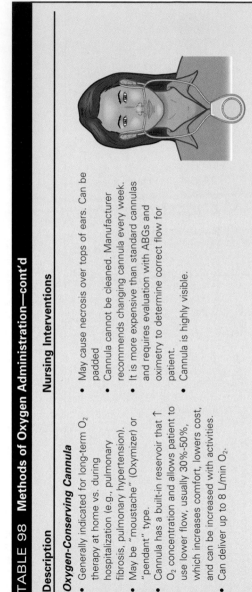

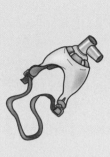

High-Flow Delivery Devices

Tracheostomy Collar

- Collar attaches to neck with elastic strap and can deliver high humidity and O_2 via tracheostomy.
- O_2 concentration is lost into atmosphere because collar does not fit tightly.
- Venturi device can be attached to flow meter and thus can deliver exact amounts of O_2 via collar.

- Secretions collect inside collar and around tracheostomy. Remove collar and clean at least q4hr to prevent aspiration of fluid and infection.
- Because condensation occurs in tubing, periodically drain distally to tracheostomy.

Tracheostomy T Bar

- Almost identical to tracheostomy collar, but it has a vent and a T connector that allow an inline catheter (e.g., Ballard catheter) to be connected for suctioning.
- Tight fit allows better O_2 and humidity delivery than with tracheostomy collar.

- Empty as necessary.
- Because T bars disconnect easily, monitor closely.
- T bar may pull on a patient's tracheostomy tube, causing irritation and potential tissue damage. Monitor this closely.
- See also Tracheostomy Collar interventions.

Continued

O

TABLE 98 Methods of Oxygen Administration—cont'd

Description	Nursing Interventions
Venturi Mask	
• Mask can deliver precise, high-flow rates of O_2. • Lightweight plastic, cone-shaped device is fitted to face. • Masks are available for delivery of 24%, 28%, 31%, 35%, 40%, and 50% O_2. • Method is especially helpful for administering low, constant O_2 concentrations to patients with COPD. • Adaptors can be applied to increase humidification.	• Entrainment device on mask must be changed to deliver higher concentrations of O_2. • Air entrainment ports must not be occluded. • Mask is uncomfortable. Remove when patient eats. • Patient can talk but voice may be muffled. • See other applicable nursing interventions listed earlier for Simple Face Mask.

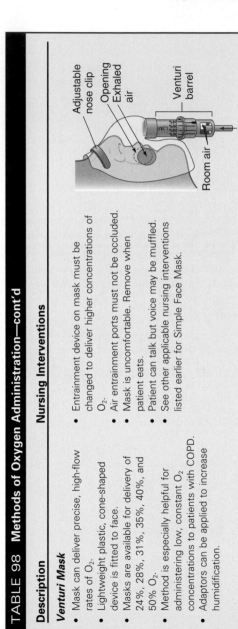

Adjustable nose clip

Opening
Exhaled air

Venturi barrel

Room air

High-Flow Nasal Cannula

- Blends O_2 with compressed air to generate FIO_2 up to 1.0 at flow rate of up to 60 L/min and PEEP of 7.4 cm H_2O.
- Active heated humidifier capable of providing 100% body humidity.
- Soft and flexible nasal prongs. More comfortable than mask.

- Nasal cannula must be smaller than 50% of nares to allow flow during exhalation and to flush out end-expiratory CO_2.
- Patient can eat and drink with device in place.
- PEEP drops about 2 cm H_2O when patient's mouth is open.

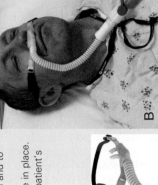

A   B

ABGs, Arterial blood gases; *BiPAP*, biphasic (bilevel) positive airway pressure; *COPD*, chronic obstructive pulmonary disease; *CPAP*, continuous positive airway pressure; *FIO₂*, fraction of inspired O_2.

The chemoreceptors in the respiratory center that control the drive to breathe respond to CO_2 and O_2. Normally CO_2 accumulation is the major stimulant of the respiratory center. Over time some patients with COPD develop a tolerance for high CO_2 levels (the respiratory center loses its sensitivity to the elevated CO_2 levels). Theoretically, for these individuals the "drive" to breathe is hypoxemia.

- Pulse oximetry and/or ABGs are used as a guide to determine what FIO_2 level is sufficient and can be tolerated. Safe administration of O_2 can be achieved by gradually increasing the concentration of oxygen, with close monitoring of both PaO_2 and $PaCO_2$. Assess the patient's mental status and vital signs before starting O_2 therapy and frequently thereafter.

Pulmonary oxygen toxicity may result from prolonged exposure to a high level of O_2 (PaO_2). High concentrations of O_2 can result in a severe inflammatory response because of oxygen radicals and damaged alveolar-capillary membranes, resulting in severe pulmonary edema, shunting of blood, and hypoxemia.

- To prevent toxicity, the amount of O_2 administered should be just enough to maintain the PaO_2 within a normal or acceptable range for the patient.

Infection can be a major hazard of O_2 administration. Heated nebulizers present the highest risk. Constant use of humidity supports bacterial growth, with *Pseudomonas aeruginosa* the most common infecting organism. Disposable equipment that operates as a closed system should be used. Each hospital has a policy on the required frequency of equipment changes based on the type of equipment used.

Chronic Oxygen Therapy at Home

Improved survival occurs in patients with COPD who receive LTOT (more than 15 hr/day) to treat hypoxemia. The benefits of LTOT include improved mental acuity, lung mechanics, sleep, and exercise tolerance; decreased hematocrit; and reduced pulmonary hypertension.

- Generally the patient should be reevaluated every 30 to 90 days during the first year of therapy and annually after that, so long as the patient remains stable.

▼ **Patient and Caregiver Teaching**
A home care guide for teaching the patient and family about home O_2 use is given in Table 99.

TABLE 99 Patient & Caregiver Teaching

Home Oxygen Use

The company that provides the prescribed O_2 therapy equipment will instruct the patient on equipment care. The following are some general instructions that you may include when teaching the patient and caregiver about the use of home O_2.

Decreasing Risk for Infection
- Brush teeth or use mouthwash several times a day.
- Wash nasal cannula (prongs) with a liquid soap and thoroughly rinse once or twice a week.
- Replace cannula every 2-4 weeks.
- If you have a cold, replace the cannula after your symptoms pass.
- Always remove secretions that are coughed out.
- If you use an O_2 concentrator, every day unplug the unit and wipe down the cabinet with a damp cloth and dry it.
- Ask the company providing the equipment how often to change the filter.

Safety Issues
- Post "No Smoking" warning signs outside the home.
- O_2 will not "blow up," but it will increase the rate of burning because it is a fuel for the fire.
- Do not allow smoking in the home, and do not smoke while wearing an O_2 cannula or other device. Nasal cannulas and masks can catch fire, causing serious burns to face and airways.
- Do not use flammable liquids such as paint thinners, cleaning fluids, gasoline, kerosene, oil-based paints, or aerosol sprays while receiving O_2.
- Do not use blankets or fabrics that carry a static charge, such as wool or synthetics.
- Inform your electric company if you are using a concentrator. In case of a power failure, the company will know the medical urgency of restoring your power.

Adapted from *www.YourLungHealth.org.*

P

PACEMAKERS

Description

The artificial cardiac pacemaker is an electronic device used to pace the heart when the normal conduction pathway is damaged.

The basic pacing circuit consists of a power source (battery-powered pulse generator), one or more conducting leads (pacing leads), and the myocardium. The electrical signal (stimulus) travels from the pacemaker, through the leads, to the wall of the myocardium. The heart muscle is stimulated to contract.

Demand pacemakers, which are the most common, sense the heart's electrical activity and fire only when the heart rate (HR) drops below a preset rate. Demand pacemakers have two distinct features: (1) a sensing device that inhibits the pacemaker when the HR is adequate and (2) a pacing device that triggers the pacemaker when no QRS complexes occur within a preset time.

Permanent pacemakers are implanted entirely within the patient's body. The power source is implanted subcutaneously, usually over the pectoral muscle on the patient's nondominant side. It is attached to pacer leads, which are threaded transvenously (through a vein) to the right atrium and one or both ventricles. Indications for insertion of a permanent pacemaker are listed in Table 100.

New technology and research are focused on miniaturized, leadless permanent pacemakers. Most candidates for these devices are patients who need single-chamber pacing for atrial fibrillation with atrioventricular (AV) block. The device is placed in the right ventricle. The lack of a transvenous lead and subcutaneous pulse generator is a major shift in cardiac pacing.

A *temporary pacemaker* is one that has the power source outside the body. There are three types of temporary pacemakers: transvenous, epicardial, and transcutaneous. Table 101 lists common reasons for temporary pacing.

TABLE 100   Indications for Permanent Pacemakers

- Acquired AV block
- Second-degree AV block
- Third-degree AV block
- Atrial fibrillation with a slow ventricular response
- Bundle branch block
- Cardiomyopathy
  - Dilated
  - Hypertrophic
- Heart failure
- SA node dysfunction
- Tachydysrhythmias (e.g., ventricular tachycardia)

AV, Atrioventricular; *SA,* sinoatrial.

TABLE 101   Indications for Temporary Pacemakers*

- Maintenance of adequate HR and rhythm during special circumstances such as surgery and postoperative recovery, during cardiac catheterization or coronary angioplasty, with drug therapy that may cause bradycardia, and before implantation of a permanent pacemaker
- As prophylaxis after open heart surgery
- Acute anterior MI with second- or third-degree AV block or bundle branch block
- Acute inferior MI with symptomatic bradycardia and AV block
- Electrophysiologic studies to evaluate patient with bradydysrhythmias and tachydysrhythmias

*List is not all-inclusive.
AV, Atrioventricular.

- A *transvenous pacemaker* consists of a lead or leads that are threaded transvenously to the right atrium and/or right ventricle and attached to the external power source.
- In *epicardial pacemakers,* atrial and ventricular pacing leads are attached to the epicardium during heart surgery in case pacing is required during the surgical recovery period. The leads are passed through the chest wall and attached to the external power source.
- A *transcutaneous pacemaker* is used to provide adequate heart rate and rhythm to the patient in an emergency situation. This type of pacemaker involves the use of external electrode pads that are connected to the external power source.

Patient Monitoring

Patients with temporary or permanent pacemakers are monitored by ECG to evaluate the status of the pacemaker. Pacemaker malfunction primarily involves a failure to sense or a failure to capture.

- *Failure to sense* occurs when the pacemaker fails to recognize spontaneous atrial or ventricular activity and fires inappropriately. Failure to sense is caused by fibrosis around the tip of the pacing lead, battery failure, sensing set too high, or electrode displacement.
- *Failure to capture* occurs when the electrical charge to the myocardium is insufficient to produce atrial or ventricular contraction. This can result in serious bradycardia or asystole. Failure to capture may be caused by pacer lead fracture, battery failure, electrode displacement, electrical charge set too low, or fibrosis at the electrode tip.

Nursing Management

After the pacemaker has been inserted, the patient can be out of bed once stable. Have the patient limit arm and shoulder activity on the operative side to prevent dislodging the newly implanted pacing leads.

- Observe the insertion site for signs of bleeding, and check that the incision is intact. Note any temperature elevation or pain at the insertion site and treat as ordered. Stable patients are discharged the same day or the following day.
- After discharge, patients need to check pacemaker function on a regular basis. This can include outpatient visits to a pacemaker clinic or home monitoring using telephone transmitter devices.
- The goals of pacemaker therapy include enhancing physiologic functioning and quality of life. Emphasize these goals to the patient and the caregiver, and provide specific advice on activity restrictions. Table 102 outlines patient and caregiver teaching about pacemakers.

TABLE 102   Patient & Caregiver Teaching
Pacemaker

Include the following information in the teaching plan for a patient with a pacemaker and the patient's caregiver.

1. Maintain follow-up care with your health care provider (HCP) to begin regular pacemaker function checks. This is often done by interrogating the device using a telephone.
2. Report any signs of infection at incision site (e.g., redness, swelling, drainage) or fever to your HCP immediately.
3. Keep incision dry for 4 days after implantation, or as ordered.
4. Avoid lifting arm on pacemaker side above shoulder until approved by your cardiologist.
5. Avoid direct blows to pacemaker site.
6. Avoid close proximity to high-output electric generators, since these can interfere with the function of the pacemaker.
7. You should not have a magnetic resonance imaging (MRI) scan unless the pacemaker is approved as MRI-safe or there is a protocol in place for patient safety during the procedure.
8. Microwave ovens are safe to use and do not interfere with pacemaker function.
9. Avoid standing near antitheft devices in doorways of department stores and public libraries. You should walk through them at a normal pace.

TABLE 102   Patient & Caregiver Teaching
Pacemaker—cont'd
10. Travel is not restricted. Inform security (e.g., airport, train station, public buildings) of presence of pacemaker because it may set off the metal detector. If hand-held screening wand is used, it should not be placed directly over the pacemaker. Manufacturer information may vary regarding the effect of metal detectors on the function of the pacemaker.
11. Monitor pulse and inform HCP if heart rate drops below predetermined rate.
12. Carry pacemaker information card and a current list of your medications at all times.
13. Obtain and wear a medical identification (e.g., Medic Alert) device at all times.
14. Consider joining a pacemaker support group (e.g., *https:// www.facebook.com/ICD.pacemaker*).

PARENTERAL NUTRITION

Description

Parenteral nutrition (PN) is a nutrient solution delivered directly into the bloodstream. PN is used when the gastrointestinal (GI) tract cannot be used for the ingestion, digestion, and absorption of essential nutrients (Table 103).

Administration of PN

PN may be administered by central or peripheral techniques. Both central and peripheral forms of PN are used in the patient who is not a candidate for enteral nutrition (EN). The patient receiving PN must be able to tolerate a large volume of fluid.

- *Central PN* is indicated when long-term nutritional support is necessary or when the patient has high protein and caloric requirements. Central PN may be administered using a central venous catheter that originates at the subclavian or jugular vein and whose tip lies in the superior vena cava. Central PN may also be administered using peripherally inserted central catheters (PICCs) that are placed into the basilic or cephalic vein and then advanced into the distal end of the superior vena cava.
- *Peripheral PN* (PPN) is administered using a large-bore catheter in a large peripheral vein. PPN is used when (1) nutritional support is needed for only a short time, (2) protein and caloric

P

> ### TABLE 103 Common Indications for Parenteral Nutrition
>
> - Chronic severe diarrhea and vomiting
> - Complicated surgery or trauma
> - GI obstruction
> - Intractable diarrhea
> - Severe anorexia nervosa
> - Severe malabsorption
> - Short bowel syndrome
> - GI tract anomalies and fistulas

requirements are not high, (3) the risk of a central catheter is too great, or (4) to supplement inadequate enteral intake.

Commercially prepared PN base solutions that contain dextrose and protein in the form of amino acids are available. The pharmacy adds the prescribed electrolytes (e.g., sodium, chloride, calcium, magnesium, phosphate), vitamins, and trace elements (e.g., zinc, copper, chromium, manganese) to meet the patient's needs. A three-in-one or total nutrient admixture containing an IV fat emulsion, dextrose, and amino acids is widely used.

Refeeding syndrome is a complication of PN that is characterized by fluid retention and electrolyte imbalances (hypophosphatemia, hypokalemia, hypomagnesemia). Conditions predisposing patients to refeeding syndrome include long-standing malnutrition states such as chronic alcoholism, vomiting and diarrhea, chemotherapy, and major surgery.

- Refeeding syndrome can occur any time a malnourished patient is started on aggressive nutritional support. Hypophosphatemia is the hallmark of refeeding syndrome and is associated with serious adverse outcomes, including cardiac dysrhythmias, respiratory arrest, and neurologic disturbances (e.g., paresthesias).

Other complications of PN are listed in Table 104.

Home Nutritional Support

Home PN nutrition is an accepted mode of nutritional therapy for the person who does not require hospitalization but who needs continued nutritional support. Patients have been successfully treated at home for many years.

- Teach the patient and caregiver about catheter or tube care, proper technique in handling the solutions and tubing, and side effects and complications.

TABLE 104   Complications of Parenteral Nutrition

Metabolic Problems

- Refeeding syndrome
- Hyperglycemia, hypoglycemia
- Altered renal function
- Essential fatty acid deficiency
- Liver dysfunction
- Hyperlipidemia

Catheter-Related Problems

- Air embolus
- Pneumothorax, hemothorax, and hydrothorax
- Hemorrhage
- Dislodgment
- Thrombosis of vein
- Phlebitis
- Catheter-related sepsis
- Occlusion

- Tell the family about support groups such as the Oley Foundation *(www.oley.org)* that provide peer support and advocacy.

Home nutritional therapies are expensive. Specific criteria must be met for expenses to be reimbursed. The discharge planning team needs to be involved early on to help address such issues. Home nutritional support may be a burden for the patient and caregivers and affect quality of life.

RADIATION THERAPY

Description

Radiation therapy is one of the oldest methods of cancer treatment. Delivery of high-energy beams, when absorbed into tissue, produces ionization of atomic particles. The energy in ionizing radiation acts to break the chemical bonds in DNA. The DNA is damaged, resulting in cell death.

Different types of ionizing radiation are used to treat cancer, including electromagnetic radiation (i.e., x-rays, gamma rays) and particulate radiation (alpha particles, electrons, neutrons, protons).

- Historically, the radiation dose was expressed in *rad* (radiation absorbed dose) units. In current nomenclature, *gray* (Gy) or *centigray* (cGy) units are used. One cGy is equivalent to 1 rad, and 100 cGy equal 1 Gy.

R

TABLE 105 Tumor Radiosensitivity*

High Radiosensitivity
- Ovarian dysgerminoma
- Testicular seminoma
- Hodgkin's lymphoma
- Non-Hodgkin's lymphoma
- Wilms' tumor
- Neuroblastoma

Moderate Radiosensitivity
- Oropharyngeal carcinoma
- Esophageal carcinoma
- Breast adenocarcinoma
- Uterine and cervical carcinoma
- Prostate carcinoma
- Bladder carcinoma

Mild Radiosensitivity
- Soft tissue sarcomas (e.g., chondrosarcoma)
- Gastric adenocarcinoma
- Renal adenocarcinoma
- Colon adenocarcinoma

Poor Radiosensitivity
- Osteosarcoma
- Malignant melanoma
- Malignant glioma
- Testicular nonseminoma

*Radiosensitivity is the relative susceptibility of cells and tissues to the effects of radiation.

- Once the total dose to be delivered is determined, that dose is divided into daily fractions. Doses between 180 and 200 cGy/day are considered standard for such fractionation, typically delivered once a day Monday through Friday for a period of 2 to 8 weeks (depending on the desired total dose).
- Radiation has an effect only on tissues within the treatment field. Radiation therapy is therefore not appropriate as the primary treatment for systemic disease. However, radiation therapy may be used by itself or in combination with chemotherapy or surgery to treat primary tumors or for palliation of metastatic lesions.
- Radiation can be delivered externally (known as *teletherapy* or *external beam radiation therapy*) or internally *(brachytherapy)*.

Rapidly dividing cells in the GI tract, oral mucosa, and bone marrow die quickly and exhibit early acute responses to radiation. Tissues with slowly proliferating cells, such as cartilage, bone, and kidneys, manifest later responses to radiation. Some cancers are more susceptible to radiation than others (Table 105).

Nursing Management: Chemotherapy and Radiation Therapy

See Chemotherapy, p. 694.

▼ **Patient and Caregiver Teaching**

See Chemotherapy, p. 699.

TRACHEOSTOMY

Description

A *tracheostomy* is a surgically created stoma (opening) in the trachea to establish an airway, or the procedure for creating this opening. It is used to (1) bypass an upper airway obstruction, (2) facilitate removal of secretions, or (3) permit long-term mechanical ventilation.

Most surgical tracheostomy procedures are done in the operating room using general anesthesia. These are typically done electively on patients already intubated who require prolonged mechanical ventilation. When swelling, trauma, or upper airway obstruction prevents endotracheal intubation, an emergent surgical tracheostomy may be performed at the bedside.

A *minimally invasive percutaneous tracheostomy* can also be performed using local anesthesia and sedation and analgesia. A needle is placed into the trachea, followed by a guide wire. The opening is progressively dilated until it is large enough for insertion of a tracheostomy tube.

- A tracheostomy tube provides a more secure airway, is less likely to be displaced, and allows more freedom of movement than an endotracheal tube. There is less risk of long-term damage to the vocal cords. Airway resistance and work of breathing are decreased, facilitating independent breathing. Patient comfort may be increased because no tube is present in the mouth.
- The patient can eat with a tracheostomy because the tube enters lower in the airway (Fig. 30). Speaking is also permitted once the tracheostomy cuff can be deflated.

When the patient can adequately exchange air and expectorate secretions, the tracheostomy tube can be removed. Close the stoma with tape strips and cover it with an occlusive dressing. Instruct the patient to splint the stoma with the fingers when coughing, swallowing, or speaking.

- Epithelial tissue begins to form in 24 to 48 hours, and the opening closes in several days. Surgical intervention to close a tracheostomy is not required.

Nursing Management

Before the tracheostomy, explain to the patient and family the purpose of the procedure and inform them that the patient will not be able to speak if an inflated cuff is used. A variety of tubes are available to meet patient needs (Fig. 30). Characteristics and nursing management of tracheostomies are described in Table 26-6, Lewis et al, *Medical-Surgical Nursing,* ed 10, p. 486.

T

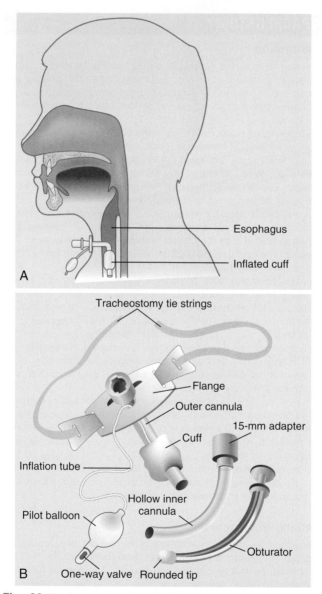

Fig. 30 Tracheostomy tube. **A,** Tracheostomy tube inserted in airway with inflated cuff. **B,** Parts of a tracheostomy tube.

Care should be taken not to dislodge the tracheostomy tube during the first 5 to 7 days, when the stoma is not healed.

- Because tube replacement is difficult, several precautions are required: (1) keep a replacement tube of equal or smaller size at the bedside, readily available for emergency reinsertion; (2) do not change tracheostomy tapes for at least 24 hours after the insertion procedure; and (3) let a physician perform the first tube change, usually no sooner than 7 days after the tracheostomy.
- If the tube is accidentally dislodged, immediately attempt to replace it. See the discussion of tube replacement techniques in Chapter 26 in Lewis et al, *Medical-Surgical Nursing,* ed 10, pp. 487 to 488.

Care of the patient with a tracheostomy involves suctioning the airway to remove secretions, cleaning around the stoma, changing tracheostomy ties, and inner cannula care if a nondisposable inner cannula is used. See Table 106 for a detailed description of tracheostomy care.

▼ **Patient and Caregiver Teaching**
- Assess ability of the patient and caregiver to provide care at home.
- Include instructions for tracheostomy tube care, stoma care, suctioning, airway care, and responding to emergencies.
- Make a referral to a home health care nurse to provide ongoing assistance and support.
- Teach patient and caregiver the signs and symptoms to report to health care professionals, such as changes in secretions (color and consistency) and elevated temperature.

TABLE 106 Tracheostomy Care

The following are general guidelines for basic tracheostomy care. Become familiar with the specific policies and/or procedures in your institution.

1. Explain procedure to patient.
2. Use tracheostomy care kit or collect necessary sterile equipment (e.g., suction catheter, gloves, water basin, drape, tracheostomy ties, tube brush or pipe cleaners, 4 × 4 gauze pads, sterile water or normal saline, and tracheostomy dressing [optional]). NOTE: Clean rather than sterile technique is used at home.
3. Position patient in semi-Fowler's position.
4. Assemble needed materials on bedside table next to patient.

T

Continued

TABLE 106 Tracheostomy Care—cont'd

5. Wash hands. Put on personal protective equipment (goggles and clean gloves).

6. Auscultate chest sounds. If wheezes or coarse crackles are present, suction the airway if the patient is unable to cough up secretions (Table 26-8, Lewis et al, *Medical-Surgical Nursing*, ed 10, p. 488). Remove soiled dressing and clean gloves.

7. Open sterile equipment, pour sterile H_2O or normal saline into two compartments of sterile container or two basins, and put on sterile gloves. NOTE: Hydrogen peroxide (3%) is no longer recommended unless an infection is present. If it is used, rinse the inner cannula and skin with sterile H_2O or normal saline afterward, to prevent trauma to tissue.

8. Unlock and remove inner cannula, if present. Many tracheostomy tubes do not have inner cannulas. Care for these tubes includes all steps except for inner cannula care.

9. If disposable inner cannula is used, replace with new cannula. If a nondisposable cannula is used:
   • Immerse inner cannula in sterile solution and clean inside and outside of cannula using tube brush or pipe cleaners.
   • Rinse cannula in sterile solution. Remove from solution and shake to dry.
   • Insert inner cannula into outer cannula with the curved part downward, and lock in place.

10. Remove dried secretions from stoma using 4 × 4 gauze pad soaked in sterile water or saline. Gently pat area around the stoma until dry. Be sure to clean under the tracheostomy flange (faceplate), using cotton swabs to reach this area.

11. Change tracheostomy tapes. Use two-person change technique or secure new tapes to flanges before removing the old ones. Tie tracheostomy tapes securely with room for two fingers between tapes and skin (Fig. 26-5, Lewis et al, *Medical-Surgical Nursing*, ed 10, p. 489). To prevent accidental tube removal, secure the tracheostomy tube by gently applying pressure to the flange of the tube during the tape changes. *Do not change tracheostomy tapes for 24 hours after the tracheostomy procedure.*

12. As an alternative, some patients prefer tracheostomy tapes made of self-gripping fabric (Velcro), which are easier to adjust.

13. If drainage is excessive, place dressing around tube (Fig. 26-5, Lewis et al, *Medical-Surgical Nursing*, ed 10, p. 489). A pre-cut tracheostomy dressing or unlined gauze should be used. Do not cut the gauze, because threads may be inhaled or wrap around the tracheostomy tube. Change the dressing as required. Wet dressings promote infection and stoma irritation.

14. Repeat care three times/day and as needed.

URINARY CATHETERIZATION

Indications for short-term urinary catheterization are listed in Table 107. Two unacceptable reasons are (1) routine acquisition of a urine specimen for laboratory analysis and (2) convenience of the nursing staff or the patient's family.

- Possible complications of long-term use (>30 days) of indwelling catheters include catheter-associated urinary tract infection (CAUTI), bladder spasms, periurethral abscess, pain, and urosepsis.

Catheterization for sterile urine specimens may occasionally be indicated when patients have a history of complicated urinary tract infection (UTI). Placement of a catheter should be the final means of providing the patient with a dry environment for the prevention of skin breakdown and protection of dressings or skin lesions.

TABLE 107 Indications for Urinary Catheterization

Indwelling Catheter
- Relief of urinary retention caused by lower urinary tract obstruction, paralysis, or inability to void
- Bladder decompression, done preoperatively and operatively, for lower abdominal or pelvic surgery
- Facilitation of surgical repair of urethra and surrounding structures
- Splinting of ureters or urethra to facilitate healing after surgery or other trauma in area
- Accurate measurement of urine output in critically ill patient
- Contamination of stage III or IV pressure ulcers with urine that has impeded healing, despite appropriate personal care for the incontinence
- Terminal illness or severe impairment, which makes positioning or clothing changes uncomfortable, or which is associated with intractable pain

Intermittent (Straight, in-and-Out) Catheter
- Relief of urinary retention caused by lower urinary tract obstruction, paralysis, or inability to void
- Study of anatomic structures of urinary system
- Urodynamic testing
- Collection of sterile urine sample in selected situations
- Instillation of medications into bladder
- Measurement of residual urine after urination (postvoid residual [PVR]) if portable ultrasound is not available

Strict aseptic technique is mandatory when a urinary catheter is inserted. See Table 108 for urinary catheter management. Address patient concerns, which may include embarrassment related to exposure of the body, an altered body image, and fear that care of the catheter will result in increased dependency.

- Catheters vary in construction materials, tip shape, and lumen size. Catheters are sized according to the French scale. Each French unit (F) equals 0.33 mm of diameter. The diameter listed is the internal diameter of the catheter. The size used varies with the patient's size and the purpose of catheterization.

The most common route of catheterization is insertion of the catheter through the external meatus into the urethra, past the internal sphincter, and into the bladder.

Suprapubic catheterization is the simplest and oldest method of urinary diversion. The two methods of insertion of a suprapubic catheter into the bladder are (1) through a small incision in the abdominal wall and (2) by the use of a trocar. A suprapubic catheter is placed while the patient is under general anesthesia for another surgical procedure or at the bedside with a local anesthetic. The catheter may be sutured into place.

- The suprapubic catheter is used in temporary situations, such as during bladder, prostate, and urethral surgery, and also used long term in selected patients.
- Tape the catheter to prevent dislodgement. The care of the tube and catheter is similar to that of the urethral catheter. A pectin-base skin barrier (e.g., Stomahesive) is effective in protecting the skin around the insertion site from breakdown.
- A suprapubic catheter is prone to poor drainage because of mechanical obstruction of the catheter tip by the bladder wall, sediment, and clots. To ensure patency of the tube include (1) preventing tube kinking by coiling the excess tubing and maintaining gravity drainage, (2) having the patient turn from side to side, and (3) milking the tube. If these measures are not effective, obtain a HCP's order to irrigate the catheter with sterile technique.
- If the patient experiences bladder spasms that are difficult to control, urinary leakage may result. Oxybutynin (Ditropan XL) or other oral antispasmodics or belladonna and opium (B&O) suppositories may be prescribed to decrease bladder spasms.

An alternative approach to a long-term indwelling catheter is *intermittent catheterization,* also referred to as "straight" or "in-and-out" catheterization. It is used in conditions such as neurogenic bladder (e.g., spinal cord injuries, chronic neurologic diseases) or bladder outlet obstruction in men. This type of catheterization may also be used in the oliguric and anuric phases of acute kidney injury

TABLE 108 Management of Patient With Urethral Catheter

U

The following measures can be used to manage the patient with a urethral catheter and prevent catheter-associated urinary tract infection (CAUTI).

1. Teach catheter care to the patient, particularly one who is ambulatory.
2. Use a sterile, closed drainage system in short-term catheterization. Do not disconnect the distal urinary catheter and proximal drainage tube except for catheter irrigation (if ordered and indicated).
3. Maintain unobstructed downhill flow of urine. Empty the collecting bag regularly, and keep it below the level of the bladder.
4. Provide perineal care (once or twice a day and when necessary), including cleansing the meatus-catheter junction with soap and water. Do not use lotion or powder near the catheter.
5. Anchor catheter using some type of securement device. Anchor catheter to upper thigh in women and lower abdomen in men, to prevent catheter movement and urethral tension.
6. Use sterile technique whenever the collecting system is open. If frequent irrigations are necessary in short-term catheterization to maintain catheter patency, a triple-lumen catheter may be preferable, permitting continuous irrigations within a closed system.
7. If ordered, aspirate small volumes of urine for culture from the catheter sampling port by means of a sterile syringe and needle. First prepare the puncture site with an antiseptic solution.
8. When the patient is catheterized for less than 2 wk, routine catheter change is not necessary. For long-term use of an indwelling catheter, replace the catheter as indicated by patient assessment and not on a routine changing schedule.
9. With long-term use of a catheter, a leg bag may be used. If the collection bag is reused, wash it in soap and water and rinse thoroughly. When it is not reused immediately, fill it with $\frac{1}{2}$ cup of vinegar and drain. The vinegar is effective against *Pseudomonas* and other organisms and eliminates odors.
10. Remove the catheter as early as possible. Intermittent catheterization and external catheters are alternatives that may be associated with fewer cases of bacteriuria and urinary tract infection (UTI) than with chronic indwelling urethral catheters.

to reduce the possibility of infection from an indwelling catheter. Intermittent catheterization is also used postoperatively, often after a surgical procedure to treat urinary incontinence.

- The main goal of intermittent catheterization is to prevent urinary retention, stasis, and compromised blood supply to the bladder caused by prolonged pressure.
- The technique consists of inserting a urethral catheter into the bladder every 3 to 5 hours. Some patients perform intermittent catheterization only once or twice each day to measure residual urine and ensure an empty bladder.
- Instruct patients to wash and rinse the catheter and their hands with soap and water before and after catheterization. Lubricant is necessary for men and may make catheterization more comfortable for women.
- The catheter may be inserted by the patient, caregiver, or HCP.
- In the hospital or long-term care facility, sterile technique is used for catheterizations. For home care, a clean technique that includes good hand washing with soap and water is used.

Teach the patient to observe for signs of UTI so that treatment can be instituted early.

PART THREE

Reference Appendix

ABBREVIATIONS

ABG	arterial blood gas
ACE	angiotensin-converting enzyme
ACLS	advanced cardiac life support
ACS	acute coronary syndrome
ACTH	adrenocorticotropic hormone
ADH	antidiuretic hormone
AED	automated external defibrillator
AIDS	acquired immunodeficiency syndrome
AKA	above-knee amputation
AKI	acute kidney injury
ALL	acute lymphocytic leukemia
ALS	amyotrophic lateral sclerosis
AMI	acute myocardial infarction
ANA	antinuclear antibody
ANS	autonomic nervous system
AORN	Association of periOperative Registered Nurses
APD	automated peritoneal dialysis
aPTT	activated partial thromboplastin time
ARDS	acute respiratory distress syndrome
ATN	acute tubular necrosis
BCLS	basic cardiac life support
BKA	below-knee amputation
BMI	body mass index
BMR	basal metabolic rate
BMT	bone marrow transplantation
BPH	benign prostatic hyperplasia
BSE	breast self-examination
BUN	blood urea nitrogen
CABG	coronary artery bypass graft
CAD	coronary artery disease; circulatory assist device
CAPD	continuous ambulatory peritoneal dialysis
CAVH	continuous arteriovenous hemofiltration
CBC	complete blood count
CCU	coronary care unit; critical care unit
CDC	Centers for Disease Control and Prevention
CIS	carcinoma in situ

Continued

ABBREVIATIONS—cont'd

CKD	chronic kidney disease
CLL	chronic lymphocytic leukemia
CML	chronic myelocytic leukemia
CMP	cardiomyopathy
CN	cranial nerve
CNS	central nervous system
CO	cardiac output
COPD	chronic obstructive pulmonary disease
CPAP	continuous positive airway pressure
CPR	cardiopulmonary resuscitation
CRRT	continuous renal replacement therapy
CRNA	certified registered nurse anesthetist
CSF	cerebrospinal fluid
CT	computed tomography
CVA	cerebrovascular accident; costovertebral angle
CVAD	central venous access device
CVI	chronic venous insufficiency
CVP	central venous pressure
D&C	dilation and curettage
DDD	degenerative disc disease
DI	diabetes insipidus
DIC	disseminated intravascular coagulation
DJD	degenerative joint disease
DKA	diabetic ketoacidosis
DM	diabetes mellitus; diastolic murmur
DRE	digital rectal examination
DVT	deep vein thrombosis
ECF	extracellular fluid
ECG	electrocardiogram
ED	emergency department; erectile dysfunction
EEG	electroencephalogram
EMG	electromyogram
ENT	ear, nose, and throat
ERCP	endoscopic retrograde cholangiopancreatography
ERS	emergency response system
ESR	erythrocyte sedimentation rate
ESRD	end-stage renal disease

ABBREVIATIONS—cont'd

ET	endotracheal
FEV	forced expiratory volume
FRC	functional residual capacity
FUO	fever of unknown origin
GCS	Glasgow Coma Scale
GERD	gastroesophageal reflux disease
GFR	glomerular filtration rate
GH	growth hormone
GTT	glucose tolerance test
GU	genitourinary
GYN, Gyn	gynecologic
H&P	history and physical examination
HAV	hepatitis A virus
HBV	hepatitis B virus
HCP	health care provider
Hct	hematocrit
HCV	hepatitis C virus
HD	hemodialysis; Huntington's disease
HDL	high-density lipoprotein
HF	heart failure
Hgb	hemoglobin
HIV	human immunodeficiency virus
HPV	human papillomavirus
HSCT	hematopoietic stem cell transplantation
I&D	incision and drainage
IABP	intraaortic balloon pump
IBS	irritable bowel syndrome
ICP	intracranial pressure
IE	infective endocarditis
IFG	impaired fasting glucose
IGT	impaired glucose tolerance
INR	international normalized ratio
IOP	intraocular pressure
IPPB	intermittent positive pressure breathing
ITP	idiopathic thrombocytopenic purpura
IUD	intrauterine device

Continued

ABBREVIATIONS—cont'd

IV	intravenous
IVP	intravenous push
JVD	jugular venous distention
KUB	kidney, ureters, and bladder (x-ray)
KS	Kaposi sarcoma
KVO	keep vein open
LAD	left anterior descending
LDL	low-density lipoprotein
LLQ	left lower quadrant
LMN	lower motor neuron
LMP	last menstrual period
LOC	level of consciousness
LP	lumbar puncture
LUQ	left upper quadrant
LVH	left ventricular hypertrophy
MAP	mean arterial pressure
MD	muscular dystrophy
MDS	myelodysplastic syndrome
MG	myasthenia gravis
MI	myocardial infarction
MICU	medical intensive care unit
MODS	multiple organ dysfunction syndrome
MRB	manual resuscitation bag
MS	multiple sclerosis
MVP	mitral valve prolapse
NAFLD	nonalcoholic fatty liver disease
NANDA-I	North American Nursing Diagnosis Association–International
NASH	nonalcoholic steatohepatitis
NG	nasogastric
NHL	non-Hodgkin's lymphoma
NPO	nothing by mouth
NS	normal saline
NSR	normal sinus rhythm
OA	osteoarthritis
OD	right eye; optical density; overdose
OS	left eye

ABBREVIATIONS—cont'd

OOB	out of bed
OR	operating room
ORIF	open reduction and internal fixation
OSA	obstructive sleep apnea
OTC	over-the-counter
PA	posteroanterior; physician's assistant
PAC	premature atrial contraction
$PaCO_2$	partial pressure of carbon dioxide in arterial blood
PaO_2	partial pressure of oxygen in arterial blood
PACU	postanesthesia care unit
PAD	peripheral artery disease
PAP	pulmonary artery pressure
PAWP	pulmonary artery wedge pressure
PCA	patient-controlled analgesia
PCI	percutaneous coronary intervention
PCO_2	partial pressure of carbon dioxide
PCWP	pulmonary capillary wedge pressure
PD	Parkinson's disease; peritoneal dialysis
PE	pulmonary embolism; physical examination
PEEP	positive end-expiratory pressure
PEFR	peak expiratory flow rate
PERRLA	pupils equal, round, and reactive to light and accommodation
PET	positron emission tomography
PICC	peripherally inserted central catheter
PID	pelvic inflammatory disease
PKD	polycystic kidney disease
PMH	past medical history
PMI	point of maximal impulse
PMS	premenstrual syndrome
PN	parenteral nutrition
PND	paroxysmal nocturnal dyspnea
PNS	peripheral nervous system
PO, po	orally
PO_2	partial pressure of oxygen
POC	point-of-care

Continued

ABBREVIATIONS—cont'd

PPD	purified protein derivative
PSA	prostate-specific antigen
PT	prothrombin time
PTT	partial thromboplastin time
PVC	premature ventricular contraction
PUD	peptic ulcer disease
R/O	rule out
RA	rheumatoid arthritis
REM	rapid eye movement
RF	rheumatic fever
RHD	rheumatic heart disease
RLQ	right lower quadrant
RLS	restless legs syndrome
ROM	range of motion
ROS	review of systems
RUQ	right upper quadrant
SA	sinoatrial
SCI	spinal cord injury
SCD	sickle cell disease; sudden cardiac death
SDB	sleep-disordered breathing
SICU	surgical intensive care unit
SIRS	systemic inflammatory response syndrome
SLE	systemic lupus erythematosus
SNS	sympathetic nervous system
SOB	shortness of breath
STI	sexually transmitted infection
SVR	systemic vascular resistance
SVT	superficial vein thrombosis
TAH	total abdominal hysterectomy
TB	tuberculosis
TBSA	total body surface area
TCDB	turn, cough, and deep breathe
TENS	transcutaneous electrical nerve stimulation
THR	total hip replacement
TIA	transient ischemic attack
TJC	The Joint Commission
TKO	to keep open

ABBREVIATIONS—cont'd

TNM	tumor, node, metastasis
TPR	temperature, pulse, and respirations
TURP	transurethral resection of the prostate
UA	unstable angina
UAP	unlicensed assistive personnel
UGI	upper gastrointestinal
UI	urinary incontinence
UMN	upper motor neuron
URI	upper respiratory infection
UTI	urinary tract infection
VAD	venous access device; ventricular assist device
VDH	valvular disease of the heart
VF	ventricular fibrillation
VS	vital signs
VT	ventricular tachycardia
VTE	venous thromboembolism
WHR	waist-to-hip ratio
WNL	within normal limits

THE JOINT COMMISSION OFFICIAL "DO NOT USE" LIST[1]

Do Not Use	Potential Problem	Use Instead
U (unit)	Mistaken for "0" (zero), the number "4" (four) or "cc"	Write "unit"
IU (International Unit)	Mistaken for IV (intravenous) or the number 10 (ten)	Write "International Unit"
D., QD, q.d., qd (daily)	Mistaken for each other	Write "daily"
Q.O.D., QOD, q.o.d., qod (every other day)	Period after the Q mistaken for "I" and the "O" mistaken for "I"	Write "every other day"
Trailing zero (X.0 mg)*	Decimal point is missed	Write X mg
Lack of leading zero (.X mg)		Write 0.X mg
MS	Can mean morphine sulfate or magnesium sulfate	Write "morphine sulfate"
MSO_4 and $MgSO_4$	Confused for one another	Write "magnesium sulfate"

[1]Applies to all orders and all medication-related documentation that is handwritten (including free-text computer entry) or on pre-printed forms.
*Exception: A "trailing zero" may be used only where required to demonstrate the level of precision of the value being reported, such as for laboratory results, imaging studies that report size of lesions, or catheter/tube sizes. It may not be used in medication orders or other medication-related documentation.

Additional Abbreviations, Acronyms, and Symbols

(For *possible* future inclusion in the Official "Do Not Use" List)

Do Not Use	Potential Problem	Use Instead
> (greater than) < (less than)	Misinterpreted as the number "7" (seven) or the letter "L" Confused for one another	Write "greater than" Write "less than"
Abbreviations for drug names	Misinterpreted due to similar abbreviations for multiple drugs	Write drug names in full
Apothecary units	Unfamiliar to many practitioners Confused with metric units	Use metric units
@	Mistaken for the number "2" (two)	Write "at"
cc	Mistaken for U (units) when poorly written	Write "mL" or "ml" or "milliliters" ("mL" is preferred)
µg	Mistaken for mg (milligrams), resulting in one thousand-fold overdose	Write "mcg" or "micrograms"

BLOOD GASES

Normal Values

	Arterial (Sea Level)
pH	7.35-7.45
PaO_2*	80-100 mm Hg
$PaCO_2$	35-45 mm Hg
HCO_3	22-26 mEq/L
O_2 saturation	>95%

*In a patient >60 years of age, normal PaO_2 is equal to 80 mm Hg minus 1 mm Hg for every year over 60. When supplemental oxygen is provided, expected PaO_2 = $FIO_2 \times 5$.

Interpreting Arterial Blood Gases (ABGs)

1. Check pH
   $\uparrow$ = Alkalosis; $\downarrow$ = acidosis
2. Check $PaCO_2$
   $\uparrow$ = CO_2 retention (hypoventilation); respiratory acidosis or
   compensating for metabolic alkalosis
   $\downarrow$ = CO_2 blown off (hyperventilation); respiratory alkalosis or
   compensating for metabolic acidosis
3. Check HCO_3
   $\uparrow$ = Nonvolatile acid is lost; HCO_3 is gained (metabolic alkalosis
   or compensating for respiratory acidosis)
   $\downarrow$ = Nonvolatile acid is added; HCO_3 is lost (metabolic acidosis
   or compensating for respiratory alkalosis)
4. Determine imbalance
5. Determine if compensation exists

Determining the Imbalance in ABGs

If pH $\uparrow$ and $PaCO_2$ $\downarrow$
         or   } **then** respiratory disorder
   pH $\downarrow$ and $PaCO_2$ $\uparrow$

If pH $\uparrow$ and HCO_3 $\uparrow$
         or   } **then** metabolic disorder
   pH $\downarrow$ and HCO_3 $\downarrow$

If $PaCO_2$ $\uparrow$ and HCO_3 $\uparrow$
         or   } **then** compensation is occurring
   $PaCO_2$ $\downarrow$ and HCO_3 $\downarrow$

If $PaCO_2$ $\uparrow$ and HCO_3 $\downarrow$
         or   } **then** mixed imbalance
   $PaCO_2$ $\downarrow$ and HCO_3 $\uparrow$

BLOOD PRODUCTS*

Description	Special Considerations	Indications for Use
Packed RBCs		
Packed RBCs are prepared from whole blood by sedimentation or centrifugation. One unit contains 250-350 mL. RBCs can be stored up to 35 days, depending on processing.	Use of RBCs for treatment allows remaining components of blood (e.g., platelets, albumin, plasma) to be used for other purposes. There is less danger of fluid overload. Packed RBCs are preferred RBC source because they are more component-specific. Leukocyte depletion (leukoreduction) by filtration, washing, or freezing is frequently used. Decreases hemolytic febrile or mild allergic reactions in patients who receive frequent transfusions.	Severe or symptomatic anemia, acute blood loss. One unit of RBCs can be expected to increase Hgb by 1 g/dL or Hct by 3% in a typical adult. One unit of RBCs can replace a blood loss of 500 mL.
Frozen RBCs		
Frozen RBCs are prepared from RBCs using glycerol for protection and frozen. They can be stored for 10 yr.	Must be used within 24 hr of thawing. Successive washings with saline solution remove majority of WBCs and plasma proteins.	Autotransfusion Stockpiling or rare donors for patients with alloantibodies.

Continued

BLOOD PRODUCTS—cont'd

Description	Special Considerations	Indications for Use
Platelets		
Platelets are prepared from fresh whole blood. One donor unit contains 3×10^{11} platelets in 30-60 mL of platelet concentrate (from whole blood). Platelets may also be pooled from multiple donors (1 apheresis unit is roughly equivalent to 4 to 6 random-donor pooled platelets). An apheresis single donation contains 200-400 mL of platelets.	Multiple units of platelets can be obtained from one donor by plateletpheresis. They can be kept at room temperature for 1-5 days, depending on type of collection and storage bag used. Bag should be agitated periodically. For patients who become refractory to frequent transfusions, may give leukocyte-reduced or HLA type-specific to prevent alloimmunization to HLA antigens.	Bleeding caused by thrombocytopenia May be contraindicated in thrombotic thrombocytopenic purpura and heparin-induced thrombocytopenia, except in life-threatening hemorrhage Expected increase of 5000/μL/U. Failure to achieve increase may be due to fever, sepsis, splenomegaly, or DIC or development of antibodies *(refractory).*

Fresh Frozen Plasma

Liquid portion of whole blood is separated from cells and frozen. One unit contains approximately 250 mL. Plasma is rich in clotting factors but contains no platelets. May be stored for up to 1 yr, depending on storage. Must be used within 24 hr after thawing.

Use of plasma in treating hypovolemic shock is being replaced by pure preparations such as albumin and plasma expanders.

Bleeding caused by deficiency in clotting factors (e.g., DIC, hemorrhage, massive transfusion, liver disease, vitamin K deficiency, excess warfarin).

Albumin

Albumin is prepared from plasma. It can be stored for 5 yr. It is available in 5% or 25% solution.

Albumin 25 g/dL is osmotically equal to 500 mL of plasma. Hyperosmolar solution acts by moving water from extravascular to intravascular space. It is heat-treated and does not transmit viruses.

Hypovolemic shock, hypoalbuminemia.

Cryoprecipitates and Commercial Concentrates

Cryoprecipitate is prepared from fresh frozen plasma, with 10-20 mL/bag. It can be stored for 1 yr. Once thawed, must be used within 5 days.

See Table 30-18 in Lewis et al, *Medical-Surgical Nursing*, ed 10, p. 628.

Replacement of clotting factors, especially factor VIII, von Willebrand factor, and fibrinogen.

*Component therapy has replaced the use of whole blood, which is infrequently used.
DIC, Disseminated intravascular coagulation; *Hct,* hematocrit; *Hgb,* hemoglobin; *HLA,* human leukocyte antigen.

BREATH SOUNDS

Normal Sounds

Type	Normal Site	Duration, I/E Ratio	Characteristics
Vesicular	Peripheral lung	I > E 3 : 1	• Soft, low-pitched, gentle, rustling sounds • Heard over all lung areas except major bronchi • Abnormal when heard over the large airways
Bronchovesicular	Sternal border of the major bronchi	I = E 1 : 1	• Medium pitch and intensity • Heard anteriorly over the main bronchi on either side of the sternum and posteriorly between the scapulae • Abnormal if heard over peripheral lung fields
Bronchial	Trachea and bronchi	I < E 2 : 3	• Louder, higher-pitched • Resembles air blowing through a hollow pipe • Abnormal if heard over peripheral lung

BREATH SOUNDS

Abnormal (or Adventitious) Sounds

Characteristics	Possible Clinical Condition(s)
Fine Crackles	
Series of short-duration, discontinuous, high-pitched sounds heard just before the end of inspiration; similar sound to that made by rolling hair between fingers just behind ear	Interstitial edema (early pulmonary edema), alveolar filling (pneumonia), loss of lung volume (atelectasis), early phase of heart failure, idiopathic pulmonary fibrosis
Coarse Crackles	
Series of long-duration, discontinuous, low-pitched sounds caused by air passing through airway intermittently occluded by mucus, unstable bronchial wall, or fold of mucosa; evident on inspiration and, at times, expiration	Excessive fluid within the lungs, heart failure, pulmonary edema, pneumonia with severe congestion, COPD
Wheezes	
Continuous high-pitched squeaking or musical sound caused by rapid vibration of bronchial walls; first evident on expiration but possibly evident on inspiration as obstruction of airway increases	Bronchospasm (caused by asthma), airway obstruction (caused by foreign body, tumor), COPD
Pleural Friction Rub	
Creaking or grating sound from roughened, inflamed surfaces of the pleura rubbing together; evident during inspiration, expiration, or both	Pleurisy, pneumonia, pulmonary infarct

COPD, Chronic obstructive pulmonary disease; *E*, expiration; *I*, inspiration.

COMMONLY USED FORMULAS

Parameter	Formula	Normal Range
Anion gap	$Na - (HCO_3^+ + Cl)$	8-16 mEq/L
Body mass index (BMI)	$\dfrac{\text{Weight in pounds}}{\text{Height in inches}^2} \times 703$	18.5-24.9 kg/m^2
Cardiac index (CI)	$\dfrac{CO}{\text{Body surface area (BSA)}}$	2.2-4.0 L/min/m^2
Cardiac output (CO)	$HR \times SV$	4-8 L/min
Cerebral perfusion pressure (CPP)	$MAP - ICP$	80-100 mm Hg
Ejection fraction (EF)	$\dfrac{SV}{\text{End-diastolic volume}} \times 100$	60% or greater
Mean arterial pressure (MAP)	$\dfrac{2(DBP) + SBP}{3}$	70-105 mm Hg
Stroke volume (SV)	$\dfrac{CO}{HR}$	60-150 mL/beat

DBP, Diastolic blood pressure; *ICP,* intracranial pressure; *SBP,* systolic blood pressure.

CHARACTERISTICS OF COMMON DYSRHYTHMIAS

Normal Rhythm/ Dysrhythmia	PATTERN			
	Rate and Rhythm	P Wave	PR Interval	QRS Complex
Normal sinus rhythm (NSR)	60-100 beats/min and regular	Normal	Normal	Normal
Sinus bradycardia	<60 beats/min and regular	Normal	Normal	Normal
Sinus tachycardia	101-200 beats/min and regular	Normal	Normal	Normal
Premature atrial contraction (PAC)	Usually 60-100 beats/min and irregular	Abnormal shape	Normal	Normal (usually)
Paroxysmal supraventricular tachycardia (PSVT)	150-220 beats/min and regular	Abnormal shape, may be hidden in the preceding T wave	Normal or shortened	Normal (usually)
Atrial flutter	*Atrial:* 200-350 beats/min and regular *Ventricular:* > or <100 beats/min and may be regular or irregular	Flutter (F) waves (sawtoothed pattern); more flutter waves than with QRS complexes; may occur in a 2:1, 3:1, 4:1 (etc.) pattern	Not measurable	Normal (usually)

Continued

CHARACTERISTICS OF COMMON DYSRHYTHMIAS—cont'd

Normal Rhythm/ Dysrhythmia	PATTERN			
	Rate and Rhythm	P Wave	PR Interval	QRS Complex
Atrial fibrillation	*Atrial:* 350-600 beats/min and irregular *Ventricular:* > or <100 beats/min and irregular	Fibrillatory (f) waves	Not measurable	Normal (usually)
Junctional dysrhythmias	40-180 beats/min and regular	Inverted; may be hidden in QRS complex	Shortened, if present	Normal (usually)
First-degree AV block	Normal and regular	Normal	>0.20 sec	Normal
Second-degree AV block				
• Type I (Mobitz I, Wenckebach heart block)	*Atrial:* Normal and regular *Ventricular:* Slower and irregular	Normal	Progressive lengthening	Normal QRS width, with pattern of one nonconducted (blocked) QRS complex
• Type II (Mobitz II heart block)	*Atrial:* Usually normal and regular *Ventricular:* Slower and regular or irregular	More P waves than QRS complexes (e.g., 2:1, 3:1)	Normal or prolonged but consistent for every QRS	Widened QRS, preceded by ≥2 P waves, with nonconducted (blocked) QRS complex

Third-degree AV block (complete heart block)	*Atrial:* Regular but may appear irregular due to P waves hidden in QRS complexes *Ventricular:* 20-60 beats/min and regular	Normal, but no connection with QRS complex	Inconsistent	Normal or widened, no relationship with P waves
Premature ventricular contraction (PVC)	PVCs occur at variable rates Underlying rhythm can be regular or irregular	Not usually visible, hidden in the PVC	Not measurable	Wide and distorted
Ventricular tachycardia (VT)	150-250 beats/min and regular or irregular	Not usually visible	Not measurable	Wide and distorted
Accelerated idioventricular rhythm	40-100 beats/min and regular	Not usually visible	Not measurable	Wide and distorted
Ventricular fibrillation (VF)	Not measurable and irregular	Absent	Not measurable	Not measurable

AV, Atrioventricular.

ELECTROCARDIOGRAM (ECG) MONITORING

ECG Waveforms and Normal Sinus Rhythm

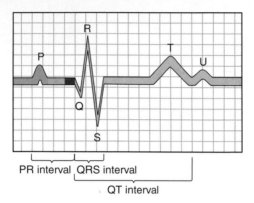

PR interval QRS interval

QT interval

ECG Waveforms and Intervals and Sources of Potential Variations*

Description	Normal Duration (sec)	Source of Possible Variation
P Wave		
Represents time for the passage of the electrical impulse through the atrium causing atrial depolarization (contraction). Should be upright.	0.06-0.12	Disturbance in conduction within atria
PR Interval		
Measured from beginning of P wave to beginning of QRS complex. Represents time taken for impulse to spread through the atria, AV node and bundle of His, bundle branches, and Purkinje fibers, to a point immediately before ventricular contraction.	0.12-0.20	Disturbance in conduction usually in AV node, bundle of His, or bundle branches but can be in atria as well
QRS Complex		
Q wave: First negative (downward) deflection after the P wave, short and narrow, not present in several leads.	<0.03	MI may result in development of a pathologic Q wave that is wide (≥0.03 sec) and deep (≥25% of the height of the R wave)
R wave: First positive (upward) deflection in the QRS complex.	Not usually measured	
S wave: First negative (downward) deflection after the R wave.	Not usually measured	

Continued

766 Electrocardiogram (ECG) Monitoring

ECG Waveforms and Intervals and Sources of Potential Variations—cont'd

Description	Normal Duration (sec)	Source of Possible Variation
QRS Interval Measured from beginning to end of QRS complex. Represents time taken for depolarization (contraction) of both ventricles (systole).	<0.12	Disturbance in conduction in bundle branches or in ventricles
ST Segment Measured from the S wave of the QRS complex to the beginning of the T wave. Represents the time between ventricular depolarization and repolarization (diastole). Should be isoelectric (flat).	0.12	Disturbances (e.g., elevation, depression) usually caused by ischemia, injury, or infarction
T Wave Represents time for ventricular repolarization. Should be upright.	0.16	Disturbances (e.g., tall, peaked; inverted) usually caused by electrolyte imbalances, ischemia, or infarction
QT Interval† Measured from beginning of QRS complex to end of T wave. Represents time taken for entire electrical depolarization and repolarization of the ventricles. Normal adult women have slightly longer QT intervals than men.	0.34-0.43	Disturbances usually affecting repolarization more than depolarization and caused by drugs, electrolyte imbalances, and changes in heart rate

AV, Atrioventricular; *MI*, myocardial infarction.

*Heart rate influences the duration of these intervals, especially the PR and QT intervals (e.g., QT interval shortens in duration as heart rate increases).

†A corrected QT interval (QTc) is calculated to account for the influence of heart rate.

GLASGOW COMA SCALE

Appropriate Stimulus	Response	Score
Eyes Open		
Approach to bedside	Spontaneous response	4
Verbal command	Opening of eyes to name or command	3
Pain	Lack of opening of eyes to previous stimuli but opening to pain	2
	Lack of opening of eyes to any stimulus	1
	Untestable*	U
Best Verbal Response		
Verbal questioning with maximum arousal	Appropriate orientation, conversant— correct identification of self, place, year, and month	5
	Confusion—conversant, but disorientation in one or more spheres	4
	Inappropriate or disorganized use of words (e.g., cursing), lack of sustained conversation	3
	Incomprehensible words, sounds (e.g., moaning)	2
	Lack of sound, even with painful stimuli	1
	Untestable*	U

Continued

GLASGOW COMA SCALE—cont'd

Appropriate Stimulus	Response	Score
Best Motor Response		
Verbal command (e.g., "raise your arm," "hold up two fingers")	Obedience of command	6
Pain (pressure on proximal nail bed)	Localization of pain, lack of obedience but presence of attempts to remove offending stimulus	5
	Flexion withdrawal,* flexion of arm in response to pain without abnormal flexion posture	4
	Abnormal flexion, flexing of arm at elbow and pronation, making a fist	3
	Abnormal extension, extension of arm at elbow usually with adduction and internal rotation of arm at shoulder	2
	Lack of response	1
	Untestable*	U

*Added to the original scale by some centers.

HEART SOUNDS

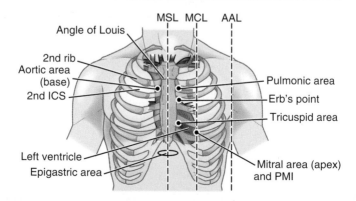

Sound	Auscultation Site	Clinical Occurrence
S_1 (M_1 T_1)	Apex	Closing of mitral and tricuspid valves; signals the beginning of systole
S_2 (A_2 P_2)	A_2 at second ICS, RSB; P_2 at second ICS, LSB	Closing of aortic and pulmonic valves; signals the beginning of diastole
S_2 physiologic split	Second ICS, LSB (pulmonic area)	Can be normal and is a split sound that corresponds with the respiratory cycle caused by a normal delay of pulmonic valve during inspiration; can be abnormal if heard during expiration or if it is constant during the respiratory cycle; accentuated during exercise or in individuals with thin chest walls; heard most often in children and young adults
S_3 (ventricular gallop)	Apex	Low-intensity vibration of the ventricular wall usually associated with decreased compliance of the ventricles during filling; heard closely after S_2; common in children and young adults and during last trimester of pregnancy
S_4 (atrial gallop)	Apex	Low-frequency vibration caused by atrial filling and contraction against increased resistance in ventricle; precedes S_1 of next cycle; may be normal in infants, children, and athletes; pathologic in patients with heart disease
Murmurs	Apex Second ICS, LSB, or RSB	Produced by turbulent blood flow across diseased heart valves. They are graded on a 6-point Roman numeral scale of loudness and recorded as a ratio. The numerator is the intensity of the murmur, and the denominator is always VI, which indicates that the six-point scale is being used. Grade I/VI indicates a murmur that is barely audible, heard only in a quiet room and then not easily; grade VI/VI indicates a murmur that can be heard with stethoscope lifted off chest wall.
Pericardial friction rubs	Usually heard best at the apex, with patient upright and leaning forward, and after expiration	Caused by friction that occurs when inflamed surfaces of pericardium (pericarditis) move against each other. They are high-pitched, scratchy sounds that may be transient or intermittent and may last several hours to days.

ICS, Intercostal space; *LSB,* left sternal border; *RSB,* right sternal border.

INTRACRANIAL PRESSURE MONITORING

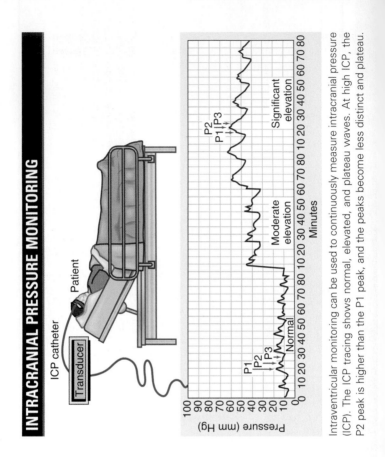

Intraventricular monitoring can be used to continuously measure intracranial pressure (ICP). The ICP tracing shows normal, elevated, and plateau waves. At high ICP, the P2 peak is higher than the P1 peak, and the peaks become less distinct and plateau.

LABORATORY VALUES

Test	Conventional Units	SI Units
Complete Blood Count		
Red blood cells (RBCs)	*Male:* 4.3-5.7 × 10⁶/μL *Female:* 3.8-5.1 × 10⁶/μL	*Male:* 4.3-5.7 × 10^{12}/L *Female:* 3.8-5.1 × 10^{12}/L
White blood cells (WBCs)	4.0-11.0 × 10³/μL	4.0-11.0 × 10^9/L
Hemoglobin (Hgb)	*Male:* 13.2-17.3 g/dL *Female:* 11.7-15.5 g/dL	*Male:* 132-173 g/L *Female:* 117-155 g/L
Hematocrit (Hct)	*Male:* 39%-50% *Female:* 35%-47%	*Male:* 0.39-0.50 *Female:* 0.35-0.47
Chemistry		
Alanine aminotransferase (ALT)	10-40 U/L	0.17-0.68 μkat/L
Albumin	3.5-5 g/dL	35-50 g/L
Alkaline phosphatase	38-126 U/L	0.65-2.14 μkat/L
Aspartate aminotransferase (AST)	10-30 U/L	0.17-0.51 μkat/L
Ammonia	15-45 mcg N/dL	11-32 μmol N/L
Amylase	30-122 U/L	0.51-2.07 μkat/L
Bilirubin		
• Total	0.2-1.2 mg/dL	3.4-21.0 μmol/L
• Direct	0.1-0.3 mg/dL	1.7-5.1 μmol/L
• Indirect	0.1-1.0 mg/dL	1.7-17 μmol/L
Blood urea nitrogen (BUN)	10-30 mg/dL	1.8-7.1 mmol/L
Calcium (total)	8.6-10.2 mg/dL	2.15-2.55 mmol/L
Cholesterol	<200 mg/dL	<5.2 mmol/L
• HDL	*Male:* >40 mg/dL *Female:* >50 mg/dL	*Male:* >1.04 mmol/L *Female:* >1.3 mmol/L

Continued

LABORATORY VALUES—cont'd

Test	Conventional Units	SI Units
• LDL	*Recommended:* <100 mg/dL *Near optimal:* 100-129 mg/dL (2.6-3.34 mmol/L) *Moderate risk for CAD:* 130-159 mg/dL (3.37-4.12 mmol/L) *High risk for CAD:* >160 mg/dL (>4.14 mmol/L)	*Recommended:* <2.6 mmol/L *Near optimal:* 2.6-3.34 mmol/L *Moderate risk for CAD:* 3.37-4.12 mmol/L *High risk for CAD:* >4.14 mmol/L
Chloride	96-106 mEq/L	96-106 mmol/L
CO_2	23-29 mEq/L	23-29 mmol/L
Creatinine	0.5-1.5 mg/dL	44-133 µmol/L
Glucose	70-120 mg/dL	3.89-6.66 mmol/L
Iron	50-175 mcg/dL	9.0-31.3 µmol/L
Lactate dehydrogenase (LDH)	140-280 U/L	0.83-2.5 µkat/L
Lipase	31-186 U/L	0.5-3.2 µkat/L
Magnesium	1.5-2.5 mEq/L	0.75-1.25 mmol/L
Osmolality	275-295 mOsm/kg	275-295 mmol/kg
Phosphorus (phosphate)	2.4-4.4 mg/dL	0.78-1.42 mmol/L
Potassium	3.5-5.0 mEq/L	3.5-5.0 mmol/L
Protein (total)	6.4-8.3 g/dL	64-83 g/L
Sodium	135-145 mEq/L	135-145 mmol/L
Triglyceride	<150 mg/dL	<1.7 mmol/L
Coagulation		
Platelets	150-400 × 10^3/µL	150-400 × 10^9/L
PT	11-16 sec	Same as conventional unit
aPTT	25-35 sec	Same as conventional unit
FSP	<10 mcg/mL	<10 mg/L

aPTT, Activated partial thromboplastin time; *CAD,* coronary artery disease; *FSP,* fibrin split products; *HDL,* high-density lipoprotein; *LDL,* low-density lipoprotein; *PT,* prothrombin time; *SI,* Système International [i.e., International System of Units].

LUNG VOLUMES AND CAPACITIES

Parameter	Definition	Normal Value*
Volumes		
Tidal volume (VT)	Volume of air inhaled and exhaled with each breath Only a small proportion of total capacity of lungs	0.5 L
Expiratory reserve volume (ERV)	Additional air that can be forcefully exhaled after normal exhalation is complete	1.0 L
Residual volume (RV)	Amount of air remaining in lungs after forced expiration Air available in lungs for gas exchange between breaths	1.5 L
Inspiratory reserve volume (IRV)	Maximum volume of air that can be inhaled forcefully after normal inhalation	3.0 L
Capacities		
Total lung capacity (TLC)	Maximum volume of air that lungs can contain (TLC = IRV + VT + ERV + RV)	6.0 L
Functional residual capacity (FRC)	Volume of air remaining in lungs at end of normal exhalation (FRC = ERV + RV) Increase or decrease possible with lung disease	2.5 L
Vital capacity (VC)	Maximum volume of air that can be exhaled after maximum inspiration (VC = IRV + VT + ERV) Higher VC for men (generally)	4.5 L
Inspiratory capacity (IC)	Maximum volume of air that can be inhaled after normal expiration (IC = VT + IRV)	3.5 L

*Normal values vary with patient's height, weight, age, race, and gender.

MEDICATION ADMINISTRATIONS

Equivalent Weights and Measures

Metric	Apothecary	Household
Weight		
1 kg	2.2 pounds	
1000 mg = 1 g	gr xv	
60 or 65 mg	gr i	
30 mg	gr ss (one half)	
0.4 mg	1/150 gr	
1 mcg = 0.0001 mg		
Volume		
1000 mL = 1 L	Approx. 1 quart	Approx. 1 quart
1 L distilled water weighs	1 kg	
500 mL	Approx. 1 pint	16 ounces
240 or 250 mL	viii (8 ounces)	1 cup
30 mL	i (1 fluid ounce)	2 tablespoons
15 mL	iv (4 fluid drams)	1 tablespoon
4 to 5 mL	i (1 fluid dram)	1 teaspoon
1 mL	Minims xv or xvi	

Drug Calculations

Ratio and Proportion

1. To set up a ratio and proportion, put on the right-hand side what you already have, or what you already know (e.g., 1000 mg : 1 mL).
2. On the left-hand side put X, or what you want to know (e.g., 750 mg : X).
3. The equation should look like this:

$$750 \text{ mg} : X = 1000 \text{ mg} : 1 \text{ mL}$$

4. Multiply the two inside numbers. Multiply the two outside numbers.

$$1000X = 750$$

5. Solve for X:

$$X = \frac{750}{1000} = 0.75 \text{ mL}$$

IV Drip Rate

$$\frac{\text{Total number of milliliters to be infused}}{\text{Total number of minutes infusion}} \times \text{Drop factor} = \text{Rate (Drops per minute)}$$

Techniques of Administration
Angles of Injection

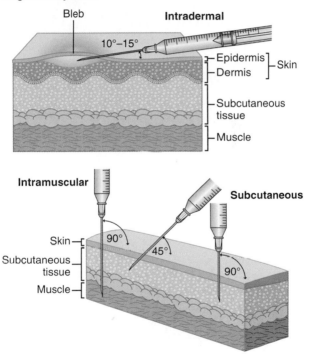

Injection Sites
Subcutaneous

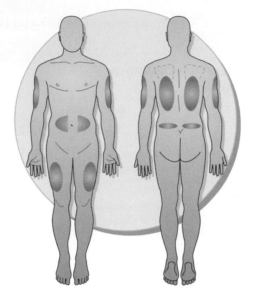

Intramuscular: Deltoid Muscle

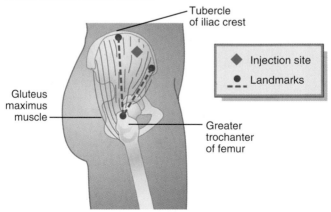

Intramuscular: Dorsogluteal Muscle

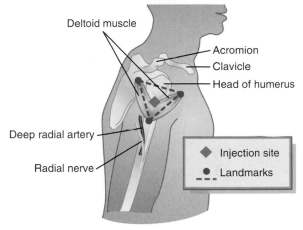

Intramuscular: Vastus Lateralis Muscle

Intramuscular: Ventrogluteal Muscle

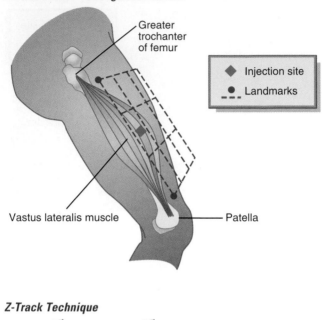

Greater trochanter of femur

Injection site ◆

Landmarks ●-----

Vastus lateralis muscle

Patella

Z-Track Technique

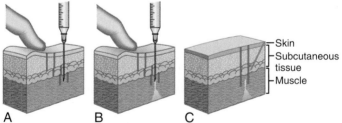

Skin
Subcutaneous tissue
Muscle

A   B   C

Intermittent IV Drug Administration
Peripheral Vein Intermittent Infusion Device
1. Irrigate device with 1 mL of normal saline.
2. Administer prescribed medication.
3. Irrigate device with 1 mL of normal saline after medication administration is completed.
4. If policy, perform a final irrigation with 1 mL of heparin solution (100 units of heparin per milliliter).

Central Vein Intermittent Infusion Device
1. Irrigate device with 2 to 5 mL of normal saline (volume depends on type of infusion catheter and agency policy).
2. Administer prescribed medication.
3. Irrigate device with 2 to 5 mL of normal saline when medication administration is completed.
4. Irrigate device with 2 to 5 mL of heparin solution (100 units of heparin per milliliter).

IV Site Complications

	Infiltration	Phlebitis
Assessment		
Color	Pale	Red
Temperature	Cool to cold	Warm to hot
Swelling	Rounded	Cordlike vein path
Pain	Yes, usually	Yes
Flow	Slowed or stopped	No change or may be slowed
Nursing Actions		
	Tourniquet proximally (flow continues—infiltration)	Discontinue IV infusion; usually call IV team
	Lower bag (blood in tubing—no infiltration)	Note irritating solution (diazepam [Valium], cephalothin sodium, potassium chloride [KCl] running too fast)
	Discontinue IV infusion	
	Call IV team	
	Get order for warm compresses and elevate part	Warm compresses; elevate and immobilize part

TEMPERATURE EQUIVALENTS

°C	°F	°C	°F	°C	°F
34.0	93.2	37.2	99.0	40.2	104.4
34.2	93.6	37.4	99.3	40.4	104.7
34.4	93.9	37.6	99.7	40.6	105.2
34.6	94.3	37.8	100.0	40.8	105.4
34.8	94.6	38.0	100.4	41.0	105.9
35.0	95.0	38.2	100.8	41.2	106.1
35.2	95.4	38.4	101.1	41.4	106.5
35.4	95.7	38.6	101.5	41.6	106.8
35.6	96.1	38.8	101.8	41.8	107.2
35.8	96.4	39.0	102.2	42.0	107.6
36.0	96.8	39.2	102.6	42.2	108.0
36.2	97.2	39.4	102.9	42.4	108.3
36.4	97.5	39.6	103.3	42.6	108.7
36.6	97.9	39.8	103.6	42.8	109.0
36.8	98.2	40.0	104.0	43.0	109.4
37.0	98.6	—	—	—	—

°C, Celsius (centigrade) degrees; *°F,* Fahrenheit degrees.

Conversion Factors

To convert from °C to °F:
$$(°C \times \tfrac{9}{5}) + 32 = °F$$

To convert from °F to °C:
$$(°F - 32) \times \tfrac{5}{9} = °C$$

TNM CLASSIFICATION SYSTEM

Primary Tumor (T)

T_0 No evidence of primary tumor

T_{is} Carcinoma in situ

T_{1-4} Ascending degrees of increase in tumor size and involvement

T_x Tumor cannot be measured or found

Regional Lymph Nodes (N)

N_0 No evidence of disease in lymph nodes

N_{1-4} Ascending degrees of nodal involvement

N_x Regional lymph nodes unable to be assessed clinically

Distant Metastases (M)

M_0 No evidence of distant metastases

M_{1-4} Ascending degrees of metastatic involvement, including distant nodes

M_x Cannot be determined

NOTE: For examples of the TNM classification system applied to diseases, see Fig. 30-14 on p. 642 and Table 27-17 on p. 516 in Lewis et al, *Medical-Surgical Nursing*, ed 10.

ENGLISH/SPANISH COMMON MEDICAL TERMS

Hints for Pronunciation of Spanish Words

- **h** is silent.
- **j** is pronounced as **h**.
- **ll** is pronounced as a **y** sound.
- **r** is pronounced with a trilled sound, and **rr** is trilled even more.
- **v** is pronounced with a **b** sound.
- A **y** by itself is pronounced with a long **e** sound.
- Accent marks over the vowel indicate the syllable that is to be stressed.

Common Words/Phrases for Clinical Situations

Introductory

I am _____.	Soy _____.
What is your name?	¿Cómo se llama usted?
I would like to examine you now.	Quisiera examinarlo(a) ahora.

General

How do you feel?	¿Cómo se siente?
Good	Bien
Bad	Mal
Do you feel better today?	¿Se siente mejor hoy?
Where do you work?	¿Dónde trabaja? (Cuál es su profesión o trabajo?) (¿Qué hace usted?)
Are you allergic to anything?	¿Es usted alérgico(a) a algo?
Medications, foods, insect bites?	¿Medicinas, alimentos, picaduras de insectos?
Do you take any medications?	¿Toma usted algunas medicinas?
Do you have any drug allergies?	¿Es usted alérgico(a) a algún médicamento?
Do you have a history of:	¿Ha sufrido antes:
Heart disease?	Del corazón?
Diabetes?	De diabetes?
Epilepsy?	De epilepsia?
Bronchitis?	De bronquitis?
Emphysema?	De enfisema?
Asthma?	De asma?

Pain

Have you any pain?	¿Tiene dolor?
Where is the pain?	¿Dónde le duele?
Do you have any pain here?	¿Le duele aquí?
How severe is the pain?	¿Qué tan fuerte es el dolor?
Mild, moderate, sharp, or severe?	¿Ligero, moderado, agudo, severo?
What were you doing when the pain started?	¿Qué estaba haciendo cuando le comenzó el dolor?
Have you ever had this pain before?	¿Ha tenido este dolor antes?
Do you have a pain in your side?	¿Tiene usted dolor en el costado?

Common Words/Phrases for Clinical Situations—cont'd

Is it worse now?	¿Es peor ahora?
Does it still pain you?	¿Le duele todavía?
Did you feel much pain at the time?	¿Sintió mucho dolor entonces?
Show me where.	Muéstreme dónde.
Does it hurt when I press here?	¿Le duele cuando aprieto aquí?

Head

Head	La cabeza
Face	La cara
Eye	El ojo

Ears/Nose/Throat

Ears	Los oídos
Eardrum	El tímpano
Laryngitis	La laringitis
Lip	El labio
Mouth	La boca
Nose	La naríz
Tongue	La lengua

Cardiovascular

Heart	El corazón
Heart attack	El ataque del corazón
Heart disease	La enfermedad del corazón
Heart murmur	El soplo del corazón
High blood pressure	Presión alta

Respiratory

Chest	El pecho
Lungs	Los pulmones

Gastrointestinal

Abdomen	El abdomen
Intestines/bowels	Los intestinos
Liver	El hígado
Nausea	Náusea
Gastric ulcer	La úlcera gástrica

Continued

Common Words/Phrases for Clinical Situations—cont'd

Stomach	El estómago, la panza, la barriga
Stomachache	El dolor de estómago
Genitourinary	
Genitals	Los genitales
Kidney	El riñón
Penis	El pene, el miembro
Urine	La orina
Musculoskeletal	
Ankle	El tobillo
Arm	El brazo
Back	La espalda
Bones	Los huesos
Elbow	El codo
Finger	El dedo
Foot	El pie
Fracture	La fractura
Hand	La mano
Hip	La cadera
Knee	La rodilla
Leg	La pierna
Muscles	Los músculos
Rib	La costilla
Shoulder	El hombro
Thigh	El muslo
Neurologic	
Brain	El cerebro
Dizziness	El vértigo, el mareo
Epilepsy	La epilepsia
Fainting spell	El desmayo
Unconsciousness	Pérdida del conocimiento (inconsciente, sin sentido)
Reproductive	
Uterus	El útero, la matríz
Vagina	La vagina

URINALYSIS

Test	Normal	Abnormal Finding	Possible Etiology and Significance
Color	Amber yellow	Dark, smoky color	Hematuria
		Yellow-brown to olive green	Excessive bilirubin
		Orange-red or orange-brown	Normal side effect of phenazopyridine
		Cloudiness of freshly voided urine	Urinary tract infection (UTI)
		Colorless urine	Excessive fluid intake, kidney disease, or diabetes insipidus
Odor	Aromatic	Ammonia-like odor	Urine allowed to stand
		Unpleasant odor	UTI
Protein	Random protein (dipstick): 0-trace	Persistent proteinuria	Characteristic of acute and chronic kidney disease, especially involving glomeruli
			Heart failure
	24-hr protein (quantitative): <150 mg/day		In absence of disease: high-protein diet, strenuous exercise, dehydration, fever, emotional stress, contamination by vaginal secretions

Continued

URINALYSIS—cont'd

Test	Normal	Abnormal Finding	Possible Etiology and Significance
Glucose	None	Glycosuria	Diabetes mellitus, low renal threshold for glucose reabsorption (if blood glucose level is normal) Pituitary disorders
Ketones	None	Present	Altered carbohydrate and fat metabolism in diabetes mellitus and starvation; dehydration, vomiting, severe diarrhea
Bilirubin	None	Present	Liver disorders May appear before jaundice is visible
Specific gravity	1.003-1.030 Maximum concentrating ability of kidney in morning urine (1.025-1.030)	Low High Fixed at about 1.010	Dilute urine, excessive diuresis, diabetes insipidus Dehydration, albuminuria, glycosuria Renal inability to concentrate urine; end-stage kidney disease
Osmolality	300-1300 mOsm/kg (300-1300 mmol/kg)	<300 mOsm/kg >1300 mOsm/kg	Tubular dysfunction Loss of renal ability to concentrate or dilute urine (not part of routine urinalysis)

pH	4.0-8.0 (average, 6.0)	>8.0	UTI Urine allowed to stand at room temperature (bacteria decompose urea to ammonia)
		<4.0	Respiratory or metabolic acidosis
RBCs	0-4/hpf	>4/hpf	Calculi, cystitis, neoplasm, glomerulonephritis, tuberculosis, kidney biopsy, UTI, trauma
WBCs	0-5/hpf	>5/hpf	UTI or inflammation.
Casts	None Occasional hyaline	Present	Molds of the renal tubules that may contain protein, WBCs, RBCs, or bacteria Noncellular casts (hyaline in appearance) occasionally found in normal urine
Culture for organisms	No organisms in bladder <10^4 organisms/mL result of normal urethral flora	Bacteria counts >10^5/mL	UTI Most common organisms: *Escherichia coli*, enterococci, *Klebsiella, Proteus*, and streptococci

hpf, High-power field.

Page numbers followed by *f* indicate figures; *t*, tables; and *b*, boxes.